W0043625

INFORMATION PROCESSING IN MEDICAL IMAGING

INFORMATION PROCESSING IN MEDICAL IMAGING

Proceedings of the 9th conference, Washington D.C., 10–14 June 1985

Sponsored by The Clinical Center and The Fogarty International Center of the National Institutes of Health, Bethesda, Maryland, U.S.A.

edited by

Stephen L. Bacharach, Ph.D.
Department of Nuclear Medicine
The National Institutes of Health
Bethesda, Maryland
U.S.A.

1986 **MARTINUS NIJHOFF PUBLISHERS**
a member of the KLUWER ACADEMIC PUBLISHERS GROUP
DORDRECHT / BOSTON / LANCASTER

Distributors

for the United States and Canada: Kluwer Academic Publishers, 190 Old Derby Street, Hingham, MA 02043, USA
for the UK and Ireland: Kluwer Academic Publishers, MTP Press Limited, Falcon House, Queen Square, Lancaster LA1 1RN, UK
for all other countries: Kluwer Academic Publishers Group, Distribution Center, P.O. Box 322, 3300 AH Dordrecht, The Netherlands

Library of Congress Cataloging in Publication Data

Information processing in medical imaging.

"Information Processing in Medical Imaging
Conference"--Foreword.
Includes bibliographies.
1. Diagnostic imaging--Data processing--Congresses.
I. Bacharach, Stephen L. II. National Institutes of
Health (U.S.). Clinical Center. III. John E. Fogarty
International Center for Advanced Study in the Health
Sciences. IV. Information Processing in Medical
Imaging Conference (9th : 1985 : Washington, D.C.)
[DNLM: 1. Diagnosis, Computer Assisted--congresses.
2. Nuclear Magnetic Resonance--congresses.
3. Radiography--congresses. 4. Radionuclide Imaging--
congresses. 5. Technology, Radiologic--congresses.
WN 200 I43 1985]
RC78.7.D53I55 1986   616.07'57'0285   85-30977

ISBN-13: 978-94-010-8392-8   e-ISBN-13: 978-94-009-4261-5
DOI: 10.1007/978-94-009-4261-5

Copyright

© 1986 by Martinus Nijhoff Publishers, Dordrecht.

All rights reserved. No part of this publication may be reproduced, stored in a retrieval system, or transmitted in any form or by any means, mechanical, photocopying, recording, or otherwise, without the prior written permission of the publishers,
Martinus Nijhoff Publishers, P.O. Box 163, 3300 AD Dordrecht,
The Netherlands.

TABLE OF CONTENTS

FOREWORD

The Information Processing in Medical Imaging Conference is
a biennial conference, held alternately in Europe and in
the United States of America. The subject of the conference
is the use of computers and mathematics in medical imaging,
the evaluation of new imaging techniques, image processing,
image analysis, diagnostic decision making and related fields.
The conference brings together leading researchers in the field
(both scientists and physicians) and other participants doing
active research in the subject areas of the conference.

The success of the meeting depends primarily upon the enthusiasm
and interest of the participants. It also depends greatly upon
the personal efforts of many individuals and collaborating
organizations. To all of those who helped to make this conference
a success, the members of the organizing committee express
their sincere thanks.

In particular, the organizers wish to acknowledge the efforts
of:

The Scientific Program Committee:

    S.L. Bacharach
    A.B. Brill
    F. Deconinck
    R. Di Paola
    M.L. Goris
    L. Kaufman
    S.M. Pizer
    A. Todd-Pokropek

and

The Clinical Center and Fogarty International Center of the
National Institutes of Health,

and

Georgetown University Medical School

From Medical Images to the Biometrics of Form

Fred L. Bookstein
Center for Human Growth and Development
University of Michigan
Ann Arbor, Michigan 48109

Within biometrics there is a subfield, morphometrics, for analyzing the geometric forms of organisms. Throughout biology and medicine it is useful to know whether two samples of organs or organisms have the same typical form, and, should they differ, to describe their differences; to indicate the shape changes involved in a cycle such as respiration or heartbeat, or accompanying growth over a lifespan; and to characterize the typical deformation that is a deformity or disease, and its response to therapeutic intervention.

Morphometric studies like these draw information from two sources: biological homology and geometric location (Bookstein, 1982). A biological **homology** is a spatial or developmental correspondence between individuals, a correspondence among definable structures or "parts"—separate bones, nerves, muscles, and the like. In the context of morphometrics it becomes a homology **map**, a correspondence not of parts to parts but of points to points. For any choice of point or curve upon or inside any particular form, the homology map associates biologically acceptable counterparts, the **homologues** of the point or curve, on all the other geometric forms in the data set. Morphometrics studies the empirical geometry of homology—variation in the relative locations of sets of homologous points over a sample of forms.

We generally sample this homology map at **landmarks**, points whose correspondence from form to form is determined with relative ease. The particular nature of the landmarks used in a study varies with the biometric context: the abutment of two bones, the origin of a valve, a reliable "corner" of sharp curvature, or a metallic implant or marker.

In this essay I shall review recent work (Bookstein, 1984-1986; Bookstein et al., 1985) dealing with the analysis of changes in landmark configurations interpreted as homology maps. This thrust, the construction of shape change as **deformation**, was first suggested by D'Arcy Thompson in 1917, but its practical application required high-speed computation (Bookstein, 1978). There are two themes to be elaborated. The comparative information we seek can be extracted in a particularly efficient way by the algebraic manipulation of **symmetric tensors**. And this information may be displayed intuitively, even aesthetically, by computer-generated quantitative diagrams faithful to the data.

Prospectus. I begin by discussing the basic unit of morphometric analysis—the shape change of a triangle of landmarks—and demonstrate its use for describing a normal human heartbeat. This approach is extended to landmark configurations more complex than triangles by the method of biorthogonal grids, which aids in the interpretation of some canine coronary data. Passing from consideration of single shape changes to the statistical analysis of large groups, I explain how to study populations of shape changes by multivariate statistical procedures. Examples include a simulation of texture change and studies of growth and of deformity in the human head. My concluding remark emphasizes the unexpected simplicity of the biometric information that we ought to be extracting from images.

Principal Strains Computed from Triangles of Landmarks

The basic unit for the study of biological shape change is a homologous pair of **triangles** of landmarks, Figure 1a. In the absence of other information we may take the homology map sampled by these limited data to be geometrically uniform, as indicated clearly in the **transformation grid** after the style of D'Arcy Thompson (1961), Figure 1b.

The visual impression this leaves depends on the orientation of the square grid upon the starting form; but this orientation is arbitrary and irrelevant. We draw the transformation more judiciously by its effect upon a collection of lines in all directions, Figure 1c. The deformation we are studying, driven by the displacements of those landmarks at the corners, deforms these segments into others which divide the edges in the same fractions. That is, the deformation takes edges to edges, median lines (dividing the opposite sides in the ratio 50:50) to medians, and so on.

To fully describe a change of form, it is sufficient to know ratios of lengths of corresponding lines in the two triangles. These dimensionless ratios are called **strains** or **extensions**. It is easiest to compute them implicitly: they are the lengths into which originally equal lengths—diameters of a circle—are deformed. Let us draw a circle, then (Figure 1d), and the oval into which the uniform shear takes it. Under the assumption of homogeneous (linear) transformation, this oval is an ellipse, precisely. Being an ellipse, the image of the circle has two axes of symmetry, which lie at 90 degrees. One is the largest diameter of the ellipse, one the smallest. The diameters of the circle which transform into them are likewise at 90 degrees.

Recall that the diameters of the ellipse embody the strain ratio as a function of direction. One of the axes of the ellipse is therefore the direction of *greatest* strain, the greatest rate of change of length, and one is the direction of *least* strain. The diameters that were mapped into them are determined by corresponding fractions of intersection along edges of the triangles. In Figure 1e we have drawn these diameters, and in Figure 1f a sketch of their straightforward measurement as transects across the triangles. These axes are called the **principal axes** of the deformation, and the rates of change of length along them are the **principal strains**. Together they completely describe the change in form of this triangle of landmarks. The area of the triangle changes by the product of the strains—1.14x0.62 = 0.707—while the most

3

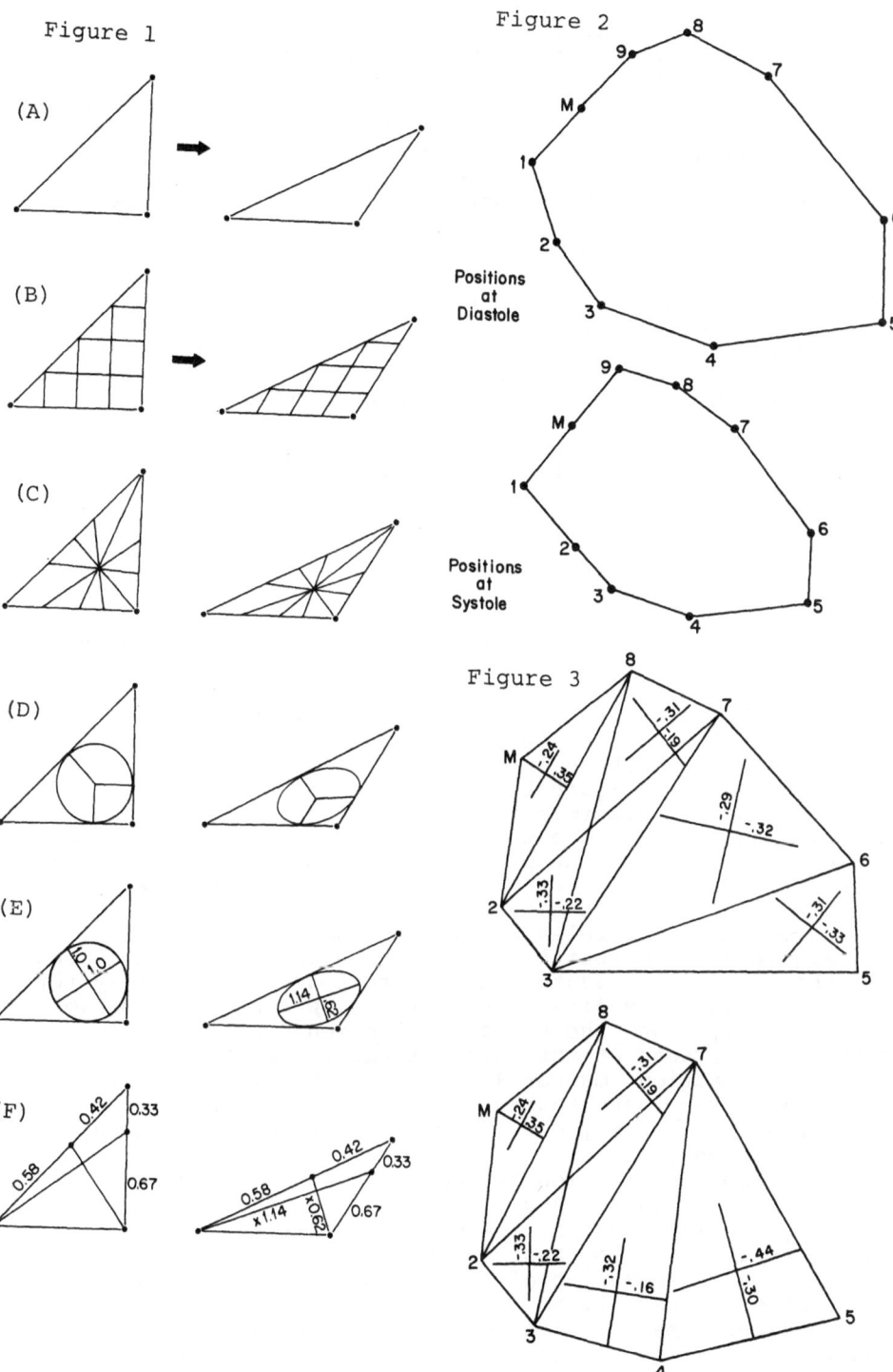

Figure 1

(A)

(B)

(C)

(D)

(E)

(F)

Figure 2

8
9
M
1
2
Positions
at
Diastole
3
4
5
6
7

9
8
M
7
1
6
2
Positions
at
Systole
3
5
4

Figure 3

sensitive descriptor of shape change is the proportion between
lengths measured in these two directions, which changes by the
factor 1.14/0.62 = 1.84. Note that we are not "measuring" the
triangles separately at all. The shapes themselves have merely
been archived; no preconceptions of specific variables have
interfered with the technique's construction of optimal
descriptions of change.

The analysis of shape change in this way is not new. The
geometrical object just introduced is a representation of
homogeneous deformation that is familiar to the mathematician
or engineer: a **symmetric tensor** formally independent of any
choice of coordinate system a priori. In this form it appears
frequently in mathematical discussions of growth and in
cartography, geology, and other sciences of position. In the
present application, the "interior" of a morphometric triangle
is not a homogeneous biological substance but an arbitrary
mosaic of tissues, fluid, or air. The shape change of this
abstract interior provides the most useful description of
changes in the configuration of its vertices, the real
biometric data.

Two Analyses of One Cardiac Cycle

The description of shape change by symmetric tensors
provides a very interesting visualization of a single human
heartbeat. The data for this example (Figure 2), taken from a
published figure (Ingels et al., 1981, Figure 3), locate nine
tantalum screws implanted in an otherwise normal human left
ventricle during coronary bypass surgery. The view is 30
degrees right anterior oblique; the apex (bottom) of the heart
is at marker 5; the base (where the left ventricle empties into
the aorta) spans markers 1 and 9.

The method of Figure 1 was used to describe the
deformations from diastole to systole of various triangles of
these implants. From the computed tensors derives the report
of Figure 3, in which the principal strains for the deformation
of the triangles shown are drawn within their forms at
diastole. The coordinate systems of the separate
configurations are irrelevant to the conclusions we draw.

Figure 3 shows that triangles 3-7-6 and 3-6-5, totalling
half the area of the ventricle, contract nearly uniformly (by
some 31%±2% in every direction). The displacement of marker 4
from marker 7, along the normal to the ventricular contour at
marker 4, contracts at the same 30% rate. Relative to the
uniform contraction, marker 4 is displaced only tangentially,
away from marker 3 and toward marker 5. (Some of this
heterogeneity is surely due to twisting of the heart about the
projection plane.)

This same contraction of about 31% persists quite far from
the apex. In triangles 2-3-7 and 8-3-7, which overlap in
Figure 3, the maximum contraction is at this same rate. The
minimum contraction in these triangles, 19% or 22%, can be
thought of as a weakening of the 32% by a superimposed
extension of markers 2 and 8 outward.

Consider a basal triangle joining markers 2 and 8 to the
midpoint of the aortic valve, M in the figures. As the apex of
the ventricle contracts, the base expands under hydrodynamic

pressure. This top triangle contracts across its base by 24%
(the same 30%, perhaps, corrected for the apparent divergence
of the translations at 2 and 8 just noted); but its projection
along the axis of the heart *increases* by 35% from end-diastole
to end-systole. In proportion to the general change of scale
by .68, this height has doubled.

These aspects of the description may be abstracted into
the nearly symmetric scheme of Figure 4. Superimposed on a
uniform contraction of 31% are outward displacements at markers
2, 1, 9, and 8 as shown, together with a lateral adjustment at
marker 4. Note the rotation of the axis of the heart relative
to the aortic valve ring.

Biorthogonal grids for the same data. The method of
triangles computes one tensor per three landmarks, a tensor
supposed to apply homogeneously to every point inside the
triangle. However, these triangles overlap—they represent a
single coherent set of points, a polygon. The method of
biorthogonal grids (Bookstein, 1978; Bookstein et al., 1985) is
appropriate for such extended configurations.

The method begins (Figure 5a) by computing a smooth
deformation—a version of D'Arcy Thompson's **Cartesian
grids**—extending the boundary correspondence inward so as to
homologously relate the interiors of our two polygons of
implants. The deformation is displayed by its effect upon a
mesh of points which is square in the top (diastolic) form; the
positions imputed to these points after the "deformation" which
is the heartbeat make up the distorted mesh inside the bottom
form. These two meshes correspond point for point, as can be
seen by comparing their relationships to the implants, points
whose homology from diastole to systole we know quite reliably.
The position and orientation of that starting square grid,
although arbitrary, do not affect the subsequent computations.
Like the deformations of triangles, this is an abstract
mathematical model of homology. It does not describe what is
"really there" but instead expresses the change of boundary
form in a convenient diagram.

From the derivative of this map a principal strain tensor
can be computed at every point (Figure 5b). These are the
infinitesimal directions corresponding to those in Figure 1e as
applied to "very small" triangles. Just as for triangles,
these directions, perpendicular inside both the diastolic and
the systolic polygons, bear the greatest and least local rates
of contraction of mathematical myocardium. Curves can be
constructed (Figure 5c) which run parallel to one arm or the
other of the crosses at every point through which they pass.
These curves constitute a grid orthogonal in both forms, before
and after deformation: a coordinate system not beholden to
features of the forms separately but customized for the
particular shape change which is cardiac contraction. Like the
mesh points of Figure 5a, the locations at which similarly
placed curves of the grids intersect, top and bottom, are
computed homologues: they correspond exactly under the map.

The gross deformation which is the heartbeat is described
by the lay of these curves upon the forms, by the principal
strains (rates of contraction of length) and their gradients
along the curves, and by the products and quotients of the pair

6

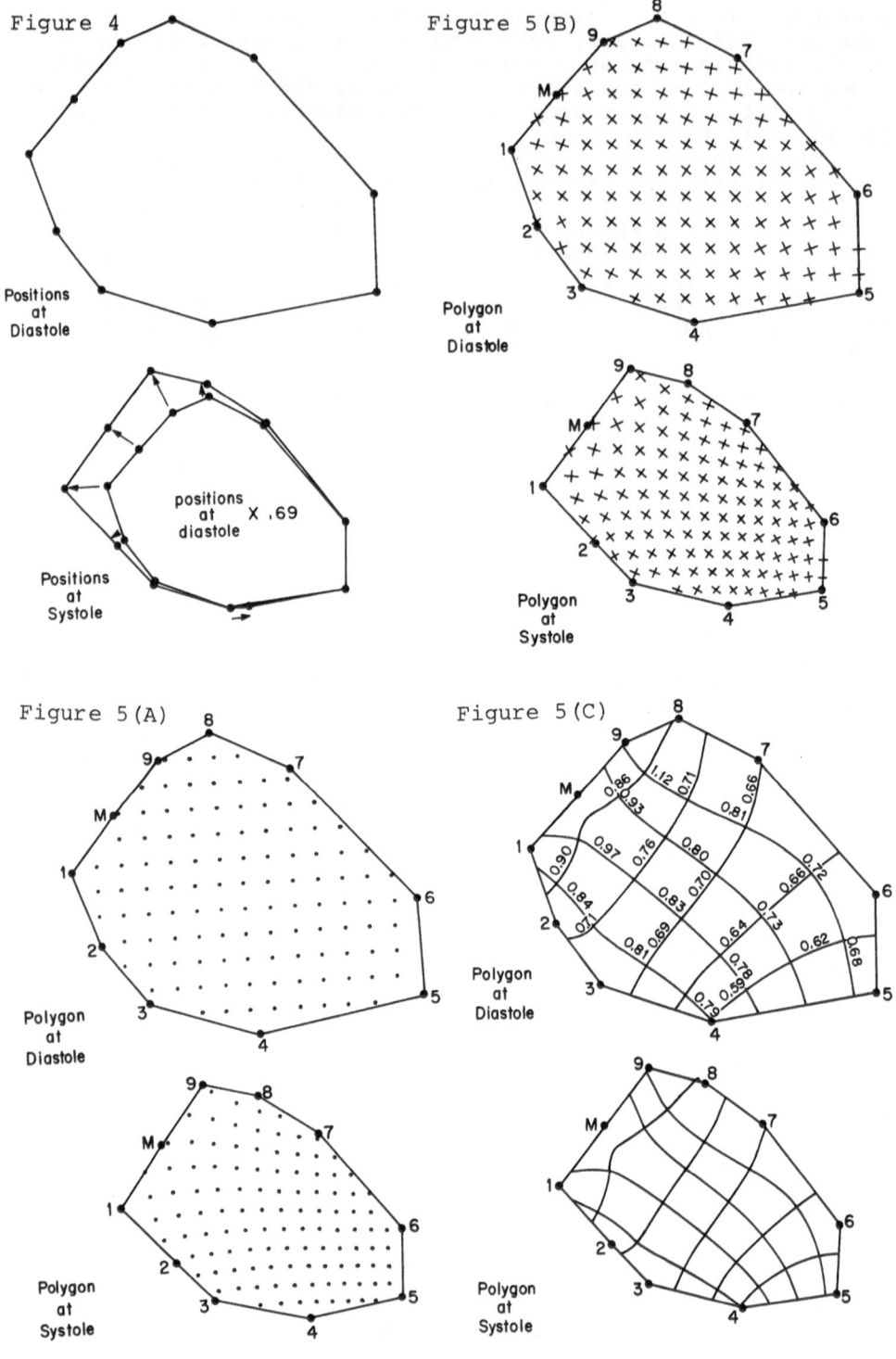

Figure 4

Positions at Diastole

positions at diastole X .69

Positions at Systole

Figure 5(B)

Polygon at Diastole

Polygon at Systole

Figure 5(A)

Polygon at Diastole

Polygon at Systole

Figure 5(C)

Polygon at Diastole

Polygon at Systole

of principal strains at every point (every intersection of curves). In Figure 5c, these strains, indicated within the diagram of diastolic form, are the actual contraction ratios, length in systole divided by length in diastole, for the abstract line-elements upon which they are drawn.

With marker 4 treated as equivalent to all the others, the heartbeat no longer presents the aspect of uniform contraction anywhere. Rather, there is clearly indicated a long axis of least contraction, from M at the base to a point between markers 4 and 5. As we saw in Figure 2, the strain in this direction is graded by a factor of 2, from a compression of some 30% near the apex to expansion near the base. This long axis is one of a system of parallels filling the interior, all showing this same gradient, all slightly curved. Perpendicular to this system are the short-axis curves of greatest contraction, likewise graded from 15%-25% near the base to better than 40% near marker 4, as in Figure 3. Everywhere the little grid rectangles become narrower faster than they become shorter.

The smooth biorthogonal description in Figure 5c is as simple as the discrete analysis of Figure 4. It expresses the same observed change of configuration using a different geometric idiom. For instance, marker 4 now appears to participate homogeneously in a shortening of the septal wall 2-4, a shortening less marked than the long-axis shortening along the free wall from marker 7 to marker 5; this asymmetry is equivalent to the rotation of the valve ring with respect to the heart axis noted in Figure 4.

Localizing Occlusion in Two Experimental Dogs

A principal theme of experimental cardiology is the measurement of coronary occlusion or myocardial infarction from images of the cardiac cycle. In the course of research into the regional analysis of these phenomena, we implanted sets of seven lead shot about the left ventricle (LV) of two experimental dogs. The shot lay in a plane perpendicular to the left anterior oblique (LAO) projection. Each dog was fitted with a balloon occluder of the left circumflex (LCx) coronary artery; dog B bore a second occluder, upon the left anterior descending (LAD) coronary artery. Our biometric polygon is sketched in Figure 6.

Dog A. We imaged dog A in his baseline condition and after sixty seconds of LCx occlusion. For each of the following grids, three consecutive contractions, diastole to systole, were averaged. The contraction at baseline, Figure 7, is represented by a nearly homogeneous grid. In the direction of maximum contraction, the ratio of final to initial length is nearly constant at 0.80 (that is, 20% shortening). Perpendicular to this is the nearly homogeneous direction of least contraction, here at a rate graded from 0.85 (near the apex) to 0.97 near the aortic valve ring.

Figure 9 shows the effect on the heartbeat of occluding the LCx artery. Although the shape of the chamber at diastole has not altered, that at systole has, and so the grids have changed. The occlusion has slightly warped the principal strains of contraction. Far from the region of presumed

8

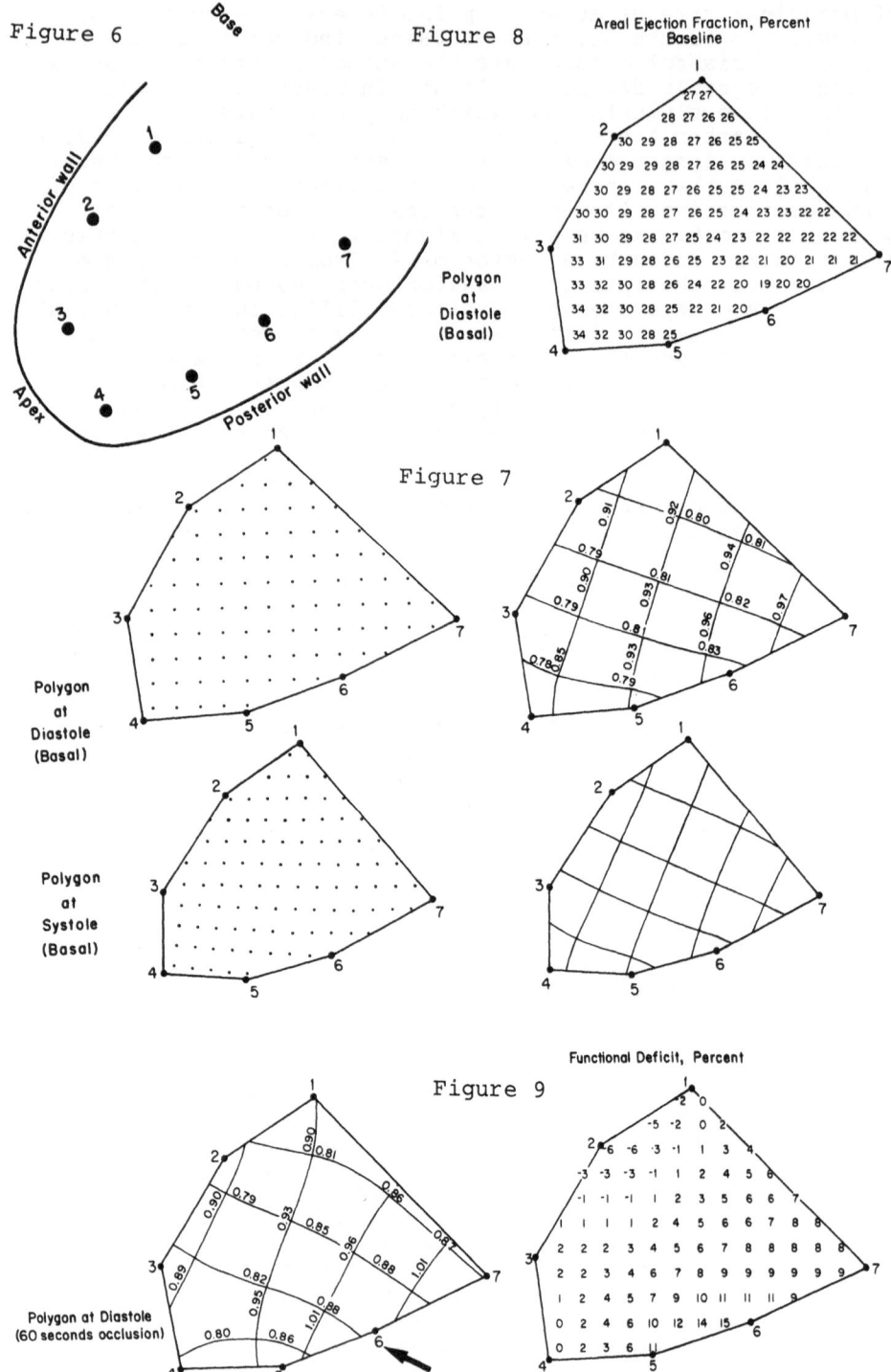

Figure 6

Base

Anterior wall

Apex

Posterior wall

Figure 8

Figure 7

Figure 9

Areal Ejection Fraction, Percent
Baseline

Polygon
at
Diastole
(Basal)

Polygon
at
Diastole
(Basal)

Polygon
at
Systole
(Basal)

Functional Deficit, Percent

Polygon at Diastole
(60 seconds occlusion)

occlusion (arrow), the rates and directions of contraction appear unaltered. Nearby, they seem to be systematically weakened in both principal directions.

Each of these contraction patterns may be represented by its Areal Ejection Fraction (AEF), the difference between 1.0 and the product of the two principal strains at every point. That for the baseline contraction, Figure 8, is quite even except in the vicinity of the apex. The other AEF, for the mean contraction under LCx occlusion, bears a steep gradient from upper left to lower right.

Because the shape of the polygon of implants at diastole has not altered substantially, we are able to map the effect of occlusion as an **AEF deficit** computed as the numerical difference between the baseline AEF and its value under occlusion, mesh point by mesh point. The map of AEF deficit for this occlusion, Figure 9 right, bears a clear maximum at the center of the myocardium served by the LCx artery.

Dog B. A second dog was affixed with seven shot in comparable positions and with occluders of both the LCx and LAD arteries. The shot were imaged in LAO projection in a baseline condition, during LAD occlusion and recovery, in a second baseline condition, and in LCx occlusion.

This dog's baseline contraction, Figure 10a, while as homogeneous as of dog A, shows a more robust contraction throughout the image. The biorthogonal grids for contraction during occlusion, Figure 10bc, are disorganized relative to that at baseline. Each grid bears a **singularity** at which contraction is by the same fraction (a mere 7-8%) in all directions. The singularity for the LAD-occluded beat is near the septal wall of the chamber; that for the LCx-occluded beat, in the middle of the free wall. Far from the occluded region, the tensors look like those at baseline.

The Areal Ejection Fractions for the two occluded conditions again demonstrate steeper gradients than the baseline AEF. The AEF deficit plot for the LCx occlusion, Figure 10b, is the same as for dog A, indicating the same focus for the myocardial disturbance. The deficit plot for dog B, Figure 10c, shows the wholly different regional emphasis of the LAD occlusion.

Statistical Analysis

To this point I have spoken of form-change as if it were studied one comparison at a time, visualized as a symmetric tensor, and reported. But one can exploit the tensor formalism much more systematically: it can be made to support all the themes of ordinary biometrics. One can compute averages of shape changes, and investigate their variances and covariances or their dependence upon outside factors. Any of these may be tested for statistical "significance" in the face of the chance variation inevitable in biological studies.

The tie between tensors and biometrics is based upon an aspect of Figure 1e already noted in passing. Recall that the ratio of measured lengths in the principal directions of a shape-change tensor is the shape variable that alters most over the course of a deformation. To pursue the implications of this assertion, let us agree to superpose all the homologous

10

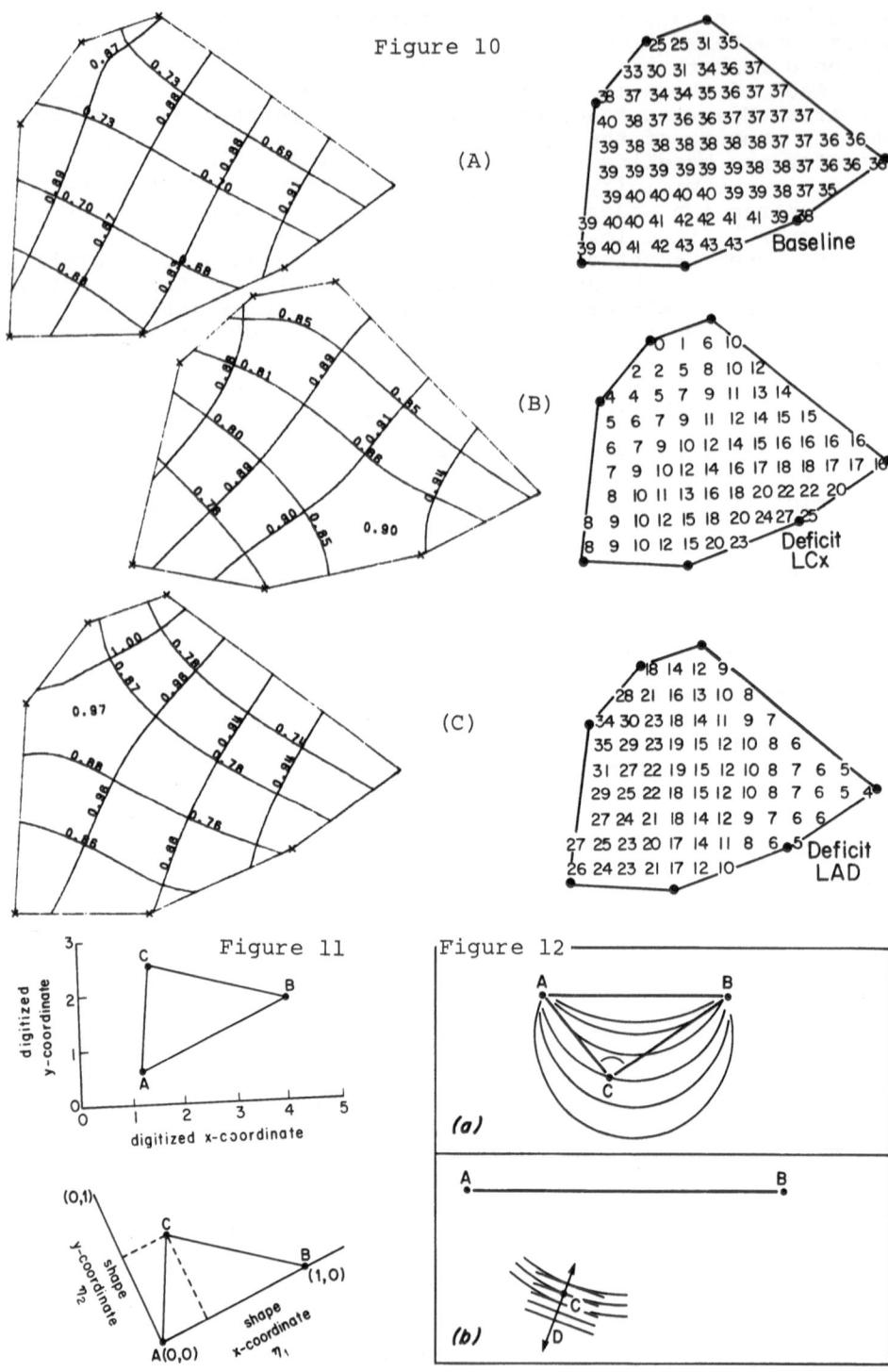

Figure 10

(A)

Baseline

(B)

Deficit
LCx

(C)

Deficit
LAD

Figure 11

Figure 12

(a)

(b)

triangles $\triangle ABC$ of a population in a common position. By change of scale whenever necessary, we shall arrange that landmark A is always put down at the point with Cartesian coordinates $(0,0)$ and landmark B at $(1,0)$, as in Figure 11. In effect we are plotting the triangle $\triangle ABC$ in a **shape coordinate space** composed of real and imaginary parts of the complex number $(C-A)/(B-A)$.

Consider any shape variable that can be computed from this triangle of landmarks $\triangle ABC$. Figure 12, for instance, illustrates the variable $\angle ACB$. Considering A and B to be fixed in position, any shape variable is constant on some curve through C; the angle $\angle ACB$ happens to be constant along the circle through A, C, and B. Neighboring curves, in this case other circles through A and B, correspond to neighboring, nearly equally spaced values of the shape measure.

In a small region of this plot, this set of curves can be approximated by a family of parallel, equally spaced straight lines, Figure 12b. The shape variable varies fastest perpendicular to these curves, in the direction of the axis D, the *gradient* of the shape variable. The smaller the variation in a population of triangles, the better a shape variable is characterized by the direction of its gradient.

Now consider two points Q and $Q+dQ$ in this space, Figure 13, corresponding to the distinct shapes of two triangles. If every shape variable is a direction in this space, we must be able to find the particular shape variable optimal for describing the difference of these two triangles—the ratio of distances along the two directions of principal strain. This shape variable, which is a *pair of directions* in the original landmark space, is a *vector* in shape coordinate space, the vector connecting the shape coordinate pairs locating the triangles.

One can easily pass back and forth between the representation of shape change by principal axes and this new representation by vectors. The construction (Bookstein, 1984a) is shown in Figure 13. Draw the circle H to pass through Q and $Q+dQ$ with center on the real axis. Let the points at which H intersects the x-axis be denoted $(W,0)$ and $(X,0)$. The angles $\angle WQX$ and $\angle W(Q+dQ)X$ are each inscribed in a semicircle; hence both are right angles. Because the X's are on the real axis, the linear transformation represented here, which leaves $(0,0)$ and $(1,0)$ fixed, also leaves the X's fixed. Then under this transformation the lines WQ and XQ correspond to the lines $W(Q+dQ)$, $X(Q+dQ)$. Because these directions (i) correspond under the transformation, and (ii) are perpendicular in both forms, they must be the principal directions of the transformation to which the construction refers—axes of the ellipse, directions of greatest and least ratio of change of size.

For small changes of shape, the circle through Q and $Q+dQ$ may be approximated by the circle through Q with tangent along the direction dQ there. Then the directions we seek through Q are at ± 45 degrees to the bisectors of the angle between dQ and the real axis, Figure 14. Furthermore, if s and t are the strain ratios in the two principal directions, we have, to first-order terms, $s-t = |dQ|/\text{Im } Q$. This is the **anisotropy** of the transformation, the greatest divergence of specific rates of change (difference of loadings) in any pair of distances.

In this way, tensor biometrics can be applied to whole populations of triangles. The statistical analysis of triangular shapes becomes the statistical analysis of scatters of points in the plane, for which ordinary multivariate maneuvers are quite adequate. It is easy to prove that this algebraic machinery is practically independent of the choice of baseline; it is also straightforward to restore to this analysis the information about size that was divided out when we reduced the triangles to their shape coordinate pairs. See Bookstein (1984b, 1986).

Example 1: Simulation of Change in Texture

As a first demonstration of the statistical analysis of deformations, consider the texture in Figure 15—a scatter of ellipses lacking all landmark information. The ellipses are randomly oriented with axis-lengths varying randomly and independently about a ratio of 2:1. The display in the figure was simulated, but might as easily have represented second-order moments of detected cells or other inclusions in an extended scene.

Each ellipse may be characterized by its shape—the ratio of lengths of its axes—and its orientation. Instead of thinking of them as shapes, however, let us treat each one as the deformation of a circle, so that it may be represented by a vector: its effect on one vertex of an arbitrary but fixed triangle. In effect we are inverting the construction of Figure 1: given the axes and the ratio of strains, to find the vector of displacement of a third point when size is adjusted so as to hold fixed the two other vertices of the triangle. By this tactic, an ellipse of anisotropy δ and principal axis at angle θ to the real axis is plotted as a vector having polar coordinates $(\delta, 2\theta)$. The scene of ellipses is thereby translated into the scatter of vectors shown in Figure 16. The design of the original simulation is plain here: the ellipses lie near a circle of radius corresponding to the expected anisotropy and independent of orientation.

Figure 17 is a modification of Figure 15 by a uniform stretch of 25% in the horizontal direction. The transformation has modestly changed both the shape and the orientation of every ellipse in the scene. Although the result does not appear notably different in directionality, the deformation involved in its construction can be unambiguously detected in Figure 18, the scatter analogous to Figure 16. In this new scatter, the circle is plainly off-center: the average vector of deformation representing the ellipses has been displaced from (0,0). This means that there is a *correlation* between orientation and shape in this new population of ellipses. Ellipses which were aligned up-and-down are now fatter; those which were aligned left-and-right are now longer, hence skinnier. The correlation thus explicitly embodies the additional deformation we have applied to each individual ellipse of the scene.

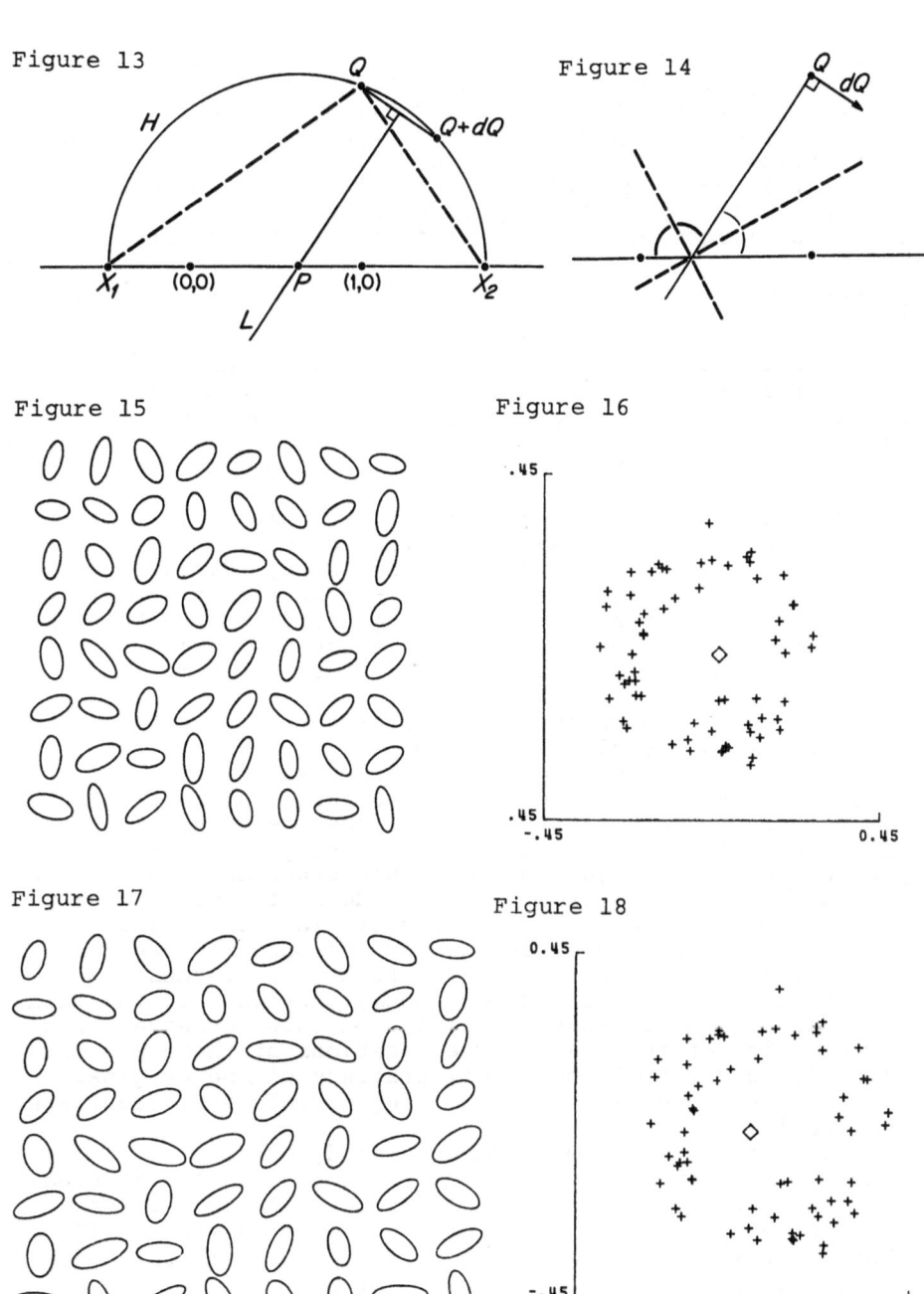

Figure 13

Figure 14

Figure 15

Figure 16

Figure 17

Figure 18

Example 2: Craniofacial Growth, Craniofacial Deformity
        Naturally our interest is concentrated in deformations of
real landmarks rather than simulated ellipses. In this same
manner we may analyze populations of deformations of landmarks
by conventional statistical methods applied to constructed
points in the shape coordinate plane. The examples following
are extracted from previously published analyses of
radiological images of human craniofacial form (Bookstein,
1984b).
        Cephalometric data. Most craniofacial biometrics begins
with x-ray images of bony crania and jaws positioned for
exposure in a standard fashion. The subject's head is placed
some six feet from the x-ray tube and a few inches from a film
cassette; the central beam of x-rays, perpendicular to the
film, passes through his ear holes. In the images which
result, edges of anatomical structures can be reliably traced
in a conventional abstraction of normal anatomy, schematized in
Figure 19.
        The data for these examples involve landmark locations
from cephalograms taken annually in the course of the
University of Michigan University School Study (Riolo et al.,
1974). The full sample is of about one hundred Ann Arbor
schoolchildren followed over various age ranges in the 1950's
and 1960's; for a subset of 36 males, there are serial records
of the four landmark locations at ages 8 years ± 6 months and
14 years ± 6 months.
        The landmarks to which I shall be referring are **Sella**, the
seat of the pituitary gland in the middle of the base of the
brain; **Nasion**, the deepest point in the curvature of the
profile at the bridge of the nose; **Anterior Nasal Spine** (ANS),
tip of the bony palate, just under the nose; **Menton**, point of
the chin; **Gonion**, the lateral corner of the jaw, often visible
in photographs of jut-jawed males; **Sphenoethmoidal Registration
Point** (SE), the intersection of two shadows (the greater wing
of the sphenoid bone and the anterior cranial base); and
Basion, the frontmost point on the foramen magnum where the
spinal column enters the skull. The first six of these
landmarks straddle the *splanchnocranium*, that part of the head
which deals with breathing, smelling, and chewing rather than
with protection of the brain. The locations of these points
are manually digitized from pencil tracings of the original
x-rays; I know of no means for locating cephalometric landmarks
automatically.
        Normal growth. The morphometric study of normal
craniofacial growth can begin with the large triangle joining
the landmarks Basion, Nasion, Menton for the 36 normal Ann
Arbor males observed at ages 8 and 14. We fix Basion at (0,0)
and Nasion at (1,0), representing the shape of this triangle in
these boys by the shape coordinates Q of Menton. The shape
change of this triangle from age 8 to age 14 is read in
displacements dQ of these coordinates. There results the
scatter of vectors dQ in Figure 20. (The "pinheads" locate the
earlier of the two positions.) The heavy black vector,
connecting the centroid of the earlier shapes to the centroid
of the later shapes, represents the mean shape change over this
six-year period.

This mean shift of shape coordinates corresponds by the construction of Figure 13 to a pair of distances, along the directions of principal strain, that might have been measured directly upon the x-rays as indicated in Figure 21. The baseline of this triangle, along the cranial base, grows least—by a mean fraction of 9.1% over this six-year period. Perpendicular to it is the direction of greatest average growth, by 17.5% over the same period. This difference of rates—evidence of a mean shape change—is hugely statistical significant. It is, furthermore, substantially correlated with net size change—the more one of these boys grew, the more his chin tended to grow "vertically," away from the cranial base.

There is some statistical regularity to the vectors of change in Figure 20. Chins beginning toward the left or the right (that is, relatively back or forward of the average position) tend to stay left or right; chins beginning relatively high or low (short faces or long faces) do not appear so predictably stable in position. Analogous to the tensor of shape change we have just been discussing, there is a tensor for directional dependence of shape stability, with principal axes of its own. Variation along the horizontal shape coordinate of Q is most predictable, with an autocorrelation of 0.89 from age 8 to age 14; variation along the vertical shape coordinate is least predictable, with an autocorrelation of 0.62 only. That different shape variables may be forecast with different degrees of accuracy is important in studies assessing the effects of orthodontic therapy. That it is so-called *vertical* change which is least predictable is a consequence of the dependence of vertical change upon size change noted in the preceding paragraph. Because the size change of an adolescent boy is essentially unpredictable, those aspects of shape most dependent upon size change will naturally be themselves the most variable. This analysis is extended to additional landmarks in Bookstein (1986).

Characterizing Apert's syndrome. The same design we applied to the longitudinal data of the heartbeat can be used for any other matched design. In particular, we may construe craniofacial deformity as deformation. Any instance of a syndrome may be measured not as a form but as a deformation of the "normal," specifically, of the age- and sex-matched University School Study normative mean. For example, consider Apert's syndrome, exemplified in Figure 22. It is one of the craniofacial *synostoses*, which generally manifest premature closure of the intracranial bony sutures about the maxilla and frontal bone. Apert's syndrome, or acrocephalosyndactyly, shows deformities of the extremities as well. Facially, the syndrome typically include a high, bulging forehead and a short maxilla (upper jaw positioned much higher and further back than normal. Landmark configurations for patients afflicted by this syndrome were lent to me by Dr. Joseph McCarthy from the data bases he maintains at the Institute for Reconstructive Plastic Surgery, New York University.

Six landmarks bound the facial region of interest in the study of Apert's syndrome. Assemble them into a polygon: Sella-SER-Nasion-ANS-Menton-Gonion. We averaged coordinates of

16

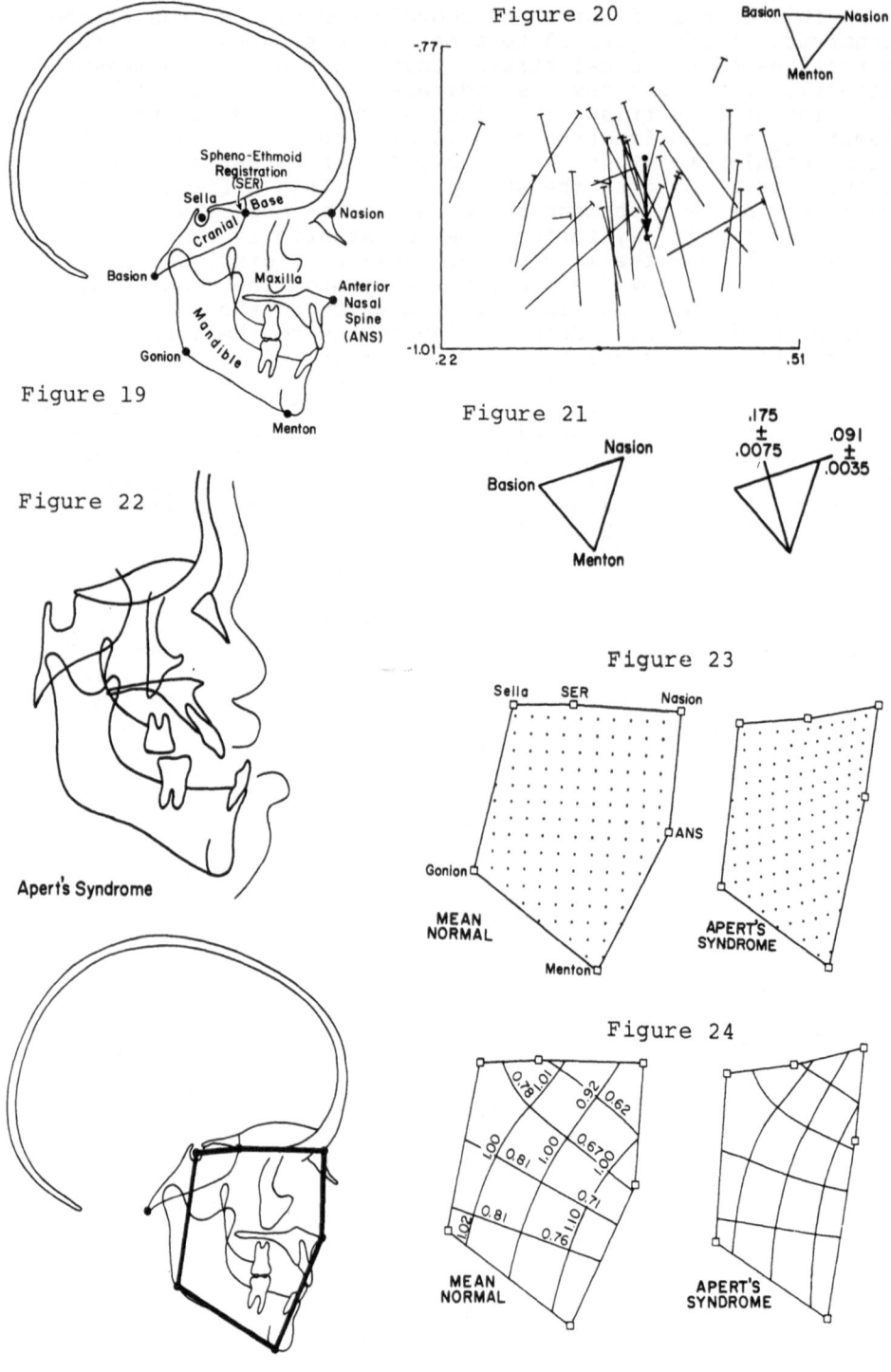

Figure 20

Basion — Nasion
Menton

Figure 19

Spheno-Ethmoid
Registration
(SER)
Sella Base
Cranial
Basion Maxilla Nasion
Mandible Anterior
Nasal
Spine
(ANS)
Gonion
Menton

Figure 22

Apert's Syndrome

Figure 21

Nasion
Basion
Menton

.175
±
.0075

.091
±
.0035

Figure 23

Sella SER Nasion

ANS

Gonion

MEAN
NORMAL

Menton

APERT'S
SYNDROME

Figure 24

0.78 1.01 0.92 0.62
1.00 0.81 1.00 0.67 0.71
1.02 0.81 1.10 0.76

MEAN
NORMAL

APERT'S
SYNDROME

the landmarks in the cephalograms of the patients and of the matched Ann Arbor normal children.

Figures 23 and 24 display the mean deformity of these 11 Apert's cases as the mean *deformation* into the typical case from the normal mean form. Figure 23 uses the diagrammatic style of the interpolated Cartesian grids, while Figure 24 summarizes the same homology map by its biorthogonal grid pair. Some dilatations are indicated, too. In this context, they are ratios of *abnormality of length* segment by segment: deformed length divided by homologous normal length.

The grids show an anteroposterior compression in the typical Apert's form that dominates relative normality of vertical dimension. Lower face height is slightly *larger* than normal, in consequence of the open-bite induced by the syndromes. There results, throughout the front of the face, a disproportion of some 30% with respect to normal shape. The grids are slightly tilted in the vicinity of Nasion, where one linear dimension appears to be most abnormal: the distance from ANS to SE. A more detailed analysis (Grayson et al., 1985) demonstrates that the point SE is nearly the seat of the syndrome; it is displaced within the shadow of the cranial base by more than half its normal distance to the line Basion-Nasion, perhaps in response to hydrostatic pressure from the developing brain.

An assortment of such separately optimal proportions can be submitted to any protocol for multiple discriminant analysis. They are particularly suited to the path-analytic discriminant model of Bookstein et al., 1985, Section 4.3.

Concluding Remark

The medical study of human anatomy, whether in the atlas or in the clinic, used to pursue two purposes jointly: the depiction of the "normal," its mean and its variants, and the authoritative specification of anomaly. Each of these is explicitly a comparative theme. In the modern equation of medical image analysis with computerized image processing, unfortunately the theme of comparison has evaporated, replaced by display of a purely *geometric* scene. The *biological* component of these images is suppressed, especially the information needed for morphometrics: the locations of named (homologous) parts or points in a series of forms.

Without this information, *we cannot compare forms intelligently.* We cannot make up for its omission by any manner of enhanced display. Rather, once a gray-scale image is processed for the extraction of modest biometrical information—the locations of a few carefully selected landmarks—the pixels or voxels are best entirely scrapped, replaced by a pair of abstract polygons, or polyhedrons, and their geometric and statistical derivatives. Tensor morphometric analysis of geometric data supports all the great themes of clinical anatomy—normal means, normal variation, characterization of anomalies—whereas the gray images, however much more realistic, wholly fail to do so.

In my view, there are two or three orders of magnitude too much information in medical images as they are currently displayed. The main need in medical image analysis today is

not for image *processing* at all. Rather, we should concentrate
our professional energies upon algorithms for the detection of
landmarks (aids to human search, or prescans for human
corroboration) and for the flagging of abnormal parts of an
extended scene. For studies of form, the remaining gray-scale
information is simply to be discarded; for studies of function,
it can be analyzed only in the coordinate system supplied by
the biometrics of form, the tensor morphometrics proposed in
this essay.

Acknowledgement. Preparation of this essay was supported
by N.I.H. grants DE-05410 to F. L. Bookstein and DE-03610 to
R. E. Moyers. The canine experiment of which one fragment is
described here was executed by A. J. Buda and Kim Gallagher
under grant HL-29716 to A. J. Buda. The data regarding
patients with Apert's syndrome were gathered under grant
DE-03568 to J. G. McCarthy.

Literature Cited

Bookstein, Fred L. *The Measurement of Biological Shape and
    Shape Change.* Lecture Notes in Biomathematics, v. 24.
    Springer-Verlag, 1978. 191 pp.
Bookstein, Fred L. Foundations of morphometrics. *Annual
    Reviews of Ecology and Systematics* 13:451-470, 1982
Bookstein, Fred L. A statistical method for biological shape
    comparisons. *J. Theoretical Biology* 107:475-520, 1984a
Bookstein, Fred L. Tensor biometrics for changes in cranial
    shape. *Annals of Human Biology* 11:413-437, 1984b
Bookstein, Fred L. A geometric foundation for the study of
    left ventricular motion: some tensor considerations. In
    Digital Cardiac Imaging, eds. A. J. Buda and E. J. Delp. The
    Hague: Martinus Nijhoff, 1985, pp. 65-83
Bookstein, Fred L. Size and shape spaces for landmark data in
    two dimensions. *Statistical Science*, accepted for
    publication, 1986
Bookstein, Fred L., B. Chernoff, R. Elder, J. Humphries,
    G. Smith, and R. Strauss. *Morphometrics in Evolutionary
    Biology. The Geometry of Size and Shape Change, with
    Examples from Fishes*. Academy of Natural Sciences of
    Philadelphia, to appear, 1985
Grayson, B., N. Weintraub, F. L. Bookstein, and J. McCarthy. A
    comparative cephalometric study of the cranial base in
    craniofacial syndromes. *Cleft Palate J.* 22:75-87, 1985
Ingels, Neil B., Jr., G. T. Daughters II, E. B. Stinson, and
    E. L. Alderman. Left ventricular midwall dynamics in the
    right anterior oblique projection in intact unanesthetized
    man. *Journal of Biomechanics* 14:221-233, 1981
Riolo, M. L., R. E. Moyers, J. S. McNamara, and W. S. Hunter.
    An Atlas of Craniofacial Growth. Monograph No. 2,
    Craniofacial Growth Series, Center for Human Growth and
    Development, University of Michigan, 1974

HUMAN VISUAL SIGNAL DETECTION AND IDENTIFICATION PERFOMANCE

A.E. BURGESS, Radiology Dept., University of B.C., Vancouver, Canada

1. ABSTRACT

The final step of the medical imaging process is display to a human for interpretation. In many cases the detectability of the visual signals is limited by statistical fluctuations. Under these circumstances it is possible, in principle, to calculate the best possible signal detection performance. We find that under some conditions humans can closely approach this limiting performance.

2. INTRODUCTION

The advent of digital imaging techniques in Radiology gives equipment designers, manufacturers, and users considerable latitude in the processing and display of medical images. Since the images are produced for human consumption, one would like to know how to optimize the coupling between the data and the radiologist's brain. This is not a new problem. A great deal of effort has been expended attempting to define "image quality" and to "enhance" medical images. There is certainly no consensus that any of these attempts has been successful. We have chosen to approach the problem from a different point of view. The most basic problem is that medical images are inherently noisy. This noise sets fundamental detection limits for large, low-contrast objects in the patient (1,2). Given this situation one can, in principle, calculate the best possible signal detection performance.

The question we ask is "How well do human observers perform in comparison with the best possible signal detection or discrimination device?". This is an obvious first step in the search for improved image display. In this paper we will describe how one defines an ideal observer and how one defines and measures human signal detection efficiency by comparison with this ideal. We will present experimental results for a variety of tasks.

Observer statistical efficiency (3,4,5) has proved to be a useful measure for studying, quantifying and understanding human observer performance of tasks involving noise-limited images. Basically the concept is as follows. Statistical decision theory allows one to calculate the best possible performance of a specified task. The hypothetical observer reaching this limit is referred to as the IDEAL OBSERVER. The ideal observer performance depends of course on the signal and noise properties, the nature of the task and the amount of a priori information about signal parameters. The dependence on prior information should be carefully noted because it is neglected in many discussions about signal detection. This fact forces one to acknowledge that SNR by itself does not completely determine task performance accuracy.

The efficiency concept is extremely powerful since it gives a measure of human performance on an absolute scale. Efficiency is commonly used as a measure of performance for mechanical and thermal devices - it is hard to argue with the second law of thermodynamics. Efficiency (DQE) is used to define the performance of photoreceptors (6) and image receptors (7) and radiologic imaging processes (8). The power of this approach lies in the fact that one can unambigously determine the maximum possible improvement in performance by image processing.

3. IDEAL OBSERVER PERFORMANCE

The fundamental limit of signal detectability is determined by two things - statistical fluctuations due to noise and uncertainty about signal parameters such as size, shape, and location. A considerable literature deals with the problem of calculating the best possible performance for given conditions (9,10). This ideal is achieved by a device called a maximum a posteriori probability detector (or alternatively a maximum likelihood detector). This device uses Bayes Theorem (eqn.1) to calculate the conditional probability of a signal being present given signal properties and image data:

$$P(\text{sig given data}) = P(\text{sig}) * P(\text{data given sig}) / P(\text{data}) \tag{1}$$

The probability of the data given the signal is determined using a cross-correlation (or matched filtering) strategy which leads to the concept of a detection SNR (2). In this case SNR refers to a statistical property given a particular signal and a particular noise distribution. Suppose the signal has a Fourier transform $S(u,v)$ and the noise has known power spectrum, $N_0 P(u,v)$, where u and v are spatial frequencies and N_0 is a constant. One can define the SNR for the ideal observer (which can re-whiten noise) using:

$$(SNR)^2 = \frac{1}{N_0} \iint_{-\infty}^{\infty} \frac{S^2(u.v)}{P(u,v)} \, dudv \tag{2}$$

If the noise is white (i.e. $P(u,v) = 1$ within the signal spectrum) human observer performance is close to ideal under some circumstances and this definition of SNR is suitable for characterizing the detectability of the signal.

4. MEASURING HUMAN PERFORMANCE

For noiseless images the visual system is limited, in principle, only by photon flux statistics and human performance is far from ideal (DQE is on the order of 1 per cent under photopic conditions as found in a normally illuminated display). The situation changes dramatically for noisy images. Many experiments involving noisy images have been interpreted as indicating that humans have internal variability (i.e. noise) that is statistically independent of image noise so that variances add. If the image noise is very small, internal noise predominates and is involved in setting signal detection limits. If the image noise is large enough, then external noise predominates and human signal detection is very good indeed.

We characterize human performance using a measure called statistical efficiency, $F = [SNR_i/SNR_h]^2$ where the subscripts refer to the SNR required by the ideal and human observer, respectively, to perform the same task with the same accuracy. Human performance is determined by running a large number of M-alternative forced-choice (MAFC) trials, determining the percentage of correct responses, finding the SNR for the ideal observer under the same conditions, and then calculating efficiency.

5. SIGNAL LOCATION UNCERTAINTY (AN EXAMPLE TASK)

In most visual psychophysics experiments the observer is given complete a priori information about the expected signal (size, shape, and location). This is not very representative of real tasks where one usually has considerable uncertainty about signal parameters. There has been a very limited investigation of this problem. Starr et al (11) investigated detection and localization of disc signals in noise with 4 alternative orthogonal locations. The results were analyzed using an ROC method. They presented a theoretical model based on statistical decision theory and concluded that the model gave adequate predictions of human observer behaviour. Swensson and Judy (12) used the MAFC method to investigate the effect of search for small numbers of possible orthogonal locations (M=1,2,4, and 8). They found that data for M=1 could be used together with statistical decision theory to predict the results for M equal to 2 and 4. However this agreement did not hold for their M equal to 8 results.

We (13) have measured the effect of signal location uncertainty on the detectability of simple signals in uncorrelated noise with values of M from 2 to 1800. An example search task is shown in Figure 1. A disc signal is present in one of the 98 alternative positions as indicated by the hash marks. The image is shown on a high quality TV monitor and the observer uses a trackball and cursor to identify the most probable location. The variation in percentage of correct localization responses for the disc detection task is shown in figure 2. It is clear that varying the amount of signal location uncertainty has a marked effect on the probability of correct response. The solid lines are for a 50% efficient observer performing the same task with the same a priori location information. Visual inspection suggests a reasonably good fit between the experimental data and these psychometric functions.

6. SUMMARY AND CONCLUSIONS

Statistical efficiencies for a number of other tasks are shown in table I. The efficiencies range mainly from 15 to 50%. This means that humans require 1.4 to 2 times higher SNR than the ideal observer to achieve a specified detection performance.

All results to date suggest that humans can be modelled as a sub-optimal Bayesian decision maker. The list of human limitations includes the following - internal noise (14), inability to precisely use location information (15), reduced (cross-correlation) sampling efficiency because of spatially and temporally local comparisons (quasi-differentiation) of image amplitudes, limited range of integration in space and time, inability to compensate for correlations in image noise (i.e. cannot "rewhiten" coloured noise) (2,16), and losses due to masking by deterministic structure (17). These limitations have surprisingly small effects on task performance and sophisticated image users are able to adopt a variety of strategies for minimizing their effects. Given complete control of display conditions, humans are able to get within factors of 2 to 4 of ideal performance. The experimental work continues.

REFERENCES
1. Hanson KM: Detectability in Computed Tomography Images. Med. Phys. 6,441-451, 1979.
2. Wagner RF, Brown DG, and Pastel MS: Application of Information Theory to the Assessment of Computed Tomography. Med. Phys. 6, 83-94, 1979.
3. Tanner WP and Birdsall TG: Definitions of d' and η as psycholophysical measures. J. Acoust. Soc. Am. 30, 922-928, 1958.
4. Barlow HB: The Efficiency of Detecting Changes in Density in Random Dot Patterns. Vision Res. 18, 637-650, 1978.
5. Burgess AE: Statistical Efficiency of Perceptual Decisions. S.P.I.E. Proc. 454, 18-26, 1984.
6. Rose A: The Sensitivity Performance of the Human Eye on an Absolute Scale. J. Opt. Soc. Am. 38, 196-208, 1948.
7. Shaw R: Evaluating the Efficiency of Imaging Processes. Rep. Prog. Phys. 41, 1103-1155, 1978.
8. Wagner RF and Jennings RJ: The Bottom Line in Radiologic Dose Reduction. SPIE Proc. 206, 60-66, 1979.
9. Green DB and Swets JA: Signal Detection Theory and Psychophysics. New York: John Wiley, 1966.
10. Van Trees HL: Detection, Estimation, and Modulation Theory Vols I,II, and III. New York: John Wiley, 1968.
11. Starr SJ, Metz CE, Lusted LB, and Goodenough DJ: Visual Detection and Localization of Radiographic Images. Radiology 116, 533-538, 1975.
12. Swensson RG and Judy PF: Detection of Noisy Visual Targets: Models for the Effects of Spatial Uncertainty and Signal-to-Noise Ratio. Perception and Psychophysics 29, 521-534, 1981.
13. Burgess AE and Ghandeharian H: Visual Signal Detection II: Effect of Signal Location Uncertainty. J.Opt.Soc.Am. A1, 906-910, 1984.
14. Nagaraja NS: Effect of Luminance Noise on Contrast Thresholds. J. Opt. Soc. Am. 54, 950-955, 1964.
15. Burgess AE and Ghandeharian H: Visual Signal Detection I: Ability to use phase information. J.Opt.Soc.Am. A1, 900-905, 1984.
16. Myers KJ, et al: Effect of Noise Power Spectra on Detectability of Low Contrast Objects. Presented at Opt.Soc. America Annual Meeting. San Diego (1984).
17. Ravesz G, Kundel HL, Graber MA: The Influence of Structured Noise on the Detection of Radiological Abnormalities. Invest.Rad. 9, 479-486, 1974.

TABLE 1. Summary of statistical efficiencies for a variety of tasks.

Task	Efficiency
2AFC detection	30 to 50%
2AFC amplitude discrimination	40 to 80%
2AFC form discrimination	15 to 40%
MAFC location identification (discs)	50%
MAFC (Hadamard) signal identification	40%
Edge location identification	25 to 40%
MAFC location in background structure	20 to 50%

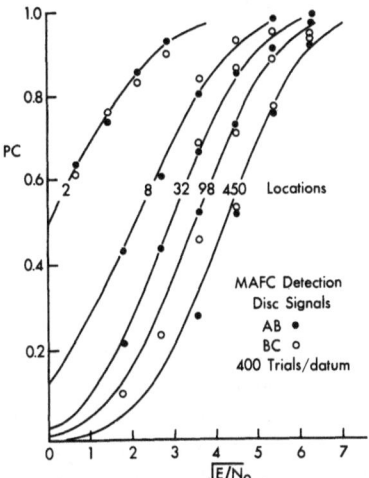

FIGURE 1. An example display for MAFC signal location identification. The disc signal (illustrated in two places above the noise field) is located in exactly one of 98 non-overlapping locations as indicated by the hash marks along the perimeter. The observer uses a trackball to move a cursor to the most probable location.

FIGURE 2. The percentage of correct location identifi-cations as a function of SNR for 5 different numbers of possible locations. The solid lines are for an observer operating at 50% statistical efficiency.

AN IMAGE DESCRIPTION FOR OBJECT DEFINITION, BASED ON EXTREMAL REGIONS IN THE STACK

Stephen M. Pizer * +, Jan J. Koenderink ~ , Lawrence M. Lifshitz * ,
Leendert Helmink ~ , Antonie D. J. Kaasjager ~

Dept. of Computer Science* and Dept. of Radiology +,
University of North Carolina, Chapel Hill, NC, USA
and
Department of Medical and Physiological Physics ~ ,
Rijksuniversiteit Utrecht, Utrecht, Netherlands

ABSTRACT

A promising image description is produced by dividing an image into nested light spots and dark spots by considering the image simultaneously at many levels of resolution [Koenderink, 1984]. These spots each include an image extremum and are thus called *extremal regions*. The nesting can be specified by a tree indicating the containment relationships of the extremal regions. This tree description, with each region described by intensity information, size, shape, and most significantly a measure of the importance, or *scale*, of the spot, absolutely and relative to its containing spot, ought to be usable in finding meaningful image objects when it is used together with *a priori* information about the expected structure of the image or its objects. This paper will describe work in the development of a computer program to compute such a description and its application to the display and segmentation of images from x-ray computed tomography and nuclear medicine.

1. PATTERN RECOGNITION AND DISPLAY VIA IMAGE DESCRIPTION

1.1. <u>Introduction</u>

Pictorial pattern recognition involves finding and labeling image objects. User interaction with and appreciation of an image frequently requires finding and labeling image objects, for example to allow the measurement of properties of the object or to provide a display which enhances the object. Indeed 3D display by shaded graphics depends on first defining the object to be displayed.

Most of the techniques attempted for defining objects work locally, directly with pixel intensity values. For example, both edge following and conventional region growing are done pixel by pixel. These methods have achieved only limited success, because the pixel values are too local to be easily combined into objects that are defined to a significant degree by their global properties. The first stage of a more attractive approach is to produce an *image description* that is more global. The creation of such a description should use only information from the image and not semantic information (from expectations about the scene or the viewing task). The second stage would use semantic ("real world") *a priori* knowledge together with the image description to define meaningful objects.

This approach of object definition based on a precomputed image description can be used for either automatic or interactive scene analysis. In automatic object definition the real world *a priori* knowledge is provided by predefined structures which are matched to the image description. In interactive object definition information is provided in addition by the human observer about objects he or she sees so that the computer can "perceive" the same object. The idea is that the observer can specify global properties of the object that is seen on some display, e.g. its location, intensity, scale, or name, and since the image has been reduced to a description reflecting global properties, fast interactive selection of image objects that match the observer's indications can be accomplished. The result can be displayed to the observer, who can accept the definition, edit it, or modify the defining parameters. The resulting object can be used to provide measurements, e.g. of volume or shape, or to serve as the basis for display or display interactions.

An attractive image description in this spirit [Koenderink, 1981] focuses on decomposing the image into light and dark spots, each, except for the spot representing the whole image, contained in others. Thus a face might be described as a light spot containing a light spot (a reflection from the forehead) and three dark spots (the mouth and the regions of the two eyes). In turn the eye regions would be described as containing a dark spot (the eyebrow), a light spot (the eyelid), and a dark spot (the eye), with the latter containing a light spot (the eyeball) which itself contains a dark spot (the iris) which finally contains a yet darker spot (the pupil). We call these light and dark spots, at whatever scale, *extremal regions*, since they each include a local intensity maximum or minimum.

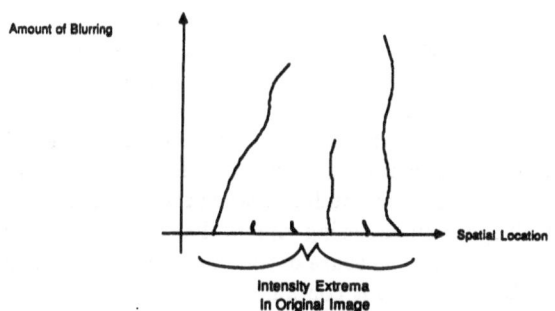

FIGURE 1. Extremal paths through the stack

1.2. Hierarchical descriptions from multiresolution processing

The image description in terms of extremal regions can be produced by following the paths of extrema in a stack of images in which each higher image is a slightly blurred version of the previous one. As illustrated in figure 1 and explained in Koenderink [1984], progressively blurring an image causes each extremum to move continuously, and eventually to annihilate as it blurs into its background. An *extremal path* is formed by following the locations of an extremum across the stack of images.

Intensity must be monotonic (increasing for dark spots and decreasing for light spots) as one moves along an extremal path from the original image towards images of increased blurring. As illustrated in figure 2, while following each extremal path

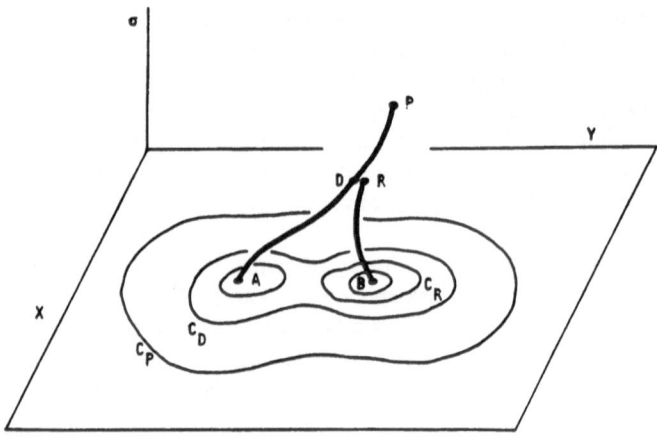

FIGURE 2. Extremal paths and associated iso-intensity contours

one can associate each path point with the iso-intensity contour that is at that point's intensity and that surrounds that extremum in the original image [Koenderink, 1984]. The points (pixels) in the original image on the contours thus associated with each extremal path then form an extremal region (see figure 3).

Each contour point in the original image can be associated with its extremal path by following the point to another with its intensity level at the next level in the stack, continuing through the levels until the extremal path is reached (see figure 4). This process defines an *iso-intensity path*.

It has been shown that all extremal paths must start in the original image if gaussian blurring is used. Extremal paths cannot be initiated at higher stack levels. However, as indicated above, extrema annihilate when the blurring is sufficient to make the light or dark spot blur into an enclosing region. The amount of blurring necessary for an extremum to annihilate is a measure of the importance or scale of the extremal region, including the subregions that it contains.

The intensity of the topmost point on an extremal path is its annihilation intensity. This is the intensity of the iso-intensity contour that forms the boundary of the associated extremal region. Remember that the annihilation intensity bounds from below (above) the intensities in the extremal region if the associated extremum is a maximum (minimum).

1.3. A tree of extremal regions for image description

As illustrated in figure 2, when an extremum annihilates at some annihilation intensity, another region's iso-intensity contour at that intensity encloses the region associated with the annihilating extremum [Koenderink, 1984]. Thus, a containment relation among extremal regions is induced by the process. This set of extremal regions together with their containment relations can be represented by an *image description tree* in which nodes represent extremal regions and a node is the child of another if the extremal region that it represents is immediately contained by the extremal region represented by the parent (see figure 5). The root of the image description tree represents the entire image.

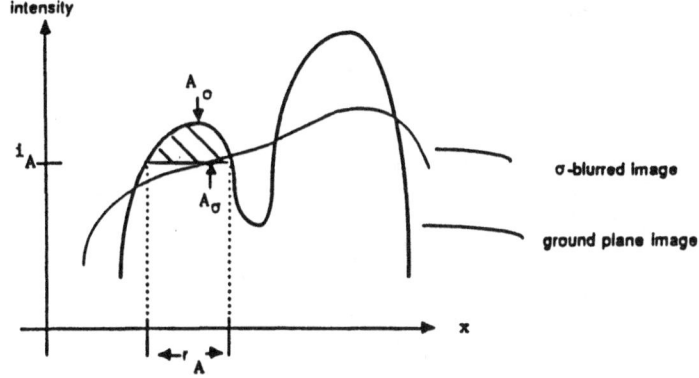

If extremum at A_o has moved to A_σ for the degree of blurring σ at which the extremum annihilates, then r_A gives the extremal region and i_A its characteristic intensity.

FIGURE 3. Extremum annihilation by blurring and consequent extremal region

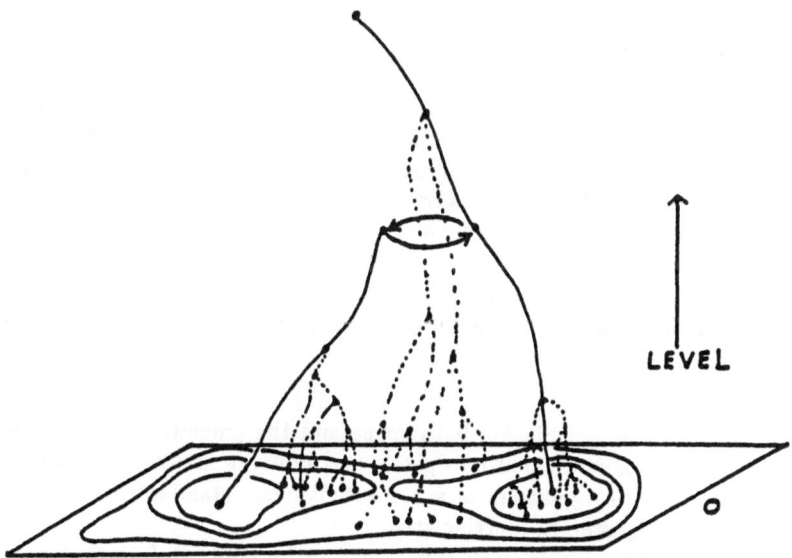

FIGURE 4. Extremal paths (indicated by solid lines) and iso-intensity paths (indicated by broken lines). Iso-intensity contours are indicated in the original image (level 0). The relation of an extremal region enclosing another region is indicated by arrows.

28

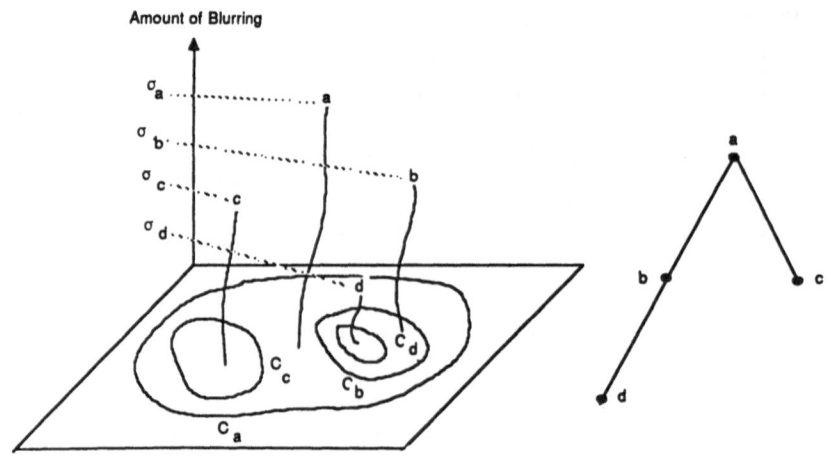

Amount of Blurring

σ_a
σ_b
σ_c
σ_d

a
b
c
d

C_d
C_c
C_b
C_a

Extremal Paths and Regions

a
b
c
d

Image Description Tree

FIGURE 5. Extremal paths, with their regions and scales, and the associated image description tree

Each node in the image description tree can be labeled with its scale, i.e. the total amount of blurring necessary for its extremum to annihilate. Furthermore, each node can be labeled with the annihilation intensity of the associated extremum. Finally, the node can be labeled with the size, shape, orientation, location, or other spatial characteristics of its extremal region.

It is possible that the description process described above can be beneficially preceded by some preprocessing, e.g. to enhance contrast or edges. In fact, Crowley [1984] has developed a similar scheme of extremum following in a multiresolution pile of images that are edge-enhanced by a sort of unsharp masking, and he has applied it with promising results. We have tried such preprocessing a few times with some benefit but will not discuss it in greater detail in this paper. However, it is worth noting that a noncognitive component of human visual perception may possibly be well modeled by an edge-enhancing preprocessing followed by the production of a stack-based image description.

2. SAMPLING

With computer implementation both space and the amount of blurring become discrete. That is, space is divided into pixels and blurring is not done continuously but by convolution with a gaussian of a non-infinitesimal standard deviation, which may vary from blurring step to blurring step.

The amount of blurring in each step needs to be controlled so that confusion in following extremal paths and associated iso-intensity paths across stack levels is avoided, while limiting the number of steps so that reasonable efficiency is achieved. When there are many extremal paths, we have taken this criterion to imply an inter-level blurring that is just large enough to ensure that real changes dominate changes due to arithmetic error. When there are few extremal paths, an inter-level blurring is chosen that produces significant progress toward annihilation of one of the paths.

Progress toward annihilation depends on taking steps related to the distance between paths. We keep count of the number of remaining paths as we move up the stack, and when there are fewer extremal paths than some threshold (in present use, 6), we blur at each level by averaging over a region whose diameter is the distance between the closest paths at that level.

For levels below the point where efficiency considerations lead to the blurring just described, we need to interpret when "real changes dominate changes due to arithmetic error." Koenderink [1984] and Pizer [van Os, 1984] have both interpreted this to mean that the attenuation of the height of some basic function is a small integer multiple of the arithmetic error, but these two investigators have chosen a different basic function. Koenderink chose a sinusoid at the Nyquist frequency associated with the total amount of blurring at any given level, while Pizer chose a gaussian which was a spike in the scene (but not the original image, which already is a blurred version of the scene) on a flat background, where the ratio of the height of the spike to the background has some value chosen as a parameter.

Koenderink's choice leads to

$$\frac{\delta\sigma^2}{\sigma^2} = k\frac{\sqrt{2\rho}}{-log_e\rho},$$

where σ^2 is the variance of the total blurring in the image at the present stack level, $\delta\sigma^2$ is the variance of the blurring to be applied to that image, ρ is the bound on the relative error in the computer representation of intensity, and k is a small integer. This has the attractive property that the amount of additional blurring ($\delta\sigma^2$) is proportional to the total blurring done to create this level.

Pizer's choice leads to

$$\frac{\delta\sigma^2}{\sigma^2} = \frac{k'\rho(1 + \beta\frac{\sigma^2}{\sigma_0^2})}{1 - k'\rho\beta\frac{\sigma^2}{\sigma_0^2}},$$

where ρ is as before, k' is a small integer, β is the ratio of background to peak height in the scene, and σ_0^2 is the blurring due to imaging. Eventually the peak height relative to the background becomes so small that no blurring can reduce it to the criterion degree. At this point the blurring at each step is chosen to allow a decrease in spatial sampling of 2 in each dimension, a common approach in multiresolution methods. To achieve this goal, $\delta\sigma^2$ must be proportional to σ^2 with a constant of proportionality of 3; the result is that the total blurring standard deviation increases by 2 at each step.

Studies by van Os and Pizer [1984] indicate that Pizer's choice leads to fewer levels of blurring with no major loss in the quality of the result, when the blurring used in the very first step of the two approaches is the same.

The sampling in space should, by normal sampling practice, decrease as you move up the stack, i.e. as the amount of blurring increases. More precisely, the interpixel distance should be proportional to the standard deviation of the total amount of blurring due to imaging together with the stack blurring. Using an argument based on the aliasing error at the Nyquist frequency, Pizer suggests a proportionality constant of approximately $\pi/\sqrt{1 - log_e\rho}$.

However, changing the spatial sampling as you move up the stack complicates the extremum and iso-intensity path following processes. As a result, in this early stage of our research, we have left the spatial sampling in all stack levels the same as in the original image. Part of the efficiency of resampling is achieved in our method, since only pixels that are on an iso-intensity or extremum path are followed to the next level.

3. AN ALGORITHM FOR PRODUCING A STACK-BASED IMAGE DESCRIPTION TREE

3.1. Algorithm description

It is our plan to use the image description region tree presented above for both automatic and interactive object definition. However, this object definition work is still in its early stages, and most of the remainder of this paper will focus on computing the image description and on properties of the resulting description.

Programs to compute the image description tree by successive blurring, extremal path following, and iso-intensity pixel linking have been written at Rijksuniversiteit Utrecht and The University of North Carolina. These programs differ slightly in the implementation details. Some of these differences will be presented later. The initial description will be of the UNC version. The programs are applicable in one, two, and three dimensions, in the last case not slice by slice but fully in 3D.

The tree described in section 1.3 represents the nesting structure of extremal regions. On the way to producing this structure it is useful to create an *intermediate description tree* which contains more detailed information about individual pixels. Each node in this tree corresponds to one pixel in the image stack, but only some pixels in the stack have a node in the tree. In particular, pixels that are either on an extremum path or an iso-intensity path make up the nodes in the tree.

A node corresponding to a non-extremum pixel is called a *normal node*, while one representing an extremum is an *extremum node*. Extremum nodes are linked by extremal path links to form a representation of an extremal path. Similarly, normal nodes are linked by normal path links to represent an iso-intensity path. A link to a normal node parent is called a normal path link, regardless of whether the child is a normal or extremum node, and an extremum node can be linked to an extremum parent by a normal path link if the connection is not part of an extremal path. Annihilation is represented by the connection of an extremum node via a normal path link to either a normal parent, or an extremum parent on a different extremal path.

An overview of the algorithm is as follows. The program links pixels in each level of the stack to pixels in the level above them. During this process it also creates nodes in the intermediate description tree. To accomplish this linking, the program works on the two adjacent images at the two stack levels being linked.

Each pixel in an image can be thought of as a potential node in the intermediate description tree. All pixels in the original image form leaf nodes of the tree; each will be either on an extremal path or an iso-intensity path. After acting on the two images as described below, the lower image is discarded (but any nodes created are kept in the tree); the upper image becomes the lower image; and the next slightly more blurred image becomes the new upper image. This process continues until only one extremal path remains. The remaining nodes are linked to this path, and the tree is then written to a file.

A skeleton of the procedure in pseudo-code is as follows:

find extrema in the original (currently "lower") image
while more than one extremum remains do
    blur "lower" image to create "upper" image
    find extrema in the upper image
    link pixels in the lower level to those in the upper level, creating nodes in the
        intermediate description tree as appropriate
    discard lower image; upper image becomes new lower image
link remaining paths to last extremal path. output tree to a file.

An explanation of the main elements of this algorithm follows.

3.1.1. Extrema identification.

Each of the two active planes is examined separately to find the existence and location of extrema. A point in an image is considered a maximum (minimum) if it is of greater (lesser) intensity than all of its eight surrounding pixels. The entire image is examined, and each of the extrema are marked as such. All other pixels are called "normal" pixels. Once this is done for the upper plane (it having previously been done for the lower plane), the linking routine is invoked.

3.1.2. Linking.

The linking routine examines each pixel in the lower plane that is on an extremum or iso-intensity (normal) path, i.e., that is a node in the tree. It finds an appropriate pixel in the upper plane to link to. The linking strategy for extremum pixels differs slightly from that for normal pixels.

The algorithm tries to link an extremum pixel in the lower image to a similar type (maximum or minimum) of extremum in the upper image. If it fails to be able to do so, then it invokes the linker for normal pixels, which has less stringent criteria for linking. The general strategy is to search for a parent in the small neighborhood surrounding the pixel directly above it in the upper image. The pixel in this neighborhood with intensity value closest to that of the child's in the lower image is picked as its parent. There is a maximum intensity difference allowed between a pixel in the lower plane and its parent. If no pixel in the selected upper plane neighborhood is close enough in intensity to the lower pixel, the neighborhood is enlarged slightly and the search continues. If no viable candidate is found then, the maximum intensity difference allowed is incremented and the neighborhood search is repeated. If this process fails to find a viable parent, the pixel is linked to the pixel directly above it.

Many extremum nodes can link to the same extremum father even though the theory for the continuous case does not allow an extremum to merge directly with another extremum, but instead requires it to merge with a saddle point, with both the saddle point and the extremum annihilating. If more than one extremum pixel is linked to the same extremum father, the extremum son with the closest intensity on the appropriate side of the father's intensity (above for a maximum, below for a minimum) is connected via an extremal path link. All of the others are connected by normal path links.

3.1.3. Node creation.

Conceptually any pixel in the upper level which has at least one child becomes a node in the intermediate description tree. Space is saved by representing the frequently occurring chains of pixels linked to the pixel directly below them with a single node holding the range of levels of the chain. A node may have many children. Both normal and extremum nodes may have normal and extremum children.

3.1.4. Extremum annihilation and object definition. Extremum nodes lie on extremal paths. That is, they have at least one child which is an extremal node, and they usually have a father which is an extremal node. This extremal path is considered to have annihilated if the extremum node is not linked to an extremum father or if it is linked via a normal path link.

The extremal node which is has been identified as annihilating is at the root of a subtree in the intermediate description tree. All nodes in this subtree belong to the extremal region associated with its extremal path. The nodes in the original image form the extremal region associated with this annihilation. This region frequently includes other extremal regions; that is, some of the subtree's nodes are annihilating extrema in their own right.

3.1.5. Termination. When only one extremum remains in the upper plane, the program is near completion. Links are created from the lower to upper plane in the usual fashion. Following this, one additional node is created. This becomes the root node of the intermediate description tree, and all nodes from the upper image plane are forced to link to this root node, in the process creating new subregion to region connections. The tree data structure, now complete, is written out to a file which can be read in and traversed by a display or pattern recognition program at a later time.

3.2. Implementation complications

The theory behind the stack technique was developed in continuous space. This means that intensity quantization (floating point), extremum and iso-intensity path following across discrete levels with discrete pixels, and finiteness of image size are all aspects which are not explicitly addressed in the basic theory.

The most significant problem arises from the non-infinitesimal blurring between each level in the stack. The major complication that this introduces is an uncertainty as to which pixel in the upper plane a pixel in the lower plane should link. In the continuous case, there is always a pixel in the upper plane with precisely the same intensity as the pixel in the lower plane, and it is always "close" to the same position as the lower pixel (in fact the path taken by the pixel from level to level is an integral curve of a vector field [Koenderink, 1984]). In the discrete case no pixel in the upper plane will have exactly the same intensity as its child, and the distance to be traversed for the link may be several pixels. Decision criteria must be developed to determine which possible linking candidate for parent pixel is the one to be chosen.

Linking criteria developed at UNC and at Rijksuniversiteit Utrecht differ somewhat. The main difference is in the way extremal points are handled. As mentioned above, at UNC each of the two active images is examined separately to locate extremal points. The points in the lower plane are then linked to an extremal point in the upper plane if possible, first by checking a close neighborhood and then a larger one. If no extremum father is found, the point is linked to a normal point.

At Rijksuniversiteit Utrecht extrema are identified only if an extremum son links to it. As at UNC the algorithm attempts to link each extremum in the lower image to an extremal point in the neighborhood just above it. If a match is not found, then hill climbing (or pit sliding) is performed until a maximum or a minimum, as appropriate for the extremal path in question, is reached. The pixel is linked to this. An extremal path is said to annihilate if a second extremal path links to the same parent pixel, in which case a decision is made as to which of the two is considered to be annihilating based on geometric and intensity differences between the father and the extremum sons.

The UNC approach requires more searching for extrema than the Utrecht approach, and it allows new extremal paths to begin at levels above the bottom. However, for evaluation of the method it allows the user to see which extrema have been missed, and extrema which are in fact due to arithmetic error do not cause problems because they annihilate quickly. The hill climbing (or pit sliding) heuristic used in Utrecht is not guaranteed to find correct links, but it may infrequently find a link that is missed by the UNC method and thus avoid creating a false annihilation.

Some other complications include determination of appropriate boundary conditions for the finite image and creation of extrema due to quantization effects. These complications can be dealt with by standard approaches without much difficulty.

3.3. Implementation performance

The current implementations have not been optimized for speed of execution or minimization of space. Some indications of the speed and size of the current UNC algorithm are nevertheless in order. The program has been applied to between five and ten CT images of the upper abdomen. It has also analyzed several synthetic images of one, two, and three dimensions. The Utrecht program has been applied to over ten 2D and 3D images from scintigraphy, MRI, radiography, and normal photography; the third dimension in the 3D images has sometimes been spatial depth and sometimes time. Most of the images have been reduced to 64 by 64 images to reduce time and space requirements of the algorithm in its testing and initial evaluation stage. Running on a moderately loaded VAX 780, the UNC program takes approximately 45 seconds to 1 minute to create each level in the stack, together with all its associated structures (marking extrema, linking to the new level, etc.). The 64 by 64 images tend to need about 20 levels of blurring before only one extremum remains. Thus the program runs for about 20 minutes. The intermediate description tree created takes about 250 kbytes, of which about half is blank inter-entry separators. Considerable space and display time could be saved by reducing the intermediate description tree to the simpler image description tree.

All of the above numbers scale approximately linearly with image area. Of course, an image with a lot of noise or very many objects will tend to take longer and create a larger data structure and so forth. If it is known in advance that the structures of interest in an image are of small scale, the processing may be terminated before only one extrema remains, saving much time.

4. INTERACTIVE DISPLAY BASED ON AN IMAGE DESCRIPTION TREE

The subdivision into regions labeled by scale and intensity provides the opportunity for the user to explore the extremal regions in the tree and select ones that are clinically meaningful and of interest. With previously available methods, defining such objects frequently involves drawing the boundary point by point. This is time consuming in two dimensions. In three dimensions not only is it unacceptably time consuming, but the normal approach of working slice by 2D slice impedes the use of interslice relations in defining the boundary.

In the approach that we have investigated, the user specifies dynamically a range of intensities and a range of scales, as well as a spatial window, and all original image pixels in regions with intensity or scale labels in these ranges are displayed if they are in the appropriate spatial window. When the user sees an object that is meaningful, the selected pixels can be taken to define the object or the result can be edited by the user. Then display or measurement operations on that object can commence.

Whenever it is desired to view the image, the display program reads in the image description tree from a file. The user is then able interactively to control which extremal regions in the image are displayed. This is done by means of various A/D devices. Two sliders are used to specify a scale range for objects to be viewed. For example, only big or high contrast objects could be displayed. Similarly, two sliders specify the intensity range of objects to be displayed. This would be used, for example, to select bright objects (like the spinal column). Four knobs are used to control the spatial locations in the image that are to be displayed (maximum and minimum x and y dimensions).

Currently the display program takes approximately two or three seconds to update the image displayed. This number is highly variable depending upon the number of objects in the image, their inter-relationships, the system load, and the speed of writing to the display device.

Below is a series of images displayed on our system. The original image that was analyzed is shown in figure 6a. This is a CT image of the upper abdomen, scaled down to a size of 64 by 64 pixels. It is displayed by adjusting the interactive knobs and sliders so as to ask for objects of all possible resolution sizes, intensity ranges, and spatial positions. The light area in the center bottom of the image is the spinal column. The roundish objects, one on either side of the spinal column, are the kidneys. On the left, about halfway up is the liver, which seems to be merging with the chest wall in this image. On the right side, above the kidney is the jejunum, and above that the transverse colon. The very dark regions are gas.

In figure 6b we have adjusted the sliders to ask only for those objects of larger scale, thus eliminating the noise. Notice that the darker regions around the kidneys are displayed as objects, even though medically they are not organs. This is an example of the program finding something which is not semantically meaningful, even though it is understandable why it did so. The major organs are clearly visible.

In figure 6c the spinal column has been eliminated by changing the intensity sliders to specify that bright objects not be displayed. It should be emphasized that these regions have been eliminated because they are regions associated with extremal paths whose annihilation intensities did not fall within the specified range. The display program is *not* simply looking at individual pixel intensities in the image. Only *extremal regions* can be displayed or removed.

In figure 6d the scale range requested specifies only the biggest objects, and all intensities are selected, resulting in a selection of the liver.

In figure 6e we have specified objects of slightly smaller scale only and have limited intensity to a middle range, thus obtaining the kidneys and jejunum. The liver is now gone.

5. EFFECTIVENESS AND FUTURE DIRECTIONS

The image descriptions produced when this stack method is applied to medical

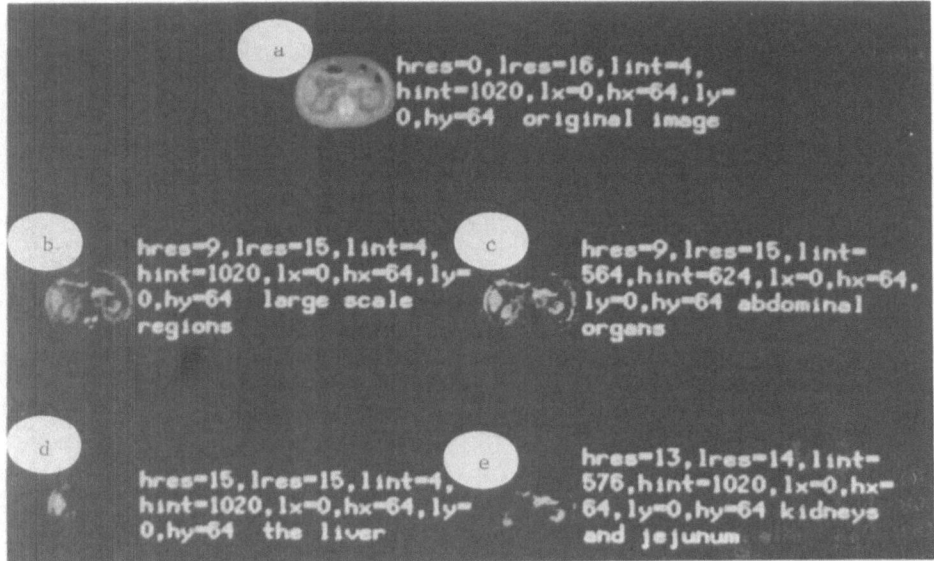

FIGURE 6. Interactive display based on image description of CT of the upper abdomen (at UNC)

images frequently contain regions that seem well related to meaningful image segments. This is true even in images with a low signal to noise ratio, such as those from nuclear medicine (see figure 7). There is therefore indication that segmentation methods based on this description will obtain far better segments than more common segmentation methods of edge detection or region growing. However, regions sometimes break up in semantically unnatural ways. For example, a blood vessel may break up into a number of pieces, and one piece may be a subregion of the organ in which it is contained, and another piece, say on the edge of the organ, may be a subregion of the region adjacent to the organ.

Structural pattern recognition techniques seem appropriate to bring semantic information to bear to correct this situation and at the same time label the objects, e.g. the blood vessel as such. These techniques operate by matching descriptions of known objects, e.g. an image description tree for a typical structure for a particular organ, to the description of our image, or a portion thereof. The multiresolution approaches have already shown themselves to be very well suited to this requirement [Rosenfeld, 1984; Crowley, 1984], as they allow one to operate at large scale (high in the description tree) first and to use matches there to guide matches at lower scale.

The results of such a matching process is the labeling of objects in the image description or the reorganization of the description tree to combine subobjects into previously undefined objects and then label the results. However, because the labeling

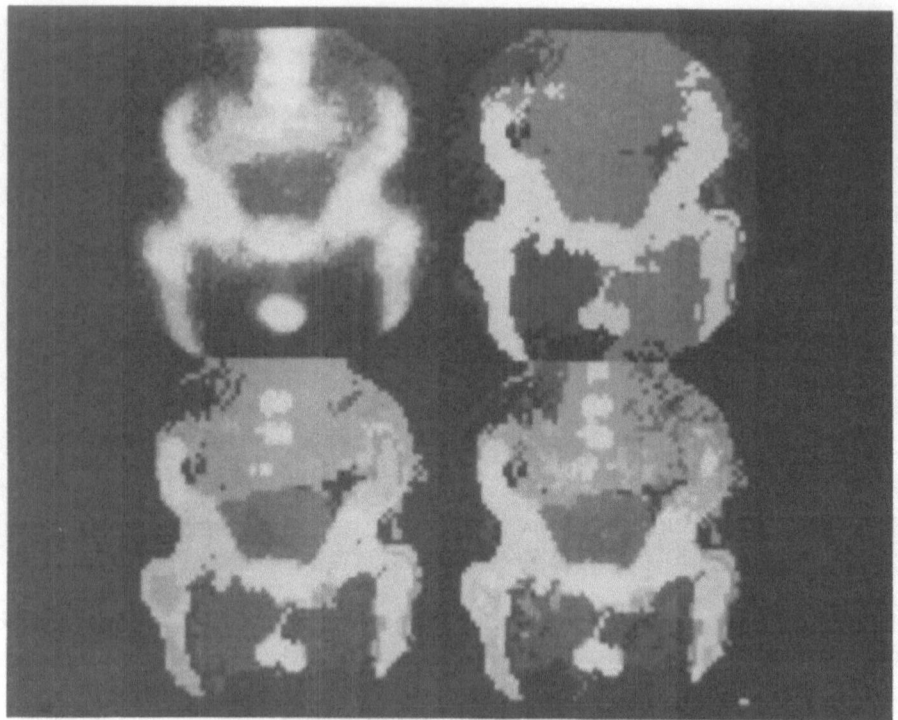

FIGURE 7. Extremal regions from image description of scintigram of the pelvis (at Rijksuniversiteit Utrecht). Upper left: original image. Other quadrants: each extremal region of scale smaller than some specified value is displayed with all its pixels at its average intensity.

depends on an image description that in the semantic sense is in error, it is likely that matching errors will result. We hypothesize that the labeling produced to date by image description followed by matching can be taken as tentative and used to produce an improved image description, which in turn could be used to produce an improved object definition and labeling. Therefore, we are presently working on

(1) creating improved image descriptions by letting the blurring used in producing the stack at any step depend on the previous tentative segmentation, and

(2) developing methods for matching the image description tree to *a priori* description trees for images or image objects to produce a labeled segmentation into image objects.

The modified blurring is nonstationary and nonisotropic, depending in scale in each direction on the scale and orientation of nearby objects that are at the stack level in question in the tentative segmentation.

We also anticipate using display based on the image description tree for defining objects in three dimensions. We plan to allow the user to select extremal regions by scale and intensity ranges, plus a 3D window, with the result displayed on the varifocal mirror or another self-luminous 3D display. When a meaningful object is seen, its surface can be directly calculated and used as the basis of a display that is more appropriate for therapy planning, such as a shaded graphics display.

ACKNOWLEDGEMENTS

We thank Alexander Toet, Cornelis de Graaf, and Matthew Mauro for useful discussions and the latter two for providing images used in this study. We are indebted to Joan Savrock for manuscript preparation and to Bo Strain and Karen Curran for photography. The research reported here was done partially with the support of grant number 1-R01-CA39060 from the U.S. National Institutes of Health and partially with the support of the Dutch Institute for Pure Scientific Research (ZWO).

REFERENCES

1. Crowley, J.L. and A.C. Sanderson, "Multiple Resolution Representation and Probabilistic Matching of 2-D Gray-Scale Shape", Tech. Rept. No. CMU-RI-TR-85-2, Carnegie-Mellon Univ., 1984. Also see Crowley, J.L. and A.C. Parker, "A Representation for Shape Based on Peaks and Ridges in the Difference of Low-Pass Transform", *IEEE Trans. PAMI*, March, 1984.
2. Koenderink, J.J. and A. van Doorn, "A Description of the Structure of Visual Images in Terms of and Ordered Hierarchy of Light and Dark Blobs", *Proc. 2nd Int. Conf. on Vis. Psychophysics and Med. Imaging*, IEEE, Cat. No. 81CH1676-6, 1981.
3. Koenderink, J.J., "The Structure of Images", *Biol. Cybernetics, 50:* 363-370, 1984.
4. Rosenfeld, A., ed., *Multi-resolution Image Processing and Analysis,* Springer-Verlag, New York, 1984.
5. van Os, C.F.A., "The Inca-Pyramid Algorithm", Tech. Rept. No. VMFF 30-84, Institute of Medical Physics, Rijksuniversiteit Utrecht, Utrecht, Netherlands, 1984.

SOME ASPECTS OF MR IMAGE PROCESSING AND DISPLAY: SIMULATION STUDIES, MULTIRESOLUTION SEGMENTATION, AND ADAPTIVE HISTOGRAM EQUALIZATION

Cornelis N. de Graaf, Christianus J.G. Bakker, Jan J. Koenderink, Peter P. van Rijk

0 Introduction

In the years 1982-1984 we have designed and built a software system for the quantitative processing, analysis and display of magnetic resonance 2D and 3D images and timeseries of images. This system supports two research projects in our university, "NMR in Oncology", and "MRI Processing and Simulation Studies".

The aim of this paper is to discuss three topics that are of particular interest. By means of simulation studies one can obtain information concerning optimal pulse sequences in certain clinical indications. Multiresolution segmentation was already previously subject of our research, now it is investigated how this technique can be utilized in simulation studies, and in quantitative tissue characterization. Finally it was investigated how the adaptive histogram equalization technique could be used to display (e.g. in a PACS console) MR images with as few interactive parameters as possible.

1 Simulation studies

In the present day practise of MR imaging the acquisition parameters (pulse sequences) are set according to the physician's experience or to data (e.g. obtained from the literature) concerning the particular clinical indication. By simulation studies the knowledge on optimal acquisition parameters for a range of clinical indications can be improved. The method is based on the fact that once NH (proton density), T1 (spin-lattice relaxation time), and T2 (spin-spin relaxation time) images of a tomographic slice are known, this information is sufficient to compute ("simulate") the images for any acquisition pulse sequences imaginable [1].

NH, T1 and T2 images can be computed from a combined multidelay inversion recovery (IR) and multiecho spin-echo (SE) acquisition [2,3]. However, previous to the computation of these three parametric images, usually several corrections have to be carried out.

There are many, but principally two types of spatial distortions that can occur with acquisitions that produce multiple images of a single slice. The first is related to offset-errors or drift in the ADC's during the course of the study. Figure 1 shows two succesive IR images at different TI (inversion time), from which it can be appreciated that

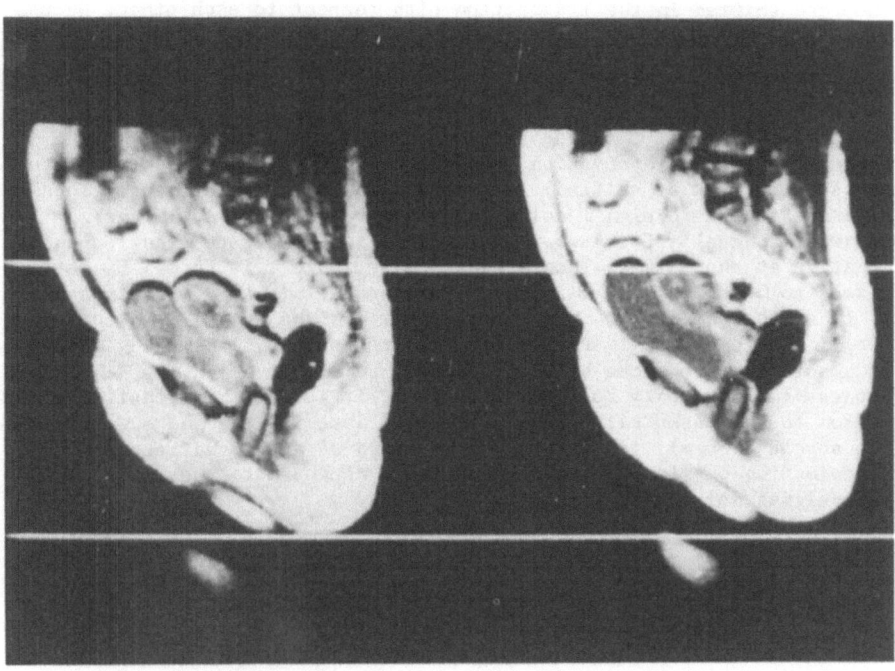

Figure 1. Two successive images from a multidelay IR measurement, at TI = 750 and 1000 msec, respectively. Notice the upward shift in the righthand image, relative to the lefthand one.

they are shifted in the Y direction with respect to each other. We use a pixelshift method to match such images to each other. Figure 2 demonstrates how this method works for two successive images s and s'. Notice that s may already have been shifted with respect to its successors. First of all s is histogrammed to print-out, and the standard deviation σ of the zero-signal peak is determined. On the basis of a priori information (the noise distribution in regions outside the structure to be shifted) a threshold factor f is set, that globally separates the zero-signal noise bandwidth from the tissue signal bandwidth. Usually f is 1.5. Notice that, in IR, tissue signals can be negative at short TI's. Then a binary mask image t is formed by setting pixels to 0, unless [s]>fσ, then pixels are set to 1. Similarly a mask t' of s' is formed. Now Δx, Δy to shift t' in the X- and Y-directions (or, in the case of figure 1, only y) are found by minimizing the sum of absolute differences between t and t' shifted over Δx,Δy. Since this process includes only boolean operations, it is extremely fast. The reason to use masks rather than the image data itself (and e.g. minimize the absolute norm), is that IR images s and s' are of different distribution outside +fσ signals, but are approximately equal in the zero-signal noise bandwidth.

A second type of spatial distortion can be corrected for less easy. Figure 3 shows the result of the above mentioned shift correction. The body contours are now in place (see lower line). However, since multiple-TI IR-measurements may last from minutes to tens of minutes, the structures within the body have changed their relative locations: the bladder is filling, and pushes some tissues in the cranial direction. An appropriate correction for this distortion should imply a subimage warping technique or rubber sheet matching [4] which we have not yet implemented.

In IR imaging pixel intensities are often related to the magnitude of the recorded signals [5]. This loss of sign information may be avoided by adjusting the phase during reconstruction, however, this is no trivial task, and is usually left undone. Hence, signals of the same magnitude but with opposite sign cannot be distinguished in an IR image unless additional information is available. The inability to discriminate between positive and negative signals may involve serious errors when quantitative T1 images are to be extracted from multi-TI images including relatively low TI's. We reported previously on a method to correct for sign-errors in IR image-series [6]. The method starts from the observation that the IR curve is monotonically increasing with TI, and comes down to a pixel-by-pixel determination of the zero-crossing TI0. In Figure 4 it can be observed that the first two of the five recorded signals clearly must be inverted, and that the last two must remain positive. It can easily be shown that there is always only one point of which the sign is uncertain (here the third). Now a weighted (on the inverse square of the signal values) second order polynomial is fitted through the inverted first two and the last two points of the curve, and the sign of the third point is easily found from the zero-crossing TI0 of the polynomial fit (here negative). See Figure 5. If an accurate TI0 value is required, the polynomial fit can be repeated on all restored signals.

We have investigated two methods for the computation of quantitative NH, T1 and T2 images, starting from several sequences of SE and IR images,

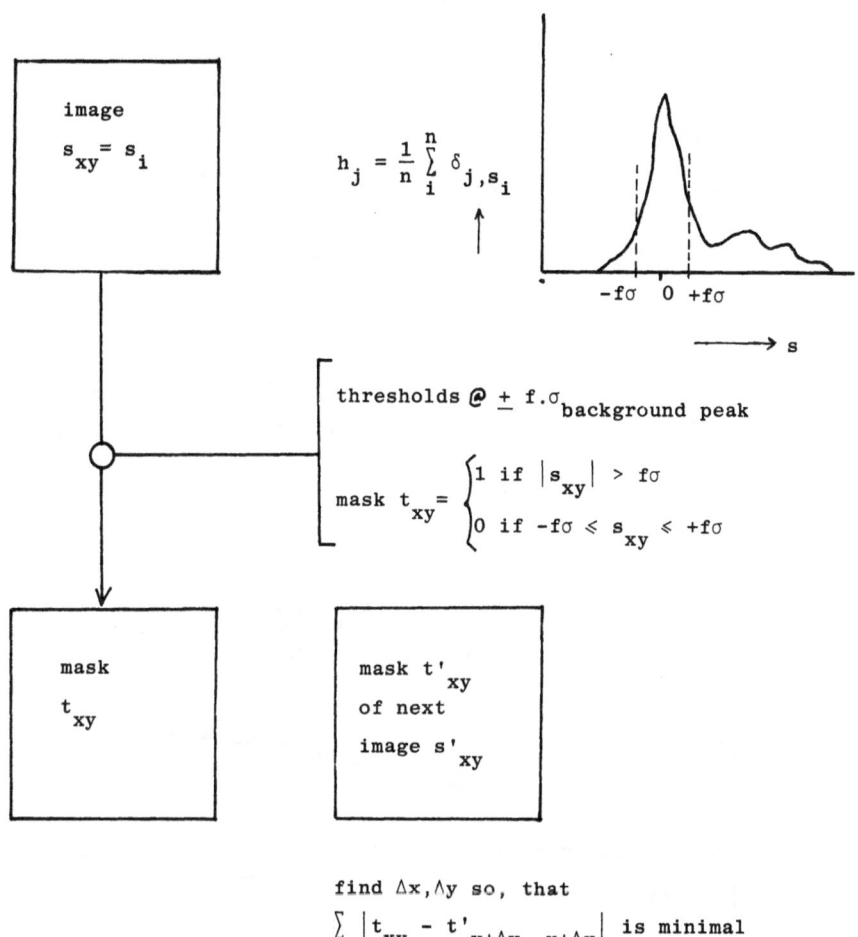

Figure 2. Pixel shift method. Image s is histogrammed to h. Mask t is created by thresholding s, and similarly t' from s'. Then s' is shifted along x and y so, that the absolute norm of t-t' is minimal.

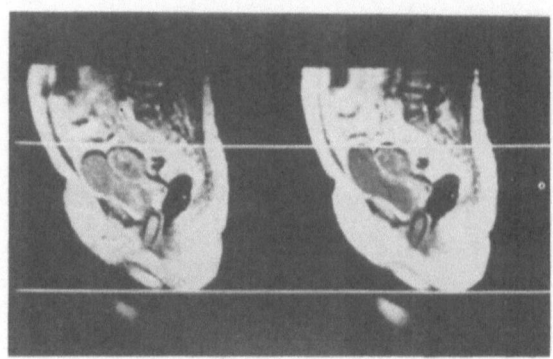

Figure 3. The righthand image (compare to Figure 1) is shifted in the Y direction. The body contour is now in place, but still some dissimilarities remain, see upper line.

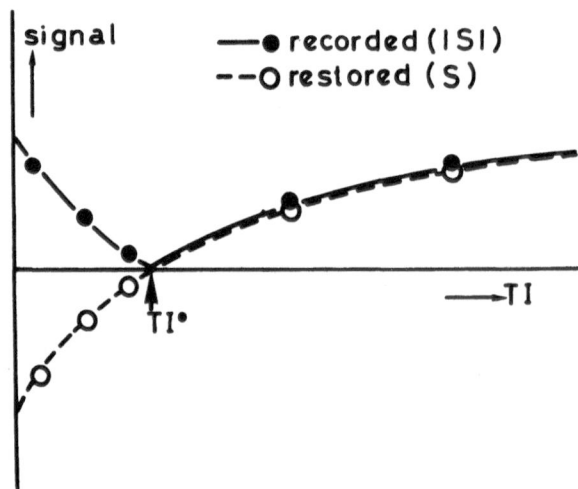

Figure 4. Graphical representation of the NMR signal as a function of the inversion time TI in an inversion recovery experiment, demonstrating the relationship between the recorded and the polarity restored IR curve. TI0 indicates the zero-crossing of the IR curve.

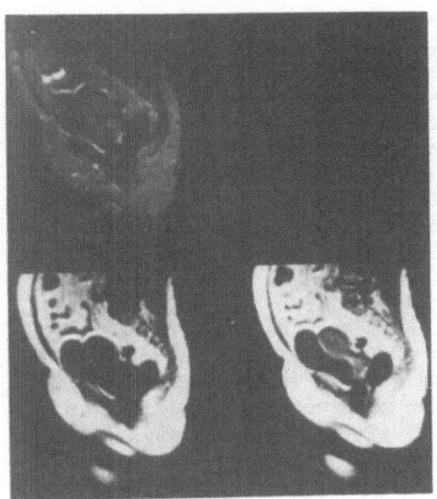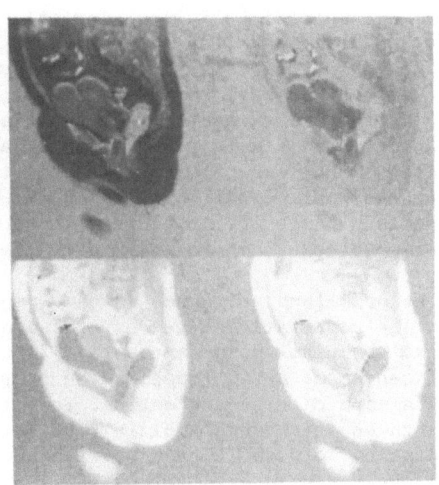

Figure 5. Four images out of an IR sequence, left: before, right: after sign correction. The images were taken at TI's 33, 150, 300, and 1500 msec, respectively.

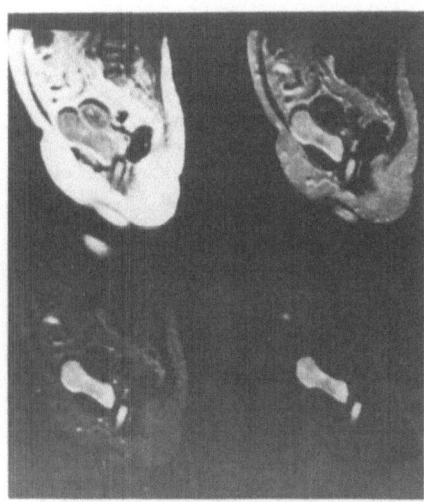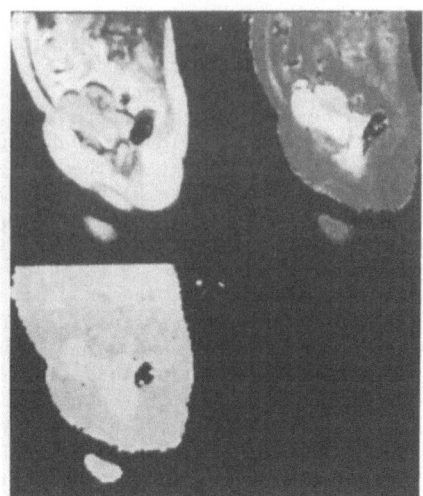

Figure 6. Right: computed T1, T2, and NH images (individually scaled to maximum intensity). Left: SE-images, at TE = 52, 104, 156, and 208 msec, used for T2 and NH computation. The IR-images of Figure 5 were used for zero-crossing, T1, and NH computation.

and the related full (not simplified) Bloch equations. The first method employed an iterative evaluation of NH, Tl and T2 simultaneously on a pixel-by-pixel basis. This method suffers from the complexity of the equations (in both SE and IR there are sums of exponential terms in the numerator and products of exponential terms in the denominator [7]), and the noise in single pixel signals. Although a robust iteration scheme was used (Levenberg-Marquardt), it turned out that either the initial guesses must be well chosen, or the data must be quite noiseless for a succesfull result. Apart from that, the computation time was awfully long. We come back to this in chapter 2.

Another method, on which we have reported earlier [3] is more efficient, in the computational sense. A T2 image can simply be computed by pixel-by-pixel mono-exponential fitting of the signals in a multi-echo SE sequence. A TIO image can be computed as described before in the paragraph on sign-correction. Then it was observed that at t=TIO the Bloch-equation for a multi-TI IR-sequence simplifies to an analytical relation between TIO and Tl without dependence of NH and T2. Hence Tl can be computed easily from TIO. Further on it turns out that NH can be simply calculated from Tl and the intercept that is set aside at the exponential fitting for T2 computation. See Figure 6.

Some postprocessing of the computed NH, Tl and T2 images is required. We removed the noise in regions outside the body (and of air inside the body) by thresholding upon a fraction of the maximum in an average absolute signal image (AASI) for the SE and the IR sequences, usually 10%. That is, NH, Tl, and T2 values for a pixel were set to zero, if its value in either the SE-AASI or the IR-AASI was less than 0.1 of the maximum.

The actual simulation implied the following processing. In one of the measured or computed images a region of interest (ROI) was manually drawn around the tissue structure of clinical interest (Figure 7). Since the aim is to simulate acquisitions that visually separate this structure best from its surroundings, also ROI's were drawn in the surrounding tissues, one for each region of approximately uniform values, that is adjacent to the center ROI. For each pixel that belonged to any of the ROI's, the Bloch equations were applied to its NH, Tl, and T2 values, to compute signals corresponding to the pulse sequences to be simulated. For each simulated pulse sequence, and within each of the ROI's the average S and the standard deviation σ of simulated pixel signals was determined. Then a contrast map was computed. A contrast map for an SE (1 echo) simulation is a 2D image, with echo times (TE) plotted on the X-axis, and repetition times (TR) on the Y-axis. A "pixel"-intensity at a certain (TE,TR) in a contrast map is the smallest of the contrast values of the center ROI with respect to the neighbour ROI's (we call this "worst case contrast"). Similarly, a contrast map for an IR simulation (1 echo) is a 3D image, with TE plotted on the X-, TR plotted on the Y-, and inversion times (TI) plotted on the Z-axis (See Figure 8). From the Bloch-equations it can be easily demonstrated that the SE contrast map is identical to the slice in the IR contrast map at TI=0.

We computed contrast-to-noise (CNR) values rather than the contrast measures that have been used by others [8, 9, 10]. The contrast perceived from two adjacent regions A and B with average signals S_A and

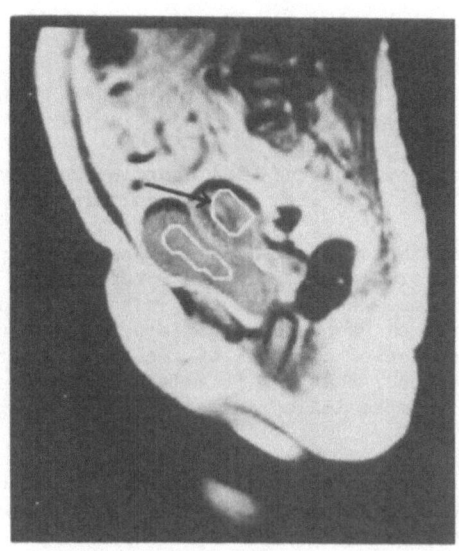

Figure 7. A first-echo SE image with ROI's drawn for contrast measurements. The "central ROI" is drawn over the tumour (arrow). There are 3 "peripheral ROI's", drawn over the bladder (lower left), the uterus (lower right), and the gut (upper right). The actual ROI's used for computations were somewhat bigger than they are shown here.

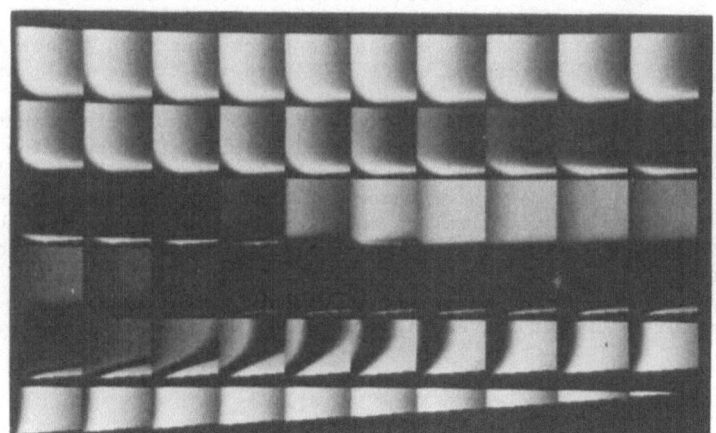

Figure 8. 3D contrast map of an IR-simulation of the patient study shown in Figures 6 and 7. The 3D map is displayed here as a series of (TE,TR) maps at exponentially increasing TI's, from 0 to 6000 msec. TE (X-axis) ranges from 8 to 512 msec. TR (Y-axis) ranges from 100 to 6400 msec. There are two highest CNR-values (here displayed as intensities) throughout the map: at TI=0, TE=144, TR=2300, and at TI=2256, TE=152, TR=2700.

S_B and noise (variance) levels σ_A^2 and σ_B^2 is globally given by:

$$CNR(A,B) = |S_A - S_B| \,/\, (\sigma_A^2 + \sigma_B^2)^{\frac{1}{2}}$$

In this way we don't have to worry about the nature of the noise that is present in ROI's (instrumental, biological, other).

The highest CNR value thoughout the (3D) contrast map gives us (TE,TR,TI) for the acquisition with optimal contrast (Figure 9).

We have simulated only the simplest SE and IR sequences possible. This is for practical reasons. The physician is interested to know what, in a given clinical indication, the fastest way is to obtain a first picture with a high probability on usefulness. If he were to acquire a complicated pulse sequence or a series of sequences to start with, he could as well acquire such, that NH, T1 and T2 images can be computed, or, even better, one or more images can be obtained by optimalization in feature space.

The latter consideration implies also, that the attractiveness of (TE,TR,TI) combinations should play a part in the judgement of the contrast map. Long TR's are inattractive, although the desire for short TR's (in order to minimize noise) may be offset by the need for long TR values in order to collect multiple slices. Furthermore there are some machine limitations like shortening TE below 10 msec. Although interesting from an academical point of view, we did not look at physically impossible sequences.

It may be advisable to simulate, apart from the CNR-optimized image, also an image at a (TE,TR,TI) for which a measured image is available, and visually compare them. Even better would it be to measure an image at optimal (TE,TR,TI) after the simulation has been carried out. In some situations the simulation fails because the Bloch equations do not apply as such, such as in the presence of flow (Figure 10) or chemical shift.

Some investigators have looked at the propagation of noise in computed [1] and synthetic [11] images. We have been wondering [12] what the effect would be of "extrapolated simulation". That is, simulating images with pulse sequence parameters of which the values extend more or less beyond the range of parameter values that were applied to measure the data from which NH,T1,T2 were computed. We did a couple of extrapolated simulations of which one is shown in Figure 11. For extrapolation outside the measured TI-range all of them showed an increasing underestimation of CNR at increasing TI's beyond the measured range.

2   Multiresolution segmentation

We have previously reported on the applicability of multiresolution image analysis schemes [13,14], such as the stack and the pyramid, on in-vivo medical imaging. The stack [13 - 16] is a general multiresolution scheme that allows for image segmentation, image feature description in database-like structures, extremum following, etc. The pyramid represents a less general multiresolution scheme, but is ideally suited for fast image segmentation [17]. Within the scope of our projects, just segmentation was of issue, so we restricted ourselves to the pyramid, in the first instance.

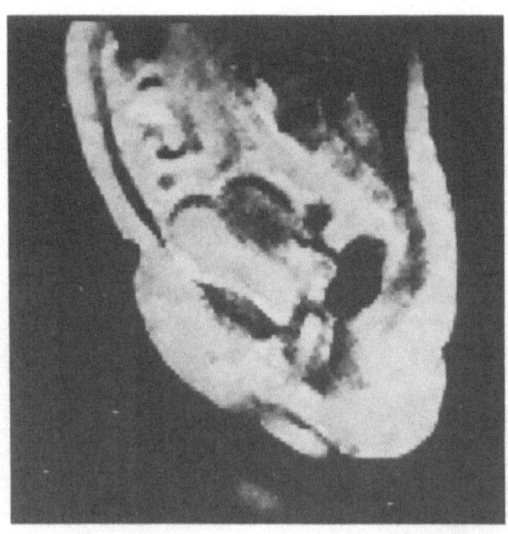

Figure 9. IR-image computed from NH,T1,T2 data in Figure 6, according to the (optimum) pulse sequence TI=2256,TE=152,TR=2700. The optimum computed SE-image (TE=144,TR=2300, see legend of Figure 8) turns out to be almost identical. Notice the high constrast of the tumour (see also Figure 7) with respect to its surroundings.

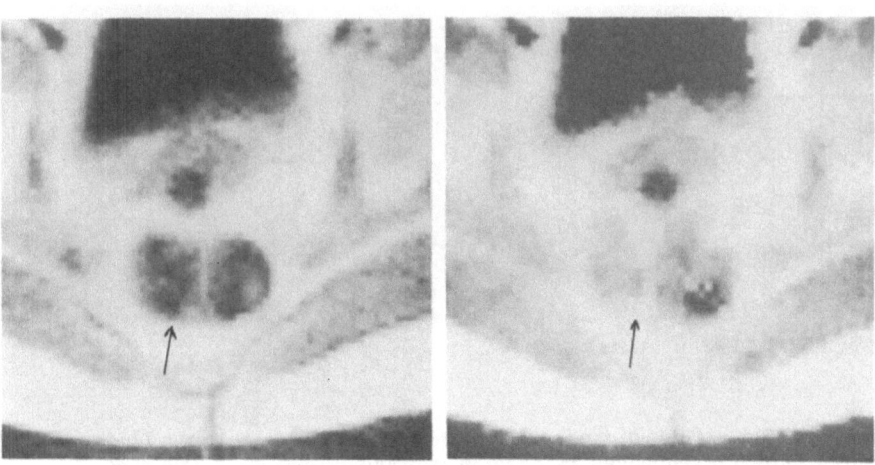

Figure 10. Measured (left) and computed (right) MR images at the same (IR) pulse sequences. The signal distributions match fairly, except in the region of the colon (arrow). The contents of the colon have moved during the measurements.

A   B

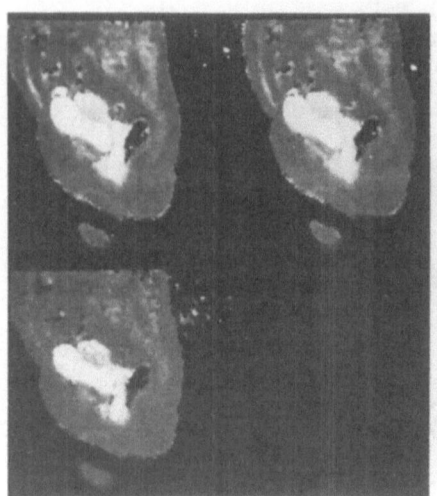
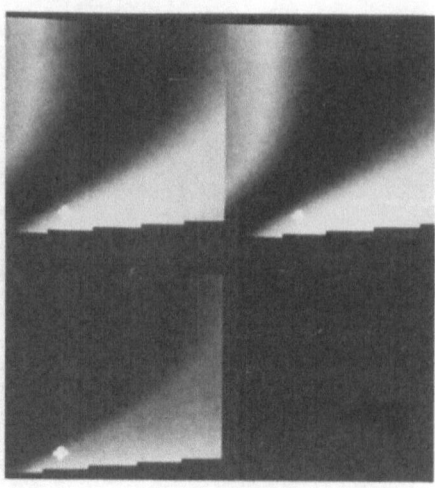

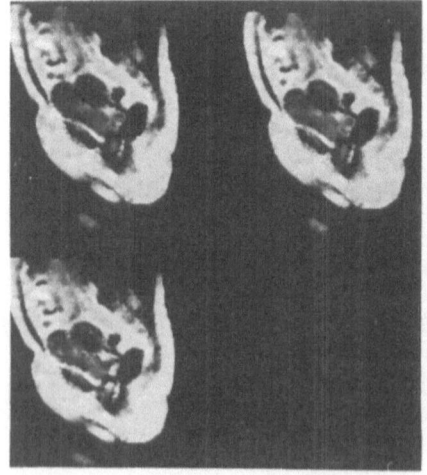
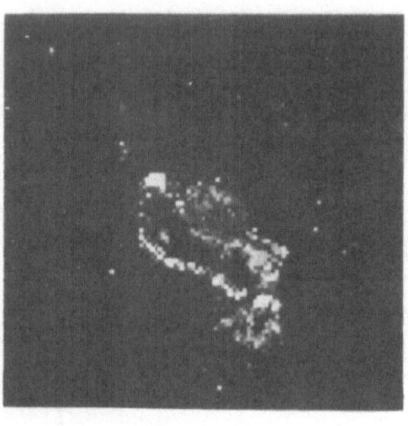

C

D

Figure 11. The effect of "extrapolated simulation". A: three T1-images,
computed from IR-sequences ranging up to 3000, 1500, and 750 msec,
respectively. B: contrast maps for an IR-simulation at TI=970, using the
T1-images in frame A, and the NH and T2 images from Figure 6. The cursor
points at TE=160,TR=1600. C: simulated images at TI=970,TE=160,TR=1600,
computed from T1,T2,NH as described above for the contrast maps. D:
absolute difference image in comparing the simulated images computed on the
basis of IR-ranges up to 3000 and 750.

A pyramid for 2D images is an layered arrangement of square arrays in which each array is half as long and wide as the next array below it (Figure 12). The pixels in the pyramid array are all indexed by triplets (x,y,u), in which x and y are spatial coordinates, and u is the height in the pyramid. In a given layer each pixel holds the average of some of the nearby pixels in the layer below. The bottom layer contains the image to be processed.

A son-father relationship is defined between pixels in adjacent layers, such that all descendants of a pixel are considered to be in the same segment. Thus the son-father relationship is based on closeness in intensity. In particular, each pixel has 4 candidate fathers (a sub-array of 2x2) and chooses the one with the closest intension as its father. The sets of candidate fathers of two adjacent pixels in a pyramid layer overlap by 50%. As a result a father can have between 0 and 16 (a subarray of 4x4) sons. The father-son links form tree structures within the pyramid (Figure 12B). The father-son relationships (segments) are not fixed, but are redefined at each iteration. At each iteration all pixels in layers other than the bottom layer are computed as the average of the bottom layer pixels that belong to their descendants according to the father-son links at the previous iteration. Based on these new within-segment averages, the father-son linkages are recomputed. At the zeroth iteration the averages are taken over all candidate bottom layer descendants.

Changes in son to father links in a given iteration step result in changes of values of pyramid pixels, which in a next iteration can lead to alteration in the links of those pixels, so that after down projection new segments may differ both in value and size from the old ones. Since such alterations shift segments in directions so, that their contents become more homogeneous, this iteration process is guaranteed to converge [18]. For the segmentation of a 256^2 image usually 6-14 iterations are needed.

In order to control the amount of segmentation (in the extreme case all pixels in the pyramid are linked to the single pixel at the top) we established linkage criteria as follows (see Figure 13). If D is the maximum possible difference of pixel values, and f is a threshold criterion, than a (son) pixel within the pyramid is not assigned a son-father link, if the intensity difference with the most likely of its candidate fathers is greater than fD. Hence such a pixel becomes the "root" (= upper pixel) of a segment. A subcriterion connected to this is to allow the linkage criterion to act only above a certain layer, so as to avoid the development of roots of many little segments in lower layers. See Figure 14. Notice that this criterion is imbedded in the bottom-up iterative process, such in contrast to a similar top-down criterion that has been suggested by Ortendahl [19].

The segmentation method described so far, has great potentials in clustering pixels together (also those that are spatially separated in the image - this is called "remote linking") for whatever reason. An obvious and powerful application is in tissue characterization [19], but also other types of MR image processing and analysis may benefit from multiresolution segmentation. We used the pyramid both in the quantitative determination of NH,T1,T2 images and as a tool to speed up

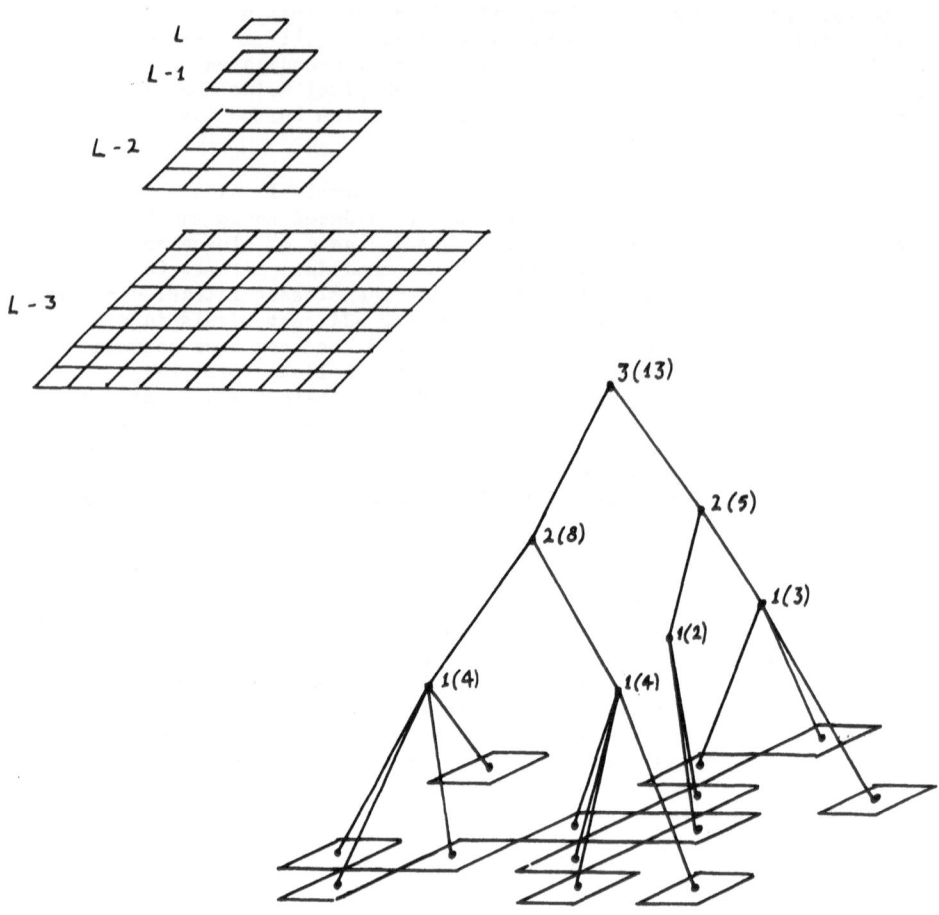

Figure 12. Left: top of a multiresolution pyramid with the 4 upper layers of 1x1, 2x2, 4x4, and 8x8 pixels. Right: a tree structure formed within a pyramid, all indicated nodes here belong to one segment.

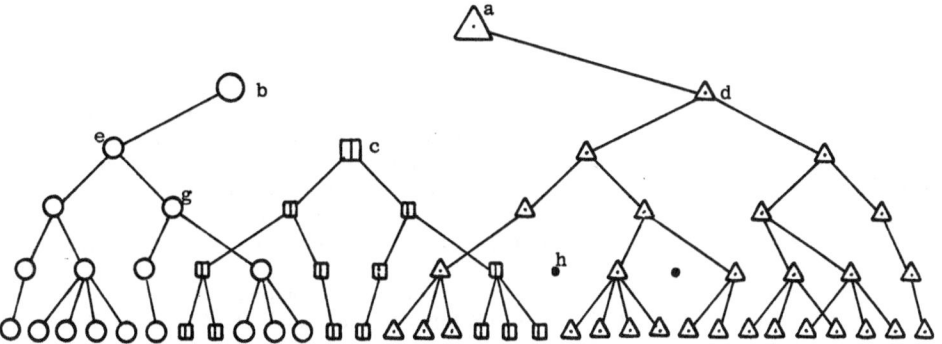

nodes a, b and c are roots:

$$|\bar{b} - \bar{a}| > f.D$$

$$|\bar{c} - \bar{b}| > f.D \; ; \; |\bar{c} - \bar{d}| > f.D$$

node g links to e: $f.D > |\bar{g} - \bar{e}| < |\bar{g} - \bar{c}|$

node h isn't linked to and doesn't link

Figure 13. Linkage criteria (see text). D = maximum possible difference of pixel values. f = criterion: fD = linkage threshold.

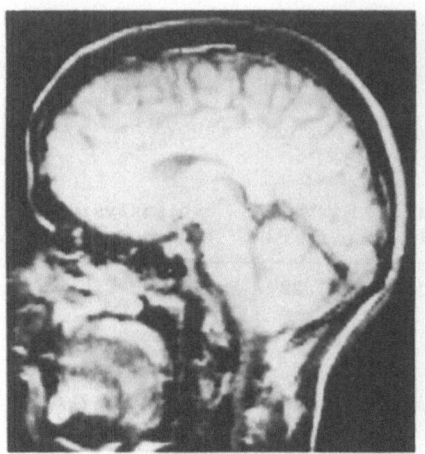 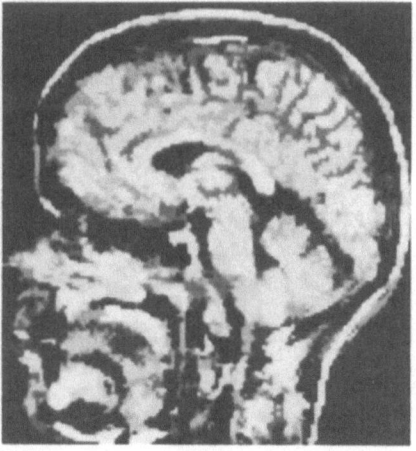

Figure 14. Original (left) and segmented (right) 128x128 MR image. The threshold above which no linkages were established was 15% of the pixel intensity range, and acted only at layers 2 (32x32 resolution) and above in the pyramid. The number of iterations required was 9, the number of different segments produced was 18.

MR image processing in a more general sense: pixel-by-pixel computations are brought down to segment-by-segment (or region-by-region) computations.

As mentioned in chapter 1, the pixel-by-pixel iterative evaluation of the Bloch equations related to a combination of multi-TE SE-measurements and multi-TI IR-measurements in an attempt to estimate NH,T1,T2 has its drawbacks. Either the initial guesses for the parameters must be extremely well chosen, or the data must be nearly noiseless, otherwise the iteration scheme (Figure 15) is likely to converge to false minima, if convergence is achieved at all. We devised a "vector-pixel pyramid", of which the pixels are multi-valued: each with as many values as IR + SE measurements were carried out during acquisition. Differences between pixel-vectors (sons to fathers) were computed as the Euclidian norm (or, square root of the sums of squares of invidual value-differences). The fact that these vectors do not exist in a strictly orthogonal system was ignored. Scaling of the various dimensions (several IR's, SE's) was not necessary, since all values were already equally scaled RF signals.

This vector-pixel pyramid was run until convergence of the linkage-tree was achieved. Then, instead of downprojection of the segments, the before described Bloch evaluation iteration scheme (Figure 15) was downprojected. Starting at the top of the pyramid (where there is very little noise, and one can afford rough initial guesses) this iterative evaluation was applied, and the outputs, NH,T1,T2 values, were downprojected along the linkages as new initial guesses for the lower layer, and so on, until the bottom layer was reached. So far we have applied this scheme to several 16x16 sub-images obtained from actual MR measurements, as a preliminary test. The resulting NH, T1 and T2 images (also of 16x16) happened to be almost identical to those which were computed via the before mentioned zero-crossing method. The computation time measurements are summarized in Table I.

TABLE I: NH,T1,T2 COMPUTED FROM 2 SE + 3 IR

	iterative		
	without pyramid	with pyramid	exp.analysis + zero-crossing
computation time	161(20)	39(22)	2.7
number of fails	11%	0,3%	0%

() = when EA + ZC used as initial guess

This effort to iteratively evaluate the pure Bloch-equations, while the zero-crossing method works fine and quick, was done in order to illustrate the usefulness of the pyramid to speed-up iterative processes in general (also in non-MR medical imaging). Amongst other applications, we plan to incorporate Venot's method [4] for image warping (also an

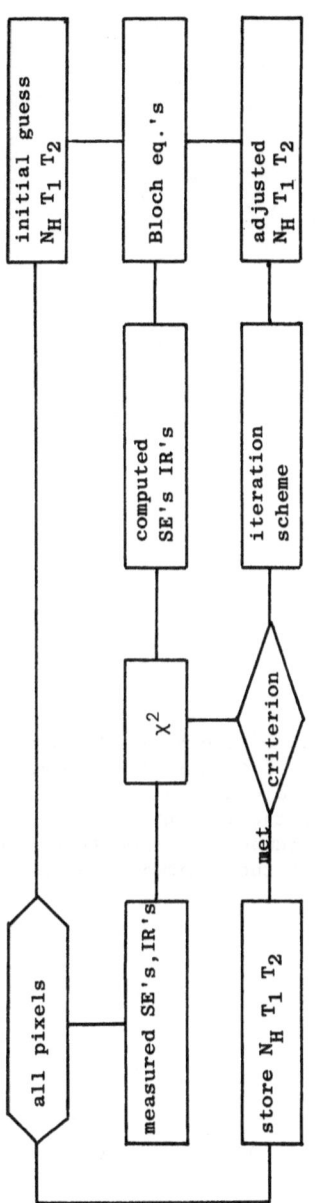

Figure 15. Iterative Bloch equation evaluation. For all pixels of the image initial values (guesses) NH,T1,T2 are set, and the signal values of the SE and IR measurements are stored. Within the iteration loop the current NH,T1,T2 parameters are combined with the Bloch equations for the actual measurements, and new signal values are computed. These are compared with the measured signals using (for example) chi-square. If the convergence criterion is not met, the current NH,T1,T2 parameters are adjusted by an iteration scheme for the solution of nonlinear equations.

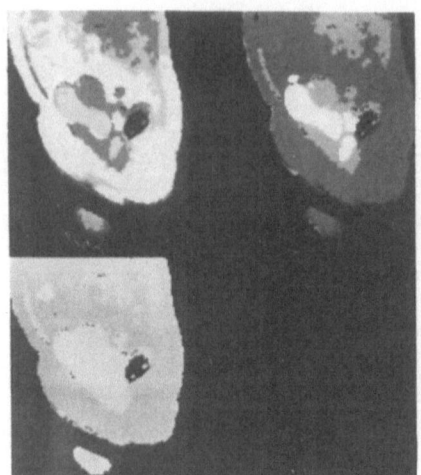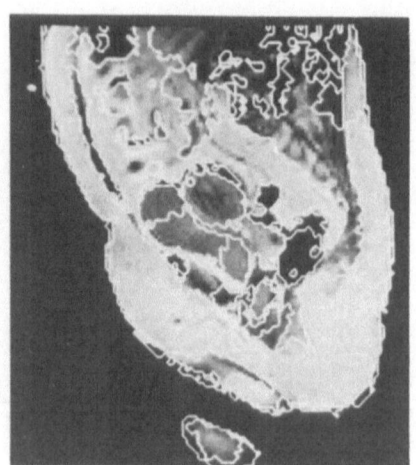

Figure 16. Result of vector-pyramid processing of the NH,T1,T2 data shown
in Figure 6. Left: the individual NH, T1, and T2 images after segmentation,
right: a measured first-echo SE image of the same patient with segment
edges drawn. The linkage threshold was 20% of the maximum difference
vector, the number of iterations was 11, the number of segments produced
was 19. The input images were scaled so, that: the maximum NH = 1000 msec
T1 = 250 msec T2.

iterative scheme) into the pyramid. Also iterative tomographic reconstruction algorithms are likely candidates for vector-pixel pyramid processing (but then in 3D).

Another nice example of the usefulness of the vector-pyramid starts off with NH,T1,T2 image data. In tissue characterization by using the pyramid as a tool [19], up till now the NH, T1, and T2 images (or other combinations of measured or computed images) were segmented individually, and following the pyramid processing the image segments were combined with each other. We have done some experiments (Figure 16) on the segmentation of images with (NH,T1,T2)-valued pixels as vectors. It turns out that tissue structures with different (NH,T1,T2) are honestly separated from each other, also if two of the three parameters are about equally valued.

3 Adaptive histogram equalization

In displaying CT and MR images human interaction is needed to set the proper intensity window for the optimal display of image features that are of diagnostic interest. Often multiple window settings are needed, when these features happen to manifest themselves on quite different intensity levels. In such cases usually multiple hard-copies of the displayed image are made, one for each of the window settings. With the advent of PACS display consoles, such interaction, for each of the many (multimodality) simultaneously displayed images individually, should be limited wherever possible.

A general approach would be to look at the amount of a priori information needed for the optimal mapping of an image on a display. Sometimes this a priori information pertains to a class of images, for example multiple gated scintigraphic bloodpool images (e.g. displayed as a movie), where a window offset of 40% of the maximum intensity nearly always gives a satisfactory display. Here the a priori information consists of one parameter, and is associated with a class of images. In other instances the a priori information is associated with the individual images within a class, and is to be entered interactively, like the window position and width (two parameters) in displaying CT or MR images. Notice that when multiple features on different intensity levels must be highlighted, the number of parameters is even higher, a multiple of two.

Pizer [20] noticed that in the absence of a priori information it is reasonable to suppose that the more pixels there are that have intensities in an given range, the more likely it is that changes in that range are important. This observation leads to a mapping scheme called "histogram equalization": the mapped image has the property that each of its intensities are used by an equal number of pixels. The difficulty with this method is that it adapts to the whole image, whereas the image is not visually perceived as a whole, but instead the eye adapts to local context when attempting to discern information at a particular image location.

The method that deals with this problem is called "adaptive histogram equalization" (AHE) [20]. In principle each pixel's intensity should be mapped by a different mapping that optimizes the information

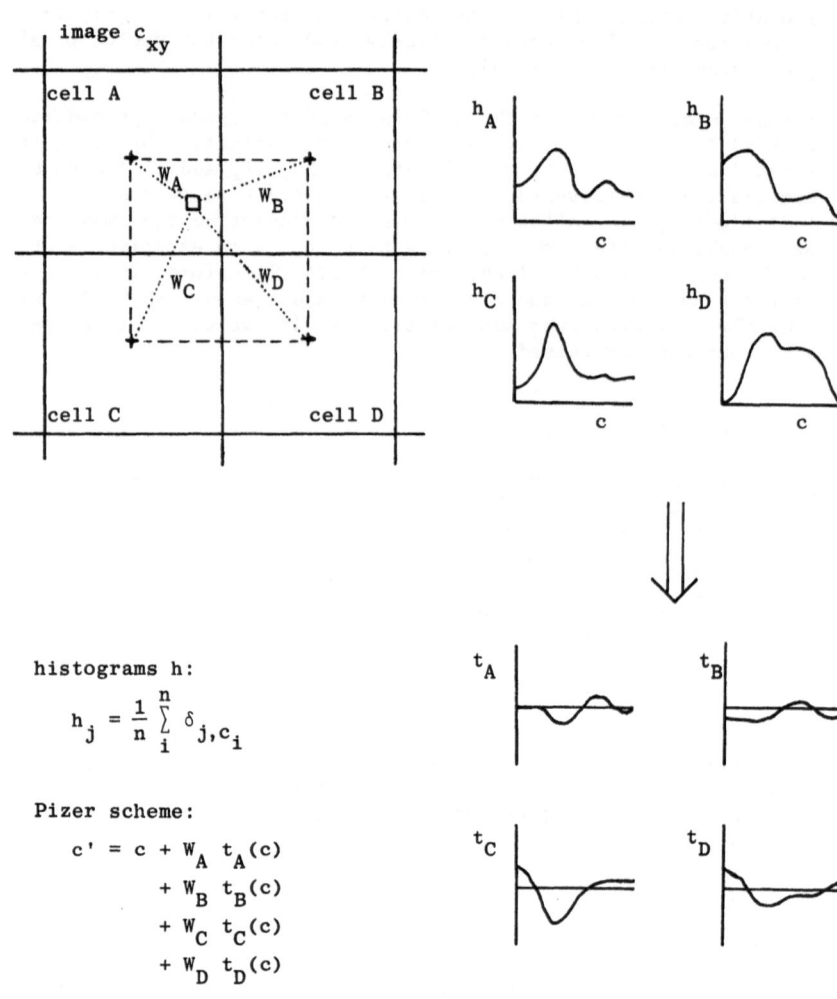

histograms h:

$$h_j = \frac{1}{n} \sum_i^n \delta_{j,c_i}$$

Pizer scheme:

$$c' = c + W_A\, t_A(c)$$
$$+ W_B\, t_B(c)$$
$$+ W_C\, t_C(c)$$
$$+ W_D\, t_D(c)$$

Feature weighting: $t' = f(t,\ \text{cell feature})$

E.g. to avoid noise augmentation:

$$t' = t \cdot \frac{\text{local SNR}}{\text{max SNR}}$$

Figure 17. Diagram of adaptive histogram equalization. See text.

transmission in the region surrounding that pixel, or its "contextual region". This method, implemented as such [21], however, takes an awful lot of computation time. Pizer devised a computation scheme that is several orders of magnitude faster, based on division of the image into non-overlapping regions of the size of a contextual region, called "basic contextual regions", here called "cells". See Figure 17. In each of the image cells the histogram h is determined, and from the histogram the "intensity shift table" t, which is a table that gives for each recorded pixel value, the value to be added so as to equalize the mapped intensities in the cell. t Is computed by integration of h over the intensities, normalizing to the maximum intensity, and·subtracting the unit intensity line. The AHE is carried out by, for each image pixel, finding the four cells of which the centers are nearest to the pixel, and adding to the pixel value the average of the corresponding entries in the four cells' intensity shift tables, weighted on the geometrical distances of the pixel to the cells' centers (Figure 17).

The method described here is completely parameter-free, insofar a priori information is at issue. However, there are some problems [22]. One is, see Figure 18, that in relatively large areas with relatively low contrast the noise is augmented considerably. In background areas outside the body contour this problem can be overcome by an image edge growing technique to set this area to zero, but inside the body contour this problem remains. Another problem is that fine structures with sharp edges (such as thin blood vessels in a DSA image, or thin ligaments in an MR image) become thickened, due to the effect, inherent to AHE, that the values of pixels on edges become less sparse.

Our aim was to bring the two parameters needed for individual image display mapping (viz. window position and width) back to one or two parameters for the display of a class of images, the class here being measured MR signal images of the IR-type (other classes are e.g. computed MR-images, CT-images, scintigraphic bone scans, etc.). We noticed that the above described problems are associated with local image features. We implemented "feature weighting" in the AHE process: the intensity shift table of a cell is multiplied with a factor (weight) between 0 and 1 so, that it corresponds with a feature to be extracted from the cell.

Obviously the presence of a relatively large area of uniform values in a cell represents itself as a small deviation of the pixel values throughout the cell. Figure 19 gives an example of AHE weighted with the inverse of cell deviation, normalized from 0 to 1 for the maximum deviation throughout the image. Notice that this example represents image mapping with one parameter, for the class of measured MR images not containing thin structures.

Figure 20 shows an MR image that does contain thin structures. A second weighting was introduced that lowers the effect of AHE at high cell deviations, corresponding with a high probability of sharp edges. Another approach (Figure 21) is a weighting scheme using the amount of gradient in a cell as a feature.

Needless to say that further investigations into the merit of feature weighted AHE are to be carried out. We are convinced, however, that indeed it will be possible to accomplish feature weighting schemes so,

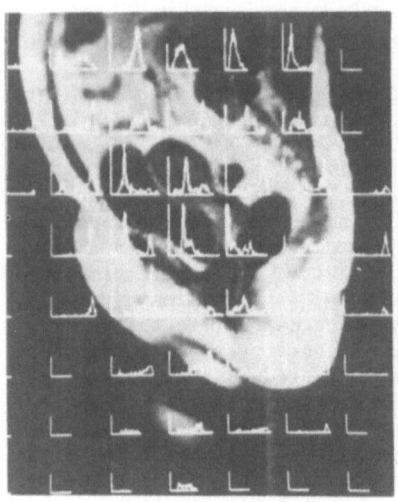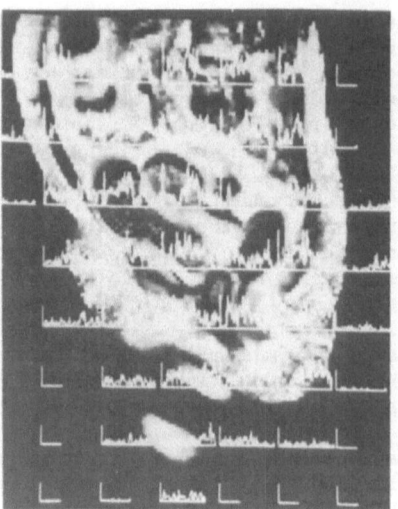

Figure 18. Original (left) and AHE'd (right) MR image, both with cell histograms drawn in. Noise outside the body contour had already been removed.

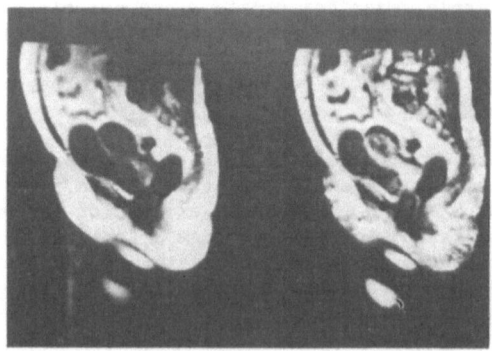

Figure 19. Original image and result of feature weighted AHE, the feature being the standard deviation of pixel values within cells. The weighting factors for the cells' intensity shift tables run linearly from 0 for zero deviation (uniform distribution) to 1 for the maximum deviation value throughout all cells.

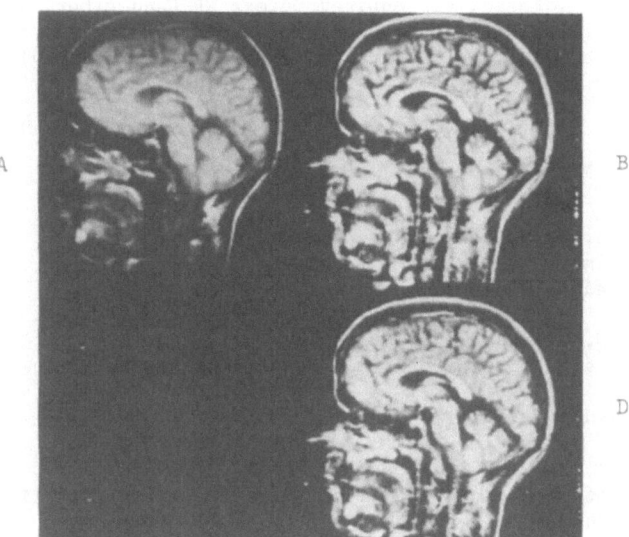

Figure 20. A: original MR image. B: feature-weighted AHE, the feature being the standard deviation. The weighting factor runs linearly from 0 for zero deviation to 1 for half maximum deviation, and is 1 for deviations over half maximum. D: as above, but for deviations over 0.75 of the maximum, the weighting factor runs linearly down to 0 for the maximum.

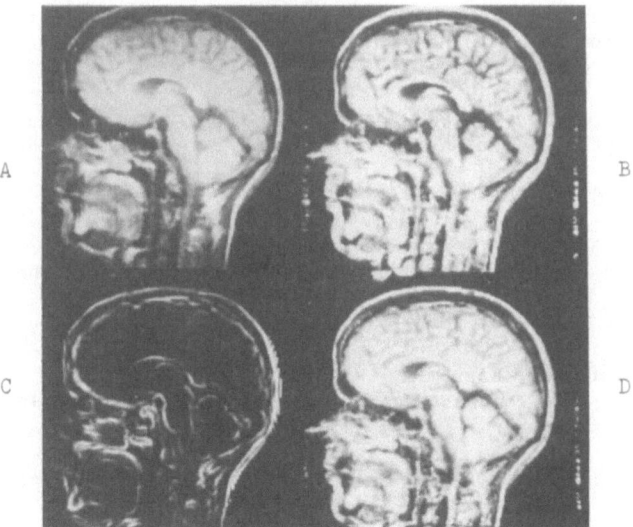

Figure 21. A and B: as Figure 20. C: gradient image of image in A. D: AHE as in B, but the weighting factor is itself inversely weighted on the average amount of gradient in cells.

that the a priori information required to map MR (and other) images in an PACS display is related to classes of images, rather than to individual images. One final remark: no JND linearization [20] of images shown in Figures 15-21 had been carried out, since it was not known what the delinearization effect of the reproduction process would be.

4 References

1. D.A. Ortendahl, N.M. Hylton, L. Kaufman, L.E. Crooks:
   Signal to noise in derived NMR images.
   Magn Reson Med 1 (1984) 316-338

2. P.L. Davis, D. Ortendahl, N. Hylton, et al:
   Optimal spin echo images for liver lesions by retrospective calculations.
   Magn Reson Med 2 (1984) 140-141

3. C.J.G. Bakker, C.N. de Graaf, P. van Dijk:
   Calculation of zero-crossing and spin-lattice relaxation time pictures in inversion recovery NMR imaging.
   IEEE Trans Biomed Eng (1985) in press

4. A. Venot, J.L. Golmard, J.F. Lebruchec, L. Pronzato, E. Walter, G. Frija, J.C. Roucayrol:
   Digital methods for change detection in medical images.
   In: "Information Processing in Medical Imaging", Ed. F. Deconinck, Brussels, Vol 8 (1984) 1 - 16

5. L.E. Crooks, J. Hoenninger, M. Arakawa, J. Watts, B. McCarten, P. Sheldon, L. Kaufman, C.M. Mills, P.L. Davis, A.R. Margulis:
   High resolution magnetic resonance imaging.
   Radiology 150 (1984) 163-171

6. C.J.G. Bakker, C.N. de Graaf, P. van Dijk:
   Restoration of signal polarity in a set of inversion recovery NMR images.
   IEEE Trans Med Im 3 (1984) 197 - 202

7. C.J.G. Bakker, C.N. de Graaf, P. van Dijk:
   Derivation of quantitative information in NMR imaging: a phantom study.
   Phys Med Biol 29 (1984) 1511-1526

8. W.A. Edelstein, P.A. Bottomley, H.R. Hart, et al:
   Signal, noise, and contrast in nuclear magnetic resonance imaging.
   J Comput Assist Tomogr 7 (1983) 391-401

9. F.W. Wehrli, J.R. MacFall, D. Shutts, R. Breger, R.J. Herfkens:
   Mechanisms of contrast in NMR imaging.
   J Comput Assist Tomogr 8 (1984) 369-380

10. W.H. Perman, S.K. Hilal, H.E. Simon, A.A. Mandsley:
    Contrast manipulation in NMR imaging.
    Magn Reson Med 2 (1984) 23-32

11. N.M. Hylton, D.A. Ortendahl, L. Kaufman, L.E. Crooks:
    Simulation techniques for evaluating magnetic resonance imaging.
    In: "Information Processing in Medical Imaging", Ed: S.L. Bacharach,
    Proc 9th Internat Conf, Washington DC (1985), this book

12. D.A. Ortendahl, personal communications (1985)

13. A. Toet, J.J. Koenderink, P. Zuidema, C.N. de Graaf:
    Image analysis - topological methods.
    In: "Information Processing in Medical Imaging", Ed: F. Deconinck,
    Brussels, Vol 8 (1984) 306 - 342

14. C.N. de Graaf, A. Toet, J.J. Koenderink, P. Zuidema, P.P. van Rijk:
    Some applications of hierarchical image processing algorithms.
    In: "Information Processing in Medical Imaging", Ed: F. Deconinck,
    Brussels, Vol 8 (1984) 343-369

15. J.J. Koenderink:
    The structure of images.
    Biol Cybern 50 (1984) 363-370

16. S.M. Pizer, J.J. Koenderink, L.M. Lifshitz, L. Helminck, A.D.J.
    Kaasjager:
    Image description through extremal regions via the stack.
    In: "Information Processing in Medical Imaging", Ed: S.L. Bacharach,
    Proc 9th Intern Conf, Washington DC (1985), this book

17. P. Burt, T.H. Hong, A. Rosenfeld:
    Segmentation and estimation of image region properties through
    cooperative hierarchical computation.
    IEEE Trans SMC 11 (1981) 802-809

18. S. Kasif, A. Rosenfeld:
    Pyramid linking is a special case of Isodata.
    IEEE Trans SMC 13 (1983) 84-85

19. D.A. Ortendahl, N.M. Hylton, L. Kaufman, L.E. Crooks:
    Tissue type identification by MRI using pyramidal segmentation and
    intrinsic parameters.
    In: "Information Processing in Medical Imaging", Ed.: S.L. Bacharach,
    Proc 9th Internaat Conf, Washington DC (1985), this book

20. S.M. Pizer:
    An automatic intensity mapping for the display of CT scans and other
    images.
    In: "Medical Image Processing", Proc 7th IPMI Conf, Stanford Un 1981,
    Ed: M.L. Goris, Stanford Un Publ (1983) 276-309

21. J. Cormack, B.F. Hutton:
    Minimisation of data transfer losses in the display of digitised
    scintigraphic images.
    Phys Med Biol 25 (1980) 271-282

22. B.M. ter Haar Romeny, K. Zuiderveld, personal communications (1985)

TISSUE TYPE IDENTIFICATION BY MRI USING PYRAMIDAL SEGMENTATION AND INTRINSIC PARAMETERS

Douglas A. Ortendahl and Nola M. Hylton
Radiologic Imaging Laboratory, University of California, San Francisco,
400 Grandview Drive, South San Francisco, CA 94080

INTRODUCTION

In Magnetic Resonance Imaging (MRI) the signal intensity depends indirectly on particular physical and chemical characteristics of the tissues being imaged. These tissue properties influence the behavior of the nuclei undergoing resonance, and their behavior is what directly affects the MRI signal. The parameters of interest that describe this behavior are the relaxation times T1 and T2, the spin density (for hydrogen, N(H)), and the microscopic (diffusion) and macroscopic (flow, motion) motional states of the nuclei. Different imaging techniques result in different responses to these MRI parameters. These parameters exist, in turn, because of certain properties of the tissues: water content, fat content, macromolecules, paramagnetic ions and flow being among the significant variables.

The interest in tissue characterization by MRI is in part due to early in vitro research which suggested that MR imaging might differentiate malignant from benign processes. In vitro measurements in rats (1) and humans (2) showed differences in T1 and T2 between malignant and benign tissues. Extensive animal work at our institution has studied the MR characteristics of normal and abnormal tissue in vivo (3,4). This work has shown substantial differences in MR parameters among normal and abnormal tissues. A sample of this work is shown in Figure 1. Significant differences are observed in the T1 and T2 values. These differences provide the excellent soft tissue contrast of MRI since hydrogen concentrations in these tissues differ by less than 15%. Note that neither T1 or T2 would be sufficient by themselves to provide contrast in all cases, but with both parameters available, all the tissues may be distinguished. There is considerable scatter in the T1 and T2 values of the tumors, but it is still possible to discriminate tumor from normal host tissue with high sensitivity, although certainly this variation makes specificity much more difficult. Figure 1 plots only T1 vs T2; in addition, there is also hydrogen density which although not providing as much contrast as the relaxation times, provides additional information.

Image contrast may be adjusted over a wide range by varying the acquisition parameters TE and TR. This is one of the advantages of MRI, but at the same time it presents a problem in terms of the amount of data which must be analyzed. Even from a minimally sufficient set of images (TR = 0.5 and 2.0 sec and TE = 28 and 56 ms) the physician can be confronted with a number of images from just one section. The original images allow calculation of T1, T2 and hydrogen images, which themselves permit calculation of images at other TR and TE points (5). Each of these images offers a different "view" of the object. A subset of the images which are available is shown in Figure 2 for a patient with a left parietal brain tumor. Add this to the fact that 15 to 20 sections are obtained simultaneously, and we see that more information can be available than is readily assimilable by the physician. One possible method to manage this situation is to use the intrinsic MRI parameters to identify the types of tissue present in the section. The apparent clustering of tissue in MR parameter space suggested by Figure 1 provides the motivation for such an algorithm. The computer is used to provide color maps where the locations of various tissues are painted with a color code. Previous work in our laboratory has shown that such maps may be produced (6,7).

THE TISSUE CHARACTERIZATION PROBLEM

Since in an image each pixel has associated with it a value of T1, T2 and H , it is useful to think of these three parameters as forming a set of basis vectors spanning the feature space of all possible types of tissue. In the ideal case each tissue type is associated with a single point in this space although it is possible that more than one tissue type maps to the same point. Although often thought of as an orthogonal set, this is not strictly true since T1, T2 and H can be correlated. For example, an increase in water content will increase the hydrogen density and will also lengthen the values of T1 and T2. For this reason only a portion of the feature space corresponds to the locus of observed tissue types from a patient population. Associated with each tissue type will also be a MR intensity for each sequence that we chose to use. In order to be able to calculate T1, T2 and H at least three intensities are required, at two different TE and TR values. In these calculations we use a solution to the Bloch equations which takes into account the various RF pulses required in the multi-spin-echo sequences used in our imager. In the ideal case these six values associated with every tissue type are redundant, only three are actually needed. The logical choice is T1, T2 and H. This basis is sufficient for the "standard" spin-echo or inversion recovery imaging used in routine clinical practice. More specialized sequences such as water-fat discriminators (8) or those for diffusion measurements (9) require the introduction of additional parameters. These additional parameters could be used in the algorithms which follow to supplement the T1, T2 and N(H) information and may help to separate tissues which are currently inseparable by T1, T2 and H alone.

After collection of the ideal image we can map each pixel into a multi-dimensional feature space. The dimension can be as large as the number of images which we acquire or calculate, but the number of images is redundant in the ideal case and can be reduced down to three. Each populated point in this image parameter space corresponds to a populated point in the tissue type space, providing a perfect tissue type map. Noise makes the problem much more difficult. There are two components to the noise: electronic and biologic. In a well designed and shielded system, the electronic noise is almost entirely due to random thermal currents in the patient which induce noise in the RF coil. In the reconstructed image this noise will be white (independent of spatial frequency) and will be independent of the TR and TE of the acquisition for equal number of averages or redundant data sets. The noise in the intensity images is propagated into the calculated T1, T2 and H values (10). The properties of this noise are well understood and the effects are usually random.

A much more difficult problem is faced with biologic variability. It has already been shown that tumors exhibit significant variability in T1 and T2 values. While the other types of tissue are more consistent in their T1 and T2 values, the size of the one standard deviation rectangle demonstrates considerable variation among different subjects. The parameters T1 and T2 reflect the relaxation of the spin system from its excited state back to its equilibrium value. On the microscopic level the behavior of the spin system is strongly influenced by magnetic fields produced by the local molecular environment. From our extensive work with animals we find reasonable correlations between 1/T1 and total water content and the same for 1/T2 except for the unusually short value for fat (6,7). In agreement with work by Koenig (11) we are unable to distinguish between the contribution of intra- and extracellular water. Yet, it is clear that more than water is involved, for otherwise all tissue would fall on a line in T1 - T2 space. Liver for example has a shorter T1 and a longer T2 than muscle. We are quite far from the day when relaxation times could be predicted from a knowledge of tissue composition. With this uncertainty it is not surprising that we see such variability.

Partial volume averaging where two or more types of tissue contribute to the observed intensity from a region is also a significant problem. This can be expected to appear at tissue boundaries and where a single tissue type does not fill the full section thickness. Despite these potential problems, excellent reproducibility of T1 and T2 values in human imaging has been obtained (12). It must be remembered that in such measurements great care is taken to insure that the regions over which data is obtained are as free as possible from partial volume problems. For example in the brain researchers draw precise areas of interest in the gray matter to avoid partial volume averaging with adjacent CSF. In tissue typing we can not be so selective, and in fact the definition of tissue type is somewhat loose. For example is muscle marbled with 25% fat still muscle? We must be able to accept a certain level of partial volume infiltration without changing the tissue type.

With this variation included, tissues are represented by multi-dimensional distributions within the feature space. The distributions for various tissues will overlap, the major problem is to identify tissue in the presence of this uncertainty. The strategy is one of segmentation, that is to divide the image up into areas where we believe that every element in this area belongs to the same class. Admittedly there will be times when it is difficult to choose between competing classes or segments, but we do force this decision. In this sense our work is different from other multispectral techniques which attempt to handle multispectral data by encoding the different bands in different colors (13,14). In earlier work a template was constructed consisting of the means and standard deviations of T1, T2 and H for the various tissues expected in the section (6). The T1, T2 and H values for each pixel in the image were compared against the template and assignments were made using a maximum likelihood method. While this technique produced acceptable tissue type maps, the signatures had to be hand tuned for each patient. There were also serious problems with partial volume artifacts, especially at the boundaries of tissues. Similar techniques have been applied by other investigators using multispectral analysis techniques from satellite imaging (15).

HIERARCHICAL SEGMENTATION

In an attempt to overcome some of these problems, we turned to hierarchical processing. Within the past few years considerations concerning the structure of the human retina and the perceptual system have led to increasing interest in hierarchically organized image description schemes (16). Such algorithms allow the simultaneous analysis of images at multiple levels of spatial resolution. This is a natural way of looking at images since although we appreciate high resolution images, the interpretation of a scene or image requires information obtained at many different levels of resolution. In these and related techniques the resolution decreases with increasing height in the hierarchy. As a side-effect the amount of noise may be reduced or superfluous detail suppressed.

The particular algorithm chosen for this work is the pyramid (17). The pyramid is defined as a stacked series of linked representations of an image each with 1/4 the number of pixels as the one below. The link structure is established from the bottom up, with the links connecting pixels on level k called the sons with pixels on level k+1, the fathers. In our implementation a son chooses the father which is most similar in terms of value. The length of the links laterally in space is limited by requiring that the choice be made from among the four pixels immediately above the son. In this process each son must be assigned a father, but it is not required that each potential father have a son. A father pixel may have zero to sixteen sons. Once all the links from level k-1 to level k have been found, the pixels on level k are recomputed to be the average of their son pixels on level k-1. This computation is weighted by the total area of each son's descendants. The process continues until the top of the pyramid is reached. Since the recomputation of the father values occurs after the links are established, some links will no longer be optimum. The process is iterated until no links change. Convergence is guaranteed (17). For MR images we find that 8-12 iterations are required.

Each pixel in the upper levels of the pyramid is linked to a series of pixels at lower levels. Because of their common lineage, these pixels form a group or segment. Segmentation is obtained by down-projecting the values of the kth level, that is to assign to each pixel in the levels below k the value of its linked ancestor in level k. The number of different segments at the bottom of the pyramid will be determined by the number of valid elements in level k, hence the choice of k is critical. Figure 3 shows how the segmentation is affected by the choice of this level. As the level of the segmentation increases the image appears smoother, and some resolution is lost as is expected since the total number of independent segments in the image is decreasing. When segmented from level seven in the pyramid, only four segments are left. Pyramidal segmentation is much more attractive than conventional smoothing since edges remain sharp. Note that gray and white matter remain sharply differentiated. This is especially desirable since we recognize that areas of potential partial volume averaging can be difficult to analyze because of their parameter values intermediate to the two involved tissues. The problem of partial volume averaging will be ameliorated as long as the number of partial volume averaged pixels is not large compared to the number of total pixels in the segment. This follows the philosophy expressed previously of forcing a decision to join one segment or the other.

The objective of segmentation is to group together pixels of similar characteristics and smooth out insignificant variation, but it is clear that at the upper levels of the pyramid dissimilar lineages will ulti-mately be forced together (gray and white matter for example). The level at which this occurs will not be the same throughout the image, so setting a lower level at which to begin the down-projection is not completely satisfactory. Moving up one level in the pyramid reduces the number of segments by approximately a factor of 4. If the number of desired segments is known and is smaller than that provided by level k and more than the number for level k+1, then at initialization, level k may be seeded with enough zero valued segments to give the desired number of segments in the final image. This approach is suggested by deGraaf (17), but requires an a priori knowledge of the desired segmentation. An alternative is to break apart those links which combine lineages which should be expected to be different, allowing different regions of the image to start at the most appropriate level of resolution. A link from a father to a son is considered to be invalid if the difference between father and son is greater than Δ. Links below level four are not broken since these are more affected by statistical fluctuations. It was empirically determined that a value of 75 intensity units is close to optimum. This is in an image where the per pixel standard deviation of intensity is about 50.

After segmentation the segments are ranked by area and each pixel within the segment is labeled with this rank. The rank is r_i for the ith basis image. When this process has been completed for each of the three basis images, each pixel within the image is associated with an ordered triplet (r_1, r_2, r_3). A new segmentation of the image is obtained by grouping all pixels with the same ordered triplet. This is called the intersected image. Since each basis image provides a separate "view" of the section and is individually segmented, the size of the segments in the intersected image will be much smaller. Each of these new segments is homogeneous with respect to each of the basis parameters and should therefore be relatively homogeneous with respect to tissue. This is dependent on the basis images properly sampling the parameter space so that differences between tissues appear as a difference in the segmentation for at least one of the images.

An alternative to this method of producing the intersected image is to use multispectral information in the formation of a single pyramid. If more than one image is to be considered in the formation of links then a distance metric must be defined. In this implementation the distance in the feature space between the ith and jth segments is given by:

$$D^2 = \sum_k w_k (\mu_{ik} - \mu_{jk})^2 \tag{1}$$

where w_k is the weight assigned to the kth image and μ_{ik} is the mean of the ith segment of the kth basis image. In this case the segments contain exactly the same pixels for each of the basis images, however the values which are projected into these segments depend on the basis image. An example of this mode of segmentation is shown in Figure 4. Note that the segmentations appear to be similar to those of Figure 3 at low levels, but at higher levels they are very different showing the influence of the other images used to form the pyramid. The intersection is performed for the three segmented images just as in the previous case. Unlike the first method of forming the intersected image, the shapes of the segments will not change. Even so we use all three segmented images in the creation of the intersection so that two different segments which happen to have the same image value will not be combined into one segment in the intersected image.

REGION GROWING AND SEGMENT MERGING

The intersected image contains many more segments than there are different tissues within the section. These segments must be merged into larger units corresponding to tissue type. This is accomplished by looking for similarity in MRI parameters between these smaller segments.

In previous work we searched for clusters in T1, T2 and N(H) space using the larger intersected segments as seeds for this clustering (7). This was done without regard for the spatial proximity of the segments which were to be merged. This procedure required that a metric be defined for deciding whether a segment should be joined to a particular seed or whether the segment is far enough away in parameter space for it to be a seed in its own right. In present work, the merging of intersected segments is performed with more emphasis on spatial proximity with a region growing algorithm. For each segment in the intersected image a list (called the adjacent segment list) is made of all other segments which are adjacent to it. The list is updated as segments are merged. By using this adjacent segment list, it is unnecessary to return to the images themselves during the merge process. The distance between the ith and jth segments in parameter space can be defined by:

$$D^2 = \sum_k \delta_k{}^2 \tag{2}$$

where k refers to the basis element and

$$\delta_k{}^2 = (\mu_{ik} - \mu_{jk})^2 / (v_{ik} + v_{jk}) \tag{3}$$

μ_{ik} is the mean of the ith segment over the kth basis image and v is the variance. These basis images may be different from those used for the creation of the intersected image. The variance is specified before hand and serves to normalize distances within the space. While v_{ik} is in general a function of all the basis means for the ith segment, where possible we try to simplify the specification of the variance by providing a dependence only on the mean of the kth basis image over segment i. An alternative approach is to define the distance, D to be the maximum δ_k for all k. In either case, segments i and j are candidates for merging if D < M, where M is specified by the algorithm or operator.

The question being asked is whether two segments belong to the same tissue type. It is important to point out the difference between this and the common question in statistical analysis of whether two distributions belong to the same parent distribution. In such cases the usual method is the F or t-test to determine the significance of the measured difference of means. For the case of segmentation there is usually little question that the parent distributions are different, probably due to slight differences in tissue composition, partial volume averaging or perhaps due to non-uniformities of the field of view. The question is whether despite these very real differences they still belong to the same tissue type. Spatial proximity is an important determinant in this decision.

With this merge procedure we introduce additional data structures, three new types of segments refered to as type A, B and C. These form a hierarchy with the intersected segments on the bottom and type C on top. Each type C segment will be composed of one or more type B segments etc. A set of merge link lists are also created in this process. At the initial stage, all of these segment types are the same as those of the intersected image. For each type A segment A_i we compare its parameter values with its adjacent segments A_j using the above metrics. If D < M then before a match is declared, the merge link lists of the two candidate segments A_i and A_j are first examined to make sure there are no inconsistencies which would invalidate the merge. If this is satisfied then the segments will be merged, the only question is the type of merge. If the area of either of the segments is less than a value SIZE then it is considered a type A link. For a type A link, the larger segment completely absorbs the smaller one for all three types of segments A-C. The area is redefined, the new mean values are the weighted averages of the two, and the larger segment absorbs the adjacent segment list of the smaller. If both segments are larger than SIZE then the link is of type B. In this case the segments are merged only in the B and C type lists. They retain their type A identity. The rationale for this multi-tier procedure is to maintain contrast in the image. We found that if the means of segments are constantly redefined when merging occurs, then areas of the image which should show good contrast may be merged because the means of the merged segments to which these regions belong are drifting closer to each other because of the effect of other areas of the image. We find that this problem is effectively avoided by allowing larger segments which presumably have greater statistical significance to maintain their type A identity throughout the merge process. This again recognizes the fact that we do not expect that the merged segments necessarily have the same parent distributions.

The consistency check which we perform to validate the merge is also designed to prevent this loss of contrast. Whenever two segments are merged this causes the combining of their merge link lists. The question asked at this point is whether such a merger is consistent with what has been done previously. Let A_i and A_j be the two type A segments which are candidates for merging and a_{bi} and a_{bj} be type A segments which are linked by type B links to the segments A_i and A_j respectively. If segments a_{bi} and a_{bj} are adjacent to each other then they also have the opportunity to merge. Looking at the distance D1 in parameter space between these two segments, if D1 > M then these two segments are not permitted to merge directly. But the merger of the segments i and j would cause a_{bi} and a_{bj} to be combined under a common type B segment, violating the contrast which we just observed between these segments. Under this logic the merger of segments i and j would not be allowed, maintaining contrast between well defined segments.

The value of M is slowly increased in subsequent iterations, so that newly merged segments may be combined with other segments. This region growing procedure is effective for those areas which are contiguous. In order to collect those tissue types which are not adjacent, each type A segment is compared with all others. Again a consistency check is performed to prevent invalid links. Links established in this way are called type C links. This C type merging is performed only after adjacent segment merging has been completed. Again several iterations of this kind of merging are performed with the value of M slowly increasing. The value of M is not permitted to be larger than the maximum used for adjacent segment merging. If additional adjacent segment merging is desired, then all type C links are broken which reduces type C segmentation to that of type B.

At any time during this procedure images of the three types of segmentation may be produced. Each pixel in the image is associated with an intersected segment number. This is in turn linked to the type A, B and C segments. Since the A, B and C type segmentations are linked in a tree structure, the type A segmentation contains the largest number of segments with the type C segmentation containing the smallest number of different segments. The tissue type image is always of type C.

During the merging process some additional cleanup of the image is performed. Small isolated segments of four pixels or less are removed and given the value of the surrounding area. In general, we do not have the confidence to make a reliable decision about regions that small. Regions of low intensity which usually correspond to partial volume averaging with bone or air are also removed. With the current algorithm once segments are combined, it is impossible to break them apart. For this reason the algorithm is conservative about the decision to merge segments. As a final stage the operator is given the opportunity to combine additional segments. Since no training set is provided, the identities of the individual merged segments are unknown at this point. The segments are labeled 1 thru m and assigned an arbitrary color. Each pixel in the image is painted with the color of the segment of which it is a member. The average intensity, T1, T2, and N(H) for each segment are also displayed on the computer terminal. The operator rearranges the color assignments using knowledge of anatomy and the parameter values of the segments to produce a more pleasing image. For example the operator may find that normal white matter in the anterior and post-erior parts of the brain is assigned to different segments, with the computer assigned colors being grossly different. In such a case, colors similar in shade (but still distinguishable) would be selected by the user for display of the two white matter segments.

The procedure which has been described is independent of the choice of basis images so long as they span the space. Because of their lower noise, our practice is to do the pyramidal segmentation and intersection using the acquired intensity images rather than T1, T2 and H. We typically use images acquired at the following values of (TE, TR): (28,500), (28,2000), (56,2000) with all times in ms. The same value of the link breaking parameter is used for each image. For the work which follows we chose the value of SIZE which determines the difference between type A and type B links to be 50 pixels. The region growing using the adjacent segment list can use either the intensity images or T1, T2 and H. When segments are merged globally without using the adjacent segment list, we exclusively use T1, T2 and H because of the possibility of some nonuniformity of intensity across the field of view which is largely corrected by use of the relaxation times.

RESULTS

The format of this publication requires us to show the tissue type images in shades of gray, although they are best appreciated in color. In Figure 5 we show the segmentation of each of the intensity images of the patient used for Figures 2-4. Each was individually segmented and then intersected. The tissue type image shows good definition of the gray and white matter. The caudate nucleus is correctly identified as gray matter immediately below the lateral ventricle which is shown as an area of cerebrospinal fluid (CSF). Fat is seen in the area of the scalp. The tumor is seen to be surrounded by a region L1 which is most likely edema. Additional structure of the lesion is seen in L2 and L3 perhaps showing areas of a necrosis. In this particular case the segmented images had 161, 152 and 159 segments respectively with the intersection image containing 2150 segments. Operator assistance was required after the number of segments was reduced to 45 by segment merging. The inability to merge without supervision beyond this point was primarily due to segments with considerable partial volume averaging especially from CSF.

The remaining examples were segmented by the pyramid simultaneously using three intensity images. In Figure 6 we show a section 1.5 cm more cranial from the previous patient. By using this different method of segmentation we have an intersection image of only 145 segments. After region growing and global merging, the operator was presented with 29 segments. Fat was easily identified by its characteristic short T1 and areas of CSF were also merged manually. Several areas of what appeared to be gray matter based on its tissue signature and location were also combined with supervision. This gives a final image with 10 segments showing excellent definition of the gray and white matter as well as several different compartments within the tumor.

In Figure 7 we present a patient with a thalmic lesion. In this case the program automatically produced 14 segments. It was not difficult for the operator to combine regions and produce a tissue type map with 8 segments. Good delineation of the white and gray matter is seen. Note that in the intensity images, white and gray matter contrast is not as pronounced as in the previous cases. Fat is observed around the eye and in the scalp. The vitreous is seen in the eye along with the CSF in the ventricles. An indication of the right optic nerve protruding into the fat is also observed. In Figure 8 we see a patient with a tumor of the right hemisphere. The algorithm was able to produce 22 segments which the operator was able to reduce to 8 regions. As in the previous example the white and gray matter is well defined despite the somewhat reduced contrast in the intensity images. The structure of the lesion is indicated by the three separate components. For Figures 6-8 the same procedure was used for the segment merging, including the same maximum value of M. Six iterations were performed for both the region growing and the global merging.

An application to body imaging is shown in Figure 9 by a section of a patient with liver metastases. In this case the intersection image contained 191 segments. The standard merging algorithm was able to produce 41 segments. We stopped at this point and allowed the operator to complete the map. Additional merging could have been obtained by using larger values of M, but it was decided to stop the automatic program in order to prevent the merging of tissues which are known to be anatomically different even though they may have similar MR characteristics. In the tissue type image we are able to show normal liver, fat and three tumors of which two are found to have similar characteristics. The aorta, ivc and hepatic vessels are also seen. As a final example of body imaging we show sagittal images of a patient with a normal uterus. In this case we have decided to perform region of interest tissue type mapping where we only segment within the region. The region is chosen to to rectangular in this case but could be irregular. Muscle, fat and bladder are easily identified. Within the uterus we are able to identify the endometrium and the myometrium. The junctional zone between the myometrium and the endometrium is found to have similar characteristics with the vagina. The radiologist would have no trouble distinguishing between these two on the basis of anatomy.

DISCUSSION

The results show a moderate amount of success. It is very gratifying that such similar results can be obtained in the head using the same protocol as seen by the results of Figures 6-8. The consistency check which prevents the merging of two regions which would destroy the contrast in another part of the image has helped considerably in making the algorithm more predictable. Using local means rather than global means for describing segments has also been shown to be very important. Creating a single pyramid rather than several separate ones for the formation of the intersection image seems to be very advantageous. This is primarily because it avoids the problem of the many isolated small regions which are produced when separately segmented images are intersected. For example with the simultaneous segmentation, an area of CSF would be classified as a single region while the separate intersection would find many small regions. Since CSF can have widely varying values depending on the amount of partial volume averaging, it is an advantage to be able to force a classification into a single region.

This brings up the important question of the proper weight to be used for each basis image. For the simultaneous segmentation we use equal weights for each intensity image. This would be logical if electronic noise were dominant, but when biologic variability is the chief problem this may not be the optimum procedure and requires more study. The weight or variance used for the basis images during the region growing and merge process similarly needs more investigation. The current algorithm is not completely automatic, but the amount of operator time required to produce a map has been considerably reduced over our previous work, especially in the head. Some additional tools that would allow the operator to select colors more readily and find the location of particular segments would speed this up even more. Ultimately we would want the algorithm to select the colors for the tissues based on their parameter values.

The purpose of this research is not to replace the physician with a computer, nor is it to replace all the original images with computer generated tissue type maps. Rather it is an attempt to integrate the information into as concise a form as possible. In cases where the anatomy is obvious, tissue type maps will add little. But where anatomy is more complex such maps will be of use. One potential use for such algorithms is in the ellucidation of lesion structure. Here region of interest analysis will be particularly valuable. Processing time will be greatly reduced and the problems that are encountered with the global merging of segments will not be as severe in this local environment.

ACKNOWLEDGEMENTS

This work is supported in part by USPHS Research Career Development Award GM00493 from the NIGMS(DHHS); USPHS Grant CA 32850 from the NCI; and by Diasonics (MRI), Inc. The authors wish to thank Drs. Hedvig Hricak and Michael Brant-Zawadski for providing patient data for this work.

REFERENCES

1. Damadian R. Tumor Detection by NMR. Science 161:1151, 1971.
2. Medina D, Hazlewood CJ et al. NMR Studies On Human Dysplasias and Neoplasms. J Nat Cancer Inst 54:813, 1975.
3. Davis PL, Kaufman L, Crooks LE et al. Detectability of Hepatomas in Rat Livers by Nuclear Magnetic Resonance. Investigative Radiology 16:354, 1981.
4. Davis PL, Sheldon PE, Kaufman et al. Nuclear Magnetic Resonance Imaging of Mammary Adenocarcinomas in the Rat. Cancer 51:433, 1983.
5. Ortendahl DA, Hylton NM, Kaufman L, et al. Analytical Tools for MRI. Radiology 153:479, 1984.
6. Ortendahl DA, Hylton NM, Kaufman L and Crooks LE. Automated Tissue Characterization with NMR Imaging. Proceedings of the 8th International Conference on Information Processing in Medical Imaging. Martinus Nijhoff Publishers, The Hague, 392, 1984.
7. Ortendahl DA, Hylton NM, Kaufman L and Crooks LE. Tissue Characterization Using Intrinsic NMR Parameters and a Hierarchical Processing Algorithm. IEEE Trans on Nucl Sci. NS-32:875, 1985.

72

8. Dixon WT. Simple Proton Spectroscopic Imaging. Radiology (In Press).
9. Wesbey GE, Mosley ME and Ehman RL. A New Application of Proton MRI:
    Measurement of the Molecular Self-Diffusion Coefficient and Its
    Effects on Observed Spin-Relaxation Times. Investigative Radiology (In
    Press).
10. Ortendahl DA, Hylton NM, Kaufman L and Crooks LE. Signal to Noise in
    Derived NMR Images. Magnetic Resonance in Medicine. 1:316, 1984.
11. Koenig SH and Brown RD. The Importance of the Motion of Water in
    Biomedical NMR. Presented European Workshop on NMR in Medicine,
    Wiesbaden, Germany, May 1984.
12. Kjos BO et al. Reproducibility of Relaxation Times and Spin Density
    Calculated from Routine MR Imaging Sequences: Clinical Study of the
    CNS. AJNR 6:271, 1985.
13. O'Connell JW et al. Color Composites: Display of Two Independent
    Parameters in a Single Functional Image. in Emission Computed
    Tomography Current Trends ed by PD Esser. Society of Nuclear Medicine
    Inc., New York, 275, 1983.
14. Dave JV et al. Importance of Higher-Order Components to Multispectral
    Classification. IBM J Res Develop. 26: 715, 1982.
15. Vannier MW et al: Multispectral Analysis of Magnetic Resonance Images.
    Radiology 154: 221, 1985.
16. Tanimoto S and Pavlidis T. A Hierarchical Data Structure for Picture
    Processing. Comp Graph Im Proc 4: 104, 1975.
17. deGraaf CN, Toet A, Koenderink JJ et al. Some Applications of
    Hierarchical Image Processing Algorithms. Proceedings of the 8th
    International Conference on Information Processing in Medical Imaging.
    Martinus Nijhoff Publishers, The Hague, 343, 1984.

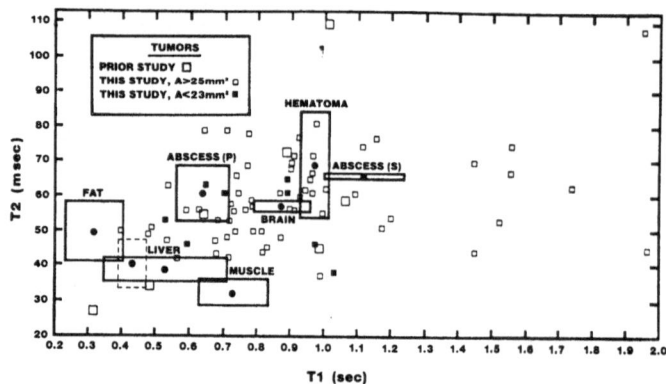

Figure 1. A plot of T1 vs T2 for various normal and abnormal tissues. The
rectangles represent one standard deviation.

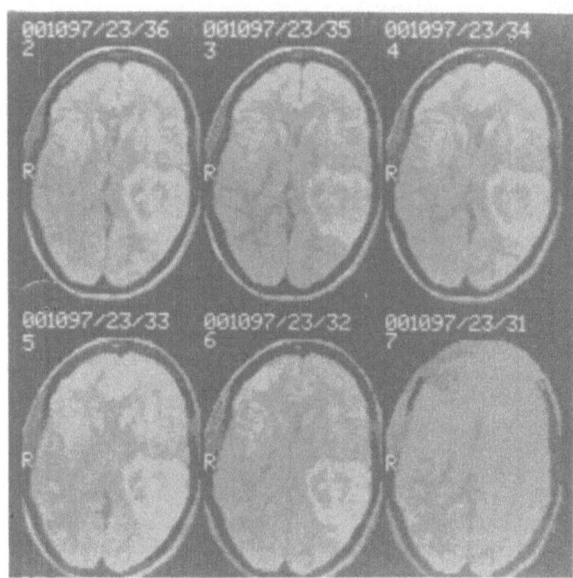

Figure 2. For a patient
with a left parietal brain
tumor we show three
acquired images along with
the calculated T1, T2 and H
images. The different
tissue contrast observed in
these images is the basis
for tissue typing.

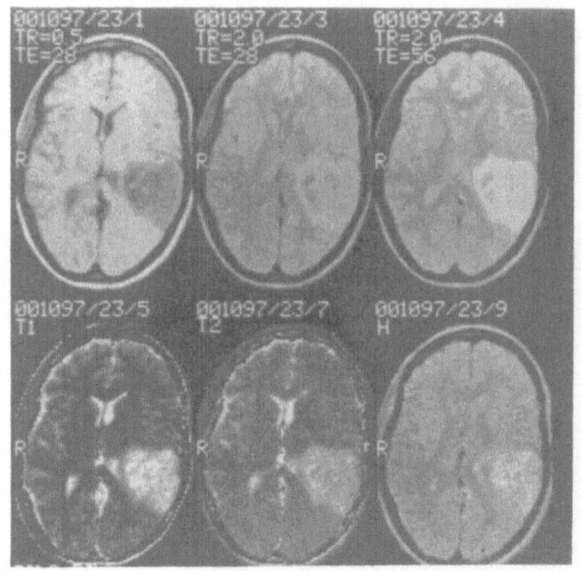

Figure 3. For the TR=2.0
sec, TE=56 ms image of
figure 2 we show 6
different pyramidal
segmentations from levels 2
thru 7. Edges remain sharp
even when segmented from
upper levels.

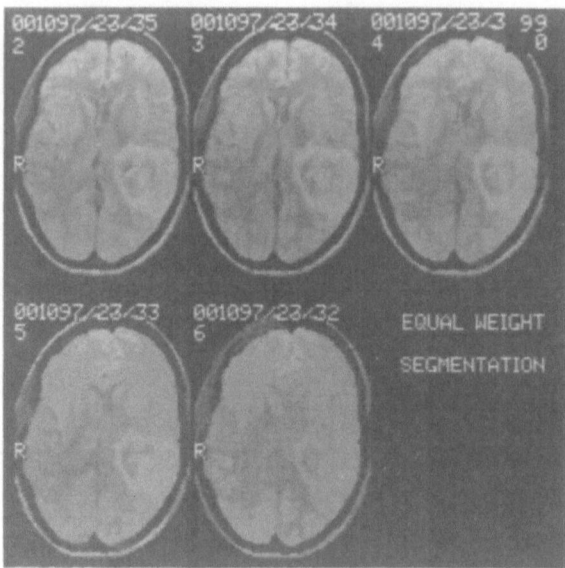

Figure 4. For the patient of Figure 3 we show the segmentation of the TR=2.0 sec, TE=56 ms image when using all three intensity images simultaneously. Segmentations from levels 2 thru 6 of the pyramid are shown. Note the differences with Figure 3 at upper levels of the pyramid.

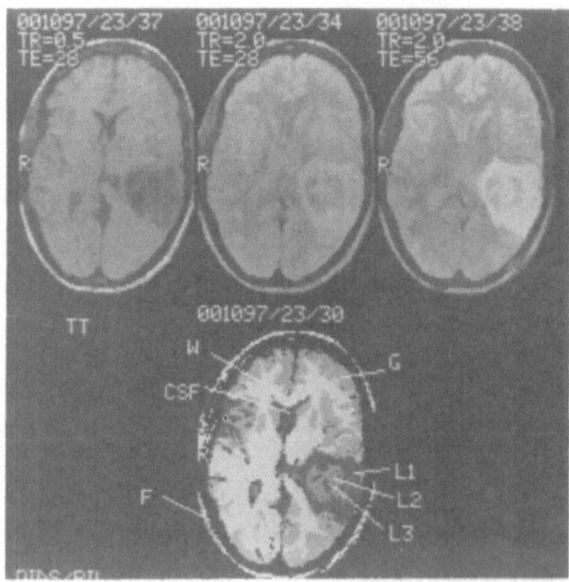

Figure 5. Level 4 segmentations are shown for the images used in the intersection image for the previous patient. The tissue type image shows good delineation of the gray and white matter, along with CSF, fat and the the structure within the lesion.

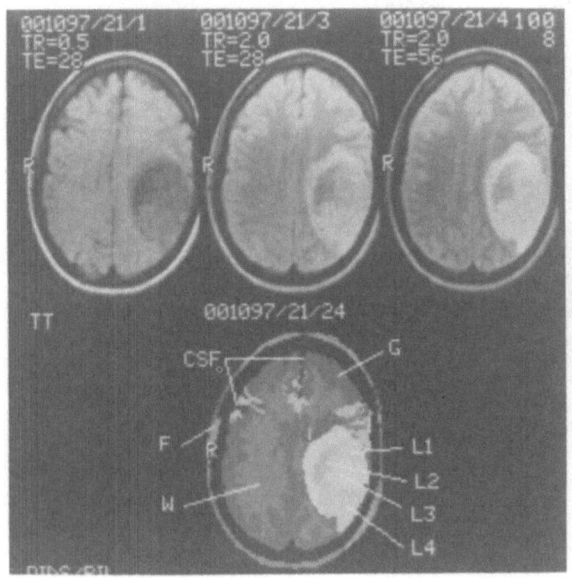

Figure 6. A section 1.5 cm higher is shown for the previous patient. Original intensity images along with the tissue type image are presented showing good definition of the anatomy as well as structure within the lesion.

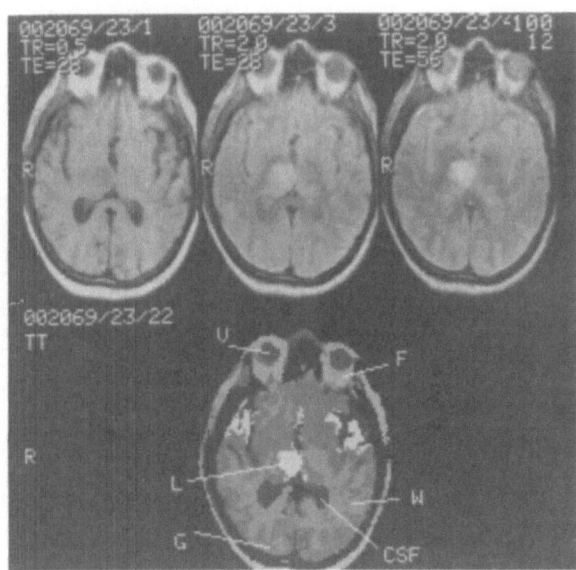

Figure 7. The intensity and tissue type images of a patient with a thalmic lesion are shown. The tumor, fat, vitreous in the eye and CSF are well seen. Gray and white matter are well defined even though the contrast is not as high as in the previous patient.

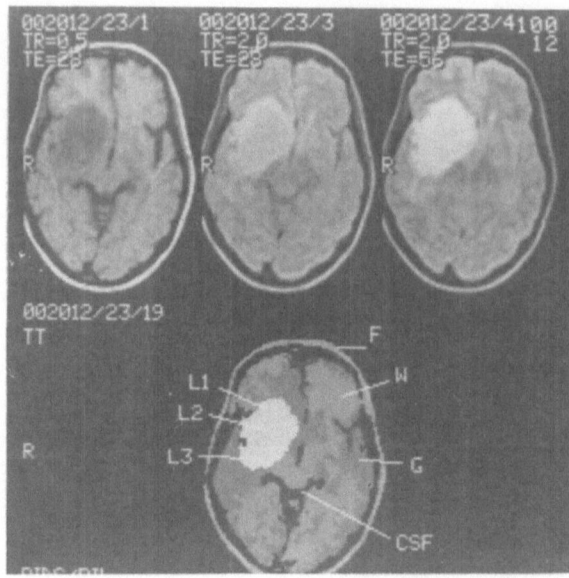

Figure 8. For a patient
with a right hemisphere
tumor the tissue type image
shows excellent definition
of the structure within the
lesion as well as the gray
and white matter in areas
of the brain where the
intensity images do not
give the contrast seen in
earlier cases.

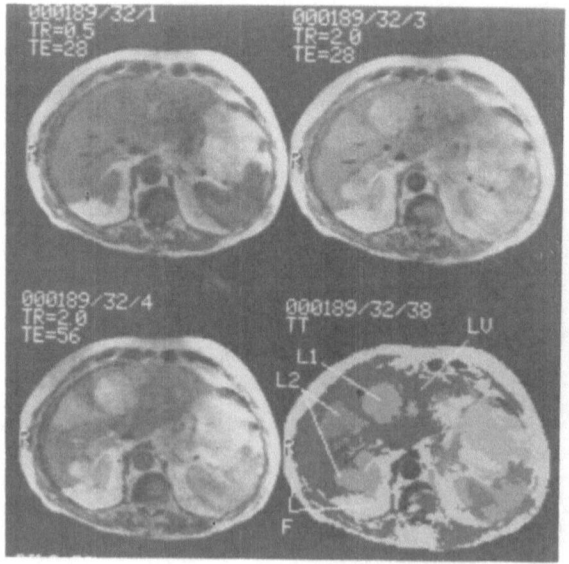

Figure 9. For a patient
with liver metastases we
show the intensity images
and the tissue type map.
Normal liver, fat and three
tumors are seen. Two of
the tumors have similar
characteristics. In
addition we see aorta, ivc
and hepatic vessels.

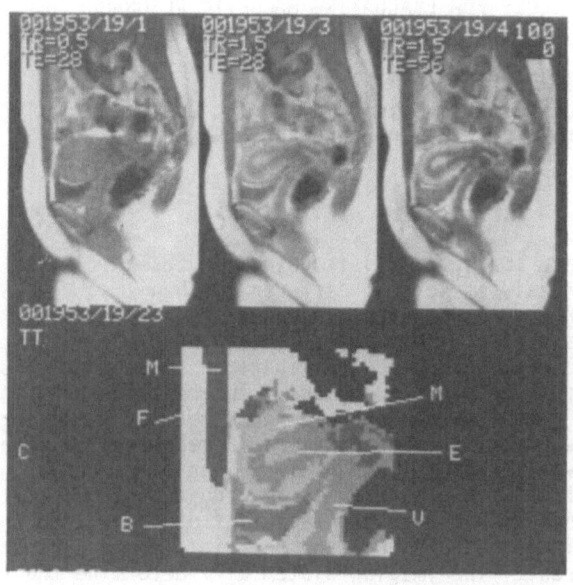

Figure 10. For a patient with a normal uterus we show the intensity images as well as the tissue map. In this case we segment only over a region of interest. Bladder, mesenteric fat, muscle, myometrium, endometrium and vagina are well seen.

SIMULATION TECHNIQUES FOR EVALUATING MAGNETIC RESONANCE IMAGING

N.M. HYLTON, D.A. ORTENDAHL
University of California, Radiologic Imaging Laboratory
400 Grandview Drive, South San Francisco, CA 94080

INTRODUCTION

Magnetic Resonance Imaging (MRI) is unique in its ability to reflect contrast on the basis of several different mechanisms. The signal is related to the hydrogen density, N(H), and the rates of relaxation, T1 and T2. Each of these factors can be exploited individually to provide contrast. The direct dependence of signal on the number of spins present, i.e., the hydrogen density, is obvious. The relationships involving T1 and T2 are less intuitive and in some sense reflect competing behaviors. T1 involves a regrowth of magnetization; T2 represents a decay.

The overall evaluation of image quality is a complex task, depending on the characteristics of the particular imaging technique, of the display system and of the human visual process. Influencing factors determined by the image will include the signal and the size, shape and contrast of the feature of interest. The imaging system will determine the spatial resolution, sensitivity and noise. Parameters of the display system, for example, brightness scale, gain, magnification and viewing conditions will also contribute to the appearance of the image. In addition, the observer's perception will be affected by the visual response of the eye as well as by psychological parameters, such as a priori knowledge or expectations (1).

ABSOLUTE SIGNAL DIFFERENCE AND FEATURE DETECTIBILITY

The concerns mentioned weigh differently for the various imaging modalities. Some attempt has been made to provide a general definition of parameters so that they may be used as yardsticks for comparison (2,3). Rose (4) has studied detectibility and the human visual process and provides a simple model for characterizing an image by determining the number of resolvable elements per unit area, T, defined as:

$$T = 1/d^2 = nC^2/k^2 \tag{1}$$

where d is the object diameter; contrast C is defined as the fraction of background brightness constituted by the signal, i.e., $C = \Delta B/B$; n is the total number of discrete events per unit area, and k is the confidence, in standard deviations, with which the identification can be made. The factor k is related to the probability that a false positive will be identified, and is chosen on the basis of the degree of accuracy required.

Rose's model assumes however, an image formed directly by individual quanta, which is not the case in MRI. It also uses a simple analysis of k as the ability to see a discrete lesion in a uniform background, a best case situation if it occurs at all.

In Rose's analysis, n is the total number of quanta per unit area, (in the case of MRI we can consider unit area to be a pixel). In a statistics-limited noise situation, the noise N is equal to the square root of n. n can be expressed as the square of $(n/\sqrt{n})$ and therefore in the statistics-limited case, as the square of (Signal/Noise) or (S/N). In MRI, the noise bears no relation to signal level S; it is constant throughout the image. Even so, the term S/N is still a valid parameter so that for MRI, expression (1) can be written as:

$$T \cong [(S/N) \times C/k]^2 \tag{2}$$

Defining contrast C as (lesion signal-background signal)/background signal, or (L-S)/S we can make the replacement,

$$T \cong [(L-S)/N \times 1/k]^2 \tag{3}$$

In order to resolve one pixel, i.e., for T = 1, we find $k \cong (L-S)/N$. Therefore, the ability to detect an object one pixel in area is proportional to the signal difference-to-noise ratio. For a larger feature, i.e., greater than one pixel in area, k will be proportional to:

$$k \cong (L-S)/N \times (1/T)^{1/2} \tag{4}$$

This proportionality justifies the use of signal difference/noise as a criteria for detectibility. The concerns in this study are those factors which can be manipulated using post-acquisition processing, i.e., signal and noise levels. Many of the other factors affecting image quality have been studied by others (1,5).

In order to systematically determine the impact of NMR imaging parameters on feature detectibility, the quantities absolute signal difference (ASD) and absolute signal difference-to-noise (ASD/N) have been evaluated as a function of changing imaging parameters. For a known sequence, it is possible to model the signal induced in the receiver coil as a function of time. Expressions have been found for a spin echo and inversion recovery sequence, each of which uses two spin refocussing pulses (180 degree pulses) to create signal echoes (6).

RETROSPECTIVE IMAGE CALCULATION

The spin echo sequence implemented in our laboratory consists of a 90 degree radiofrequency (rf) pulse followed by two 180 degree pulses at times T and 3T. This sequence of pulses is repeated after a time TR. The 180 degree pulses produce echoes at times TE1 and TE2 = 2TE1 after the 90 degree pulse, where TE1 = 2T. The voltage induced in the receiver coil is directly proportional to the y-component of the transverse magnetization. We can model this induced signal by following the evolution of the bulk magnetization vector through the sequence and then imposing steady state conditions. For signal readout coincident with either the echo at time TE1 or TE2 after t=0, the signal has decayed according to T2 to give a measurable signal intensity:

$$M_y(TE_n) =$$

$$M(0)[1-2\exp[-(TR-3T)/T1]+2\exp[-(TR-T)/T1]-\exp(-TR/T1)] \times \exp(-TE_n/T2)$$

$$\tag{5}$$

where n=1,2, and the assumption has been made TR >>T2. Similarly, we find the expression for an inversion recovery sequence in which a 180° pulse is used to invert the magnetization at a time TI before the excitation:

$$M_y(TE_n) = M(0)[1-2exp(-TI/T1)+2exp[-(TR-3T)/T1]$$
$$-2exp[-(TR-T)/T1]+exp(-TR/T1)] \times exp(-TE_n/T2) \qquad (6)$$

Noticing that these expressions are a function of the intrinsic tissue parameters T1, T2 and N(H) and of the pulse timing parameters TE, TR (and TI in the case of inversion recovery), one can calculate the signal generated at any set of pulse timing parameters if the intrinsic parameters are known. If these values are known at every position in an image, it is possible to compute a new image for any set TE, TR, and TI. Such an image will be referred to as a calculated or retrospective intensity image.

ABSOLUTE SIGNAL DIFFERENCE PLOTS

For two tissues, referred to as lesion and background, that have been characterized by their T1, T2 and N(H) values, it is possible, using the signal intensity expressions above to evaluate the difference in signal intensity between the two tissues for specified values of TE and TR and TI. By computing the spin echo intensity difference for a range of TE and TR values, a plot can be generated showing the spin echo ASD as a function of the imaging parameters. An example of such a plot is shown in Figure 1 (top) for lesion and white matter in the brain of a patient with a right temporal astrocytoma. TR ranges along the horizontal axis from 0 to 5 sec, TE is plotted along the vertical axis from 0 to 200 ms. The ASD is reflected by a color scale in which violet-white is the maximum ASD over the range shown and red-black denotes minimum ASD. The iso-contour for any given difference value is represented by the associated color and shows the realm of TE,TR pairs which will yield an equivalent degree of signal difference. It is important to note that the map describes the relationship between only the two tissues specified. While imaging anywhere on the iso-contour will produce the same degree of signal difference between these tissues, contrast relationships between other tissues in the image will most likely change significantly. For that reason it may be necessary to consider more than one pair of tissues before choosing the imaging parameters.

Another characteristic of the ASD map is the dark null band which represents the region of little or no tissue contrast, since the signal intensities from the two tissues are very similar or equal. Regions adjacent to but on opposite sides of the null band have contrast of opposite polarity. For example, points of the same shade found on either side of the null band will produce the same amount of signal difference, however in one case lesion will be brighter than background and in the other case background will be brighter.

The ASD plot can be used as a guide to retrospective image calculation. Four points corresponding to different TE and TR values are shown in Figure 2. As predicted by the ASD plot for lesion and white matter, the four acquired images using (TR = .5 sec, TE = 28 ms), (TR = .5 sec, TE = 56 ms), (TR = 2.0 sec, TE = 28 ms) and TR = 2.0 sec, TE = 56 ms) all show lesion darker than white matter. In the calculated (TR = 5.0 sec, TE = 110 ms) image, lesion/white matter contrast has reversed.

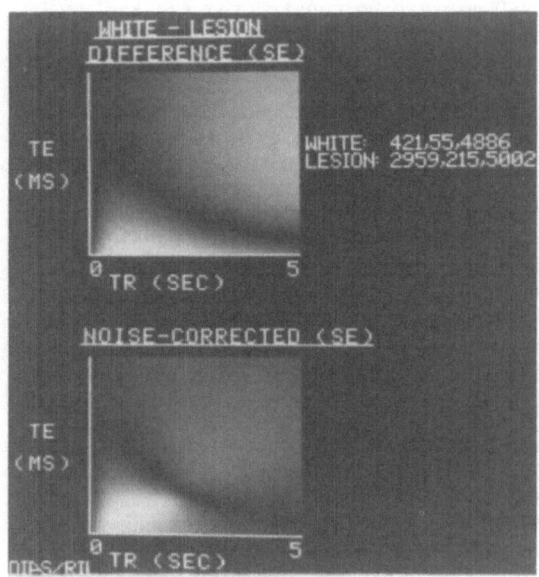

FIGURE 1. Spin Echo ASD plot (above) and ASD/N plot (below) are shown comparing white matter and lesion as a function of the pulse timing parameters TE and TR for a patient with a temporal astrocytoma. TE ranges from 0 to 200 ms, TR ranges from 0 to 5 sec. The difference plot predicts maximum signal difference between lesion and white matter for TE = 0 ms, TR = 1.0 sec. Difference-to-noise is predicted optimal at TE = 20 ms, TR = 0.8 sec.

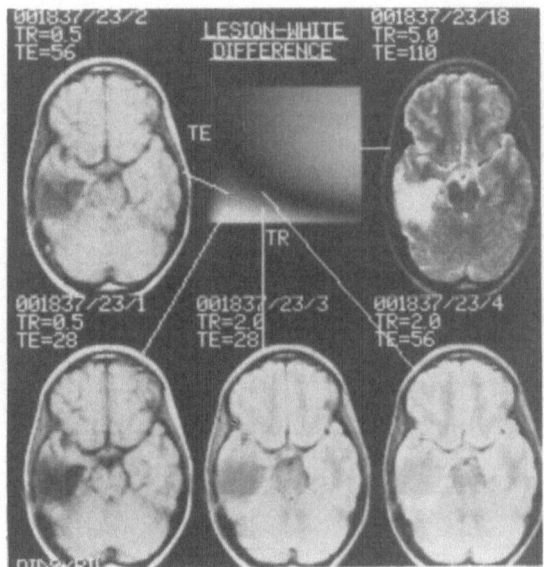

FIGURE 2. Images corresponding to five points on the difference plot of Figure 1. Upper left and lower three images result from a typical spin echo imaging protocol. Since all four fall on or below the null band, in each case lesion is of lower or equal intensity than white matter. The upper right image is calculated for the maximum difference point above the null band and shows lesion brighter than white matter. This image is affected by propagated noise however, as predicted by the ASD/N plot in Figure 1.

A map similar to the spin echo ASD map can be constructed for the inversion recovery technique. In this case the interesting relationship involves the two imaging parameters TI and TR. At a time TI prior to each rf excitation, the magnetization is inverted with a 180° pulse. This relationship implies that TI<TR. Thus the inversion recovery difference plot considers only the region for which TR>TI. The example shown in Figure 3 for the inversion recovery ASD between white matter and infarcted tissue, reveals multiple dark bands which slope upward slightly with increasing TR. The contrast mechanism for inversion recovery allows not only a disappearance of contrast when the magnetizations are equal, but also when they are equal in magnitude and opposite in sign. Compared to the single region of zero contrast for spin echo, when both magnetizations are positive and equal, inversion recovery has a more sensitive contrast mechanism. Several contrast reversals can occur as TI and TR values change. Variations in TI values of only several hundred milliseconds can result in contrast minimization rather the maximization. This high degree of sensitivity combined with large patient-to-patient variability makes sequence optimization for inversion recovery difficult to achieve. Calculated images corresponding to the labeled points (a),(b) and (c) of the inversion recovery ASD are also shown in Figure 3. A contrast reversal occurs between points (a) and (c). Relative contrast has been found to have a dramatic impact on perceived lesion size and conspicuity, making the intensity relationship an important consideration when choosing technique (7).

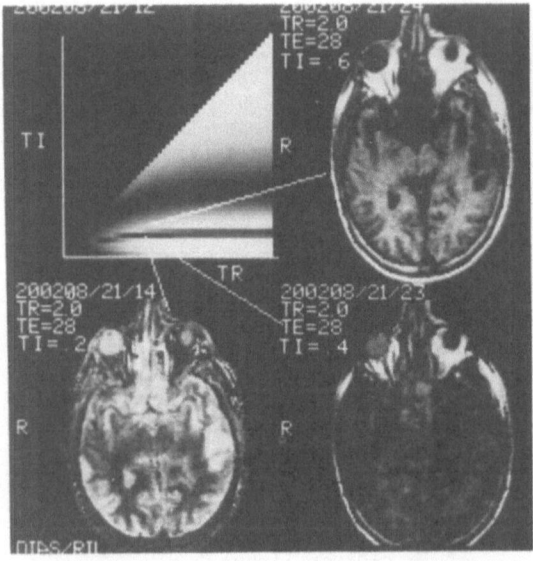

FIGURE 3. Absolute difference map for the inversion recovery technique shows the contrast relationship between lesion and white matter for a patient with an infarct as a function of TI and TR. Three simulated images corresponding to indicated points on the ASD map illustrate the large degree of contrast variation possible with small changes in TI.

Multi-tissue Footprints. Two or more of the difference plots can be intersected to find the region for optimal imaging when more than two tissues are involved. Such an intersection, which we call a 'footprint' is shown in Figure 4 for three tissues.

In the patient of Figure 4, the parieto-occipital brain tumor visible in the right side of the image has a complex structure. Three separate regions of the tumor were located and characterized by their T1, T2, and N(H) values. Each pairwise combination of these areas, labeled L1, L2 and L3 in Figure 4, was evaluated by looking at its ASD as a function of the spin echo parameters TE and TR. A multi-tissue footprint was created for the three lesion areas by requiring 50% or greater of the maximum ASD for each pair. The footprint, also shown in Figure 4 has a narrow region of relatively long TR and very short TE that provides the required 50% ASD for each pair. Pathology in the head is often characterized by lengthened T2, resulting in greater contrast and thus greater visibility in longer TE images. However, as this case illustrates in Figure 5, long echo imaging cannot always be used reliably for optimal differentiation, even with elevated T2 pathology. Calculated images at TE values of 56, 84 and 112 ms show increasing tumor/white matter contrast as TE increases, providing better definition of the entire tumor as a whole. Internal lesion structure however, is lost as echo delay increases, resulting in a tumor of homogeneous appearance in the longer echoes. The decreasing contrast between sections of the tumor as TE increases is predicted by the ASD plot shown in Figure 5.

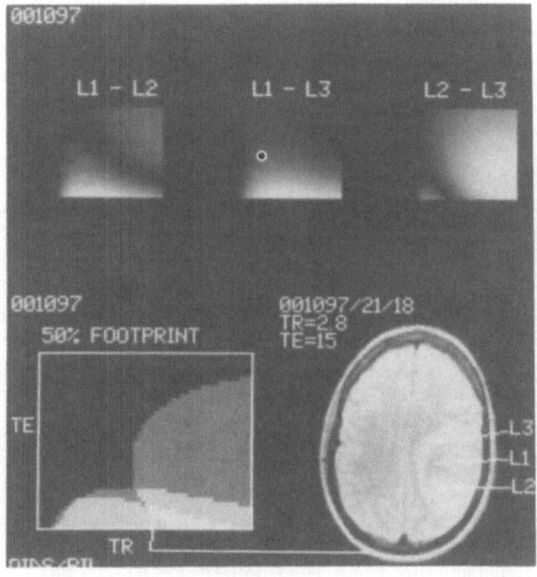

FIGURE 4. Three plots (above) show spin echo ASD for each of the pairwise combinations of the three regions of tumor identified in the lower right image. Lower left "footprint" shows in white the imaging regime in which all three pairs are of 50% or greater of their maximum possible signal difference.

Noise-Corrected Absolute Difference (ASD/N) Plots

In order to evaluate the impact that propagated noise has on calculated image quality, the ASD plots can be modified by calculating for each point (TEa,TRb), the amount of noise propagated from the original images using an error propagation analysis. It is necessary to specify the values of TE and TR for each of the three original intensity images used to derive the T1,T2 and N(H) values. Normalizing the original noise to a value of one, the ASD at each point is divided by the noise at that point. An example of such a 'noise-corrected' plot (ASD/N) is shown in Figure 1 (bottom) for the corresponding uncorrected ASD plot (top) referred to earlier. When compared to the uncorrected plot, certain characteristics are noticeable. The high intensity region has become much more localized and surrounds the area which includes the TE and TR values of the original images, i.e., TR = .5 and 2 sec, TE = 28 and 56 ms. The rate of falloff moving away from this region is large, overcoming the increasing trend shown in the ASD plot as TR increases. The ASD/N plots provide a measure of confidence with which to gauge an image calculated at the new parameters relative to the original images. These plots point out the limitations on image calculation imposed by the choice of actual imaging parameters. For image quality comparable to the original images, one is generally restricted to the calculation of images localized in TR to the region of data acquisition, although for certain T1 and T2 values an improvement can be achieved by extrapolating to short TR and long TE values (8). The effects of propagated error can be seen in the calculated image at (TR = 5.0 sec, TE = 110 ms) shown in Figure 2, which appears significantly noisier than the acquired images shown.

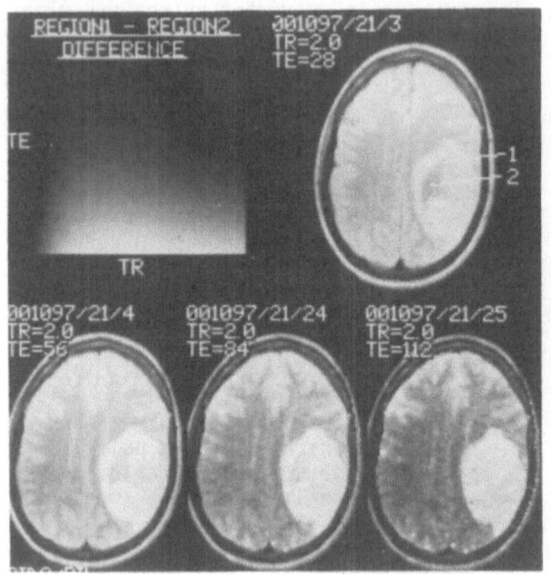

FIGURE 5. A spin echo difference map (upper left) for the two regions of tumor identified in the upper right image predicts decreasing contrast as TE increases. This decrease is illustrated by the TE = 56, 84 and 112 ms images shown along the bottom row despite improved contrast between the tumor as a whole and surrounding white matter.

The ability to calculate long TR images of reasonable quality is desirable because of the savings in imaging time that would result. We can explore the usefulness of such a technique by asking which pair of acquisition TR values would yield the best S/N in a calculated image of chosen TR. Since we are most interested in the calculation of long TR images, a TRc value of 5 seconds was chosen. It was a further restriction that the pair of acquired images result in a time savings of at least a factor of 2 over the time it would take to acquire the desired image, i.e., TR1 + TR2 must be no larger than TRc, or 2.5 seconds. Table 1 lists the ratio of the S/N of the calculated image to the S/N of the acquired image, for all possible pairs of TR values in steps of 100 ms. This was

TABLE 1

TR_1	TR_2	C/A*	T1/ΔT1	C/A*	T1/ΔT1	C/A*	T1/ΔT1
(ms)		T1 = 300		T1 = 500		T1 = 800	
100	2400	.996	.402	.837	.246	.268	.138
200	2300	.994	.884	.907	.631	.525	.380
300	2200	.990	1.000	.894	.824	.576	.533
400	2100	.985	.949	.869	.889	.568	.612
500	2000	.975	.834	.833	.871	.536	.634
600	1900	.960	.698	.785	.804	.490	.613
700	1800	.934	.564	.721	.707	.433	.560
800	1700	.890	.440	.640	.591	.367	.484
900	1600	.815	.327	.536	.467	.294	.391
1000	1500	.687	.225	.408	.336	.214	.287
1100	1400	.479	.131	.256	.203	.131	.175
1200	1300	.175	.043	.088	.068	.044	.059

TR_1	TR_2	C/A*	T1/ΔT1	C/A*	T1/ΔT1
		T1 = 1500		T1 = 2000	
100	2400	.059	.053	.037	.032
200	2300	.155	.152	.099	.094
300	2200	.204	.222	.136	.138
400	2100	.223	.266	.153	.168
500	2000	.222	.287	.156	.183
600	1900	.209	.287	.149	.185
700	1800	.187	.271	.134	.176
800	1700	.159	.240	.115	.157
900	1600	.127	.198	.093	.130
1000	1500	.093	.147	.068	.098
1100	1400	.056	.091	.041	.060
1200	1300	.019	.031	.014	.020

* C/A = [S/N$_{(calculated)}$] / [S/N$_{(acquired)}$]

generated for a range of T1 values: T1 = .3, .5, .8, 1.5 and 2.0 sec. In the case of very short T1, (i.e., .3 sec), a maximum in calculated image S/N was predicted for the combination (.1, 2.4). However, these values could be varied by as much as .8 sec and only suffer a loss of 20% in S/N. As T1 increases, the maximum in S/N becomes less broad, and shifts away from the extreme values. By T1 = .8 sec, the best S/N is obtainable using the (.3, 2.2) pair. By T1 = 2.0 sec, the maximum has shifted to the (.5, 2.0) pair and the maximum is much less broad; 20% spanning only .2 sec on either side. These results indicate that for intensity calculations when T1 is short, the choice of acquired images to use is not critical. The choice becomes more critical with increasing T1, but remains roughly between .3 and .5 sec for the shorter TR value. Since a range of T1 values will appear in most intensity images, this choice would tend to be most dependable. Our standard imaging technique using .5 and 2.0 sec TR values used to generate the calculated images of this study, falls in this region.

Also calculated and listed in Table 1 are the T1 signal/noise values obtainable for each pair of TR values. Comparison with the optimized values of TR for the calculated image shows that the T1 S/N and the calculated image S/N are not optimized at the same point. The maxima for optimized T1 S/N and calculated image S/N are sufficiently broad that a compromised choice of TR values can be chosen resulting in reasonably high S/N in both cases. For most values of T1, this value appears to be between .4 and .6 for the lower TR, over the range shown.

Modeling Field-Dependent Relaxation Time Changes

The impetus to image at higher field strengths is spurred by the theoretical dependence of S/N on field, H. This has been predicted to follow a 3/2 relationship (9), however experimental models have been found to range from a square root to a linear dependence. S/N is not the only concern in imaging however. Equally if not more important is contrast, which in MRI imaging is strongly driven by T1 differences between tissues. T1 values also change with field and have been found to increase with increasing field strength depending on tissue. Several experimental models show T1 changes with increasing fields as a function of various tissue groups, i.e. gray matter, white matter, muscle, fat, kidney, liver, cerebral spinal fluid (CSF), etc. (10,11). In each of these models the rate of increase with field varies with tissue in such a way that the T1 values tend to converge at higher field strength.

In our laboratory, T1 and T2 values were measured at several field points between 1.4 and 7 kGauss. These values were fit to a square root of field strength dependence as a function of tissue group for gray and white matter, fat, muscle and CSF. CSF was found to behave similarly to pure water and exhibited no measurable able changes in T1 with field. T2 appeared to be largely independent of field, possibly showing a slight decreasing trend with increasing field strength. T2 was initially modeled to a ln H dependence, but appeared to have no noticeable impact on image contrast.

The models of T1 vs. H for the five tissue categories were used to extrapolate T1 values from 3.5 KGauss, the operating field strength of the magnet at the time of data acquisition, to any new value of field strength. It was assumed that the T1 vs. H models remain valid outside of the range of field strengths used to establish them. It should be emphasized that the experimental models are based on very limited data and are not being purported to be precise. Rather, the method of evaluation is of significance. The models used can be easily updated as more experimental data becomes available. Nevertheless, the reflected trends in the models have been supported by published work of other authors and appear to be relatively accurate (10, 12).

T1 values were extrapolated by interpolating between the curves just above and below the T1 value at 3.5 KGauss and maintaining the same proportionality at the new field strength value. Using this method T1 images calculated from data acquired at 3.5 KGauss were extrapolated creating T1 images at new field strengths. T2 was assumed independent of field strength. The extrapolated T1 images, along with T2 and N(H) images, both assumed independent of field, were used to reconstruct simulated intensity images at new field strength values. Such images reflect the effects of field-dependent T1 changes only and not of changes in S/N that would be expected if the new field image were actually acquired. ASD plots can similarly be extrapolated to new fields to show the effects of field strength on contrast for given values of the imaging parameters. At present, imaging at more than one field point requires as many magnets and quickly becomes impractical as the number of points increases.

Figure 6 shows a set of spin echo images computed at 3.5 and 20 kGauss for a patient with an infarct. These images indicate a loss of contrast between infarct and surrounding white matter as field increases. This loss is predicted by the ASD plots created for white matter and infarct at 3.5 and 20 kGauss, also shown in Figure 6.

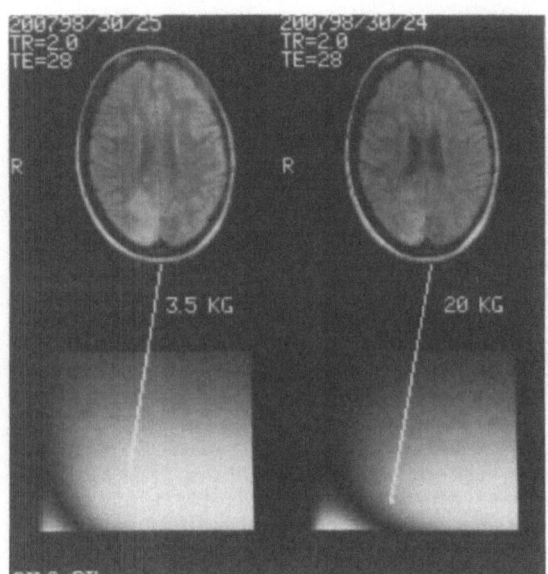

FIGURE 6. Spin echo ASD plots at 3.5 and 20 kGauss for a patient with an infarct predict the loss of lesion/white matter contrast evident in the calculated (TR = 2.0sec, TE = 28ms) images shown. Gray matter/white matter contrast has also decreased.

Computing The Integral Image

The S/N of an image will increase proportionally to the square root of the number of redundant data sets, or average taken. During the image acquisition, the doubling of the number of averages taken carries the penalty of also doubling the total imaging time. Therefore, economical and practical considerations limit the extent to which increased averages can be used to improve S/N during acquisition. Post-acquisition, in some cases S/N can be gained by averaging non-identical data sets, at the expense of some information. For example, two or more echo images, i.e., images identical except for different values of TE, can be averaged to produce an image of S/N improved by the square root of n, where n is the number of images averaged. However, the resulting image has lost T2 information.

In cases of long T2 pathology, the long echo image is often of increased value because of the improved differentiability of the lesion (6). Most regions of the long echo image, however, for which T2 is relatively short, will suffer from low S/N due to their low signal intensity at long TE. Averaging of the short and long echoes in these cases will produce an image that benefits from the long echo images which contribute heightened appearance of the lesion as well as gaining S/N from the averaging process.

It can be shown that in the limit as the number of data sets used for averaging increases, the sum can be replaced by an integral given by;

$$S = S(0) \int \exp(-TE/T2) \ dTE \tag{7}$$

where;

$$S(0) = N(H) \times [1-2\exp(-(TR-3T)/T1)+2\exp(-(TR-T)/T1)-\exp(-TR/T1)] \tag{8}$$

The integral reduces to:

$$S = S(0) \times T2 \tag{9}$$

S(0), also called the Free Induction Decay (FID) image since it represents the signal at TE = 0, can easily be obtained from the same data set required to obtain T2. Therefore both S(0) and T2 can be derived from two images only, of different TE values.

Using this relationship, it is possible to calculate the 'integral' image, as shown in Figure 7. Also shown in Figure 7 is an image obtained by averaging echoes at TE = 28,56,100,150 and 200 ms. The integral image contains equivalent detail to the average image, however it was computed using the TE = 28 and 56 ms. images only, thereby requiring a much reduced acquired data set than the averaged image. The integral image does not benefit from the improvement in S/N gained by averaging more than two images since it it obtained from two images only.

Retention of Polarity in Inversion Recovery

In an inversion recovery sequence, the 180 degree inverting flip at time TI before the 90° flip causes a negatively-directed z-magnetization. Depending on the length of time T1, and the particular TI value, at the instant of the 90° flip, the z-magnetization may still be negative, or could be zero or positive valued. Consider two tissue samples with different values of T1, i.e., T1a and T1b. Over the time interval TI, the two tissues will undergo different amounts of recovery depending on their equilibrium z-magnetization, M(0) and their T1 value. If TI is adjusted such that the two tissues have recovered to equal but opposite values of z-magnetization, the pursuant 90° pulse will flip both into the transverse axis, resulting in equal magnitude vectors of opposite polarity. Since present imaging methods map signal magnitude and do not take phase into account, the two tissues will yield identical signals and contrast between the two is lost. Methods have been suggested for retaining polarity information in inversion recovery images (13); these methods require additional acquisitions in order to extract the phase.

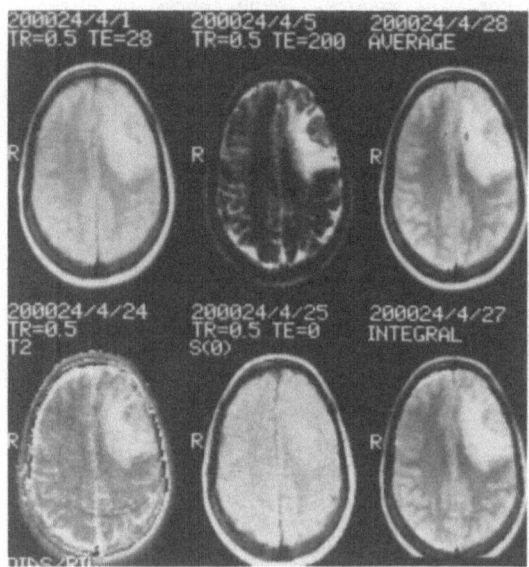

FIGURE 7. Top left and center images show high signal-to-noise of the early echo (28 ms.) and enhanced lesion contrast of the late echo (200 ms.), respectively. Top right image results from averaging echoes at 28, 56, 100 150 and 200 ms. Bottom right "integral" image results from the product of the T2 and S(0) images shown bottom left and center and closely approximates the averaged image in detail.

Another interesting effect of this phenomena occurs in partial volume averaged elements bordering the two tissues. In such a volume containing both tissues, equal but opposite contributions cancel one another causing diminished signal. This appears in the image as a dark band at the border between the two tissues which are of equal signal intensity.

Simulated inversion recovery images can be used to study both of these effects. It is also possible to retain the polarity information and display it. One way of achieving this is to translate the negative valued z-magnetization into negative valued transverse magnetization and then display zero intensity as gray with negative values ranging from gray to black and positive intensities ranging from gray to white. An example of such an image is shown in Figure 8 along with the corresponding simulated inversion recovery image for which polarity was not retained. In this way complete advantage is taken of the increased dynamic range resulting from magnetization inversion. The simulation of the retained polarity inversion recovery image requires no additional data acquisition or computation. The concern is in the simulated image case as it would also be for the acquired image, a problem of appropriate display of the additional polarity information. The disadvantage of the display method shown is that zero signal intensity has now been assigned to gray rather than black as reflected by the background of the images shown. Inversion recovery methods are often used precisely to cause a zeroing of a particular tissue, perhaps because its high signal overshadows a neighboring less intense signal. By adjusting TI to yield zero z-magnetization for that tissue at the time of the 90° pulse, no component of magnetization is rotated into the transverse plane and therefore no signal results from that tissue in the image. By choosing to display that tissue as medium gray rather than black, it may again appear as a distracting signal. Comparing the set of inversion recovery images with an equivalent set showing retained polarity, both shown in Figure 8, it is immediately noticed that the contrast reversal experienced by gray and white matter between TI values of .2 and .4 sec is not present in the retained polarity images. This can be explained by the fact that the tissue with the largest magnitude is nonetheless negative valued and therefore results as a lower intensity in the retained polarity image. In order to see a true contrast reversal it is necessary to move to a long TI value.

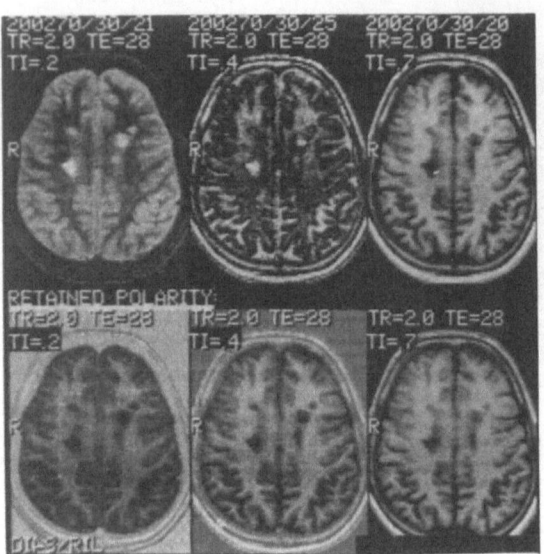

FIGURE 8. Calculated inversion recovery images for a patient with multiple sclerosis with (below) and without (above) polarity retention show contrast variability as TI changes from .2 to .7 sec.

CONCLUSIONS

Mathematical modeling and computer simulation techniques have been developed as an approach to the problem of sequence optimization. Simulation allows the in-depth study of parameter effects on image intensity and contrast that would be impractical if not impossible to achieve experimentally. It also allows the study of a patient post-imaging by generating new images via retrospective calculation without requiring additional data acquisition. New techniques can be tested prior to implementation. Impirical models showing T1 changes with field strength give early indications of the impact of increased operating field strength on contrast. These techniques are successful within the limitations of propagated noise. This noise has been quantified and attempts made to minimize its effects.

REFERENCES

1. Goodenough DJ: Assessment of Image Quality of Diagnostic Imaging System, Medical Images: Formation, Perception and Measurement, Chap. 4, Wiley, Chichester, 1976.
2. Kaufman L, Shosa DW: Generalized Methodology for the Comparison of Diagnostic Imaging Instrumentation. AFIPS Press, Vol. 49, 445-451, 1980.
3. Shosa DW, Kaufman L: Methods for Evaluation of Diagnostic Imaging Instrumentation, Phys Med Biol, Vol. 26, No. 1, 101-112, 1981.
4. Rose AA: Vision: Human and Electronic, Plenum Press, 1973.
5. Edelstein WA, Bottomley PA, et al: Signal Noise and Contrast in Nuclear Magnetic Resonance (NMR) Imaging, J Computer Assisted Tomography, Vol, 7, 391-401, 1983.
6. Feinberg DA, Mills CM, et al: Multiple Spin-Echo Magnetic Resonance Imaging, Radiology. Vol. 155, 437-442, 1985.
7. Posin JP, Ortendahl DA, Hylton NM, et al: Variable Magnetic Resonance Imaging Parameters: Effect on Detection and Characterization of Lesions, Radiology. Vol. 155, 719-725, 1985.
8. Ortendahl DA, Hylton NM, Kaufman L, Crooks LE: Optimal Strategies for Obtaining the Minimal NMR Data Set. IEEE Transactions on Nuclear Science, 1985. (In Press).
9. Hoult DI, Richards RE: The Signal-to-Noise Ratio of the Nuclear Magnetic Resonance Experiment, J of Magnetic Resonance. Vol. 24, 71-85, 1976.
10. Hart HR, Bottomley PA, et al: Nuclear Magnetic Resonance Imaging: Contrast-to-Noise Ratio as a Function of Strength of Magnetic Field, AJR, Vol. 141, 1195-1201, 1983.
11. Kaufman L, Crooks LE: Technical Advances in Magnetic Resonance Imaging, Presented at the Annual Postgraduate Course in MRI, CT and Interventional Radiology, 1985.
12. Bottomley PA, Foster TH, et al: A Review of Normal Tissue Hydrogen NMR Relaxation Times and Relaxation Mechanisms from 1-100 MHz: Dependence on Tissue Type, NMR Frequency, Temperature, Species, Excision, and Age, Med Phys, Vol. 11, No. 4, 425-448, 1984.
13. Bakker CJG, de Graaf CN, van Dijk P: Restoration of Signal Polarity in a Set of Inversion Recovery Images, IEEE Transactions on Medical Imaging. (In Press).

THE DEVELOPMENT OF A COMMAND LANGUAGE AND META-LANGUAGE IN NUCLEAR MEDI-
CINE PROCESSING SYSTEMS, USING FORTH

Michael L. Goris and Philippe A. Briandet

INTRODUCTION:

A priori, the requirements of flexibility versus ease of use seem
antagonistic in dedicated scintigraphic computer systems. This follows
from the fact that flexibility is most often achieved by multiplicity of
options. In many cases, the flow through the options is directed by decision trees or menus. which have the major disadvantage of requiring
multiple, and repetitive answers to often obscure questions. Alternatively the direct call to the program library requires that the operator
remember the name of all available programs, which are often mnemonic by
courtesy only.

Ease of use on the other hand is most often attained by a menu
structure with few levels, and rigid data structures.

In this paper, we briefly describe an attempt to reconcile the requirements, based on FORTH, in which the first access of the user is to
a two layer MENU directing to predefined and well established PROTOCOLS
but further and progressive access to stringing of simple commands and
primitives.

DESCRIPTION OF FORTH STRUCTURE:

FORTH (1,2) is a language using individual execution modules which
can be stringed or built into composite words. Variables or vectors can
be used but the operations are explicitly performed on the stack, in a
reversed polish mode: As an example, if the primitive FRAME-MAX computes the maximal value in a frame or data file (xt), and TOT computes
the total number of counts (xm), the command f#F>K : F>K dup FRAME-MAX
swap TOT. " total = ". ." maximum = " . ; prints out both values as follows:

    f# dup
    f# f# FRAME-MAX
    f# xm swap
    xm f# TOT
    xm xt .
    xm   .
    --

The data are directly loaded in memory, with their characteristics
stored in variables. As an example, an image is defined by the variable
"nbfram" the number of frames and the word "size" which places the size
of the array on the stack. The command IO-scan : IO-SCAN nbfram @ 0 DO

i F>K cr LOOP; prints out sm and tm for all the frames in the image. FRAME-MAX itself:

: FRAME-MAX frame-addr 0 size 0 DO 1 pick i GET MAX loop drop; transforms the frame number to a memory address, and uses size to define the loop. GET adds the index i to the address and places the value on the stack. MAX leaves the largest of two values on the stack.

In this example, it is important to note that all the WORDS are directly executable and addressable by the end-user; there is no layer of programs buffering the use of subroutines.

DESCRIPTION OF COMMAND LANGUAGE MODULES:

The command language is a tool for the execution of simple (in contradistinction to complex or composed of many steps) operations on scintigraphic objects. Scintigraphic objects are IMAGES (I) of which the typical example is the image of a gated cardiac cycle, and typically consist of n FRAMES (F), which are square data arrays, 64 x 64 or 128 x 128, represented by their number, going from 0 to n. Other scintigraphic objects are CURVES (C), REGIONS OF INTEREST (R) and CONSTANTS (K). An additional object is a DYNAMIC STUDY (D), which differs from an image by being too large to be stored unmodified in workzone. There are three types of utility objects: QUADRANTS (Q), or the display quadrant for images, GRAPHICS (G), or the screen location for curve displays, and disc disc STORAGE (S).

Those "objects" can be moved (copied), added, subtracted, multiplied, divided, smoothed, and displayed. Any one of those actions is called an operation. The basic rules are simple; i.e., in an HP pocket calculator, the addition of 222 and 35 is obtained by 222 "enter" 35 "enter" "+", and yields 257. In our case, however, the "enter" key is simply a "space," obtained with the space bar, and the "function" is a WORD or name, entered in alphanumerics, followed by a carriage return ("cr") for execution. All processing is preceeded by a load operation, which brings the data in memory.

SYNTAX

OPERATIONS are represented by WORDS composed of letters, operation signs and sometimes numerals and names. The operation signs are "+" (add), "-" (subtract), "*" (multiply) ":" or "/" (divide), and > (copy into or store result in). Some operations are defined by words of more than one character: SMOOTH, EDGE. . . .

OBJECTS are represented by single letters, if they are to be further defined by the variables (see below), or by a letter and a numeral , if they are totally defined. The objects characters are "F", "C", "K", "R" and "Q" for the display screen, where Q0 represents a full screen, and the quadrants of the screen are numbered 1 through 4. "S" represents the disc storage and "G" the graphic display. In "G" there are no "quadrants," but G0 forces initialization of the graph, while G1 adds a curve to the graph.

VARIABLES are numerals, and are entered before the word which defines the operation. Not all words have associated variables.

DESTRUCTIVE operations are those whose word does not end with a "'>" sign associated with an object. The destructive operations store the results over the original.

COMMANDS are generally given as follows:

V V V WORD "cr"

where V represents the variable, WORD the command and "cr" a carriage return. One can, however, make a string of commands as follows:

V V V WORD1 V V WORD2 V WORD3 WORD4

In this case, the first word required three variables, the second two, the fourth none. The string is executed only when "cr" is entered.

COMMANDS

FRAME COMMANDS

f1 F-ZERO-CLIP
All negative values in frame f1 are set to zero.

f1 f2 F>F
copies f1 into f2.

f1 f2 f3 F+F>F
adds f1 + f2 and places result in f3.

f1 f2 f3 F-F>F
subtracts f2 from f1 and places result in f3.

f1 f2 f3 F:F>F
divides f1 by f2 and places result in f3.

f1 f2 f3 F*F⊁F
multiplies f1 with f2 and places result into f3.

f1 N f2 F+NF>F
add frames f1 to f1+n-1 and stores result in f2.

f1 F-INVERT
multiplies the values in f1 by -1.

k1 k2 f1 K/K*F
multiplies f1 by k1 and divides the result by k2.

k1 f1 K/max*F
scales f1 to k1.

k1 k1 K+F
adds the value k1 (positive or negative) to all values in f1.

f1 F>K
computes and prints the total counts and maximum counts.

f1 F>Q0
displays f1 in full screen.

f1 q1 F>Q
displays f1 in quadrant q1 (1-4).

f1 F**2>Q0
displays square of f1 in full screen.

F-SCAN
displays all frames of an image in memory.

f1 F-SMOOTH
smoothes frame f1.

f1 F-MID
enhances middle range values in f1.

f1 F-EDGE
transforms f1 to its Laplacian (2d).

f1 F-TURN-
flip frame f1 over horizontal axis (rotate y to -y).

f1 F-TURN-DISPLAY
same operation, but displays result.

f1 F-TURN/
flip image along diagonal (x-y interchange).

f1 F-TURN/-DISPLAY
same, with display of result.

CURVE OPERATIONS

C-INIT
Prepares empty curves of length equal to the image length.

n1 C>G0
displays a preexisting curve n1; initializes the graph.

n1 C>G1
displays curve n1 on preexisting graph.

n1 n2 C:C>G1
display curve n1 scaled to curve n2.

n1 n2 2C>G0
display two curves scaled to the larger one. Resets the graph.

c1 c2 C>C
copies curve c1 in curve c2, but c2 must preexist.

n1 n2 n3 C-C>C
subtract curve n2 from n1, result in curve n3

n1 n2 n3 C-Cnorm>C
subtract curve n2 from curve n1 after normalization for area ROI used to create n2

n1 n2 n3 C+C>C
curve addition

c1 c2 c3 C:C>C
generates c3 as prothousand of c1 curve divided by c2. All curves must preexist.

c1 c2 c3 C*C>C
multiplies c1 by c2 (point by point) and places result in preexisting c3.

n1 C>K
give max and min and total count under curve of curve n1.

k1 n1 K+C
adds the value of the constant k1 to all points of the curve n1.

k1 k2 n1 K/K*C
multiplies curve n1 by k1 and divides result by k2.

n1 n2 C>DC
computes (three point convolution) derivative from curve n1 and places result in curve n1.

REGION OF INTEREST OPERATIONS

ROI-CR
creates a set of consecutive regions of interest and produces the corresponding curves. Starts with initialization.

r1 r2 r3 R*R>R
make a ROI # r3 from the intersection of r1 and r2.

r1 R>E
Erase ROI # r1.

r1 r2 r3 R+R>R
make a ROI # r3 from the UNION (idempotente) of r1 and r2.

r1 r2 r3 R-R>R
make a ROI # r3 from the EXCLUSION of r1 and r2.

r1 r2 R>R
copies r1 into r2.

r1 r2 dx dy MOVE-ROI
make a ROI #1 r2 by moving r2 by dx and dy (128x128).

r1 ROI-EDGE
display ROI # r1 on GO

MIXED OPERATIONS

f1 F+RO>QO
display frame f1 with all ROI's in overlay.

r1 f1 R*F>K
yields the counts within ROI r1 in FRAME f1.

r1 f1 f2 R*F>F
inclusive mask of f1 by r1, result in f2

f1 r1 F>R
creates a roi r1 from all non-zero points in f1.

f1 r1 f2 F-R>F
Interpolative background subtraction, using the borders of r1, performed on f1, results in f2.

```
f1 r1 F>R
produce ROI#r1 from all non-zero points in f1
```

```
f1 F+RO>KO
displays f1 with all roi's in overlay, and prints roi-counts.
```

STRINGING:

Custom-made protocols can easily be obtained through stringing. As an example, IO-NORM can be defined to normalize an image to total counts as follows:

```
: IO-MAX 0 nbfram @ 0 DO i max-frame drop MAX LOOP;
: IO-SCALE nbframe @ 0 DO 2dup i K/K*F LOOP 2drop;
: IO-NORM IO MAX 1000 / 1000 swap IO-SCALE ;
```

CONCLUSION:

In a system where common protocols are directly accessed through a two-layered menu, and require no multiple questions to be executed, flexibility is obtained by direct access, first to a command structure with a simple syntax, and subsequently by direct access to primitives with the possibility of stringing. Ease of use and flexibility have been combined.

REFERENCES

1. Brodie, Leo: Starting Forth. Englewood Cliffs, New Jersey: Prentice-Hall, Inc., 1981.

2. Brodie, Leo: Thinking Forth: A Language and Philosophy for Solving Problems. Englewood Cliffs, New Jersey: Prentice-Hall, Inc., 1984.

PROLOG for Symbolic Image   Analysis

ROSENBERG S., ITTI   R., BENJELLOUN L.

Department of Nuclear   Medicine   and   Ultrasound
University Hospital   Trousseau, 37044 - Tours , France

ABSTRACT

The   central theme of this paper is the use   of
non-numerical methods for image analysis. It is proposed
that   the logic programming language Prolog is a
suitable tool for this purpose. A Prolog program consists
of   a set of   facts and rules. New facts can be   deduced
by the inbuilt inference mechanism. In contrast to
classical programming it is necessary to   consider the
objects of the   domain of investigation and the
relationships between them.   A set of rules   is derived
heuristically for the classification   of   myocardial
scintigrams. Fuzzy logic and probability theory   are then
applied in a Prolog   program to the problem of prediction
of coronary artery anatomy   from a   given scintigraphic
pattern.   A generative grammar has been written in   Prolog
to either analyse or produce   coded scintigraphic patterns.

Introduction to Prolog

A Prolog   program consists of a database containing
a set of facts about a certain domain   and a set of rules
that enable conclusions to be drawn from   these facts. The
programmer creates a   mini-world in which the   only
propositions that are true are those written down explicitly
as facts and those that can be deduced by the inbuilt
inference   mechanism.
Standard Edinburgh syntax as detailed in the   text
'Programming in Prolog' of Clocksin and   Mellish shall
be used   throughout this paper. A simple   program about
family relationships might   take   the   following form:
                    female(jane).
                    male(jack).
                    sister(jane,jack).
                    brother(X,Y) :- male(X),sister(Y,X).
Translated into English this program reads as follows:
Jane   is a female, Jack is a male, Jane is the sister of
Jack, X is the brother of Y if X is a male   and Y is the
sister of X. Each fact is made up   of a predicate

(female,male,sister) followed by one or more arguments
(jane,jack) inside a pair of brackets. All words beginning
with lowercase letters are taken to be constants whereas
variables begin with capital letters. The properties of
the mini-world about family relationships can be
investigated by writing down a question after the system
prompt:

                    ?-female(X).

This is a Prolog goal which allows examination of the
database from top to bottom. If pattern matching is
successful then the variable X will take on (become
instantiated to) a certain value. In this case we would
get only one answer:

                    X=jane

since there is only one female in our mini-world.

                    ?-male(X),sister(Y,X).

is a conjunction of goals where the comma represents AND.
In English the corresponding question is "Is there a male
who has a sister?". Prolog examines the conjunction of
goals from left to right and succeeds to match both goals
with facts in the database thus proving that the conjunction is true. It is important to realise that variables
are only local in their scope. Once a variable X in a
particular conjunction or rule takes on a certain value,
then all X's in that conjunction or rule take on the
same value.

    If the head of a rule is taken as a goal

                    ?-brother(X,Y).

then the goal only succeeds if all the subgoals in the
body of the rule can be proven. "X->jack" is the author's
notation for "X is instantiated to jack". The above goal
sets off the following sequence of events:

        male(X) succeeds, or more precisely matching of the
                structure 'male(X)' succeeds.
    X-> jack.
    sister(Y,jack) succeeds.
    Y->jane.
    brother(jack, jane) is proven.

    To illustrate the backtracking mechanism here is a
little program about set theory:

                    subset(a,b).
                    subset(b,c).
                    subset(c,b).
                    equal(X,Y) :- subset(X,Y),subset(Y,X).

The three facts state that a is a subset of b, that b
is a subset of c and that c is a subset of b. The
programmer must decide a priori on the meaning of a
fact and must be consistent throughout the program. Thus
'subset(a,b)' is interpreted as meaning that a is a
subset of b and not the inverse. The rule is a
transcription of the defintion : two sets A and B are
equal if and only if A is a subset of B and B is a
subset of A. Here now is the way Prolog searches to
satisfy the goal 'equal(X,Y)'.which reads :'are there
two sets that are equal'

equal(X,Y) matches the head of the rule, thus the goals
in the body of the rule must first be proven.
subset(X,Y) succeeds.
X->a, Y->b.
subset(a,b) is proven.
Since the scope of X and Y is from the beginning until
the end of the rule, the next goal is subset(b,a).
subset(b,a) fails.
Here the resolution mechanism goes back or backtracks
to the first goal, undoes the instantiations of X and
Y, then tries again by continuing on down the database.
subset(X,Y) succeeds.
X ->b,Y ->c.
subset(b,c) is proven.
subset(c,b) is proven.
equal(b,c) is proven.
We would need to include another rule about the transit-
ivity of set inclusion to prove that a is a subset of
c.

Statement of the problem

"Create a classification scheme for myocardial
scintigrams that enables optimal prediction of coronary
artery pathology"
There is no strict correspondance between scintigraphic patterns and coronary artery pathology for a
number of reasons: normal anatomical variants of the
coronary arterial tree, collateral circulation and the
intrinsic fuzziness of scintigraphic and angiographic
subclasses. This inherent uncertainty can be dealt
with by a combination of fuzzy set theory and probability
theory. In our model the anterior and left anterior
oblique scintigrams are each divided into five regions.
Each region is considered as being either normal,hypoact-
ive or very hypoactive. These regions of interest are
coded 0 for normal, 1 for hypoactive and 2 for very
hypoactive. It is clear that 'normal','hypoactive' and
'very hypoactive' are linguistic variables that
designate fuzzy sets associated with the degree of
radionuclide uptake. The two projections are grouped
together to give a single 'scintigraphic pattern'
consisting of the ten regions in an ordered sequence.
Rules for classification of these patterns were chosen
heuristically with the aid of clinical experience
(R.Itti) and a training set of 243 myocardial
scintigrams and their matching coronary angiograms (tables
1 and 2).

First approach

In order to come to grips with possibilistic (a
matter of degree) and probabilistic uncertainty, fuzzy
reasoning is introduced. Let U, R1, ...,R10 be system

variables whose given values are denoted by fuzzy
subsets: U = normal,anterior,inferior,lateral,infero-
anterior,infero-lateral,antero-lateral and extensive
scintigraphic patterns and R1 to R10(regional parameters)
= normal,low or very low radionuclide uptake.

The database consists of such statements as:
if(R6 or R7) are very low and(R4 and R5 and R9 and R10)
are not very low then U is anterior
if (R4 or R5) are very low and (R6 or R7) are very low
and(R9 or R10) are not very low then U is infero-anterior.

A compatibility estimate is made in order to calculate
the strength of the assertion. The anterior type scintigraphic pattern shall be taken as an example. The inclusion zone is (R6,R7) and the exclusion zone is (R4,R5,R9,
R10). If the total uptake in the inclusion zone is "low"
and "high" in the exclusion zone then the strength of the
assertion that the sequence is of the anterior type
will be high. The total uptake in the inclusion zone
and that of the exclusion zone may be thought of as
fuzzy sets denoted by the names 'low','medium' and
'high'. Such a set of rules was represented as a set of
Prolog facts . This lead to conclusions of the type:
"It is concluded with a high degree of certainty that
the scintigraphic pattern is of the anterior defect
type".

Furthermore, fuzzy conditional probabilities such as:
PROB (at least | lateral)   is about 0.8
     (CX stenotic | scintigraphic)
                   | pattern
can be estimated from the data set. Hence the output
could end with "the probability that at least the
circumflex artery is stenotic is about 0.8".

The regional uptake data is input to the database in the form of Prolog facts. The top level procedures
may be thought of as a column of filters through
which the regional data are passed. If matching of the
scintigraphic pattern is successful then the program
goes on to determine the strength of the conclusion and
prints out some information about fuzzy conditional
probabilities.

It became evident that one of the great advantages
of programming in Prolog is the ease with which a
complex program can be changed. This is due to the high
degree of modularity and the absence of traditional
control structures.

Second approach

A scintigraphic pattern can be considered as an
element of a formal language defined by a generative
grammar and a lexicon. Such a grammar consists of a set
of production rules that generate well-formed strings
in the language L. Prolog provides a grammar rule notation
that greatly facilitates the writing of grammars.

A proposed set of production rules for scintigraphic patterns is:
```
     sequence(X)--> ant_proj(X),lao_proj(X).
     ant_proj(X)--> antero_apical(X),inf(X).
     lao_proj(X)--> extended_ant(X),lat(X).
     antero_apical(X)--> ant_lat_bas(X),apical(X).
     extended_ant(X)--> ant(X),apical(X).
     ant_lat_bas(X)--> antero_basal(X),antero_lateral(X).
```
The variable X enables transmission of the sequence type -
normal,anterior, . . extensive.The terminal elements of
a tree corresponding to this grammar are in fact the
coded regional uptake values:

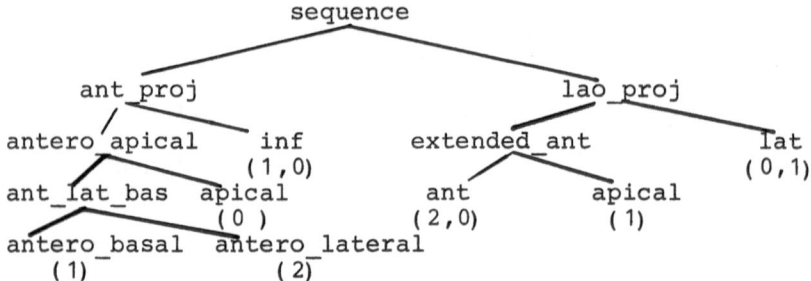

scintigraphic sequence = (1,2,0,1,0,2,0,1,0,1)

The sequence represented is of the anterior defect
type;possible configurations of the anterior segment are
(0,2) ,(2,0) , (1,2) ,(2,1) and(2,2) . The corresponding
configurations for the lateral (or inferior) segment are
(0,0) ,(0,1) , (1,0) and (1,1) .
     Semantics are included by labelling the terminal
elements in the lexicon - for instance:
```
               lat(normal) --> (1,1)
               lat(normal) --> (0,1) .
```
Numerical constraints on the sum of the sequence are
applied by a top-level procedure. The program functions
in both analysis and synthesis - a given sequence
can be analysed or the set of all poosible strings of
a given sequence type can be generated. A catchall
procedure is included to trap those sequences that
can't be analysed by the grammar (about 15%).

Conclusion

     The idea of symbolic computation probably started with
Ramon Lull in the 14th. century. In the 17th. century
Leibniz developed a calculus of reasoning. Now, in the
20th. century, we have at our disposal a number of tools
that facilitate the task. Prolog seems to be a good
candidate for the non-numerical approach to image processing. The field is in an embryonic state and many
hard and fascinating questions need to be addressed.

The wide diffusion of artificial intelligence techniques should stimulate research workers to look at the non-numerical side of the question.

References

1. Colmerauer A: Prolog, langage de l'intelligence artificielle. La Recherche, 1984, n° 158.
2. Clocksin WF, Mellish CS: Programming in Prolog, Springer Verlag, 1984.
3. Mamdani EH, Efstathiou HJ: Logic and PRUF - A Survey, IFAC Symposium, Marseille, France, 19-21 July 1983.
4. Szolovits P, Pauker SG: Categorical and probabilistic reasoning in medical diagnosis, Artificial Intelligence,11: 115-144,1978.
5.Thomas AJ: Expert systems for diagnostic imaging in digital imaging. Clinical advances in Nuclear Medicine, The Society of Nuclear Medicine,1982.
6. Zadeh LA:Fuzzy Sets, Inf. and Cont. 8 :338-353,1965.
7. Zadeh LA: The role of fuzzy logic in the management of uncertainty in expert systems. Memo. n° UCB/ERL M83/41. Electronics research lab.,College of Engineering,Univ.of California,Berkeley.

Annexe
Myocardial regions of interest.

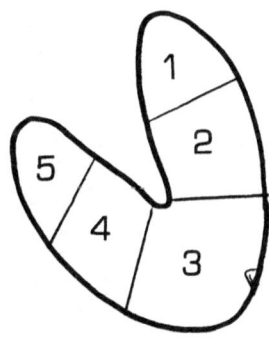

*anterior
projection*

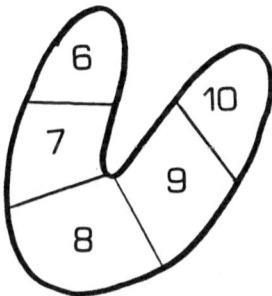

*left anterior
oblique projection*

figure 1.

SCINTIGRAPHIC REGION (Ri)

ANGIOGRAPHIC DIAGNOSIS	R1	R2	R3	R4	R5	R6	R7	R8	R9	R10	n° images in DB
NORMAL	3	2	5	1	4	18	7	0	1	4	34
LAD	11	11	41	15	13	62	44	16	3	0	43
RCA	8	7	37	49	55	26	19	28	16	17	36
CX	5	6	15	16	13	8	3	6	19	23	20
LAD-RCA	12	8	20	28	31	35	28	18	8	9	30
LAD-CX	7	5	17	12	14	14	10	12	10	14	17
RCA-CX	0	4	19	24	23	8	6	9	25	20	18
LAD-RCA-CX	12	17	53	52	53	37	32	37	28	27	45
											243

Table 1.
The numbers in the array are the sums of the regional scores for a given region and for a given angiograhhic diagnosis. The higher the number the more pronounced is the hypoactivity.
LAD = left anterior descending a.
RCA = right coronary a.
CX = circumflex a.

A HEURISTIC CLASSIFICATION OF MYOCARDIAL SCINTIGRAMS

Scintigraphic class	Inclusion criteria Regions that must be scored 2	Exclusion criteria Regions that must not be scored 2	Other constraints
ANTERIOR	(6 or 7)	(4 and 5) and (9 and 10)	sum$\leqslant$8
INFERIOR	(4 or 5)	(6 and 7) and(9 and 10)	sum$\leqslant$8
LATERAL	(9 or 10)	(4 and 5) and (9 and 10)	sum$\leqslant$8
ANTERO-INFERIOR	(4 or 5) and (6 or 7)	(9 and 10)	-
ANTERO-LATERAL	(6 or 7) and (9 or 10)	(4 and 5)	-
INFERO-LATERAL	(4 or 5) and (9 or 10)	(6 and 7)	-
EXTENSIVE	(4 or 5) and (6 or 7) and(9 or 10)	-	-
NORMAL	0 or 1 in each region	2 in any region	sum$\leqslant$4
NON-CLASSED	otherwise		

0 = normal uptake
1 = low uptake
2 = very low uptake

Table 2.

RECENT DEVELOPMENTS IN APPLIED POTENTIAL TOMOGRAPHY-APT

D.C. BARBER, B.H. BROWN

1. INTRODUCTION

The electrical resistance of various tissues are known to cover a wide range of values. Table 1 shows some typical values taken from the literature and it can be seen that even within the soft tissues differences are quite substantial. Images of the distribution of resistance within the human body should show good contrast between these tissues. It is the aim of resistance imaging to produce such images.

Table 1

Tissue	Resistivity Ohm m.
C.S.F	0.65
Blood	1.5
Skeletal muscle	5.3
Fat	20.0
Bone	160.0

The possibility of producing tomographic resistance images has been investigated by several groups over the past few years and a review of this work has been given by Barber and Brown (1984). Most groups have confined their theoretical and experimental interest to the problem of reconstructing the distribution of resistance within a two dimensional object from measurements taken on the boundary of the object. Most objects of interest are three dimensional and a full treatment of the three dimensional problem will differ significantly from the two dimensional case. Nevertheless this paper will also concentrate on the two dimensional problem but will show experimentally that a method of image reconstruction derived from an analysis of the two dimensional problem can produce useful images from data collected from three dimensional objects, including the human body.

The aim of resistance imaging is to reconstruct the distribution of resistance within an object from measurements obtained via an array of electrodes connected to the boundary of the object (Figure 1). One possible approach is to measure the resistance between all possible pairs of electrodes on the boundary (by passing current between them) and then compute a distribution of resistance consistent with these measurements. Solutions using this approach have been proposed by Dines and Lytle (1981) Schomberg and Tasto (1981) and Kim et al (1983) and some reconstructions have been attempted by these authors from simulated and laboratory data. A fundamental problem with this approach, apart from the computational complexities, is that any measurement made between electrodes connected to the body surface will inevitably contain

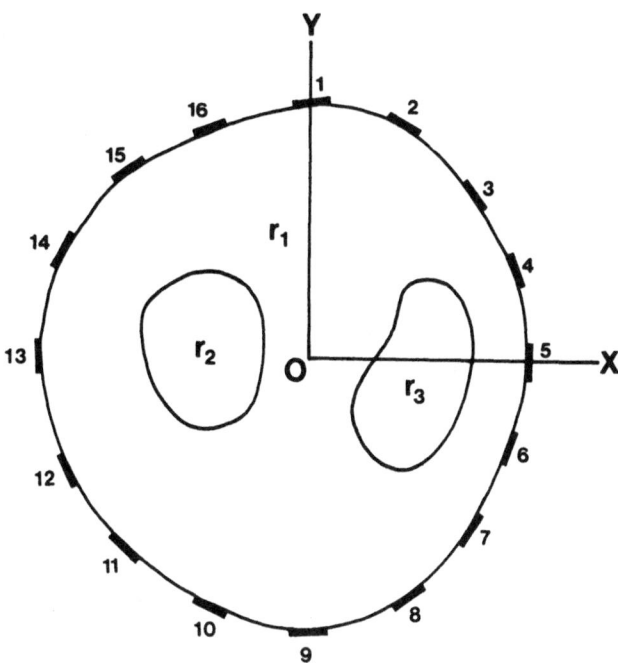

Figure 1. The measurement configuration.

a component of resistance due to the skin contact resistance which
cannot be separated from the required tissue resistance and is at least
of the same order of magnitude as this resistance. This will produce
significant errors and may well make reconstruction impossible.

An alternative approach is to make measurements of the voltage
developed at the other electrodes while current is flowing between a
pair of electrodes, called the drive electrodes in this paper. This
method has the advantage that voltage can be measured without
effectively taking any current so that skin contact resistance is not
important. Measurements may not be reliable at the electrodes through
which current is flowing. A variety of reconstruction algorithms have
been proposed for reconstructions from this data (Yamashita and
Takahashi 1981, Nakayama et al 1981, Sakamoto and Kanai 1983, Seagar
1983, Barber et al 1983a,b) and are described briefly in Barber and
Brown(1984). Only one of these has produced reconstructions from in-
vivo data (Barber et al 1983a,b) and it is the purpose of this paper to
describe in some detail the reconstruction algorithm used. The data is
generated by applying a voltage or potential to the object (and so
causing a current to flow) and the image produced is a tomographic
image, hence the name Applied Potential Tomography has been given to
this method. The term impedance imaging is also found in the
literature. Use of the term impedance implies the presence of a
capacitive component of current flow and there is little evidence of
such a component in tissue at the frequencies (50 kHz) being used
here,except perhaps in lung tissue. •Resistance imaging is probably a

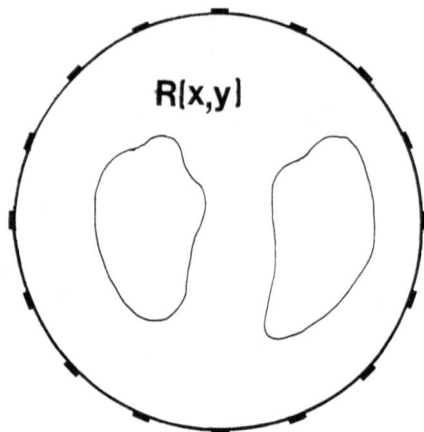

Figure 2.   The idealised measurement configuration.

accurate description.

2.THEORY
2.1 Potential distribution within an isotropic resistive medium.
     The theoretical problem to be dealt with here is the reconstruction
of the resistance distribution within a two dimensional circular region
surrounded by a medium of effectively infinite resistance.   Figure 1 is
therefore idealised to Figure 2 including the addition of equally spaced
electrodes.   Passing current between a pair of the electrodes (a drive
pair) will cause a current to flow within the region.   The distribution
of voltage within the region is given by a solution of the equation

$$c. \nabla^2 V + \nabla c. \nabla V = 0 \qquad (1)$$

consistent with the known boundary conditions, where $c=c(x,y)$ is the
distribution of conductivity within the region.   It is convenient to
replace c by R where $R = -\ln c$ in which case Equation 1 reduces to

$$\nabla^2 V = \nabla R. \nabla V \qquad (2)$$

R is log resistance and this equation suggests that images of log
resistance rather than resistance should be constructed.   If the
resistance is uniform within the region then Equation 2 reduces to
Equation 3, Laplace's equation

$$\nabla^2 V = 0 \qquad (3)$$

For current passing between a particular pair of electrodes the voltage
developed along the boundary of the region depends on the distribution
of resistance within the region.   Measurement of the boundary voltage
profile for current flowing between one pair of electrodes does not
provide sufficient information to uniquely reconstruct the required
distribution of resistance.   However other boundary profiles can be
obtained by passing current between other pairs of electrodes.   The

resulting set of measurements may permit an approximate reconstruction of the required distribution.

Equation 2 represents a non-linear relationship between V and R because of the occurrance of ∇V on the RHS of the equation. Suppose a solution to this equation is given by

$$V = V_p + V_u \qquad (4)$$

where V_u is a solution of Laplace's equation. Then substituting this solution into Equation 2 gives

$$\nabla^2 V_p = \nabla R \cdot \nabla V_p + \nabla R \cdot \nabla V_u \qquad (5)$$

since $\nabla^2 V_u = 0$. If ∇R is small we can assume that $\nabla V_p \ll \nabla V_u$ and write

$$\nabla^2 V_p = \nabla R \cdot \nabla V_u \qquad (6)$$

which is a linear relationship between R and V_p. Now V_u is a function of the applied current pattern i as is V_p so for the i th drive pair

$$\nabla^2 V_p(i) = \nabla R \cdot \nabla V_u(i) \qquad (7)$$

and this represents a set of linear equations relating R to the $V_p(i)$. Reconstructon of R requires the inversion of these equations. This paper will describe a back-projection technique which approximates the required inversion.

2.2 The drive configuration

If N electrodes are connected to the boundary of the object then current can be passed between N(N-1)/2 possible pairs of electrodes and (ignoring the difficulty of measurements at the electrodes through which current is flowing) a set of N-1 independent voltages measured per electrode pair. However only N-1 of these possible drive pairs are independent. Consider the set of measurements obtained by passing current between adjacent pairs of electrodes. Then the measurements which could be obtained by passing current between say electrodes j and k can be obtained by summing together the results from the sets of electrodes (j,j+1) ..... (k-1,k). The measurements from any of the possible drive pairs can be obtained by summation over the measurements from the set of adjacent drive electrodes. Although it is not neccessary to use adjacent drive electrodes there are only N-1 independent drive configurations in the N(N-1)/2 possible drive electrode pairs. There is some evidence (Barber et al 1984) both theoretical and experimental to suggest that the best set of drive electrodes to use is indeed the set of adjacent drive electrodes since this appears to provide the best resolution although not the highest sensitivity. So far absolute sensitivity has not proved to be a problem and the drive electrode set consisting of adjacent drive electrodes has been used in this work. N rather than N-1 drive pairs are used for convenience. Figure 3 shows the drive configuration used.

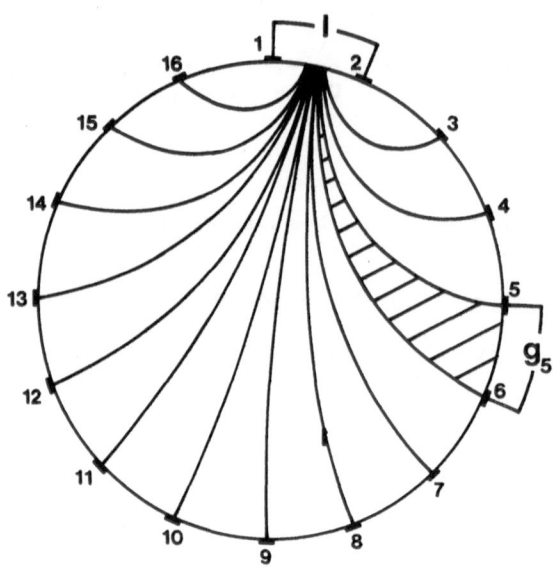

Figure 3. Equipotentials from an adjacent drive configuration.
The shaded area represents the area into which back-projection of
the normalised gradient for electrode pair 5 occurs.

2.3 Back-projection

In practice rather than measuring the voltage at the electrodes it
is more useful to measure the voltage difference between adjacent pairs
of electrodes as an estimate of voltage gradient along the boundary of
the region. Measurement of voltage difference is both practically
easier than absolute measurements of voltage and in addition it is
gradient mesurements which are required by the reconstruction algorithm.
Figure 4 shows a boundary profile of voltage differences (or voltage
gradient) for a 32 electrode configuration. The logarithm of the
gradient rather than the gradient is plotted. Consider a firstly a
boundary profile $g_u(\theta)$ taken from a region of uniform resistance and a
second boundary profile $g_m(\theta)$ taken from a region of the same boundary
shape but with a non-uniform (but isotropic) distribution of resistance
within the region . These profiles will in general differ. In order to
back-project $g_m(\theta)$ we can take the view that a back-projection is the
simplest distribution of the property being measured (in this case
resistance) which can describe the observed measurements. Figure 3
shows the equipotentials for this adjacent pair drive configuration and
the simplest distribution of resistance which can explain for example
that $g_m(5)$ is different from $g_u(5)$ is for the resistance between the
equipotentials ending on electrodes 5 and 6 to be altered in the ratio
$g_m(5)/g_u(5)$ or equivalently the log resistance to be altered to
$\ln(g_m(5))-\ln(g_u(5))$. Summarising this process, a boundary profile
$\ln(g_m/g_u)$ (Figure 5.) is formed and is back-projected along the
equipotentials. The equipotentials shown (Figure 3) are for the uniform
case and it is implicit in this method that because the changes in
resistance are assumed to be small the shape of the equipotentials are

not changed significantly from the uniform case. g_m can be written as

$$g_m = g_p + g_u \tag{8}$$

In this case

$$\ln(g_m/g_u) = \ln(1 + g_p/g_u) \tag{9}$$

and if $g_p \ll g_u$ then

$$\ln(1 + g_p/g_u) \approx g_p/g_u \tag{10}$$

In other words the normalised perturbation of gradient is back-projected to obtain a back-projected image of log resistance.

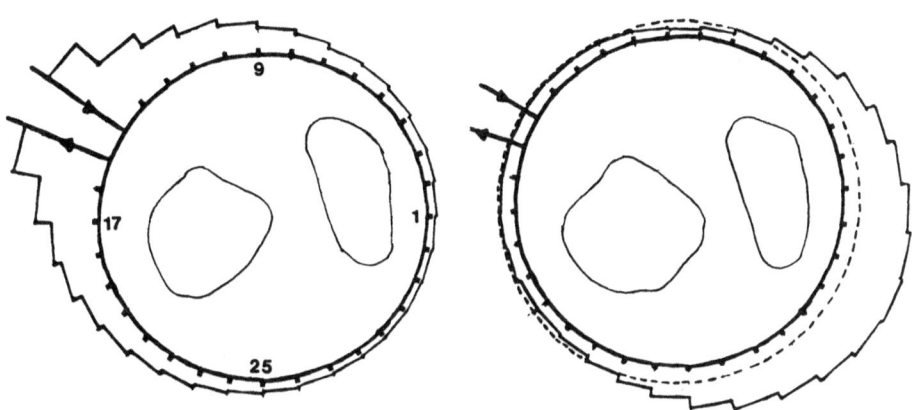

Figure 4. A boundary profile.   Figure 5. A normalised profile.

2.4 Transformation into u,v space and solution of Equation 5.

In order to identify the relationship between the boundary profile and the distribution of resistance within the region the problem needs to be transformed into a more convenient space. It may be easily shown for the circular region of Figure 2 that current flows along circular paths between the electrodes (including along the boundary of the circular region) and that the equipotentials are also arcs of circles. Equipotentials and lines of current flow are of course orthogonal to each other and this problem may be converted to a more convenient rectangular coordinate system using a bipolar transformation (Margenau and Murphy 1964). For ease of theoretical analysis however it is convenient to consider the case where the distance between the electrodes becomes very small. Then the drive pair of electrodes become a current dipole and the appropriate transformation is given by the relationships

$$x = u/(u^2 + v^2)$$

$$y = v/(u^2 + v^2)$$

$$u = x/(x^2 + y^2)$$ (11)

$$v = y/(x^2 + y^2)$$

If

$$ds^2 = dx^2 + dy^2$$

then

$$ds/du = ds/dv = x^2 + y^2 = 1/(u^2 + v^2)$$ (12)

Figure 6 shows x,y space and u,v space for this transformation.

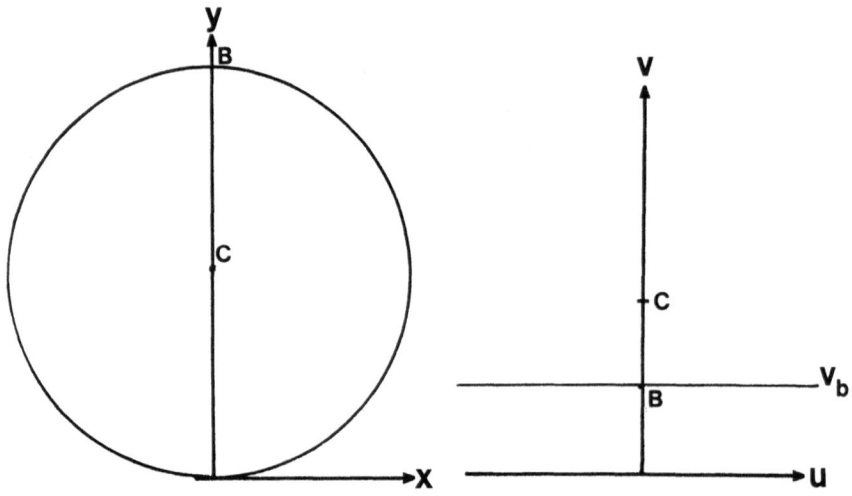

Figure 6. x,y space and u,v space. The points B and C are identified in both spaces. V_b is the boundary of the circular region transformed into u,v space.

Lines of constant u represent equipotentials and lines of constant v represent lines of current flow. The position of the boundary in u,v space is shown and is given by the value $v_b = 0.5$ for a region in x,y space of unit radius. The form of Equation 5 is unchanged by this transformation and may now be rewritten

$$\nabla^2 V_p = E \cdot dR/du$$ (13)

where E= dV/du is now a constant value and dV/dv =0. Equation 6 is much easier to solve in this space. Transforming into frequency space, with frequency variables w_u, w_v and $v_p(w_u,w_v)$ the Fourier transform of V_p, $r(w_u,w_v)$ the Fourier transform of R

$$-(w_u^2 + w_v^2) \cdot v_p(w_u,w_v) = j \cdot E \cdot w_u \cdot r(w_u,w_v) \tag{14}$$

and

$$v_p(w_u,w_v) = -j \cdot r(w_u,w_v) \cdot E \cdot w_u / (w_u^2 + w_v^2) \tag{15}$$

The Fourier transform of the gradient of V in the u direction can be obtained by multiplying both sides of Equation 15 by $j \cdot w_u$

$$j \cdot w_u \cdot v_p(w_u,w_v) = r(w_u,w_v) \cdot E \cdot w_u^2 / (w_u^2 + w_v^2) \tag{16}$$

i.e.

$$g_p(w_u,w_v) = r(w_u,w_v) \cdot E \cdot w_u^2 / (w_u^2 + w_v^2) \tag{17}$$

This gives a simple relationship between the value of the voltage gradient and the distribution of log resistance within the object. Of primary interest is the value of the gradient at the boundary of the object i.e. at $v = v_b$. Assuming the origin in u,v space is shifted to lie on the line $v=v_b$ the F.T. of the boundary gradient is given by

$$b_p(w_u) = E \cdot \int_0^\infty \frac{r(w_u,w_v) \cdot w_u^2 \, dw_v}{w_u^2 + w_v^2} \tag{18}$$

Now consider a point object at depth $q = v-v_b$ in the region. The F.T. of this object is given mirror symmetry about the origin

$$r(w_u,w_v) = \cos(w_v \cdot q) \tag{19}$$

which gives

$$b_p(w_u) = 0.5 \cdot E \cdot |w_u| \cdot \pi \cdot \exp(-q|w_u|) \tag{20}$$

This is the F.T. of the boundary profile produced from a point object a distance q from the boundary. This function can be interpreted in two ways. Firstly the complete Fourier transform of this function is given by

$$G(u) = E \cdot (q^2 - u^2) / ((u^2 + q^2)^2) \tag{21}$$

and this may easily be shown to be the field gradient produced by a small current dipole of strength E at depth q. This is a physical interpretation of Equation 20. An image reconstruction interpretation is as follows. Equation 20 can be divided into two terms. The exponential term can be thought of as a term representing the Fourier transform of a point response function (PRF) measured at the boundary for a point object at depth q. Its transform into real space is

$$s(u) = q/(q^2 + u^2) \qquad (22)$$

which means that the point response is positive and increases in width with depth into the region. The second term is $|w_u|$ which is a ramp filter. These results can be interpreted as meaning that the boundary profile is already ramp filtered i.e. back projection of boundary data can proceed without further ramp filtering. The rather severe depth dependance of the PRF as indicated by Equation 21 suggests that as with gamma camera tomography the solution will only be approximate and will require further processing.

Dividing both sides of Equation 20 by E gives an expression for $G(u)/E$. This is invariant under the transformation of Equations 11 and

$$G(u)/E = g_m(\theta)/g_u(\theta) \qquad (23)$$

Back-projecting $G(u)/E$ in u,v space along the v axis and transforming into x,y space produces the same back-projection as back-projecting $g_m(\theta)/g_u(\theta)$ in x,y space along the equipotentials.

2.5 The weighting function for back-projection.

Back-projection in the present case is back-projection along the equipotentials through the region and these are curved. Associated with each point in the image is a direction of back projection identified as the direction of the appropriate equipotential through this point. There are N back-projections through any point and it is important to appreciate that the angular distribution of these back-projections is not neccessarily uniform. For example since all equipotentials end normal to the boundary, for pixels close to the boundary there will be a marked preference for equipotentials to have a direction close to normal to the boundary. Failure to achieve angular uniformity of back-projection through each image point can produce unacceptable reconstruction artefacts. Approximate uniformity can be achieved by inversely weighting each point on each back-projection according to the local angular density of back-projections associated with that point. The method of calculating the weights is illustrated in Figure 7. For a given drive dipole (O) at angle θ to the reference direction the direction of back-projection through the point P is given by ϕ. The inverse angular density of back-projections through P is therefore given by $d\phi/d\theta$. A somewhat tedious trigonometric calculation shows that this density is given in the coordinate system of Figure 6 by either

$$W(x,y) = 2 \cdot v - 1 \qquad (24)$$

or the equivalent form

$$W(x,y) = (1-r^2)/(x^2 + y^2) \qquad (25)$$

where r is the distance from the centre of the field of view to the point (Figure 7).

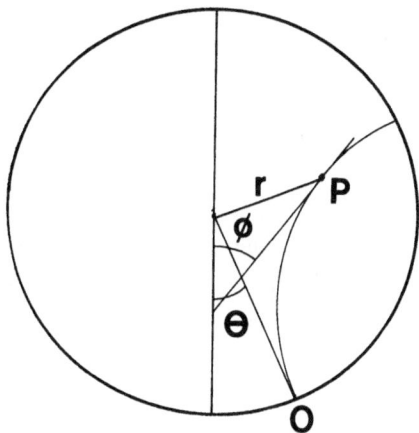

Figure 7. The method of calculating the angular density of projections is to calculate dφ/dθ.

Figure 8 shows theoretical reconstructions of point objects at distance 0.0 and 0.67 from the centre of a circular region of unit radius.

        (a)   (b)

Figure 8. Reconstructions of theoretical point objects at the centre of the field of view (a) and 0.67 from the centre (b). The field of view is of unit radius.

2.6 Image filtering

Because of the severe depth dependence of the PRF given in Equation 22 the images are still very blurred and need to be filtered. The effective overall PRF of the imaging system is seen from the above images to be very position dependent. The width of the back-projection of a point object at depth v at the position of the object is given from Equation 21 as $2 \cdot (v-v_b)$ in u,v space. Width is defined as the zero to zero distance. When transformed into x,y space (using the ds/du relationship of Equation 12) the width becomes

$$H(x,y) = 2 \cdot (v-v_b)/(u^2 + v^2) = (1 - r^2) \qquad (26)$$

where r is defined in Figure 7 and may be taken as a measure of (though not equal to) the resolution at a radius r. An approximate method of converting the filtration problem to a position-independent one is to apply a radial transformation to the image before filtering in order to produce uniform resolution, filter the image with a position independent resolution restoring filter and then apply the inverse transformation to the result. It is easily shown that an approriate transformation is given by

$$d = \tanh(r) \qquad (27)$$

where d is the radial distance in the transformed image and r the radial distance in the original space and an appropriate inverse transformation is given by

$$r = 0.5 \cdot \ln((1+d)/1-d)) \qquad (28)$$

The appropriate filter to use may be obtained empirically from the image of the object at the center of the field of view and Figure 9 shows the theoretical data of Figure 8 processed in this way. This method is not exact and some distortion can still be seen in the image in Figure 9b.

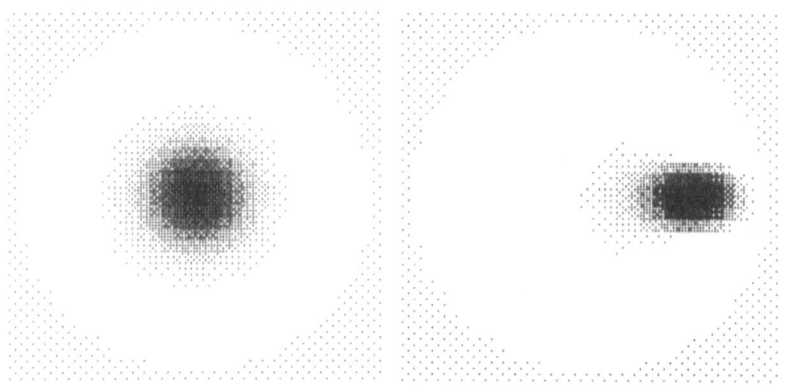

(a)   (b)

Figure 9.   The images of Figure 8 filtered as described in the text.

Figure 10 shows reconstructions of a 1 cm. cylindical perspex object imaged in a shallow dish of saline using a 16 electrode system. Some reconstruction artefacts can be seen in these images principally because the assumption of small changes in resistivity is violated. g_u is measured with the objects removed.

(a)   (b)

Figure 10. Reconstruction of experimental data. The objects are at (a) the centre of the field of view and (b) 5 cm from the centre of the field of view. The dish (field of view) is 15 cm. in diameter.

2.7 Geneneralisation to arbitrary reference distibutions.

Central to this method is the idea that what is back-projected is the ratio of the measured values to the values which would be obtained from the case of uniform resistance. This idea can be generalised to include back-projecting a ratio taken against a non-uniform reference distribution. Consider the solution of the equation

$$\nabla^2 V = \nabla R_r \cdot \nabla V \tag{29}$$

as V_r and the solution of the equation

$$\nabla^2 V = (\nabla R_r + \nabla R_p) \cdot \nabla V \tag{30}$$

as $V = V_r + V_p$. Then

$$\nabla^2 V_p + \nabla^2 V_r = \nabla R_r \cdot \nabla V_p + \nabla R_r \cdot \nabla V_r + \nabla R_p \cdot \nabla V_p + \nabla R_p \cdot \nabla V_r \tag{31}$$

and if the terms in ∇V_p are eliminated as being small compared to the terms in ∇V_r we have

$$\nabla^2 V_p + \nabla^2 V_r = (\nabla R_p + \nabla R_r) \cdot \nabla V_r \tag{32}$$

i.e.

$$\nabla^2 V_p = \nabla R_p \cdot \nabla V_r \tag{33}$$

This is analogous to Eq 6 and given that V_r is known a priori the back projection of $g_m(\theta)/g_r(\theta)$ should proceed along the equipotentials of

118

V_r. In principle it is possible to provide a transformtion which transforms the line of u and v into a rectangular space but this will no longer be as simple as Equations 11.   Nevertheless it may reasonably be assumed, given the generally good performance of the method that acceptable results can be obtained for modest deviations of R_r from uniformity.   Figure 11a shows the image of a fairly large perspex object and Figure 11b the image of an additional small object reconstructed with the data from the previous object as the reference.   Note that in this case back projection was still along the equipotentials for the uniform case.   Some distortion is present in the image of Figure   11b but this represents a fairly extreme case.   An important problem with resistance imaging is incomplete knowledge of the geometry of the object boundary or what is effectively the same incomplete knowledge of the uniform gradients .   However if the only interest is in changes in resistance then a measurement taken before changes occur can be used as the reference.   Exact knowledge of the measurement geometry is not neccessary for useful images to be produced.

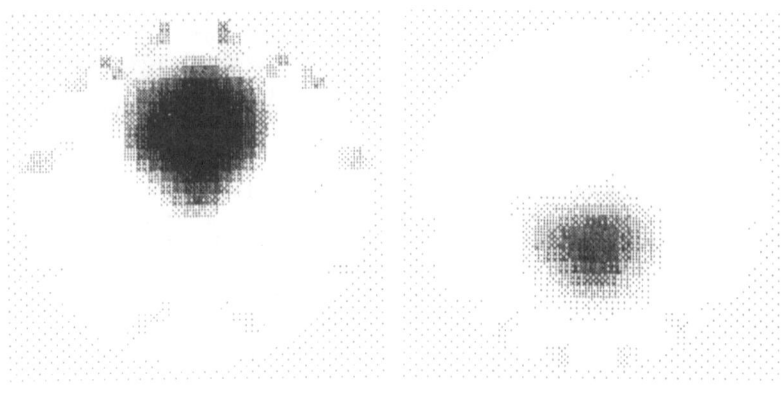

(a)   (b)

Figure 11.   (a) is the image of a 3 cm. perspex object and (b) the image of an additional 1 cm. perspex object using the data from (a) as the reference.   Note that the peak amplitude of the object in (a) is 9 times greater than that in (b).

Most applications will require the imaging of three dimensional objects.   Assuming that electrodes can be placed on the boundary of an object so that they define a plane, the two dimensional algorithm appears to give quite acceptable reconstructions. Figure 12 shows an image of a plastic rod imaged in a hemispherical bowl of saline with a 16 electrode system.   The geometric position of the object is retained quite well and suggests that acceptable results can be obtained from three dimensional objects.

3. IN-VIVO DATA

Figure 13a shows an image produced from a ring of electrodes placed around the chest of a normal volunteer.   The reference data were collected during expiration and the actual image is the difference between inspiration and expiration. The lungs are well visualised. Figure 13b shows an image from a patient which shows decreased resistance changes in the right lung consistent with known fluid in the lung.

Figure 12. The image of a 1 cm. diameter, 5 cm. long perspex object imaged in an approximately hemispherical tank of radius 30 cm. The reconstruction used the two dimensional algorithm.

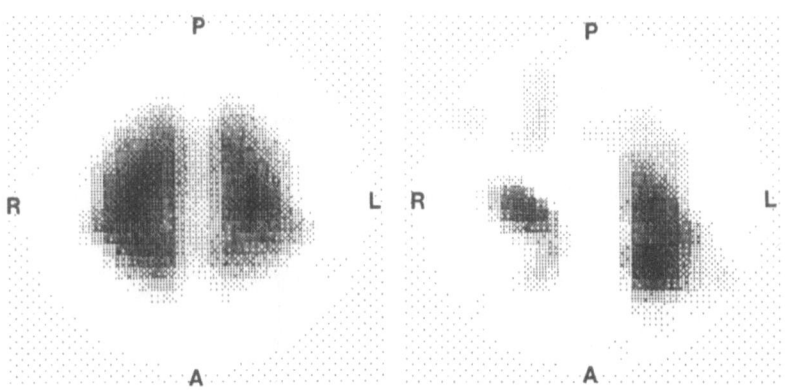

          (a)   (b)
Figure 13. An image (a) showing the difference in resistance between inspiration and expriation in a normal volunteer and an image (b) showing the lungs of a patient with known fluid in the right lung.

Figure 14 shows images reconstructed from data taken from 16 electrodes

·placed around the abdomen at a point midpoint between the navel and the left nipple. A reference frame was collected and then a series of 30 second images taken after the subject had drunk 300 ml. of tap water. The subsequent images show emptying of this meal and subsequent studies of a similar nature have shown excellent correlation between gamma camera gastric emptying data and resistance data. The 30 second collection time was chosen to reduce breathing artefacts.

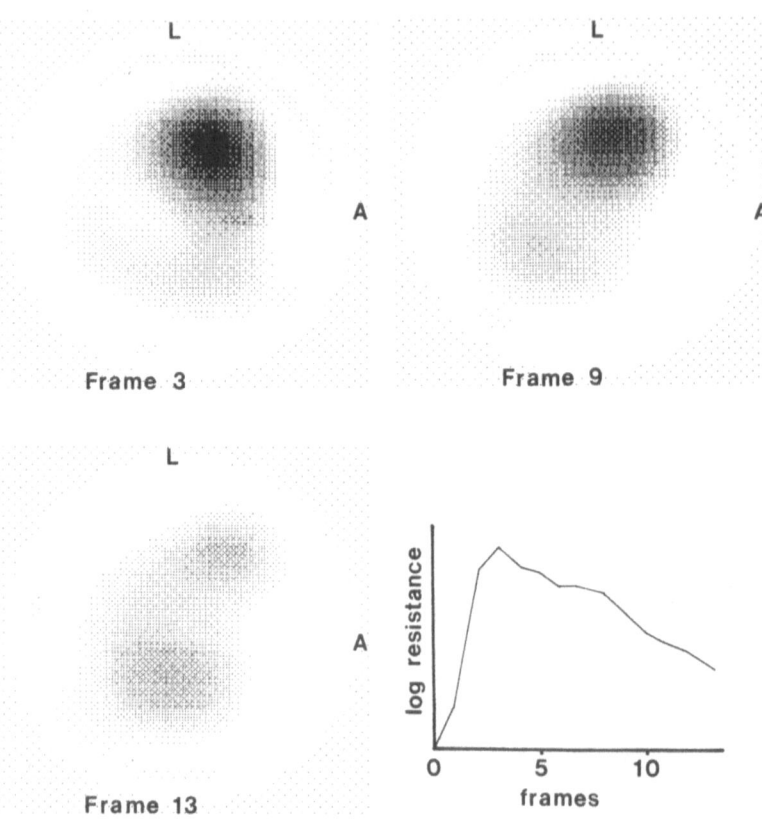

Figure 14. Three images taken from a sequence of images of the emptying of a liquid meal from the stomach. The emptying curve extracted from the complete sequence of images is shown.

4.DISCUSSION AND CONCLUSION

This work has concentrated on the use of a fairly simple algorithm for several reasons. It is unlikely that resolutions comparable with other imaging procedures will be obtainable with resistance imaging in the immediate future and it is best at this stage to concentrate on the current advantages of the system such as simplicity and speed. Using the method described above for imaging resistance changes it has proved possible to reconstruct images from a 16 electrode system in 20-30 seconds using an 8086 system (with 8087 coprocessor) which is certainly fast enough for the applications described here. Data collection is actually much faster than this (0.1 seconds) so we can collect data at a much higher speed. Using a relatively inexpensive computer system the hardware cost for a 16 electrode system cam be kept to less than $5000 which compares very favourably with other imaging systems. Improved image quality will probably require iterative solutions involving some sort of solution to Equation 6 plus knowledge of the object boundary plus some correction for the third dimension. It is planned to explore these and other possibilities in the future.

REFERENCES

Barber DC and Brown BH: Applied Potential Tomography. J. Phys. E:Sci. Instrum., 17, pp723-733, 1984.

Barber DC, Brown BH and Freeston IL: Experimental results of electrical impedance imaging. Proc VIth Int. Conf. Electrical Bioimpedance (ICEBI),Zadar, Yugoslavia pp1-5, 1983a.

Barber DC, Brown BH and Freeston IL: Imaging spatial distributions of resitivity using applied potential tomography. Electron. Lett. 19 pp933-935, 1983b.

Barber DC, Brown BH and Freeston IL: Imaging spatial distributions of resitivity using applied potential tomography-APT. Information processing in medical imaging. Martinus Nijhoff, 1984.

Dines KA and Lytle RJ: Analysis of electrical conductivity imaging. Geophys. 46 pp1025-1036, 1981.

Kim Y, Webster JG and Tompkins WJ: Electrical impedance imaging of the thorax. J. Microwave Power 18 pp 245-257, 1981.

Margenau H and Murphy GM: The Mathematics of Physics and Chemistry. Van Nostrand, pp187-190, 1964.

Nakayama K, Yagi W and Yagi S: Fundamental study on electrical impedance CT algorithm utilising sensitivity theorem on impedance plethysmography. Proc. Vth Int. Conf. Electrical Bioimpedance (ICEBI), Tokyo, pp99-102, 1981

Sakamoto K and Kanai H: A fundamental study of an electrical impedance CT algorithm. Proc. VIth Int. Conf. Elecrical Bioimpedance (ICEBI), Zadar, Yugoslavia pp349-352, 1983

Schomberg H and Tasto M: Reconstruction of spatial resistivity distributions from resistance projections. Philips, gmbH, Hamburg, MS-H, Report 2715/81, 1981.

Seagar AD: Probing with low frequency electric currents. Phd Thesis University of Canterbury, Christchurch, NZ. 1983.

Yamashita Y and Takahashi T: Methosd and feasibility of estimating impedance distributions in the human torso. Proc. VIth Int. Conf. Electrical Bioimpedance (ICEBI), Tokyo, pp87-90, 1981.

THE DESIGN AND PERFORMANCE OF A DIGITAL IONOGRAPHIC IMAGING SYSTEM

B. M.MOORES, R. BOOLER, T. DOVAS.

1. INTRODUCTION

The development and practical application of image processing procedures is a major undertaking [Andrews (1978)], and medical imaging is one of the more useful applications. Initially most effort in the field of information processing for medical imaging was applied to nuclear medicine [Lasher et al (1983)] and computed tomography [Herman (1982)].

The evolution of digital fluorography, emission tomography and magnetic resonance has opened up new avenues. More recently attempts are being made to develop processing techniques for conventional radiography [Kalender et al (1984),Cocklin and Lams (1984)].

If we assume that information processing has an important role to play in the field of medical imaging then we will need to consider its impact. In order to do this there are three factors to consider:-

i. What effect information processing has on the diagnosis and subsequent management of the patient;

ii. The prognosis for the patient following diagnosis and treatment.

iii. The number of patients involved.

The first two factors will need a great deal of investigation before definitive answers emerge. The third can, however, already be assessed. Table 1 presents the projected number of medical imaging procedures for the year 1980 in the United Sates [Johnson and Abernathy (1983)].

TABLE 1. Projected number of radiological procedures in the United States 1980

Procedure	Total Number
Plain film radiography	140,300,000
Contrast studies	22,900,000
Ultrasound	7,300,000
Nuclear Medicine	5,800,000
Computed tomography	3,300,000
Special vascular procedures	1,000,000
Diagnostic cardiac catheterization	500,000

In terms of the volume of medical imaging information, processing is at present only applied to minority modalities. This is dictated by the fact that nuclear medicine, computed tomography and digital fluorography are digitally compatible, the most frequently performed examination; plain film radiography, is not. Until a digitally compatible radiographic transducer becomes routinely available, the widespread application of information processing techniques will not be applied to the most frequent type of examinations.

A number of digitally compatible radiographic transducers are already under consideration and/or development [Smathers and Brody (1985)]. The number of different techniques receiving consideration indicates the considerable interest being shown. The advantages and disadvantages of each approach in terms of cost, dose efficiency and image quality will be an area for ongoing research over a number of years.

The method or methods which ultimately provide the future requirements for digitally compatible radiographic transducers will need to possess the right combination of cost, dose efficiency and image quality if it is to compete with the existing film based systems.

In this paper we wish to outline some of the main design aspects and initial performance capability of a digital ionographic imaging system. This technique offers a wide variety of design options and we will attempt to highlight the interplay which exists between them.

2. DIGITAL IONOGRAPHY

The main component of the digital ionographic imaging system are:-

i. An ionography chamber for the production of a latent electrostatic image.

ii. An image reading mechanism

iii. A means of storing and displaying the digital image.

2.1. The ionography chamber

The latent electrostatic image is produced by an ionographic technique similar to that described previously [Moores et al (1980)]. The chamber has a circular cross section of 55 cm diameter and spherical geometry with concentric electrodes centred on the X-ray focal spot. The lower electrode is made of aluminium and has a radius of curvature of 200 cms. The upper electrode is a thin deposit of aluminium located on the upper surface of the 100 μm thick insulating plastic sheet (Mylar) used to collect the ions. The upper electrode is formed to the correct curvature by means of a fibre glass top plate. Freon 13B1 is employed in the chamber as the X-ray absorbing medium.

In order to collect the ions liberated by X-ray absorption in the gas a voltage of 80 kV is applied to the lower electrode of the chamber. To ensure that each equipotential plane between the two electrodes is concentric about the X-ray focus and resolution is maintained at the edges of the chamber, guard rings are incorporated in the walls of the chamber. The correct voltage is applied to each guard ring by means of a voltage divider network.

The upper electrode is maintained at earth potential and the remainder of the chamber is enclosed in a stainless steel earth can. To maintain adequate resolution the chamber must be aligned with respect to the X-ray focal spot (see section 3.2). Although Freon 13B1 gas is relatively inexpensive the sizeable volume of the chamber indicates the desirablity of employing a gas recycling mechanism. The simple mechanism employed ensures rapid filling and emptying of the chamber whilst ensuring gas loss in less than 5 per cent. The foil is inserted and removed from the chamber with air at atmospheric pressure inside the chamber.

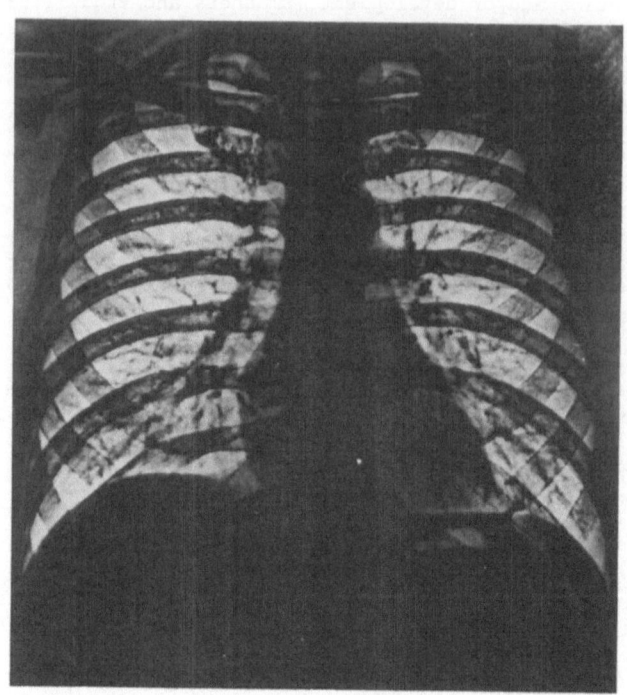

FIGURE 1. A powder cloud developed ionographic image of a chest

The performance of the ionography chamber is demonstrated in Figure 1 which shows a powder cloud developed image of a chest. The patient entrance dose employed was 500 μSv.

2.2 Image reading mechanism

The plastic foil containing the latent electrostatic image is mounted on a flat surface and scanned by means of guarded electrometers.
In a laboratory prototype unit two electrometers were employed [Moores et al (1985)] and a maximum field coverage of 12 x 12 cm^2. In the clinical prototype unit four electrometers are at present employed with a maximum field coverage of approximately 38 x 38 cm^2. The number of electrometers can easily be increased to a maximum number governed by the packing density of the supporting electronics.

The carriage assembly containing the electrometers is driven by a variable speed motor operating under microprocessor control. A stepping motor, also under microprocessor control, moves the carriage sideways at the end of each linear traverse. Carriage movements of a fraction of a milli-metre can easily be reproduced. A graticule positioned at the side of the carriage provides reference pulses for the control unit.

Stretching the foil during the reading process ensure that the separat-ion between the foil and the electrometers can be accurately maintained.

The signal detected by each electrometer is fed into a high impedance unity gain amplifier followed by further amplification stages. Signals from all of the heads are then multiplexed prior to A/D conversion.

2.3 Storage and display
Signals from the A/D converter are fed into a 1600 x 1200 display memory with 10 bit planes. Images stored in memory can be displayed at 30 frames/ sec on a wide band TV monitor capable of displaying 1600 x 1200 pixels. An example of the display capability of the system is shown in Figure 3 where an original 256 x 256 pixel image of a hand has been reproduced 30 times. Window width and height facility are employed to interrogate the full grey scale of the image data.

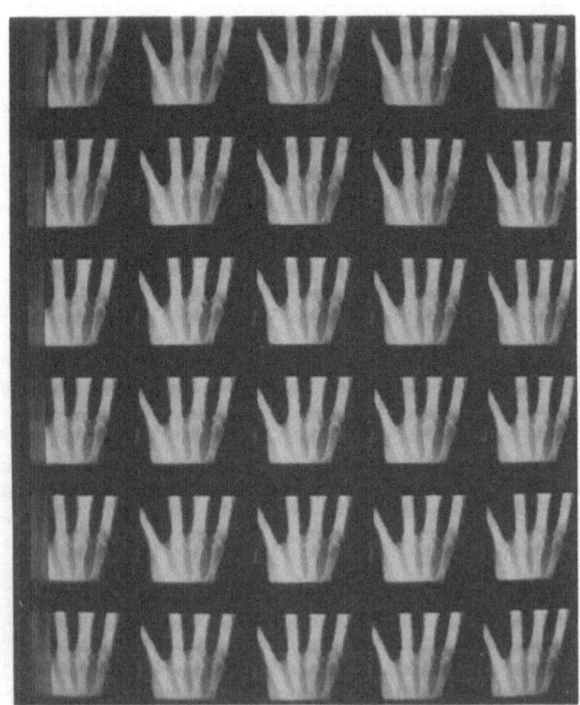

FIGURE 2. A 256 x 256 image display reproduced on a 1600 x 1200 pixel display unit

Images can be stored on Winchester disk for short term data processing requirements and full 10 bit data integrity is maintained. Image data can be offloaded onto magnetic tape for long term archival.

3. PHYSICAL PERFORAMNCE OF THE SYSTEM
Important measures of physical performance of any X-ray imaging system

are sensitivity, resolution, noise, signal-to-noise and.or contrast capability. The overall performance of a digital ionography system in terms of any of these parameters depends upon the performance of each of the main components, i.e the ionography chamber, the reading system and storage/display unit.

3.1 Sensitivity

The sensitivity of the ionographic process in producing the latent electrostatic image depends upon (i) the gas employed, (ii) gas pressure, (iii) gas thickness, (iv) voltage applied to the chamber ((v) insulating foil thickness and its permittivity, (vi) incident X-ray beam quality. The sensitivity in terms of patient dose also depends upon the thickness and composition of the front face of the chamber.

The sensitivity of the ionography process has been assessed for a number of gases, pressure-thickness values and incident X-ray spectra [Fenster et al (1974), Boag et al (1976)]. For instance with Freon 13B1 at 10 atm-cms and 65 kV_p incident X-ray beam, absorption of over 40 per cent should result. A high proportion of the energy absorbed will contribute to the final image. With the chamber employed in this work ionographic images of a chest and chest phantom have been produced at the same exposure as that required for a medium speed screen/film combination [see Figure 1 and Booler et al (1985)].

The sensitivity of the image reading process depends upon (i) electrometer probe diameter, (ii) probe-foil separation, (iii) probe and input impedance of the amplifier stages, (iv) subsequent electronic gain (v) sampling rate.

The probe and input impedance of the amplifier stages also plays an important part in determining the electronic noise. Sensivity of the image reading process is more correctly assessed in terms of the signal-to-noise ratio. It has been shown that for a probe-foil gap of 100 μm, foil thickness of 100 μm and 75 μm diameter probe,signals in the region of 1 mV can be generated at the input to the amplifiers for exposure levels in the region of 0.25 Ckg^{-1} (1 mR).

The display also affects sensitivity both directly and indirectly. The gain or brightness and contrast settings of any video display will affect visual perceptability of the final image. Also, contrast transfer can be improved by manipulating the image data in order to produce optimum display [Ishida et al (1984)]. The same contrast can, therefore, be detected at a lower exposure. It seems unlikely that manipulation of the display characteristics will be employed to reduce patient exposure directly but more likely to enhance diagnosis. This ability to separate the image forming and display aspects of radiographic images, which is not possible with film, will be one of the potential benefits of digital radiography.

Sensitivity, which is more usefully determined by design considerations at the ionographic and image reading stages is directly related to resolution.

3.2 Resolution

Resolution also depends upon the design of each component in the overall system. The most important is the ionography system since it determines the "baseline" resolution of the latent electrostatic image. The variation in resolution with gas and gas pressure has been investigated for a variety of incident X-ray beam qualities [Fenster et al (1974)]. More recently the resolution limits of low gas pressure ionography chambers has been investigated [Booler and Moores (1985)]. For low pressure chambers there are three main aspects to consider:-

i. The tolerances on centering a deep chamber, possessing spherical geometry, to the X-ray focal spot.

  ii. The ranges of the photoelectrons liberated in the gas
 iii. The effect of ante charge collection on the plastic foil.

The tolerances imposed by employing spherical chamber geometry has been investigated [Seelentag and Boag (1979)]. The most critical tolerances are the lateral displacement and the angle of tilt of the chamber away from the central radius joining focal spot and chamber centre. Since these two are related a single phantom can be used to correct for both simultaneously [Booler and Moores (1985)]. This phantom enables the chamber to be aligned to within the tolerances imposed by the X-ray source.

The effect of photoelection range upon ionographic resolution has been calculated using the continus slowing down approximation (CSDA) [Johns et al (1974)]. The additional effect of elastic scattering was recently considered in the design of a septaless high pressure Xenon detector for use in scan projection radiography [Rutt et al (1983)]. This work has been extended to include low pressure (1-2 atmospheres) ionography chambers employing Freon 13B1 as the absorbing gas [Booler and Moores (1985)]. The line spread functions and corresponding modulation transfer function calculated for Freon 13B1 gas at 1-2 atmospheres gas pressure and 65 kVp X-ray beam incident is shown in Figure 3A and B respectively.

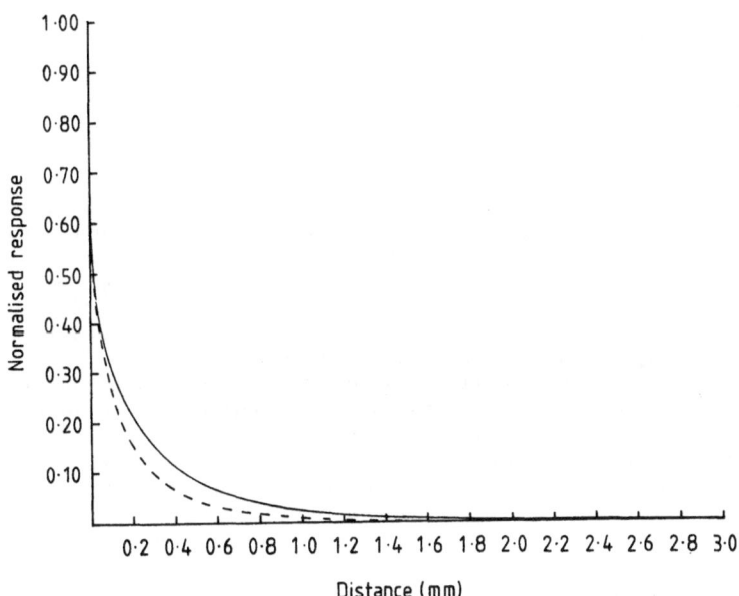

FIGURE 3A. Calculated line spread function for Freon 13B1 gas and 65 kVp
X-ray beam. 1 atmosphere ——— , 2 atmospheres - - - -

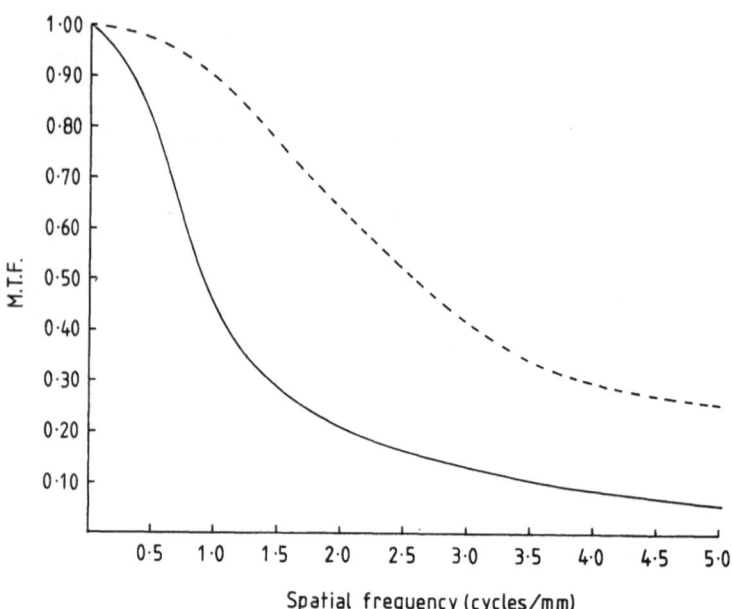

FIGURE 3B. MTF's corresponding to the linespread function shown in 3A.
1 atmosphere ————, 2 atmospheres - - - -.

This work indicates that even at atmospheric gas pressure and diagnostic X-ray beam qualities there is significant contrast transfer in the region of 3 lp/mm and this has been verified experimentally [Booler and Moores (1985)]. Increasing the gas pressure to only 2 atmospheres improves resolution markedly. Incidently,increasing the gas pressure also increases sensitivity and unlike many other X-ray imaging systems both resolution and sensitivity may be improved simulataneously.

The effect of ante charge collection, whereby charge which has already been collected on the foil influences the subsequent charge collection has been noted [Booler and Moores (1985)]. This is not a major factor at charge densities normally employed but it would need to be considered if attempts were made to collect very high charge densities corresponding to high X-ray exposures. There are techniques for charge collection which may reduce this effect even at high collected charge densities.

The reading system forms the link between the latent image and its display. The probe diameter, foil-probe separation, sampling rate, amplifier bandwidth and scanning speed all affect the resolution of this component. Probe apertures and foil-probe separations which can comfortably accommodate the resolution limits set by the ionography chamber, at least at low gas pressures, can be achieved [Moores et al (1985)].

In order to employ image reading times which compete favourably with film processing times sampling rates and amplifier bandwidths in the khz/sec range are required. AT the other end of the scale, large format X-ray images of sufficient resolution require high resolution VDU's and hence wide bandwidth video amplifiers [Moores (1984)]. A display monitor with bandwidth in the region of 100 MHz is employed on the present system. This permits a 1600 x 1200 pixel display capability which even for large format images provides adequate display resolution.

3.3 Noise

Noise, signal-to-noise and contrast detectability are all related and play an important role in defining the performance of X-ray imaging systems. The aim in designing any X-ray imaging system is to try and ensure that quantum noise due to the finite number of X-ray photons employed is the predominant noise process. This means that system noise should be as low as is reasonably achievable. The main system noise processes in a digital ionographic unit are electronic/amplifier noise, mechanical vibration, other electrical pickup and non-uniformities in the foil.

Electronic noise is dictated mainly by the input impedance at the first stage. Measurements undertaken on a laboratory prototype unit [Moores et al (1985)] indicate that noise levels in the region of 20 mV can easily be achieved for signal levels of 1 volt. Hence signal-to-noise ratios of 50 can be produced which compare favourably with values noted for screen/film combinations under similar sampling aperture conditions [Shaw and Moores (1985)]. Recent threshold contrast-detail measurements undertaken on this system clearly indicate that other electronic pickup, namely the motor driving the carriage, was the major source of noise. The large field system employs a much higher quality motor and measurements indicate that improved signal-to-noise is achievable. When all other noise sources are reduced to a sufficiently low level the variation in the foil remain. Contrast detail measurements indicate that existing foil technology is adequate, given the signal-to-noise ratios already achievable.

4. IMAGE PROCESSING

Digital imaging technique will play an increasingly important role in medical imaging. The single most important impact will be the widespread application of information technology but the potential for improved diagnosis through a more detailed interrogation of imaging data cannot be ignored.

Data processing techniques have been applied to existing digitally compatible imaging modalities. These examinations are not the most frequently undertaken. They also tend to provide structurally simple images. For instance a CT examination provides information over a wide contrast range but each slice only corresponds to information originating from a few millimeters of tissue thickness. It is perhaps no accident, therefore, that attempts are now being made to interrogate multiple slice images in three dimensions in order to increase the data base presented to the eye for diagnosis.

The majority of medical imaging examinations involve plain film and a high proportion of them are chest examinations. These provide valuable information concerning a wide variety of clinical conditions. Studies on visual search patterns of chest images indicate that radiologists may read the image in an optimum way in relation to the occurrence of abnormalities [Kundel (1974)]. However it has been shown that a high proportion of abnormalities are missed [Herman and Hessel (1975)]. Also that there is no apparent relationship between length of training and accuracy of detection and a strong correlation between the number of abnormalities or complexity of an image and inaccuracy. Obviously information processing of routine radiographs could enhance the presentation of relevant detail and improve diagnosis.

A great deal of semi quantitative information is already extracted from plain film images and physiological as well as pathological information can be derived [Trapnell (1982)]. The facility to enhance the radiologists' interpretative capability with the quantitative data already available on the radiographic image would hopefully extend this facility.

Whilst film is employed as the imaging medium the widespread application of data processing to radiographic images will not be feasible within existing budgetary constraints. Even if it did prove cost effective to digitze film, it is not the ideal detector. Its non-linear response means that data has already been processed before digitization. Also signal-to-noise transfer of film is only optimum at a particular level of exposure, it decreases rapidly above and below this value. The first requirement for the widespread application of information processing to radiography is the development of a digitally compatible transducer which ideally has a linear response over a suitable dynamic range.

Given the development of such a transducer there are three possible stages of processing which can be applied to digital radiographs [Moores et al (1985)].

i. Stage 1 processing involves manipulation of the raw data in order to produce the best possible data base. For instance in digital ionography the ability to correct signals originating from different eletrometers is an example. This would enable the tolerances on the manufacture of multiple electrometers to be relaxed whilst ensuring a uniform intensity across an image.

ii. Stage 2 processing involve the manipulation of the data to produce an image which is deemed better or enhanced in some way. Gamma correction, edge enhancement and smoothing are examples. Most effort to date has been applied to this form of processing of digital radiographs [Cocklin et al (1983)].

iii. Stage 3 processing corresponds to image analysis techniques which attempt to measure quantities associated with an image or even interpret the data directly. Data compression techniques fall into this category since an understanding of the image data base is required to ensure that following compression an image can be reproduced to within some acceptable level of "quality".

Examples of all of these stages as applied to a digital ionographic image is shown in Figure 4. Here an original 256 x 256 pixel image of a hand has undergone some preliminary processing and has then been enlarged four times to provide easier visualization. A line profile at any level horizontally or vertically in the image can be displayed in graphical form and provide the basis for quantitation.

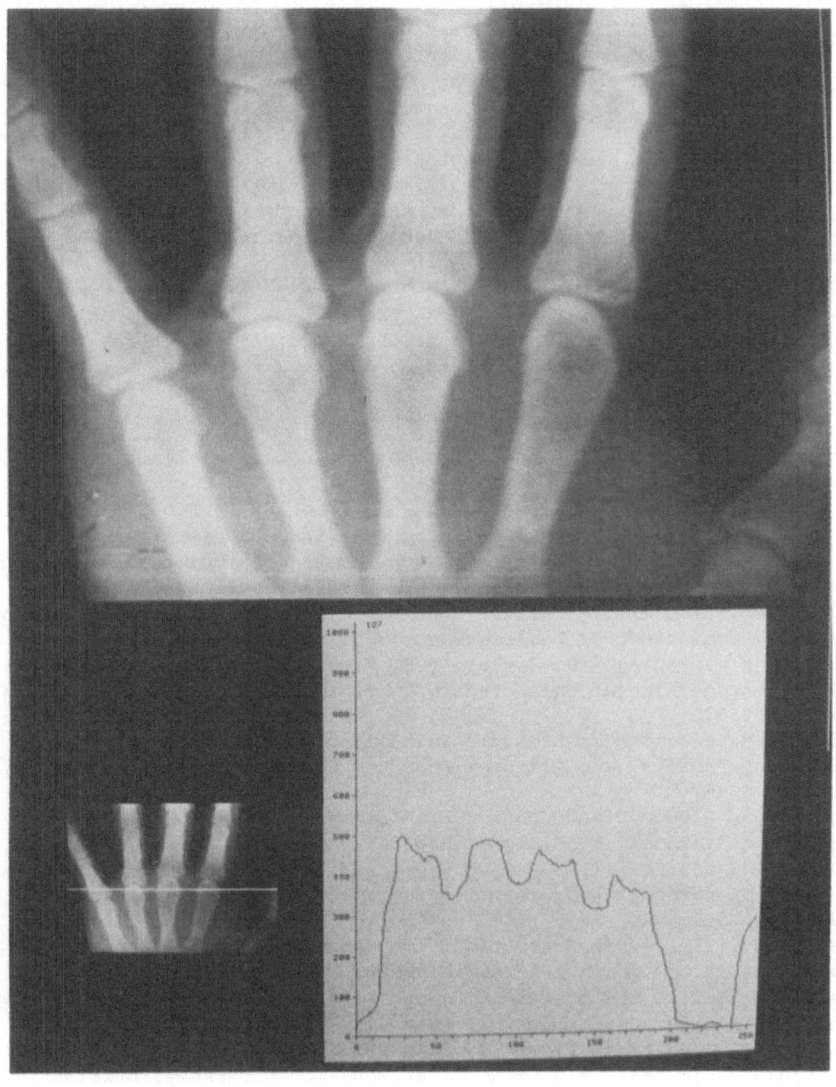

FIGURE 4. An original 256 x 256 pixel image (bottom left) enlarged four
times and a line profile displayed graphically.

132

5. SUMMARY AND CONCLUSION

The design and performance of a digital ionographic imaging system has been described. The main components of the system, namely (i) an ionographic chamber, (ii) a scanning electrode assembly, (iii) a storage and display unit are described. The interplay between the design of each and their effect of system performance in terms of sensitivity, resolution, noise, and signal-to-noise has been highlighted.

The role that data processing can play has been described. The development of useful processing techniques will form the basis of future work with the system as will the further development of the technology. Results to date indicate that digital ionography will be able to complete with screen/film combinations in terms of imaging performance. The technology is also compatible with the radiographic environment and given developments in certain areas it could enhance existing work practices.

ACKNOWLEDGEMENTS

This work was undertaken with funds provided by the North West Regional Health Authority and the Medical Research Council. The authors are grateful for the technical assistance provided by Messrs J Narcott and A Platt.

REFERENCES

1. Andrews H C: Tutorial and selected papers in digital image processing. IEEE Computer Society, New York, 1978
2. Boag J W, Barish R J and Seelentag W W: Ionography, Proceedings of the L H Gray Conference. John Wiley and Sons Ltd, Chichester, 1976.
3. Booler R V and Moores B M: Resolution limits of a low pressure ionography chamber. To be published in Physics in Medicine and Biology, 1985.
4. Booler R V, Moores B M, Asbury D L: Large area ionography - preliminary results. Submitted for publication, 1985.
5. Cocklin M L, Goulay A R, Jackson P H, Kaye G, Kerr I H, and Lams P: Digital processing of chest radiographs. Image and Vision. Computing 1, 67-78, 1983.
6. Cocklin M L, Lams P M: Digital radiology of the chest in Digital Radiology Physical and Clinical Aspects. Hospital Physicists' Association London, 1984.
7. Fenster A, Plewes D and Johns H E: Efficiency and resolution of ionography in diagnostic radiology. Medical Physics, 1, 1-10, 1974.
8. Herman P G and Hessell S J: Accuracy and its relationship to experience in the interpretation of chest radiographs. Investigative Radiology, 10, 62-67, 1975.
9. Herman G T: Image reconstruction from projections, the fundamentals of computerized tomography. Acadmeic Press, New York 1980.
10. Ishida M, Doi K, Loo L, Metz C E, and Lehr J L: Digital Image Processing: contrast radiographic patterns. Radiology, 150, 569-575, 1984.
11. Johns H E, Fenster A, Plewes D, Boag J W and Jeffrey P N: Gas ionization methods of electrostatic image formation in radiography. British Journal of Radiology, 47, 519-529, 1974.
12. Johnson J L, Abernathy D L: Diagnostic imaging procedure volume in the United States. Radiology, 146, 851-853, 1983.
13. Kalender W A, Hubener K H, and Jass W: Digital scanned projection radiography, optimization of image characteristics, Radiology, 149, 299-303, 1983.
14. Kundel H L: Visual sampling and estimates of the location of information on chest films. Investigative Radiology, 9, 87-93, 1984.

15. Lasher J C, Blumhardt R and Lancaster J L: The digital computer: the role of functional imaging in radiology. Radiology, 153, 69-72, 1984. Society of Photo Optical and Instrumentation Engineers, Vol 314 Digital radiography, 1981

16. Moores B M, Ramsden J A and Asbury D L: An atmospheric pressure iono- graphy system suitable for mammography. Physics in Medicine and Biology, 25, 893-902, 1980.

17. Moores B M: Physical aspects of digital fluorography, in Digital Radio- logy Physical and Clinical Aspects. Hospital Physicists' Association, London, 1984.

18. Moores B M, Dovas T, Pullan B and Booler R: A prototype digital iono- graphic imaging system. Physics in Medicine and Biology, 30, 11-20,1985.

19. Moores B M, Booler R V, Dovas T and Asbury D L: Production and pro- cessing of digital ionographic X-ray images. British Journal of Radio- logy, 57, 1157-1160, 1985.

20. Rutt B K, Drost D J, and Fenster A: A xenon ionization detector for scanned projection radiography: Theoretical considerations. Medical Physics, 10, 284-292, 1983.

21. Seelentag W W and Boag J W: Prototype ionographic imaging chamber. Acta Radiol Diagn, 20, 537-550, 1979.

22. Shaw A and Moores B M: Noise transfer in screen-film subtraction radiography. Physics in Medicine and Biology, 30, 229-238, 1985.

23. Smathers R L and Brody W R: Digital radiography: current and future trends. British Journal of Radiology, 58, 285-307, 1985.

24. Trapnell D H: Chest radiology - guesswork or science. British Journal of Radiology, 55, 93-107, 1982

APPLICATION OF INFORMATION PROCESSING TECHNIQUES TO OPHTHALMIC IMAGING

R.W. ROWE[*], S. PACKER[*], M. HALIOUA[†], AND H.C. LIU[†]
[*]North Shore University Hospital/Cornell University, Manhasset, NY 11030
[†]New York Institute of Technology, Center for Optics, Lasers and
Holography and NYCOM, Old Westbury, NY 11568

ABSTRACT
   A digital fundus imaging system, based on a conventional fundus camera,
and employing a charge-coupled device array is presented. The processing
steps required to convert images formed from monochromatic light reflected
from the back of the eye into quantitative maps of spectral reflectance
are discussed. Three examples of the potential of spectral reflectance
images to characterize patho-physiological processes are examined in the
context of the early diagnosis of diabetic retinopathy, choroidal
melanoma, and glaucoma respectively. Preliminary studies on the utility
of shape analysis by invariant moments for characterization of the optic
nerve in glaucoma, and texture analysis by the spatial gray-level dependency method for characterization of pigmented lesions are described.
Finally, a new and simple technique for measurement of three-dimensional
optic nerve topography is presented which promises to be much more
accurate than existing photogrammetric or optical sectioning methods.
Results of this technique on larger objects than the eye are shown and an
error analysis for the optic nerve is derived.

1. INTRODUCTION
   The human visual apparatus is perhaps the most sophisticated and
efficient information processing system known. From a physical point of
view, the process of vision is one of transduction of light energy into
electro-chemical form by a series of complex, well-regulated mechanisms
for which specialized cells, tissues, and anatomical structures exist in
the eye and brain. The anterior structures of the eye constitute an
optical system which forms images on the retina, a photo-chemical sensor
whose output is a coded, multi-channel train of electrical signals.
Multiplexing and transmission of these signals is carried out over the
neural pathways to the brain, which is the central processor responsible
for the extraction and interpretation of attributes of the recorded image
information. Disruption of the flow of information at any stage in this
extended chain of processes results in impairment or loss of vision.
Figure 1 charts in schematic form some of the better known visual
disorders and diseases in relationship to the steps in the visual process
and the associated anatomy and physiology.
   In general, the most serious ocular diseases affect the sensory and
transmission mechanisms which involve structures in the fundus or
posterior region of the eye. Non-invasive visualization of these
structures is of key importance in the diagnosis of such diseases, thus
fundus imaging systems of one kind or another form a large part of the
ophthalmologists armamentarium of diagnostic tools. In all of these
devices a fairly intense source of light is formed into an aerial image in

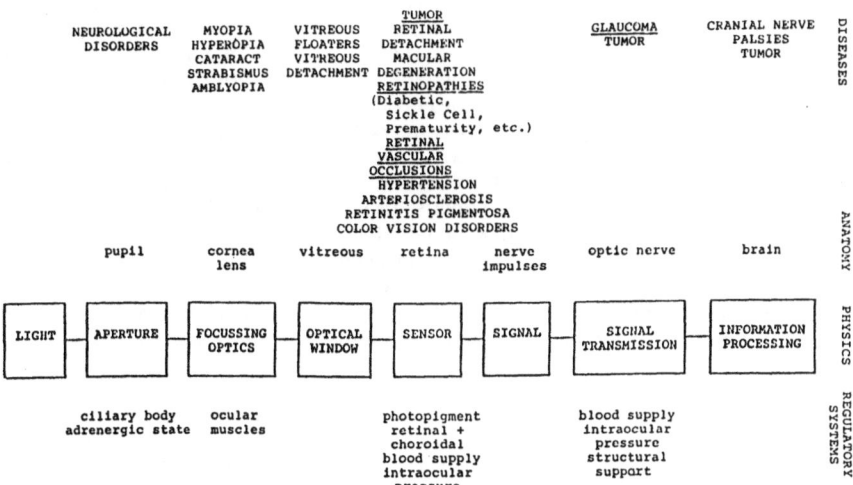

FIGURE 1. Schematic of the visual process in terms of its physics, anatomy, and pathophysiology

front of the eye where it is viewed by the observer or relayed onto photographic film. Not only do such systems permit examination of the state of health of the retina, choroid, optic nerve head and their respective blood supplies but the retinal circulation is the only part of the systemic vasculature available to direct view and can yield information on systemic diseases such as diabetes and hypertension.

Until recently, photographic film was the only means of recording fundus images. This allowed qualitative assessment of the size and shape of structures, their anatomic location, their color and the documentation of changes over time in any of these features. Vascular dynamics could be studied by rapid sequential photography of the dispersion of intravenously injected, fluorescent dye through the retinal and choroidal vascular beds (1). However, as in other imaging specialties, it has become apparent that in many cases accurate diagnosis depends on, or is aided by, the quantitative measurement of the amount of light reflected from the posterior structures of the eye and the extraction of quantitative measures from such reflectance maps. Although quantitative light measurement can be performed by densitometry of photographic film, the limited dynamic range and the difficulty of controlling and calibrating the development process does not make the photographic method readily amenable to routine clinical use. However, with the recent introduction of high resolution solid state imaging sensors, and the availability of low cost, powerful computing resources, the routine acquisition of quantitative, digital, image maps of fundus reflectance has become a reality.

Conventional fundus photography is performed in polychromatic, white, or red-free light. Since the depth of penetration of light is strongly dependent on wavelength, structures at a range of depths are imaged by such photographs. For example, blue light does not penetrate beyond the nerve fiber layer which lies above the retina, whereas green wavelengths penetrate into the retinal cells. Longer, red wavelengths reach the pigment epithelium and superficial choroid, posterior to the retina, while in the near infrared increasing wavelengths penetrate to increasing depths in the choroid and sclera. Monochromatic images therefore provide a means of isolating information from distinct anatomic planes in the back of the eye. Furthermore, there is selective absorption of certain wavelengths by different structures according to their chemical composition and structural state as evidenced by the different color of ocular structures when viewed in while light. Thus examination of spectral reflectance characteristics also provides a means of studying ocular physiology.

This paper describes a digital fundus imaging system based on a charge-coupled device (CCD) array which we have developed around a conventional fundus camera. The processing steps required to obtain quantitative spectral reflectance images are described together with new applications on information processing techniques to the diagnosis of three major ocular diseases; glaucoma, diabetic retinopathy, and choroidal melanoma.

2. THE IMAGING SYSTEM

Images of the back of the eye are formed by a conventional fundus camera (Topcon TRC-WT) shown schematically in figure 2. A tungsten filament lamp housed in the instrument provides continuous, variable intensity low-level illumination for viewing and patient positioning. Sufficient illumination for a photographic image is provided by a short, bright flash of light from a xenon arc which can be set to one of eight intensity levels.

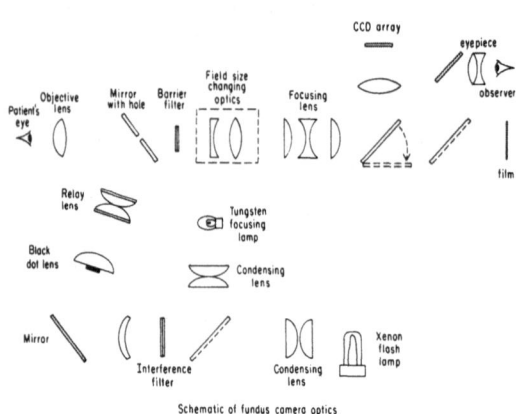

Schematic of fundus camera optics

FIGURE 2. Schematic diagram of fundus camera optics

Monochromatic light is achieved by placing a narrow band interference filter in the illumination path. A fiber optic light guide has been mounted in the fundus camera to transmit a small, fixed fraction of the filtered illuminating beam onto a calibrated photodiode energy meter in order to monitor variations in intensity. The optics in the illuminating path produces an annulus of light at the corneal surface, which, after passage through the cornea, dilated pupillary aperture, lens and vitreous, illuminates a circular region of the retinal surface. Reflected light

returning from the retina and choroid forms an aerial image which is mag-
nified and focused onto the film plane of a camera and through an eyepiece
for immediate viewing by the photographer. The angular subtense of the
field of view at the retina is selectable between 20, 30, and 45 degrees.
A further modification to the device allows the image to be deflected
along an extension tube where it is minified optically and focused onto
the surface of a 320x244 element CCD array (Hitachi KP-120). The video
output from the CCD can be viewed on a TV monitor (see figure 3) and is
digitized at a rate of 30 frames per second by a frame grabber (Colorado
Video 274C). Any chosen frame can be held in the framestore memory by
ceasing further digitization. An electronic synchronization circuit has
been constructed to ensure that digitization begins before the flash of
light from the xenon arc is triggered, and that the frame during which the
flash occured is stored. The grabbed frame is transferred to a

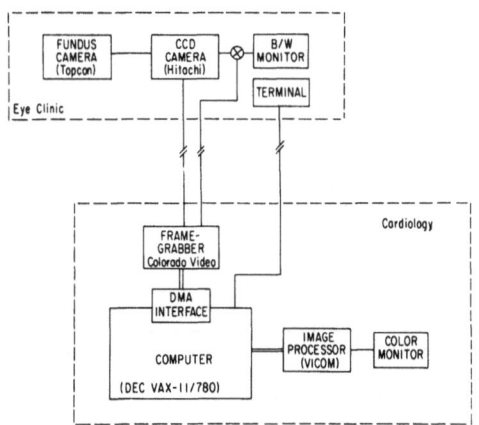

FIGURE 3. Block diagram of digital eye camera system

VAX-11/780 computer in the Cardiology Department via a parallel direct
memory access interface (DEC DR-11W) and stored on disk as a 256x256
matrix. This transfer takes about a second. Image restoration, processing and analysis tasks are performed using a specially designed, menu-
driven program package written in FORTRAN. A log is kept of every function invoked together with any numeric parameters of that operation. This
record of operations may be displayed at any point during the processing
session to keep track of operational steps, and output as hard copy at the
end of the session for permanent reference. The images are displayed through the framestore memory on a black and white monitor or can be transferred to a VICOM image processor in the Cardiology Department for more
sophisticated display options using graphics or pseudocolor.

3. SPECTRAL REFLECTANCE MEASUREMENT

The reflectance $r(x,y,z,t,\lambda)$ at any point (x,y,z) in the fundus at time t, and for wavelength λ may be written as

$$r(x,y,z,t,\lambda) = I_r(x,y,z,t,\lambda)/I_i(x,y,z,t,\lambda) \qquad \dots (1)$$

where $I_r(x,y,z,t,\lambda)$ is the intensity of light of wavelength reflected from point (x,y,z) at an instant in time t, and $I_i(x,y,z,t,\lambda)$ is the incident amount of light at that point and time. Clearly, measurements of the intensities I_i and I_r inside the eye cannot be obtained. Externally to the eye, the filtered light source emits an intensity distribution $I_s(x,y,t,\lambda)$ which is modified by the illumination optics and then again by passage through the eye to the retina. If the transmission functions of the illumination optics and eye are $t_{io}(x',y',\lambda)$ and $t_{ie}(s,y,z,\lambda)$, assumed to be independent of time, then

$$I_i(x,y,z,\lambda) = I_s(x',y',t,\lambda) \cdot t_{io}(x',y',\lambda) \cdot t_{ie}(x,y,z,\lambda) \qquad \dots (2)$$

Similarly,

$$I_d(x'',y'',z',t,\lambda) = I_r(x,y,z,\lambda) \cdot t_{re}(x,y,z,\lambda) \cdot t_{ro}(x'',y'',\lambda) \cdot s_d(x'',y'',\lambda) \qquad \dots (3)$$

describes the intensity function measured by the external detector array, with sensitivity function $s_d(x'',y'',\lambda)$, of the passage of the reflected light from the retina through the eye, with transmission function $t_{re}(x,y,z,\lambda)$, and the image forming optics of the fundus camera described by $t_{ro}(x'',y'',\lambda)$. In other words,

$$r(x,y,z,t,\lambda) = \frac{I_d(x'',y'',z,t,\lambda)}{I_s(x',y',t,\lambda)} \cdot \frac{1}{t_{io}(x',y',\lambda)t_{ie}(x,y,z,\lambda)t_{re}(x,y,z,\lambda)t_{ro}(x'',y'',\lambda)s_d(x'',y'',\lambda)} \qquad \dots (4)$$

Now suppose the retina could be replaced by a constant, uniformly reflecting surface of reflectance $\rho(z,\lambda)$. In the absence of any change in the fundus camera optics or ocular transmission, the detected light distribution would be, from (4),

$$I_{dp}(x'',y'',z,t,\lambda) = \rho(z,\lambda) \cdot I_s(x',y',t',\lambda) \cdot t_{io} \cdot t_{ie} \cdot t_{re} \cdot t_{ro} \cdot s_d \qquad \dots (5)$$

In practice, an estimate of I_{dp} is obtained by imaging an optical model eye whose retina is a uniformly reflecting surface of barium sulfate (Eastman White Coating). The resulting non-uniform image is a combined measure of the non-uniformity of illumination, the non-uniformity of transmission of the fundus camera optics, and the spatial variation of sensitivity of the detector array. Since the variation of the spatial distribution of the source intensity with time is small in comparison to the variation with time in total output (which is typically several percent), $I_s(x,y,t,\lambda)$ may be considered to be $I_s(t,\lambda)$. Then,

$$r(x,y,z,t,\lambda) = \rho(z,\lambda) \cdot \frac{I_d(x'',y'',z,t,\lambda)}{I_d(x'',y'',z,t',\lambda)} \cdot \frac{I_s(t',\lambda)}{I_s(t,\lambda)} \qquad \dots (6)$$

gives the retinal reflectance in terms of known and measured quantities. The measurements $I_s(t,\lambda)$ and $I_s(t',\lambda)$ are obtained from the calibrated photodiode energy meter. This method cannot take into account the variation in optical properties from eye to eye, nor any changes in time within a given eye such as changes in refractive state, chromatic changes of the lens with age, or development of cataracts. It should however permit the measurement of the relative spectral reflectance of different regions of the fundus. Simultaneous measurement of I_d and I_{dp} would be possible with a second detector array, cross calibrated against the first, and a replacement of the mirror next to the fundus camera objective by a beamsplitter which would send part of the illuminating beam into the model eye. Since the amount of light reaching the retina from the surface of the eye is largely determined by the area of the pupillary aperture, it is necessary to measure the pupil diameter and use a similarly sized pupil in the model eye. The linearity of the detector array is calibrated in a separate experiment which need be performed relatively infrequently.

CCD cameras have many advantages over other photo-sensors for this kind of quantitative imaging (2). They are an order of magnitude more sensitive than Vidicons or photomultiplier tubes throughout the visible region of the spectrum, and additionally respond into the near infrared out to about 1100nm. This near infrared sensitivity is of particular importance for ophthalmic imaging since it permits visualization of choroidal features which are invisible to the eye, and would require infrared film together with much higher light levels to be imaged photographically. The spectral response of CCDs is also much flatter than that of other detectors, varying by less than 50% over the wavelength range 400 to 1000nm. These spectral characteristics, together with the good linearity and high dynamic range (typically $\geqslant$ 1000:1) of CCDs make them ideally suited to multispectral imaging. In contrast to tube-based video cameras, they suffer minimal geometric distortion which eliminates the need for distortion correction for quantitative applications. As a part of a clinical instrument their small size, ruggedness, and operation at room temperature are also ideal features. Although the spatial resolution does not approach that of film, with the highest optical magnification of the fundus camera each detector element corresponds to 26nm on the retina, which is sufficient to resolve small blood vessels (though not the capillary bed) and adequate for the majority of applications. With higher resolution arrays becoming increasingly available, the spatial resolution will soon be acceptable for routine fluorescein angiography.

In order to compare the reflectance of small regions of the retina and choroid at different wavelengths and construct spectral signatures, it is necessary to register the monochromatic images to a common co-ordinate system since neither the eye nor the camera field of view remains in precisely the same orientation from frame to frame even though a fixation device is used to direct the eye's gaze to the same point in space. Provided fixation is maintained fairly well, the relationship between the coordinates of any pair of images can be considered to be related by a two-dimensional linear transformation

$$x' = \alpha + \lambda(x\cos\theta + y\sin\theta)$$
$$y' = \beta + \mu(-x\sin\theta + y\cos\theta) \qquad \ldots\ldots (7)$$

In other words, there may have been a translation in the x or y direction of α or β pixels respectively, a rotation through an angle θ, or a change of scale λ,μ respectively of the orthogonal axes between one image and the next. The five unknown parameters α,β,λ,μ and θ can be computed according to equation (7) from the respective co-ordinates of three fiducial points corresponding to common landmarks in each of the images. Easily identifiable landmarks are branchings of major blood vessels, or the intersections of blood vessels with other structures such as the optic nerve, which are marked interactively using a cursor. Since the features imaged change significantly with increasing wavelength, it is important that any image be registered with the one closest to it in wavelength in order to locate the fiducial points with the greatest accuracy, rather than registering all images to a single reference image.

4. APPLICATIONS

4.1. Spectral reflectance signatures

Light absorption spectrometry of in-vitro samples of biological materials is a standard laboratory technique for studying properties such as structural state or chemical composition. For example, measurement of the oxygen saturation of whole blood is based on the differential light absorption between oxygenated and reduced hemoglobin (3,4) which also gives rise to the observed difference in color between arterial and venous blood. At certain wavelengths, known as isobestic points, the absorption of hemoglobin is independent of its oxygen saturation and depends only on the total amount of hemoglobin present, whereas at any other wavelength the absorption is dependent on both the total amount of hemoglobin and the relative concentrations of the reduced and oxygenated forms of the pigment. A simple algebraic equation can therefore be solved to yield a linear relationship between the oxygen saturation and the ratio of the logarithms of the transmittances at the two wavelengths, one of which is an isobestic and the other being a wavelength where there is a marked difference in the absorption coefficients of reduced and oxygenated hemoglobin. This principle has been applied in-vivo in many branches of medicine including surgery (5), cardiology (6,7), pediatrics (8) and burns treatment (9).

In the eye, the retinal neurons depend for their survival on a carefully controlled environment together with a continuous supply of oxygen and nutrients derived from blood vessels in the retina itself and from the underlying, highly vascular choroid. Any interruption of the blood supply to the retina which prevents the retina from receiving sufficient oxygen, causes irreversible damage, leading ultimately to blindness. There are many diseases which compromise retinal oxygenation, the most serious of which is diabetic retinopathy, a frequent complication of long-standing diabetes and the leading cause of new blindness in adults of any age. A number of physiological factors combine in diabetes to result in retinal tissue hypoxia. However there is no evidence of this hypoxia until it has existed for some 15-20 years, after which secondary effects such as venous dilation, regions of capillary non-perfusion, existence of micro-aneurysms and neovascularization can be observed in fundus photographs and fluorescein angiograms. What is required is a non-invasive method of measuring retinal tissue oxygenation which could detect the earliest signs of diabetic retinopathy when it might still be possible to alter the outcome of the disease. Since oxygen diffuses into the retina from blood in the capillaries in the retina and choroid, measurement of capillary oxygen saturation by reflection oximetry could provide a means of monitoring retinal oxygenation. It is known that late in the disease, capillary perfusion of small regions of the retina ceases. However, in early diabetes, the retinal hypoxia is due to increased intravascular oxygen caused by an increased affinity of hemoglobin for oxygen, a reluctance of the hemoglobin to release its oxygen, and impaired diffusion from the capillary bed. Whether this can be detected by spectral reflectance, remains to be seen.

The reflection of light from blood in the eye follows an inverse relationship to the absorption, though scattering may cause shifts in the isobestic wavelengths. Monochromatic fundus images (10,11) such as those shown in figure 4 demonstrate changes in the relative reflectance of arteries and veins from wavelength to wavelength. Early attempts at fundus reflectance oximetry (12,13), using the isobestic in the blue (515nm) and a second wavelength in the green, were able to follow changes in retinal artery oxygenation in rabbit eyes but did not have much success in humans largely because the strong absorption of the short wavelengths by the ocular media and blood prevented sufficient light from returning to the sensor. Below 600nm, there are several sharp peaks and valleys in the absorption spectra which mean that a high degree of monochromaticity must be achieved for which the band-pass filters of the early studies were not adequate. Furthermore, the absorption of oxygenated and reduced hemoglobin differs by no more than a factor of four in the low wavelength region of the spectrum, so that considerable precision in measurement is required. Greater success has been achieved by using summed measurements from a scanned detector at the 569nm and 585nm isobestics and a contrast wavelength of 559nm (14). Beyond 600nm, there is a much greater separation of the reduced and oxygenated absorption curves and generally a slower change with wavelength which continues for over 100nm until finally the curves cross again at about 810nm. Not only is there greater reflectance at these wavelengths, but Rayleigh scattering from structures smaller than the wavelength is much reduced. The CCD detector has high sensitivity in this region of the spectrum and an illuminating bandwidth of 20-30nm is easily tolerated. However, beyond 700nm the reflected light is predominantly from the choroid rather than from the more superficial retina, thus the physically more suitable, longer wavelengths cannot be used for retinal oximetry. In general the two wavelengths should be as close as possible so that information from the same depth is being recorded. Although individual capillaries cannot be resolved from our system, the average reflectance from a region of the capillary bed is measurable and should be related to oxygenation inbetween blood vessel branches. The distribution of capillaries is essentially constant, and their wall thickness is the same on the arterial and venous sides. By contrast, retinal arteries and veins have significantly different wall thicknesses and flow patterns which lead to differences in reflectance between them, and along the length of a single vessel, making quantitatively accurate measurements difficult.

Another application of in-vivo blood oximetry measurements in the eye is to the diagnosis of glaucoma. Glaucoma is a disease arising from an inbalance between the rate of production of aqueous humor by the ciliary body and the rate of outflow from the anterior chamber, mostly because of an obstruction to fluid outflow. The result is an increase in intraocular pressure which causes irreversible atrophy of the optic nerve and corresponding loss of vision, leading ultimately to blindness. While there is considerable controversy over what the mechanisms are which relate poorly tolerated, or elevated intraocular pressure to the end point of destruction of the optic nerve (15,16,17), there is growing evidence that there is

142

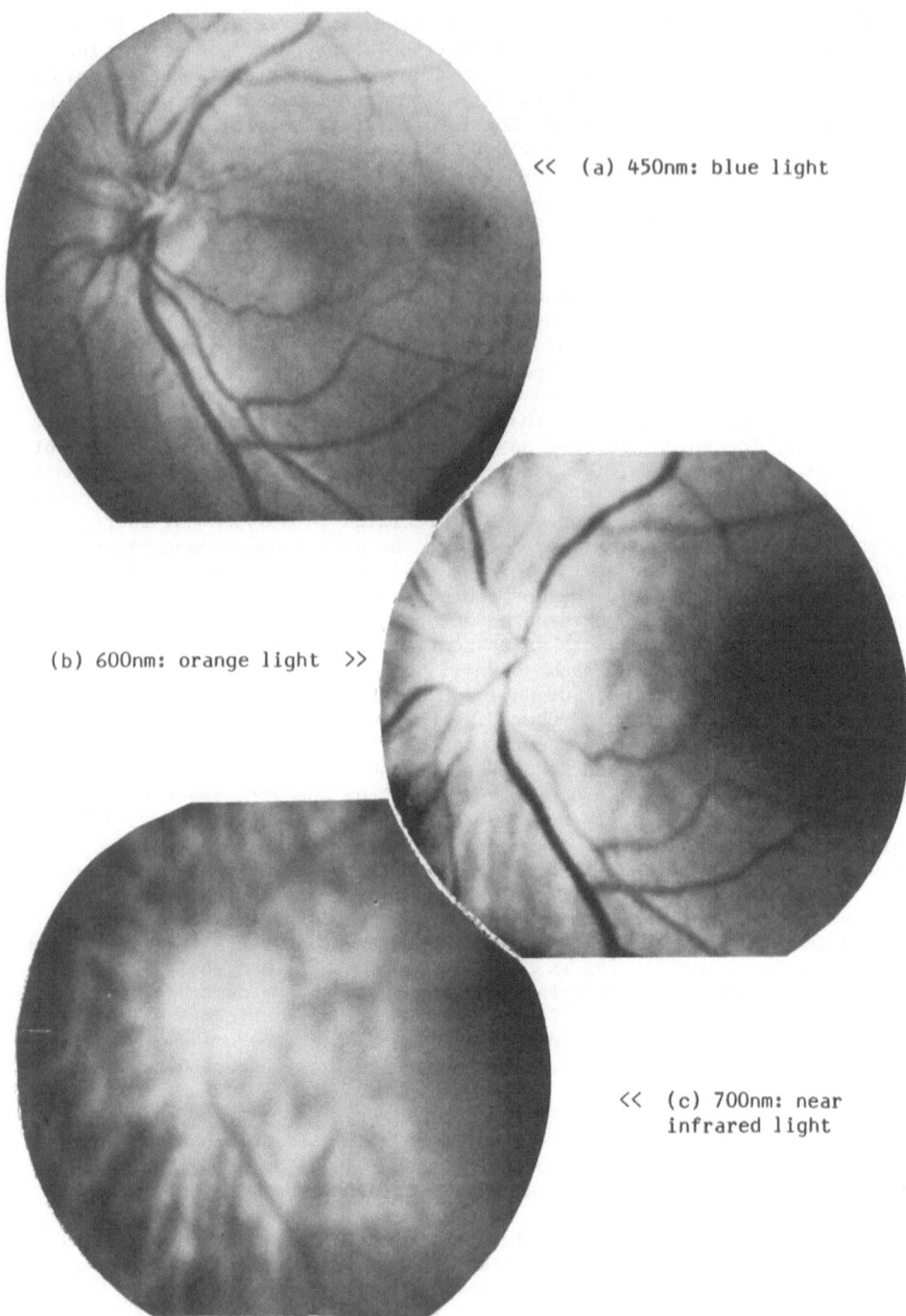

<< (a) 450nm: blue light

(b) 600nm: orange light >>

<< (c) 700nm: near
infrared light

FIGURE 4. Monochromatic spectral reflectance fundus images

that there is ischemia in the optic nerve head itself and possibly in the choroidal blood supply to the optic nerve. Fluorescein angiography shows decreased fluorescence of the optic nerve in glaucoma, and in fundus photographs there is a characteristic pallor or whitening of the optic disk which correlates well with visual field changes (18). Densitometric measurement from film of the relative amounts of red and green light reflected from regions of the optic nerve has been proposed as a means of quantifying the color changes which give rise to the observation of pallor (19). Broad wavlength bands were used in the red and green regions of the spectrum which correspond to sections of the hemoglobin absorption spectrum where there is separation of the oxygenated and reduced curves. In green light, oxygenated hemoglobin absorbs more strongly than reduced hemoglobin whereas red light is absorbed more by the de-oxygenated pigment. Thus reduced oxygenation should give rise to a decrease in the red-green reflectance ratio as observed in glaucoma. With our fundus imaging system, the use of narrow band interference filters, a sensitive, linear detector, and digital reflectance images should permit more accurate characterization of the spectral reflectance changes which signal the onset of optic nerve damage. Furthermore, the ability to measure choroidal reflectance as shown in figure 4(c) may help elucidate the role of the choroidal vasculature in glaucoma.

Spectral reflectance is also of interest for the diagnosis of malignant neoplasms of the eye. Choroidal melanoma, although a relatively rare lesion, is particularly malignant and since its ophthalmoscopic appearance in the early stages is not different from that of benign nevi, its diagnosis presents a difficult clinical problem. Usually diagnosis is not possible until the tumor has grown significantly, causing other complications such as retinal detachment, and is frequently after metastasis has begun. In the wavelength range 8 to 16 mico-meters there are differences in the absorption of infrared radiation between nevi and melanomas which are believed to be related to different concentrations of nucleic acids in the two tumors (20,21). It has further been demonstrated (22) that in the wavelength range 900-1000nm there are quantitative differences in light absorption between benign nevi and malignant melanomas which are indicative of tumor growth and may also signal malignant changes. Structural changes in certain proteins have been proposed to explain this phenomenon. In this near infrared region of the spectrum, the sensitivity of the CCD detector is well suited to the study of the spectral characteristics of pigmented lesions of the fundus. Studies are underway to examine whether spectral reflectance signatures can be identified which reliably characterize malignancy. Certainly near infrared photography with infrared film leads to excellent definition of pigmented lesions bacause of the strong absorption by melanin (23,24,25,26). This has been used to facilitate the detection of the first signs of growth of pigmented lesions which may signal malignancy, and to monitor the effect of radiotherapeutic treatments which provide less radical alternatives to enucleation.

4.2. Texture Analysis

Another potential discriminator between benign pigmented lesions of the choroid and malignant melanomas is the texture of the light intensity distribution reflected from the tumor. For example, when a melanoma grows it increases not only in area but also extends in height in a dome shape which pushes up onto the overlying retina, whereas nevi remain flat and contained in the choroid. Ultimately the upward expansion of the melanoma will cause retinal detachment which is easily observed funduscopically. Earlier in the process, fundus photographs show changes in the texture of the tumor reflectance such as a lightening in central regions, increased smoothness of the peripheral regions, and a general loss of uniformity. Differences in pigment distribution between lesions would also give rise to textural differences in the images. Such textural differences are mirrored in the spatial frequency domain by the distribution of the power spectrum (27,28). Coarse texture gives rise to high power at low spatial frequencies while fine texture contributes more to high spatial frequencies. Directional biases and periodicity in the spatial distribution result in anisotropicity in the spatial frequency domain and high density at certain frequencies respectively. However a number of algorithms operating in the spatial domain have been more successful in characterizing texture than Fourier analysis (29).

In particular, analysis of the spatial dependencies of gray levels has been fruitful. Within a chosen region the probability of a transition between gray level a and gray level b between any pair of pixels separated by a distance d in a direction θ is given by

$$p(a,b,d,\theta) = \frac{n[g_{ij} = a, \; g_{i'j'} = b]}{N} \qquad \ldots\ldots (8)$$

where n is the number of occurrences of gray level pairs (a,b) at pixel locations (i,j) and (i'j'), N is the total number of pixel pairs considered, and

$$\theta = \arctan[(j' - j)/(i' - i)$$
$$d = [(i' - i)^2 + (j' - j)^2]^{1/2} \qquad \ldots\ldots (9)$$

the set of probabilities $[p(d,\theta)]$ for all possible gray level pairings results in an NxN array known as the gray-level co-occurrence matrix which contains important texture context information. To infer visual qualities of patterns, it is generally necessary to use more than one d,θ combination and the discriminatory power of the co-occurrence matrices increases as more d,θ values are used. Five measures of texture are typically derived from each co-occurrence matrix: energy; entropy, which is a measure of homogeneity; correlation, which is a measure of gray-level local homogeneity and inertia. However, it has been shown (30) that these measures do not gauge all the important textural information contained in the co-occurrence matrices since visually distinct texture patterns can be generated which yield different co-occurrence matrices but for which the texture measures are not different. A new set of measures has therefore been proposed which better correspond to visual quality (30). We have found display of the co-occurrence matrices as images to be useful in detecting differences between the co-occurrence probabilities for different images and propose to study whether measures of changes in, and attributes of, co-occurrence matrices can be used to differentiate between benign and malignant pigmented tumors of the choroid.

4.3. Shape description

In both the diagnosis of melanoma and glaucoma, fundus photography is used to detect changes in the spatial patterns of reflected light intensity due to pathology. As well as pallor of the optic disc, glaucoma results in progressive reflectance changes of the central, most highly

reflecting area of the optic nerve known as the cup. The normal physiological cup is a small, circularly symmetric depression of the optic nerve
backwards from the retina which results in a bright, white, circular area
at the center of the disc whose diameter is usually less than half that of
the disc. With the loss of nerve fibers and the supporting glial cells
due to increased intraocular pressure, there is enlargement, preferent-
ially in the vertical direction, and backward extension of the cup giving
rise to a larger diameter, more elliptical region of high reflectance.
The deepening of the cup is also evidenced by a change in direction of the
retinal blood vessels as they pass over, and disappear into the cup, and a
nasal displacement of the vessels. While, with training, the eye and
brain are sensitive to such alterations in the spatial distribution of
light intensity, no quantitative measures result. On the otherhand there
are mathematical descriptors of two-dimensional distributions which are
appropriate for the analysis of fundus reflectance images and particularly
quantitative spectral reflectance maps. Analysis of the gray-level histograms of the optic nerve area has been performed on digitized fundus
photographs (31) which reduces the information processing to one dimension
but also destroys the information on the spatial relationship of the
imaged intensities.

Any two dimensional distribution $f(x,y)$ has an infinite set of moments
defined as

$$M_{pq} = \int_{-\infty}^{\infty}\int_{-\infty}^{\infty} x^p y^q f(x,y)dxdy \quad ; \quad p,q=0,1,2,\ldots \qquad \ldots\ldots (10)$$

which is uniquely determined by that distribution. Thus two different
intensity distributions will result in two different sets of moments which
could in principle be used as descriptors. Moments of different orders
characterize various visual attributes of the distribution. For example,
the zero order moment M_{00} gives the total 'mass' or intensity of the
distribution while the second order moments m_{20}, m_{02} and m_{22}
respectively describe the extent of the distribution in the horizontal,
vertical, and diagonal directions. Axial asymmetry is given by third
order moments; horizontal asymmetry is measured by m_{12} and m_{30},
vertical asymmetry by m_{21} and m_{03}. Quadrant asymmetry is described by the fourth order moments m_{13} and m_{31}.

However, to be of practical value such descriptors should be invariant
to translations, rotations, and changes of scale. A set of seven moment
invariants has been derived which characterize the shape of a distribution
irrespective of its scale, orientation or location in space (32) and have
been used for pattern recognition tasks (33). First the central moments

$$\mu_{pq} = \int_{-\infty}^{\infty}\int_{-\infty}^{\infty} (x-\bar{x})^p (y-\bar{y})^q f(x,y)dxdy \qquad \ldots\ldots (11)$$

$$\bar{x} = m_{10}/m_{00} \quad ; \quad \bar{y} = m_{01}/m_{00}$$

are computed which are translation invariant. A normalization step makes
these moments also invariant under scale change while rotation invariance
is achieved with seven specific combinations of the normalized central
moments up to order three. The seventh invariant moment changes sign
under improper rotations and thus distinguishes mirror images. A further

146

modified set of six moment invariants has been proposed which also remain
invariant under changes in contrast (34) but we have found these insensitive to real changes in the object distribution.

To assess the suitability of the invariant moments for measuring changes
in the reflectance pattern of the optic nerve in glaucoma, a simulation
study was carried out. The normal optic nerve distribution was modeled as
a circular region corresponding to the cup, 20 pixels in diameter and with
an intensity of 120, lying centered within a 50 pixel diameter disk of
intensity 100. Changes typical of a glaucomatous optic nerve were modeled
in three separate experiments; (a) the disk intensity was reduced in steps
of 20 intensity units to simulate pallor, (b) the cup diameter was increased successively until it filled the whole disk, and (c) the cup was
made increasingly elliptical in the vertical direction. A smooth change
in the first invariant moment and several of the higher order invariant
moments was observed in each case as reported previously (35). The invariant moments were also used to monitor changes in the reflectance pattern
due to increased cupping of the optic nerve in a modified Zeiss model eye
(36). Images were acquired for optic nerve depths increased by increments
of 0.025 inches. Since the optic nerve in this model is very small, the
changes between successive images were barely discernible to the eye, but
were followed more or less linearly by the logarithm of the first invariant moment as shown in figure 5. The reproducibility of the moment
values is indicated by the small dispersion between three measurement
points at an optic nerve head position of 1.7 mm. Intensity histograms of
the same distributions were much less sensitive to the changes in reflectance than the invariant moments. However, this sensitivity could also be
a problem in the case of considerable image noise. Fortunately the optic
nerve is a highly reflecting structure which yields a good signal to noise
ratio. Because the distribution of blood vessels over the optic nerve
varies considerably from one eye to another, this method will be restricted to following changes in a single eye. Nevertheless this could be of
considerable clinical importance in detecting the first signs of change in
the optic nerves of hypertensive eyes or in monitoring the effects of
pressure reduction therapy.

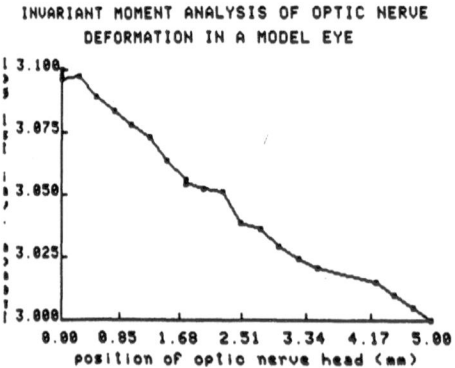

Figure 5: Variation of first invariant moment with increasing cup
depth in a model eye

4.4. Surface topography

Since the changes in reflectance of the optic nerve in glaucoma are, at least in part, due to three-dimensional changes in the configuration of the optic nerve there has been considerable interest in the measurement of the topography of the optic nerve. Stereophotography (36,37,38,39) provides a qualitative assessment of the excavation of the optic nerve and is frequently employed in clinical practice. Quantitative measures of the three-dimensional shape can be obtained from stereo photographs by using the stereophotogrammetric technique used in cartography, in which an observer moves a small floating mark in space to follow the surface in the fused stereo image (40,41). Because of the need for specialized equipment and highly trained personnel this technique is not suitable for routine clinical application. Also, the accuracy of the measurements is limited by the small convergence angle achievable through the narrow pupil. Digital photogrammetry eliminates the manual analysis of stereophotographs and is more reproducible, though probably less accurate than the best photogrammetrist (42). An alternative approach based on optical sectioning, measures the deformation of a series of parallel slit beams of light over the cup (44,45,46,47). The displacement of each stripe of light from its usual straight path is proportional to the depth of the surface below the plane of the retina and to the stereo base. An absolute measurement of cup volume is however difficult since the separation of the slits at the retina is not known precisely and depends on the refractive error of the eye unless a Goldmann contact lens is employed. Higher contrast stripe photographs can be achieved by using a striped pattern of laser light to excite fluorescence in fluorescein dye in the retinal blood vessels (48), but then the procedure becomes invasive with the associated discomfort and risks of fluorescein angiography. Moiré topography of the optic nerve has also been attempted (49) but only a few Moiré fringes could be produced on the cup thus limiting the accuracy of the method. Although a human observer can readily interpret Moiré contours, automation of the process is complicated. A method of automated measurement of three-dimensional topography based on phase measurement has been developed (50,51) which is potentially extremely accurate, and lends itself to

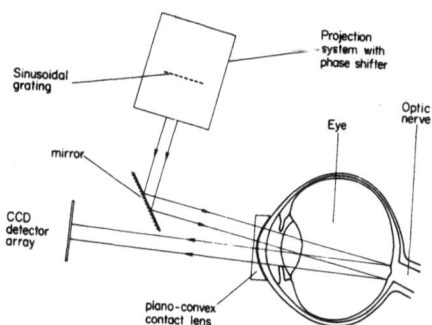

FIGURE 6. Schematic diagram of fundus topography measurement system

digital imaging. This method also seems appropriate for the study of the optic nerve and while similar to the techniques described above, offers a number of advantages.

Figure 6 shows a schematic diagram of the profilometry system. A projection system incorporating a sinusoidal transmission grating and a phase shifter illuminates a small region of the retina around the optic nerve through one side of the pupillary aperture with fringes having a sinusoidal intensity distribution. The parallel grating fringes are bent by the hills and valleys of the retina, the optic nerve, and the retinal blood vessels and this deformed pattern is recorded by a CCD array. The difference in phase between the intensity variation across the optic nerve and that across a reference plane is related to the depth or height of the optic nerve surface. A plane outside the eye may be chosen as the reference surface, or the front surface of the flat part of the retina on either side of the optic nerve where the fringes are not distorted could be used. The optical geometry is shown in more detail in figure 7. Along the reference plane the recorded intensity variation can be described as

$$I_R = a(x,y) + b(x,y)\cos\phi_R(x) \qquad\qquad \dots\dots (12)$$

where $a(x,y)$ is the background or dc light level and $b(x,y)$ is the fringe contrast. If the illumination is divergent, then the phase ϕ_R is a non-linear function of x. Every point on the reference plane is characterized by a unique phase value with respect to a point of origin such as the intersection of the imaging optical axis with the reference plane. For example the point C has a phase value

$$\phi_{RC} = 2\pi n + \phi'_{RC} \qquad\qquad \dots\dots (13)$$

where n is an integer and $0 < \phi'_{RC} < 2\pi$. Since equation (12) has three

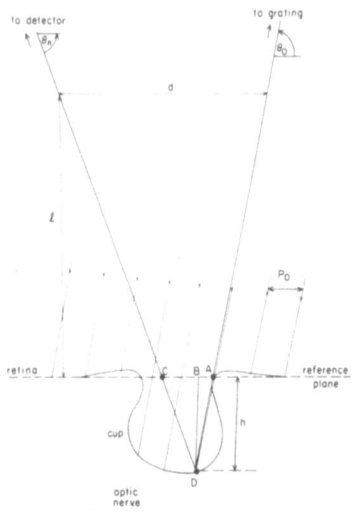

FIGURE 7. Geometry of phase-measuring profilometry of the optic nerve

unknowns, it is not possible to compute the phase ϕ_{RC} from a single intensity measurement. However, if the phase is successively shifted by $2\pi/N$ by translating the grating by distance p_0/N, then provided $N>3$, the I_i intensity measurements, (i =1,N) yield N equations which can be solved for the phase:

$$\tan\phi_{RC} = \sum_{i=1}^{N} I_i \sin(2\pi i/N) / \sum_{i=1}^{N} I_i \cos(2\pi i/N) \qquad \ldots\ldots (14)$$

As the phase function is continuous, it is possible to determine n in equation (13) by detecting sharp phase changes of nearly 2π which occur between two neighboring sample points whenever a complete grating period has been sampled. The same element of the detector which records the intensity at C, also measures the intensity at D. At the point D the intensity is the same as that which could have been observed at A on the reference plane, modified by the object reflectivity:

$$I_D = r(x,y)[a(x,y) + b(x,y)\cos\phi_D] \qquad \ldots\ldots (15)$$

The difference in phase ϕ_{CD} between points C and D is related to the geometric distance AC. In the case of parallel illumination:

$$AC = (p_0/2\pi)\ \phi_{CD} \qquad \ldots\ldots (16)$$

where p_0 is the projected grating spacing. AC is in turn related to the surface depth BD:

$$BD = h = [1(AC/d)]/[1 + (AC/d)] \qquad \ldots\ldots (17)$$

by simple geometry. Since D>>AC, then AC/d<<1 and equation (16) may be approximated by

$$h = 1(AC/d) = AC\tan\theta_0 \qquad \ldots\ldots (18)$$

where θ_0 is the angle of the grating illumination. A mapping algorithm locates the point A. In general A lies between two detector sampling points and is therefore determined by linear interpolation of the known phase values.

Figure 8 shows the surface profile (solid line) of a cylindrical test object which was measured by a three phase shift implementation of equat-

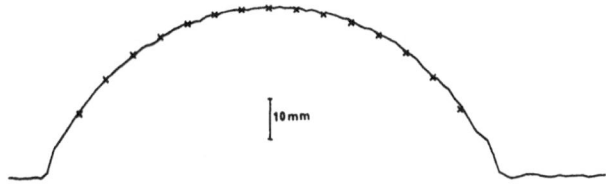

10 mm

FIGURE 8. Comparison between phase-measuring profilometry and contact measurements of a cylindrical test object

ion (14) in white light using a projected grating period of about 15mm, and a 128x128 element photodiode detector array. The cross marks indicate measurements made by a manual contact profilometer which agree to better than 1% except in the regions of steepest slope where manual contact methods are not very reliable. A mannequin face was measured by the same optical technique as an example of a more general class of object. Figure 9 shows the deformed grating pattern produced and figure 10 is a perspective plot of 97 profile lines which were reconstructed from three interferograms with one third of a period phase shift between them. All the features of the face are clearly resolved.

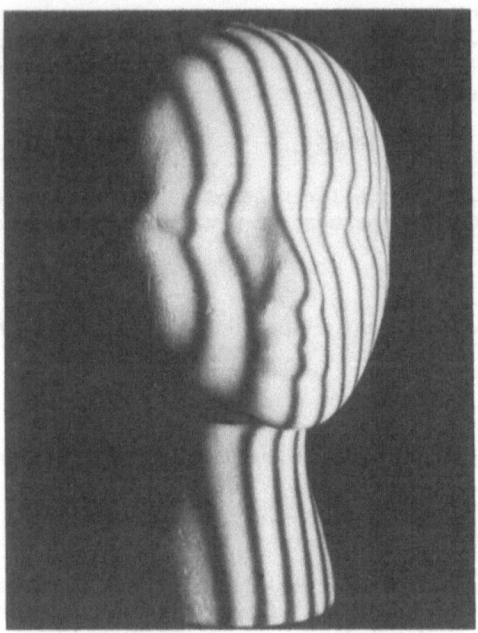

FIGURE 9. Interferogram of mannequin face

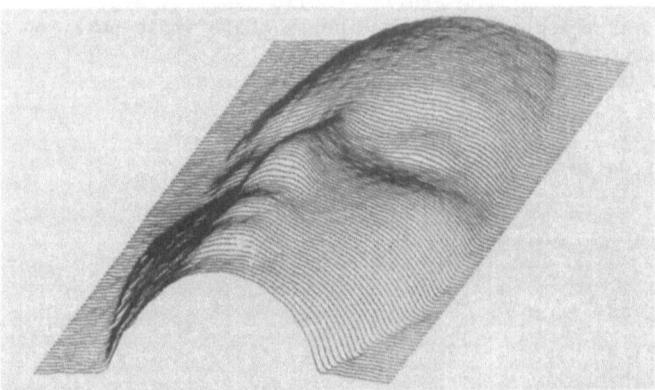

FIGURE 10. Profiles of mannequin face reconstructed from 3 interferograms

For profilometry of the optic nerve, a region of about 3mm diameter can be illuminated with about 12 fringes, giving about 8 fringes over the optic nerve itself and p_0 = 0.25 mm. With the CCD array used in the digital fundus imaging system, this would result in about 20 elements sampling each projected period. Considering the worst case of a pupil diameter of only 4mm (for example due to long term use of miotics) the projection angle θ_0 would be 83.5° which leads to an effective wavelength

$$\lambda_e = p_0 \tan\theta_0 \qquad\qquad \dots\dots (19)$$

of 2.2mm which is equal to the depth which would cause a 2π phase shift. The worst case error in phase measurement has been computed (52) to be approximately

$$\Delta\phi_{max} = 1/0.866Q \qquad\qquad \dots\dots (20)$$

where Q is the number of resolvable gray levels at the point in question on the object. Since the optic nerve reflects strongly, and the CCD quantizes with 8 bit precision (256 gray levels), a local gray level resolution of 100 should be easily achievable. Then the maximum phase error would be 1.15%. The corresponding maximum error in depth measurement Δh is then

$$\Delta h = \lambda_e(\Delta\phi/2\pi) \qquad\qquad \dots\dots (21)$$

or $4\mu m$ in this case. This is almost an order of magnitude better than the depth resolution achievable by photogrammetry and significantly better than the $20\mu m$ resolution claimed by the laser contour angiography technique. Even with only 6 projected fringes and 50 resolvable gray levels, the depth resolution would be a very acceptable $16\mu m$. The r.m.s error over the whole region is about half of the maximum error and would therfore be less than $10\mu m$.

Because this is an ac technique, variations in reflectivity across the surface of the optic nerve do not matter provided they are not non-linear functions of intensity. By selecting the grating spacing and the illumination angle appropriately, the depth resolution can be tuned to study coarse or fine detail. The same method could also be used to measure tumor growth, or the development of staphylomas in high myopes. Another potential application is to the measurement of corneal topography for fitting of contact lenses or as an aid in corneal surgery such as radial keratotomy. The computation involved requires only an arctangent function and simple linear interpolation thus a low cost microcomputer can be used to perform the image data acquisition, control of the grating translation, computation of the surface topography and display of the results. With the use of three frame buffers, the three phase images can be acquired in about a tenth of a second which should be rapid enough to prevent eye movement between frames.

5. CONCLUSION

A versatile, digital ocular fundus imaging system has been constructed for the purpose of quantitative measurement of spectral reflectance characteristics of ocular structures in various diseases. The application of several information processing techniques to the analysis of spectral reflectance maps in order to obtain new diagnostic information has been described. Spectral reflectance signatures promise to offer a means of earlier detection of diabetic retinopathy, choroidal melanoma and glaucoma. Descriptors of two dimensional attributes of reflected intensity distributions such as texture and shape have been applied to the diagnosis of malignant lesions and changes in the optic nerve in glaucoma. Finally, a new and accurate technique for measuring the topography of the optic nerve has been proposed as a further tool in the study of glaucoma.

ACKNOWLEDGMENTS
The authors wish to thank the American Diabetes Accociation - New York Affiliate for a grant in support of the development of the spectral reflectance imaging system. Research funds from New York Institute of Technology are gratefully acknowledged for permitting the development of the phase-measuring profilometry technique. We also wish to thank the Stanford University Eye Clinic for loan of the model eye, and the Medical Department of Brookhaven National Laboratory for use of its image processing facilities.

REFERENCES
1. Wong D: Techniques of Fundus Photography. Kodak Topics in Biomedical Photography, Vol. M3-718, Eastman Kodak Company, 1976.
2. Kristian J. and Blouke M.: Charge-coupled devices in astronomy. Scientific American, pp67-74, October 1982.
3. Millikan G.A.: A simple photoelectric colorimeter. J. Physiol. (London), 79:152, 1933.
4. Zylstra W.G.: Fundamentals and applications of clinical oximeters. Royal van Gorcum, Assen (Netherlands), 1953.
5. Wood E.H. and Geraci J.E.: Photoelectric determination of arterial oxygen saturation in man. J. Lab. Clin. Med., 34:387-401, 1949.
6. Enson Y., Briscoe W.A., Polanyi M.L. and Cournaud A: In vivo studies with an intravascular and intracardiac reflection oximeter. J. Appl. Physiol., 17:552-558, 1962.
7. Mook G.A., Osypka P., Sturm R.E. and Wood E.H.: Fibre optic reflection photometry on blood. Cardiovasc. Res., 2:199-209, 1968.
8. Sutterer W.F.: Optical artifacts in whole blood densitometry. Pediat. Res., 1:66-75, 1967.
9. Anselmo V.J. and Zawacki B.E.: Diagnosis of cutaneous thermal burn injuries by multispectral imaging analysis. Jet Propulsion Laboratory Research Report, JPL 79-34, 1978.
10. Behrendt T. and Wilson L.A.: Spectral reflectance photography of the retina. Am. J. Ophthalmol., 59:1079-1088, 1965.
11. Ducrey N.M., Delori F.C. and Gragoudas E.S.: Monochromatic ophthalmoscopy and fundus photography II: the pathological fundus. Arch. Ophthalmol. 97:288-293, 1979.
12. Gloster J.: Fundus oximetry. Experimental Eye Research, 6:187-212, 1967.
13. Cohen A.J. and Laing R.A.: Determination of retinal blood oxygen saturation from microdensitometer scans of ocular photographs. Photographic Science and Engineering, 20:31-35, 1976.
14. Delori F.C., Deupree D.M. and Weiter J.J.: Evaluation of the retinal vessel oximetry technique. Invest. Ophthalmol. Vis. Sci. 26(3) Suppl:37, 1985

15. Drance S.M.: Is ischemia the villain in glaucomatous cupping and atrophy? Controversies in Ophthalmology, ed. Brockhurst R.J. et al., W.B. Saunders Co., pp292-300, 1977.
16. Maumenee A.E.: The pathogenesis of visual field loss in glaucoma. Controversies in Ophthalmolgy, ed. Brockhurst R.J. et al., W.B. Saunders Co., pp301-311, 1977.
17. Anderson D.R.: Is ischemia the villain in glaucomatous cupping and atrophy? Controversies in Ophthalmology, ed. Brockhurst R.J. et al., W.B. Saunders Co., pp312-319, 1977.
18. Schwartz B.: Cupping and pallor of the optic disc. Arch. Ophthalmol. $\underline{89}$:272-277, 1973.
19. Zenker H-J, Mierdel P. and Marr E.: Quantitative evaluation of pallor-disc ratio and colour of the optic disc by a photographic method. Graefe's Archive for Clin. and Exp. Ophthalmol., $\underline{220}$:184-186, 1983.
20. Woernley D.L.: Infrared absorption curves for normal and neoplastic tissues and related biological substances. Cancer Res., $\underline{12}$:516-523, 1952.
21. Cawley E.P., Rathbun D. and Wheeler C.E.: Infrared spectroscopic studies of pigmented skin tumors. Arch. of Derm. and Syph., $\underline{70}$:748-753, 1954.
22. Packer S., Schneider K., Lin H-Z, and Feldman M.: Digital infrared fundus reflectance. Ophthalmol., $\underline{87}$:534-542, 1980.
23. Huekamp B.: Die Infrarot-Photographie in der Differentialdiagnostik von Pigmentveranderungen des vorderenaugen Abschnittes. Ber. der Deutsch. Ophthalm. Ges., $\underline{59}$:322-325, 1955.
24. Ernest J.T.: Color translation fundus photography. Am. J. Ophthalmol., $\underline{65}$:170-174, 1968.
25. Dallow R.L.: Color infrared photography of the ocular fundus. Arch. Ophthalmol., $\underline{92}$:254-258, 1974.
26. Denffer H.v. and Warth P.: Weitere Anwendungsmoglichkeiten der Infrarot-Falschfarben Fotographie in der Augenheilkunde. Klin. Mbl. Augenheilk., $\underline{171}$:959-965, 1977.
27. Chen C.H. and Young G-K.: A study of texture classification using spectral features. Technical Report, SMU-EE-TR-82-1, Dept. of Electrical Engineering, Southeastern Massachusets University, North Dartmouth, MA, 1982.
28. Lim J.S. and Malik N.A.: A new algorithm for two-dimensional maximum entropy power spectral estimation. IEEE Trans. on Acoustics, Speech and Signal Processing, ASSP-$\underline{29}$(3):401-413, 1981.
29. Wezka J. Dyer C. and Rosenfeld A.: A comparative study of texture measures for terrain classification. IEEE Trans. Systems, Man and Cybernetics, SMC-$\underline{6}$(3):204-222, 1980.
30. Conners R.W.: Towards a set of statistical features which measure visually perceivable qualities of texture. Proc. IEEE Conf. on Pattern Recognition and Image Processing pp. 382-390, Chicago, 1979.
31. Schwartz B. and Kern J.: Scanning microdensitometry of optic disk pallor in glaucoma. Arch. Ophthalmol., $\underline{95}$:2159-2165, 1977.
32. Hu M-K.: Visual pattern recognition by moment invariants. IRE Trans. Inform. Theory, IT-$\underline{8}$:179-187, 1962.

33. Sadjadi F.A. and Hall E.L.: Numerical computations of moment invariants for scene analysis. Proc. IEEE Computer Soc. Conf. on Pattern Recognition and Image Processing, Catalog No. Ch1318-5/7/0000-0181, pp181-187, 1978.
34. Maitra S.: Moment Invariants. Proc. IEEE, 67(4):697-699, 1979.
35. Rowe R.W., Packer S., Rosen J. and Bizais Y.: A charge-coupled device imaging system for examination of the ocular fundus. Proc. SPIE, 454:65-71, 1984.
36. Rosenthal A.R., Falconer D.G., and Pieta I.: Photogrammetry experiments with a model eye. Brit. J. Ophthal., 64:881-887, 1980.
37. Allen L.: Ocular fundus photography. Am. J. Ophthalmol. 57:13-28, 1968.
38. Schirmer K.E. and Kratky V.: Stereochronoscopy of the optic disk with stereoscopic cameras. Arch. Ophthalmol., 98:1647, 1980.
39. Donaldson D., Prescott R., Kenedy S.: Simultaneous stereoscopic fundus camera utilizing a single optic axis. Invest. Ophthalmol. Vis. Sci. 19:289, 1980.
40. Crock G.W.: Stereotechnology in medicine. Trans. Ophthal. Soc. U.K. XC:577, 1970.
41. Saheb N.E., Drance S.M. and Nelson A.: The use of photogrammetry in evaluating the cup of the optic nervehead for a study in chronic simple glaucoma. Canad. J. Ophthal., 7:466-470, 1972.
42. Rosenthal A.R.: Digital photogrammetry of the optic nerve head. Proc. SPIE Vol. 166, Applications of Human Biostereometrics (NATO), pp255-262, 1978.
43. Schwartz B. and Takamoto T.: Biostereometrics in ophthalmology for measurement of the optic disc cup in glaucoma. Proc. SPIE Vol. 166, Applications of Human Biostereometrics (NATO), pp. 251-254, 1978.
44. Holm O. and Krakau C.E.T.: A photographic method for measuring the volume of papillary excavations. Annals of Ophthalmol., 1:328-332, 1970.
45. Krakau C.E.T. and Torlegard K.: Comparison between stereo and slit image photogrammetric measurements of the optic disc. Acta Ophthalmologica 50:863-871, 1970.
46. Holm O.C., Becker B., Asseff C.F. and Podos S.M.: Volume of the optic disk cup. Am. J. Ophthalmol., 73(6):876-881, 1972.
47. Shapiro J.M.: Contour photography of the optic nerve head: Stereometric basis. Proc. SPIE Vol. 361, Biostereometrics '82, pp322-323, 1982.
48. Shapiro J.M.: Topographic mapping of the ocular fundus by laser contour angiography: The man-machine interaction. Proc. SPIE Vol. 166, Applications of Human Biostereometrics (NATO), pp255-262, 1978.
49. Nakatani H., Shimizu Y., Kikkiwa A. and Suzuki N.: Moir topographic method for measuring the depth of papillary excavation. Documental Ophthalmol., pp. 135-140, W. Junk Publishers, The Hague, 1977.
50. Srinivasan V., Liu H.C. and Halioua M.: Automated phase-measuring profilometry of 3-D diffuse objects. Appl. Optics, 23(18):3105-3108, 1984.
51. Srinivasan V., Liu H.C. and Halioua M.: Automated phase-measuring profilometry: a phase mapping approach. Appl. Optics, 24(2):185-188, 1985.

VISUALIZATION OF THE OXYGENATION STATE OF BRAIN AND MUSCLE IN NEWBORN INFANTS BY NEAR INFRA-RED TRANSILLUMINATION.

S.R.ARRIDGE,M.COPE,P.VAN DER ZEE,P.J.HILLSON,D.T.DELPY

Dept. of Medical Physics and Bioengineering
University College Hospital, London, England

1.0 INTRODUCTION

1.1 Clinical Aims

Inadequate oxygen supply to the brain and cerebral haemorrhage are the two main causes of death and permanent disability in infants who need intensive care [1,2]. Haemorrhage is easy to detect by ultrasound imaging, but this technique does not identify hypoxic or ischaemic changes until it is too late to intervene successfully to prevent irreversible damage. Non-invasive methods are therefore urgently needed, so that the oxygen supply to the brain can be monitored, and therapy put on a rational basis. Phosphorous Nuclear Magnetic Resonance Spectroscopy, which provides valuable information about oxidative phosphorylation, has proved to be one such method [3], but it suffers from the disadvantages that it is expensive and the baby has to be transported to the spectrometer.

Two new projects are being conducted at University College Hospital with the aim of developing equipment that will provide the clinical investigator with an indication of the degree of blood or tissue oxygenation in the brain and other organs of newborn babies. The technique employed uses light at wavelengths in the near infra-red to transilluminate tissues, and relate changes in optical density to changes in oxygenation state. The aim of one project is to make quantitative, global measurements of the oxygenation state of a volume of tissue; the second project attempts to produce images of the tissues in which intensity is related to oxygenation.

In addition to monitoring the occurence of cerebral hypoxia, another application is assessment of blood volume and peripheral perfusion. Small preterm infants often develop hypovolaemia during the first few days after birth, which is difficult to monitor non-invasively. Since cerebral perfusion is preserved above peripheral perfusion during hypovolaemia, monitoring the oxygenation state of peripheral muscle could provide a means of assessing overall blood volume.

These non-invasive monitoring techniques could have many applications in other areas of medicine. For example in general muscle studies, monitoring of tissue viability in reconstructive and amputative surgery, and perhaps via fibre optics to the monitoring of internal organs including the heart.

1.2 Background work

The body is relatively transparent to light in the wavelength region 700-1300nm. In defining the optical density (OD) of any sample an empirical definition is $OD = -\log_{10} I/I_o$ where I is the measured output intensity for I_o input intensity. A simple absorbing medium (i.e. no scattering) of length d containing concentration [c] of centres with absorption cross-section σ_a follows Beer's Law

$$I=I_o \exp - \sigma_a[c]d$$

so that OD = $(\ln 10)\sigma_a[c]d$

In blood the absorption spectrum of haemoglobin shows differences for the oxidized (HbO_2) and reduced (Hb) forms (Fig 1). In particular note that at about 805 nm, known as the isobestic point, the optical density of Hb and HbO_2 are the same. Similarly the spectrum for cytochrome aa_3 (Caa_3) shows differences in its oxidized and reduced form (fig 2). This compound is one of the components of the oxidative phosphorylation chain in the cell mitochondria, and its oxidation state is related to the rate of cellular metabolism, and cellular oxygen supply.

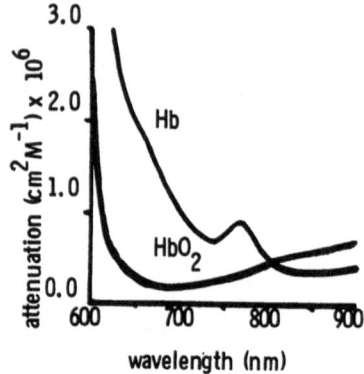

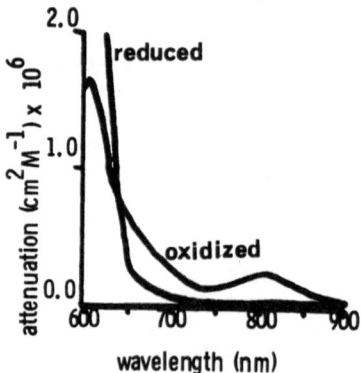

Figure 1 : Absorption spectra of oxy- and deoxy-heamoglobin

Figure 2 : Absorption spectra of cytochrome aa_3 oxidised and reduced (redrawn from [4])

In a simple analysis the optical density OD(λ) of a tissue sample at wavelength λ will contain contributions from Hb, HbO_2 and Caa_3 plus other terms assumed constant. By monitoring changes in transmitted intensity at three or more wavelengths we can in theory monitor non-invasively changes in blood volume, blood oxygenation, and tissue oxygenation. This principle, termed 'Niroscopy' by Frans Jobsis, has been used by him in **in-vivo** animal experiments, where he has found good correlation between results obtained by this method and actual oxygen measurements made in tissue and blood with electrochemical oxygen electrodes [5,6]. All work so far published has been based on a spectrophotometric non-imaging technique. The possibility, and usefulness of some form of imaging is the main subject of this paper.

2.0 PHYSICAL MODEL OF LIGHT PROPAGATION IN TISSUE

In a non-imaging system the path taken by light through the tissue under study is relatively unimportant. However, if we wish to localise the measurements of transmitted flux in order to image, we need to know how light is propogated in tissue. Beer's Law cannot be applied naively for **in-vivo** measurements because of the extensive light scattering that takes place. The infants we are concerned with are 7-14 weeks premature and have ear-to-ear, known as Bi-Parietal, head diameters (BPD) up to 8cms. We have found the optical densities involved are of the order of 7-10. Van der Hulst has pointed out [7] that for a scattering medium with OD > 0.2 the process of light propogation must be treated as one of multiple scattering. The attenuation of light in biological scattering materials has been studied in the past with reference to two main areas: Haematocrit and oxygenation determination in thin blood samples, and dosimetry calculations for Photoradiation Treatment. In the former application Radiative Transfer Theory has been applied to provide a multiple scatter theory [8,9,10] which, however, assumes detailed knowledge of particle size and shape. Several authors [11,12,13,14,15,16] have shown that, provided that the total sample length is much longer than the mean free path between scattering events, then a multiple scattering sample may be modelled by diffusion statistics. In addition the diffusion equation has been applied successfully to model flux distribution in Photoradiation Treatment [17,18], despite the seeming invalidity of applying homogeneous solutions to complex heterogeneous structures.

We derive here a formalism for using analytical techniques to model transmitted light in tissues of interest. This will be used not as a basis for analyical solutions, but as a formalism for defining the physical basis of different measurement techniques.

In a diffusing medium the photon flux $F(r)\hat{n}$ in photons per unit area per unit time at position $r = (x,y,z)$ in direction $\hat{n}$ is related to the photon density $P(r)$ by

$$F(r) = -D(r) \nabla P(r) \tag{1}$$

where D has dimensions $(length)^2 (time)^{-1}$, and is dependent on w and k, the absorption and scattering coefficients at each point. We can define terms $w = \sum_i \sigma_{ai}[i]$ and $k = \sum_i \sigma_{si}[i]$ where [i] is the concentration of centres of type i with absorption and (total) scattering cross-sections σ_{ai} and σ_{si}. The factors w and k are wavelength dependent, although for large particle incoherent scattering the dependence of k is weak.

From continuity, the net decay in photon density is due to absorption only, and photon flux input is represented by source terms $q(r)$, giving

$$\nabla .F(r) = -(wc/n)P(r) + q(r) \tag{2}$$

where c is the speed of light and n the refractive index of the medium, and

$$(\nabla D(r)).(\nabla P(r)) + D \nabla^2 P(r) = (wc/n)P(r) - q(r) \tag{3}$$

In a homogenous medium $\nabla D = 0$ so that:

$$(\nabla^2 - \alpha^2)P(r) = -(1/D)q(r) \tag{4}$$

where $\alpha^2 = (wc/n)(1/D)$. In an infinite medium solutions to (4) are of the form

$$P(\mathbf{r}) = (A/r)\exp(-\alpha r) \tag{5}$$

These describe exponentially decaying photon densities where the effective attenuation coefficient α is a combination of the scattering and absorption coefficients. Values of α have been found for different tissues [17,18,19] and examples are given in Table 1. Wilson [18] has found that for scattering dominated cases (e.g. brain) the value of α is nearly independent of wavelength above 700nm and that the photon density follows the form of (5). This implies that to first order it may be possible to assume that the diffusing properties of the tissue remain constant with changes in oxygenation. Such solutions are only valid within the tissue, away from sources of input flux.

Table 1. Attenuation coefficients and penetration depths for light in post-mortem tissue at 633nm. Taken from references [17,19]

Tissue	Attenuation coefficient α (cm^{-1})	Penetration depth $\delta = 1/\alpha$ (mm)
Brain (cow)	2.5	4.0
Muscle (cow)	5.6	1.8
Liver (cow)	13	0.8
Brain (normal adult)	7 - 13	0.8 - 1.5
Brain (neonate)	2.2 - 3.3	3 - 4.5

Some authors [12,15] have used Green's Function methods to predict transmitted and back-scattered flux densities from thin blood samples. Difficulties arise in stipulating boundary conditions, since we require zero photon density on the surface of a complex three-dimensional object. For an infinite homogeneous space the Green's Function for (4) is

$$G_1(\mathbf{r},\mathbf{r'}) = \frac{1}{4\pi} \frac{\exp-(\alpha|\mathbf{r}-\mathbf{r'}|)}{|\mathbf{r}-\mathbf{r'}|} \tag{6}$$

When considering the input fluxes incident on a surface, approximated as an infinite half-space with $z > 0$, the Method of Images can be used [12] to satisfy the boundary condition $G(\mathbf{r},\mathbf{r'}) = 0$ on the surface $z = 0$. Leading to

$$G_2(\mathbf{r},\mathbf{r'}) = \frac{1}{4\pi} \frac{\exp-(\alpha|\mathbf{r}-\mathbf{r'}|)}{|\mathbf{r}-\mathbf{r'}|} - \frac{1}{4\pi} \frac{\exp-(\alpha|\mathbf{r}-\mathbf{r}^*|)}{|\mathbf{r}-\mathbf{r}^*|} \tag{7}$$

i.e., for each source term at $\mathbf{r'} = (x',y',z')$, a negative source is imagined at $\mathbf{r}^* = (x',y',-z')$, so that the photon density is zero on the surface z=0. The extension of this analysis to the boundary conditions of a complex three-dimensional surface are not simple. G_2 is required to determine the influence of external light sources whilst G_1 can be used within the tissue, where the surface is assumed infinitely distant.

A second approach is to attempt Monte-Carlo modelling of photon survival in tissue [20,21] and results show agreement with analytical solutions in simple geometries. Monte-Carlo methods need explicit values for the differential scattering cross-section $d\sigma/d\Omega$, the absorption cross-section, and total scattering cross-section given by

$$\sigma_s(\hat{r}_1) = \int_\Omega \frac{d\sigma}{d\Omega}(\hat{r}_1,\hat{r}_2)\ d\Omega\ (\hat{r}_2)$$

where the integral is over all solid angles.

Kubelka-Munk theory [22] of the optical properties of intensely light scattering materials has been applied to give an explicit relationship for the one-dimensional case:

$$D = (c/n)\ 1/(w+2k) \tag{8}$$

with the implication that α is independent of n [23,24]. Although many authors use this relation for photon diffusion, it is not clear however that this can be readily applied to the three- dimensional case.

We can now extend some of the earlier results to a complex three-dimensional system. If we suppose that the scattering properties of the tissue are independent of wavelength, and that the diffusion parameters can be approximated by the homogeneous solution, then (7) can be used to derive the photon density $P(r)$ in the presence of source fluxes. If we now include local variations in absorbence as sink terms $f(r)$ in (4) we obtain :

$$(\nabla^2 - \alpha^2)P'(r) = -(1/D)(q(r) - f(r)P(r)) \tag{9}$$

Then (6) can be applied to give an expression for the perturbed density $P'(r)$:

$$P'(r) = \frac{1}{4\pi} \int_V \frac{f(r')P(r') - q(r')}{D}\ \frac{\exp-(\alpha|r-r'|)}{|r-r'|}\ d^3r' \tag{10}$$

where the integral is taken throughout the volume of the sample. It would be possible to attempt iterative solutions to this by putting $P'(r)$ into (4), and deriving higher order perturbations.

Expression (10), whilst in general insoluble, can be simplified by imposing specificity on the measuring systems used to detect transmitted light. We can ask to what extent such specificity reveals information on the oxygenation state of the subject under study. We will consider three types of measurement specificity:
1) Spectral - Spectrophotometric measurements
2) Spatial - Imaging
3) Temporal - Time gating of detected photons.
The type of measurement attempted leads to quite different instrumentation. The first type forms the basis for almost all previous work published in this area, and can provide quite detailed information on oxygenation state changes. The second type is only at the stage of preliminary trials and much consideration is necessary for determining its usefulness. The third type is as yet conjectural, but may provide the most accurate measurements.

3.0 SPECTROPHOTOMETRIC MEASUREMENTS

3.1 System Description

Figure 3 shows a system schematic of a spectrophotometric system developed at UCH for use on pre-term babies. High peak power semiconductor laser diodes are used to send short pulses of radiation to the head via a fibre optic. The small quantity of transmitted photons are carried via a second fibre optic to a photomultiplier tube where they are detected. The photon counts are gated sequentially for different wavelengths and analysed by microprocessor.

Here the source term in (10) is the flux of the input fibre, which has an angular dependence. The measured signal T is found by inserting $P(r')$ in (1) and integrating over the acceptance angle θ and area A of the detecting fibre.

$$T(\lambda) = \int\int_A 2\pi \, W(\theta)F(r).dS \, d\theta \tag{11}$$

where $W(\theta)$ is a weighting factor representing the angular sensitivity of the detecting fibre, and the vector dS is normal to the surface of the fibre. It would be very difficult to use the form of T to provide structural information about $F(r)$. We can, however, determine to what extent changes in oxygenation state show up as changes in T, and its dependence on wavelength.

3.2 Results

An initial test of the principle was carried out using the forearm of a normal adult volunteer. The tissue thickness was 6cms representing the equivalent in optical densities of about 8 cms of brain tissue. A rapidly inflatable cuff on the upper arm allowed blood supply to be cut off suddenly. Figure 4 shows the results of monitoring T at three different wavelengths, where change in optical density is plotted as a function of time. As the blood supply is cut off we note an increase in OD at 778nm. From Figure 1 we see that at 778nm, Hb has a higher absorption coefficient w than HbO_2. This increase in OD can therefore be interpreted as a fall in oxygenation level of the blood. Similarly at 847nm, where HbO_2 has a larger value of w than Hb, we detect a fall in OD. It is interesting to note that the rate of fall of OD at 847nm is less than the rise at 778nm. In addition we find a fall in the OD at 813nm, close to the isobestic point for haemoglobin, which should remain constant if haemoglobin was the only contributing factor. The effect may be an indication that we are detecting the drop in oxidation of Caa_3, which has a broad absorbence peak encompassing both this wavelength and 847nm in its oxidised form but not in its reduced form.

3.3 Conclusions

More detailed analysis of these results would not be justified by the simplicity of the experiment in light of the complexity of the theoretical treatment given in section 2. However the implications are firstly that sufficient photons are transmitted to be detected, and secondly that potentially good contrast is available for the parameters under investigation.

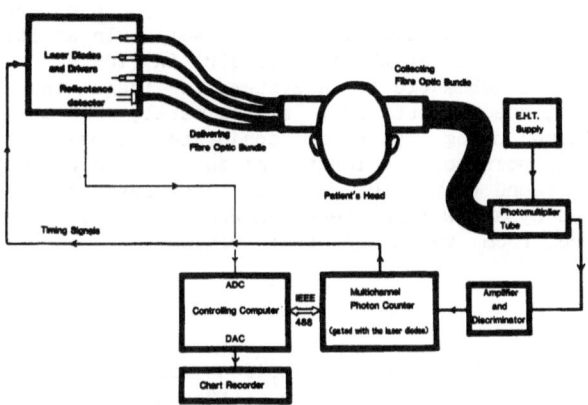

Figure 3 : Schematic of spectrophotometric measuring system

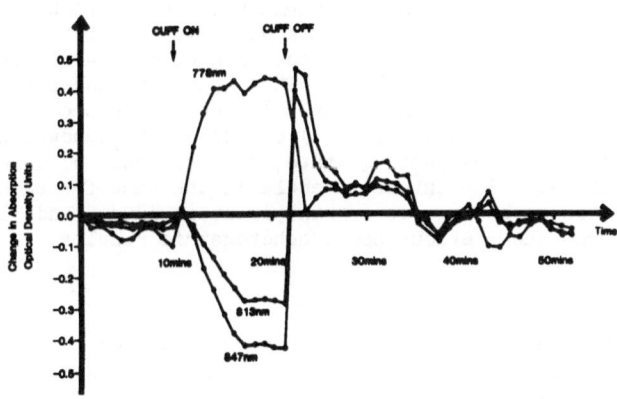

Figure 4 : Absorption changes across 6cms. of adult forearm
when the blood supply is cut off by a rapidly inflating blood
pressure cuff on the upper arm.

4.0 IMAGING MEASUREMENTS

4.1 System Description

By imaging the output flux we can eliminate the area integral from (11). By using a collimating system to select only one direction for the detected flux we remove the angular integral as well. In addition using a collimated input beam simplifies the form of q(r) in (10).

Figure 5 shows the schematic for a system to image the transmitted light from a collimated input beam approximately 5 cms in diameter. Collimation is achieved using a pair of conjugate lenses with a point source at the focal point of the input lens and a pinhole aperture at the focal point of the second (detecting) lens. The detector is an image intensifier followed by a low light level camera. The source used is a 150 Watt white light arc, from which spectral regions of interest can be selected by filtration.

4.2 Results

After losses in the delivery system the incident radiation is about 10Wm^{-2} at the surface of the illuminated organ. After attenuation in the 6-8cm thickness of tissue in the head of a typical premature baby the emergent flux is estimated as $10^{-7} - 10^{-9} \text{ Wm}^{-2}$ or about $10^3 - 10^5$ photons $\text{s}^{-1} \text{ mm}^{-2}$. Focussing by the lens increases the flux density, but selection of the collimating axis reduces the transmitted signal, so that it is at the low limit of detection by the camera. The implication of these figures is that for in-**vivo** measurements the signal to noise ratio is very poor, and narrow band spectral filtration cannot be used in the present system without reducing the signal to below detection level. Light can be imaged through the head of babies with BPD upto 8cms. but the definition of resultant images is poor as can be seen in figure 6.

By contrast, Fig 7 shows the image through the 3-4cms thickness of the palm of an adult volunteer, showing both a blood vessel as the dark line top right, and bone as a lighter central area. Figure 8 a) - d) show the effect of reduced oxygenation on the hand. The experiment was performed in the manner described in 3.2. The images in a) and b) employed a 10nm bandwidth filter centred at 840nm, and in c) and d) a 10nm bandwidth filter at 760nm; a) and c) are in the resting state, and b) and d) are after several minutes anoxia. The intensity scale is the same for each image. As can be seen, the tissue becomes more transparent at 840nm and less at 760nm, as expected from the previous spectrophotometric results.

4.3 Discussion

We are interested in determining to what degree scatter will degrade the obtainable image. In any interval Δz the change in flux along an axis $\hat{z}$ is given by (see figure 9a)

$$\Delta F_z = -(w+k)\Delta F_z \; z \; + \oint \frac{d \; \sigma(\hat{r}, \hat{z})}{d \Omega} F_r .dS \qquad (12)$$
$$+ \text{ higher order terms}$$

where the last term represents scatter into this direction from the flux in all other directions. The use of collimation eliminates those photons that are scattered out of the imaging axis, but allows those that are scattered

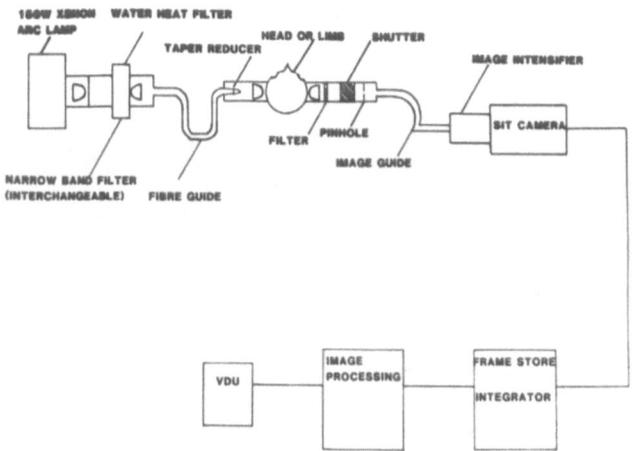

Figure 5 : Schematic of imaging system

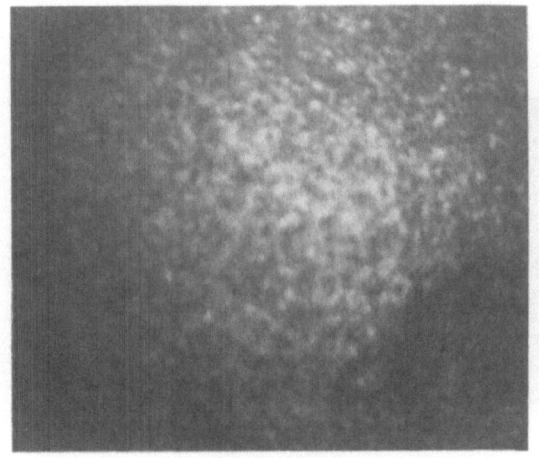

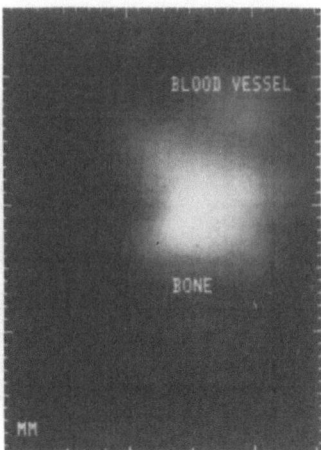

Figure 6 : Single frame image through the head of a baby of 7.5cm. BPD. 100nm bandwidth filter centred at 658nm.

Figure 7 : Average of 128 frames through adult palm of 3-4cms thickness. 100 nm bandwidth filter centred at 658nm.

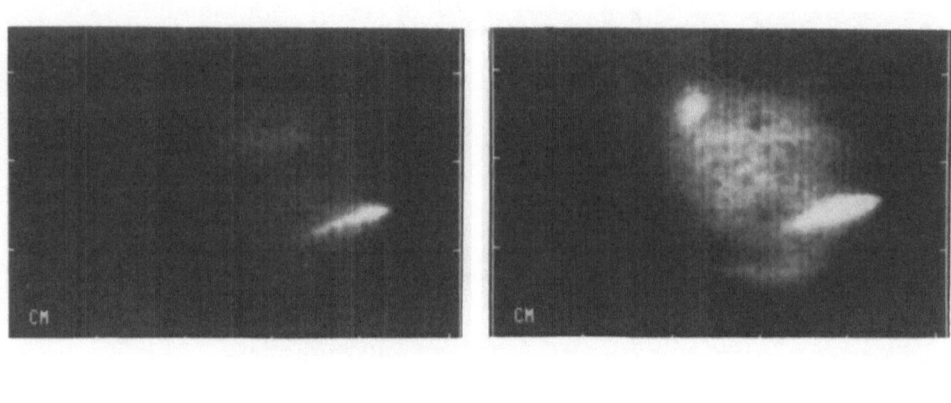

a)   840nm   b)

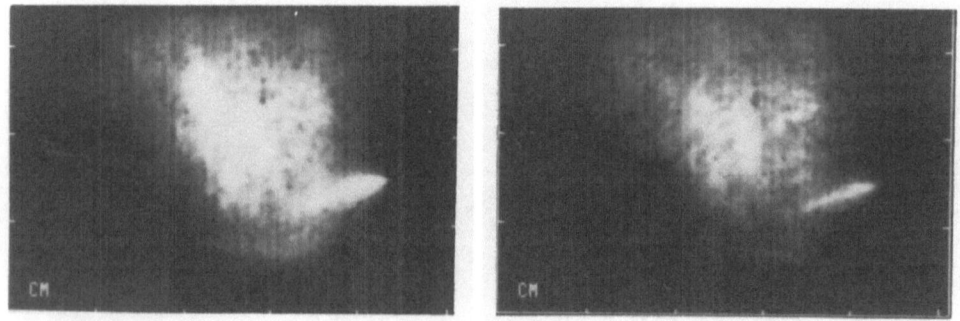

c)   760nm   d)

Figure 8 : Effect of hypoxia on the transparency of adult palm at two
different wavelengths. Figures a) and c) without hypoxia; b) and d)
with hypoxia. Note increase in transparency at 840nm and decrease
at 760nm. 10nm bandwidths for both filters. Averaged over 128 frames

twice or more, with their resultant direction back along the imaging axis; i.e. we accept terms in (12) of the form:

$$\iint_{V\,\Omega} F_z \frac{d\sigma\,(\hat{z},\hat{r})}{d\Omega} \frac{d\sigma\,(-\hat{r},\hat{z})}{d\Omega} d\Omega\,(\hat{r})\,dV$$

integrated over the volume of the sample and over all solid angles for the direction r, together with higher order terms, as illustrated in Figure 9b.

An experimental demonstration of this first order improvement is shown in figure 10. The images show a grid of wires with diameters (top to bottom), 0.23, 0.56 and 1.4 mm respectively, viewed through 15cms of scattering solution, with and without collimation. The scattering medium used was a solution of 38g l^{-1} of dried milk in water. This was added in small quantities to a cell of water containing the wire grids. Figure 10a is the image with no scattering solution present. The scattering coefficient, k, of the solution is estimated at about 0.01 - 0.05 [c] cm^{-1}, where [c] is the concentration in ml l^{-1} of added milk solution. The mean free path between scattering events is about 30 cms. (i.e. twice the overall path length) in b), 15cms. in c) and 6cms. in d). The grid is practically indiscernible at this degree of scatter. At the same scattering concentration, but using collimation, the grid is still well resolved (e). At double this concentration (f), where scattering length is 3cm. the smallest wire becomes unresolvable. Although a fairly crude experiment these results show that the effect of collimation is significant, allowing resolution of fine detail at up to five times the scattering length of the sample. A more highly absorbing phantom improves resolution because higher order scattered photons will be attenuated more by their longer path lengths. The gain is however obtained at the expense of a reduction in transmitted light intensity.

In-vitro we attempted to detect the edge of an aperture placed in the path of the input beam, when imaged through a 1cm. slice of ox-brain. From Table 1, the penetration depth in ox-brain is 4mm. Using values for absorption due to blood and cytochrome we estimate that the mean free path between scattering for brain tissue is 2mm, so that the sample length is

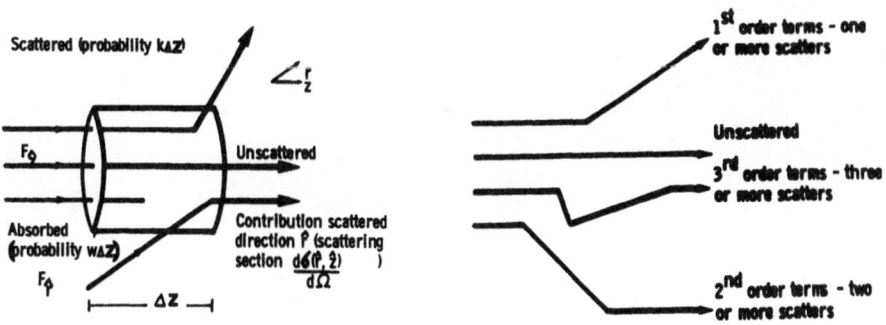

Figure 9a : Change in flux in direction $\hat{z}$ in a small interval Δz

Figure 9b : Different order terms in scattering

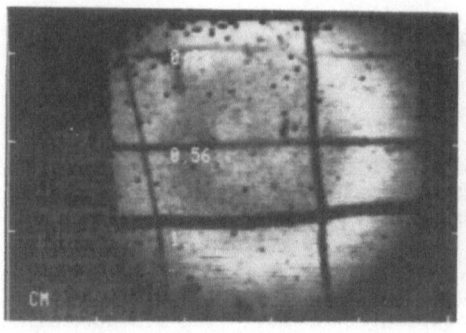

a) Phantom (no scattering)
    wire diameters in mm.

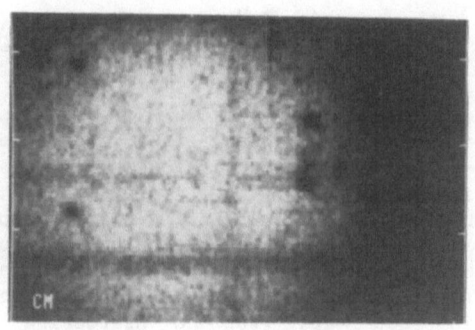

b) 1ml of scattering solution
    no collimation on detector

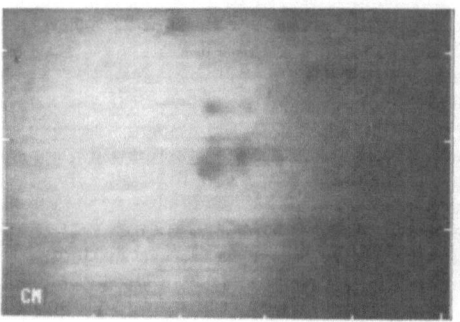

c) 2ml of scattering solution
    no collimation.

d) 5ml of scattering solution
    no collimation.

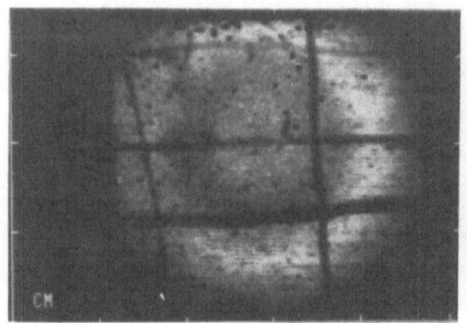

e) 5ml of scattering solution
    with collimation.

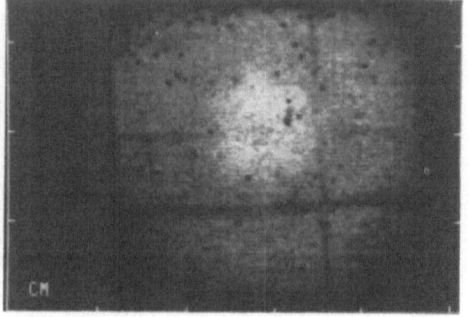

f) 10ml of scattering solution
    with collimation.

Figure 10 : Removal of first order scattering by collimation
Images averaged over 128 frames.

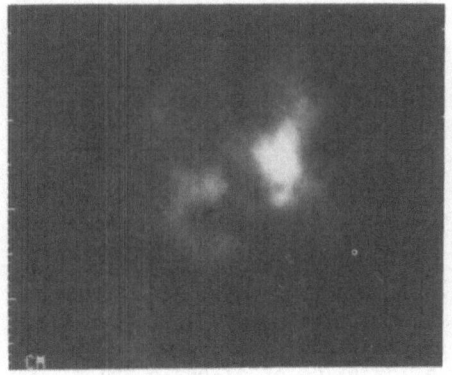

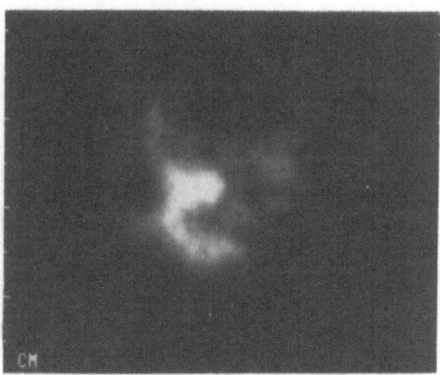

a) Cylindrical input beam.

b) Input as a) - top right half of
    beam masked by opaque aperture

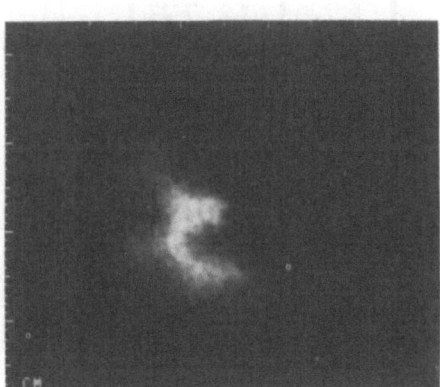

c) Result of subtracting (b-a) and
    thresholding at zero intensity

Figure 11 : Images through 1 cm ox-brain. 100nm bandwidth centred at 834nm
Images averaged over 128 frames.

about five times the scattering length. Figures 11 a)-c) show the results
of this experiment. In a) the input is a collimated cylindrical beam 5cms
in diameter. In b) the beam is divided in half obliquely from top left to
bottom right. Thus the top right half of the picture is illuminated by
light diffusing around the opaque edge. Figure 11 c) shows the result of
subtracting a) from b) and thresholding at zero intensity. The aperture
edge is quite well detected.

4.4 Point Spread Functions

The effective resolution at any depth can be characterised by the
extent to which a point source diffuses into the tissue. Figure 12
represents the object as a series of parallel planes of absorbers $f_d(r)$,
perpendicular to the imaging axis. The calculated form of the Point Spread
Function at different depths is plotted in figure 13, using equation (5)
with values for α taken from Table 1. Table 2 gives the half-maximum
widths. An experimental determination of the PSF was made using a
Helium-Neon laser as an approximation to a two-dimensional delta-function,
aligned along the imaging axis of the system shown in figure 5. The
results are shown in figure 14 a) for a 1cm slice of ox-brain and c) for
the human palm. The values measured from these images are also shown in
Table 2. As can be seen they are much lower than the estimated value,
suggesting that resolution may be better than predicted. It may be that
the values of α quoted in Table 1 were measured in tissue that had been
dead longer than our samples which were only two or three hours old. It
was certainly noticeable in our experiments that the optical properties of

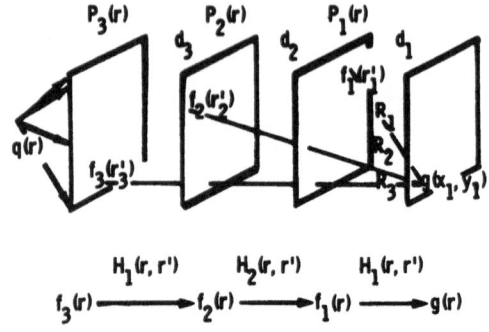

Figure 12 : Contributions to g from a depth d are thought of as convolved
with a transfer function H_d, characterised only by tissue diffusion
properties. The relation of this approach to that of section 2 may be seen
by considering the contributions to $g(r)$ as the sum of all terms $f_d(r')$
multiplied by the incident intensity $P(r')$ and the Green's Function $G(\mathbf{r},r')$
at that point. E.g. :

$$g(x_1,y_1) = P(r'_1)f_1(r'_1)\frac{exp-(\alpha R_1)}{R_1} + P(r'_2)f_2(r'_2)\frac{exp-(\alpha R_2)}{R_2}$$
$$+ P(r'_3)f_3(r'_3)\frac{exp-(\alpha R_3)}{R_3}$$

where : $R_1 = (x_1-x'_1, y_1-y'_1, z_1-z'_1)$
$R_2 = (x_2-x'_2, y_2-y'_2, z_2-z'_2)$
$R_3 = (x_3-x'_3, y_3-y'_3, z_3-z'_3)$

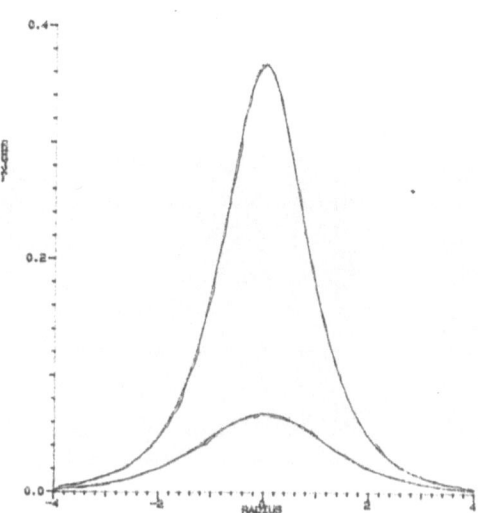

a) depth z = δ (top line), 2δ (bottom line)

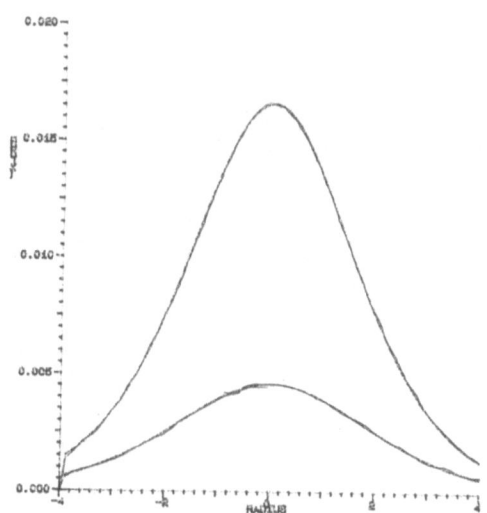

b) depth z = 3 δ(top line), 4 δ(bottom line)

Figure 13 : The function $(1/r)\exp(-\alpha r)$ where $r = (x^2 + z^2)^{-1/2}$.
x and z are in units of $\delta = 1/\alpha$.

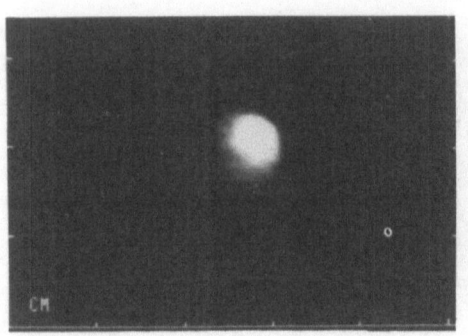 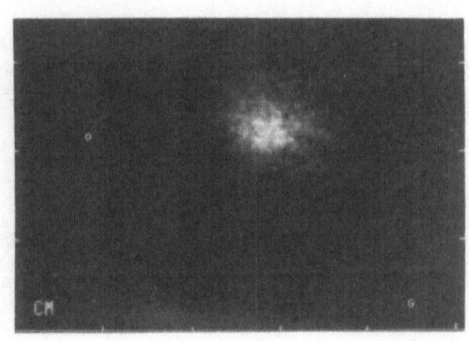

a) PSF for 1cm ox-brain   b) PSF for 2-3cms adult palm

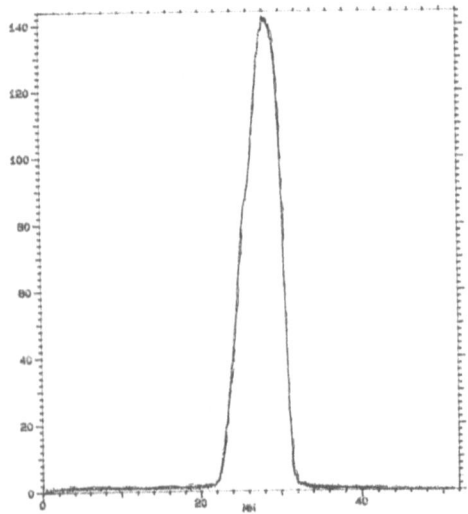 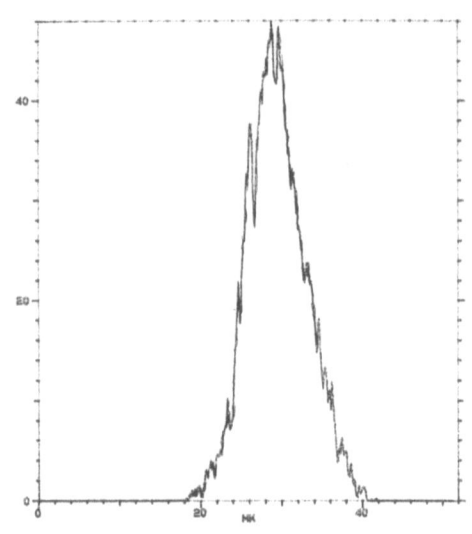

c) Density profile of a)   d) Density profile of b)

Figure 14 : Point Spread Functions (PSF) for brain and hand measured using a Helium-Neon Laser aligned on the imaging axis of the detector.

the tissue changed significantly with time.

Table 2. Half maximum widths of the Point Spread Functions for ox-brain tissue - theoretical and experimental

Tissue	Depth in tissue (mm)	PSF Half-maximum width (mm)
Theoretical :		
Ox-Brain	4.0	7.6
(derived from Eq. (5))	8.0	15.2
	12.0	22.8
	16.0	30.4
Experimental :		
Ox-Brain		
(from Figure 14a)	10.0	3.0
Human Palm (from 14b)	30-40	7.0

If the PSF can be accurately characterised for different depths of tissue, we can attempt to deconvolve the image by an appropriate function dependent on the depth of the tissue. We suppose the tissue acts as a linear transfer function H_d on the object function f_d so that

$$g = H_d f_d + n$$

where g is the detected image and n is noise. The functions f_d represent the perturbations f(r) in Equation 10, and the transfer function H_d is the effect of the Green's Function. Strictly, it is incorrect to assume spatial stationarity of H_d, so that Fourier deconvolution would be invalid.

A more generalised technique would be to use pseudo-inversion by Singular Value Decomposition. If f_d and g are represented as column vectors of size n and m respectively then H_d is an nXm matrix. The ith column of H_d is the one-dimensional representation of the PSF obtained by applying a delta- function at the ith position in f_d. Thus in principle it would be possible to apply a laser at different points on the input side of the tissue sample, and record the varying PSF functions at each position for inclusion in H_d. This analysis is attractive in that in effect it allows for a spatially variant Green's Function in (10), and releases us from the necessity of assuming constant diffusion properties. In addition, an iterative technique could be applied to re-estimate the form of H_d after an initial solution for f_d.

Pseudo inversion is very costly computationally. An example using only 64 points in f_d took five minutes to invert on an Amdahl 470 at the University of London. The future for this approach would probably lie in the ability to store singular vectors in a lookup table as tissue characteristics, and use fast parallel processing to provide crude on-line inversion. More detailed experiments are required to derive the form of H_d for different tissues at different wavelengths.

4.5 Instrumentation Improvements

By scanning a collimated source and detector synchronously we can reduce the photon density $P(\mathbf{r})$ off axis. We thus eliminate the second order terms in (12) but accept terms of the form:

$$\iiint_V\int_\Omega\int_\Omega F_z\frac{d\sigma(\hat{\mathbf{z}},\hat{\mathbf{r}}_1)}{d\Omega}\ \frac{d\sigma(\hat{\mathbf{r}}_1,\hat{\mathbf{r}}_2)}{d\Omega}\ \frac{d\sigma(\hat{\mathbf{r}}_2,\hat{\mathbf{z}})}{d\Omega}d\Omega(\hat{\mathbf{r}}_1)d\Omega(\hat{\mathbf{r}}_2)dV$$

integrated over all angles for $\mathbf{r}_1$ and $\mathbf{r}_2$ and throughout the volume of the sample, as shown in figure 9b.

Figure 15 shows a system used by Professor Kaneko at Hamamatsu University, in collaboration with Hamamatsu Photonics K.K., to test this technique [25]. The top row of pictures in figure 16 show the images obtained with a broad white light input beam and an uncollimated detector, similar to the experiment described in section 4.3. Here the scattering solution is fresh milk, so that scattering is much higher, an estimate for the mean free path between scattering events being about 0.3mm. The overall path length is only 4cms. and the size of the wire being imaged is 2.6mm in diameter - nearly twice the diameter of the largest wire in figure 10. The wire is imaged at decreasing depths from the detector. Clearly the object is unresolvable until almost at the front (detector) face of the phantom.

Using a laser and detecting slit scanned synchronously, the images in the bottom row of figure 16 were reconstructed. The resolution is good near the input and output surfaces of the phantom, but rather worse in the centre of the phantom, where the combined effect of the diffused input beam and large PSF is maximal. Clearly a considerable improvement is achieved. Some **in-vitro** and **in-vivo** work in this area has been done by Jarry et.al. [26].

A system is at present under development at UCH to perform one dimensional scanning. A narrow fibre coupled to a self-focussing lens is used to produce a collimated input beam. The line of scan can be rotated tomographically, to allow two-dimensional reconstructions of a slice. As yet no measurements have been taken.

5.0 TEMPORAL MEASUREMENTS

Advancements in ultra-high speed camera and light source technology have made pico-second time resolution possible [27]. If we used fast light pulses in synchrony with a high speed shutter and camera, it is in principle possible to select only the totally unscattered photons, by time-of-flight determinations. Then the attenuation coefficient for the measured signal will be the line integral of (w+k) along the projection line. The problem to be faced in this modality is whether such high selection will reduce the number of photons detected to a level where noise will be dominant, since the maximum level of input flux is necessarily limited by safety considerations. For example, for a BPD of 6cms attenuation would be of the order of 15_2OD. The maximum allowed radiation dose is 2000Wm^{-2} (10^{16} photons s^{-1} mm^{-2}), so that only 10 photons s^{-1} mm^{-2} would be transmitted on average. Although detectable, Shott noise alone would constitute a 30% of the signal. Thus this modality would probably require long sampling times. For thinner tissue samples, this approach may

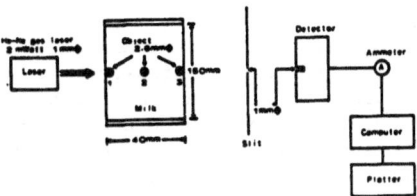

Figure 15 : Schematic of system to scan source and detector (courtesy of Hamamatsu Ltd.)

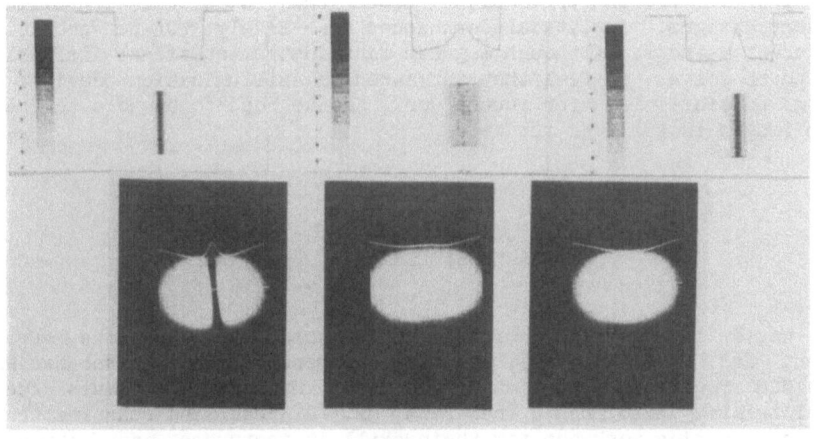

a) depth = 40mm   b) depth = 20mm   c) depth = 0mm

Figure 16 : The top picures are images of a 2.6mm wire at different depths in undiluted milk solution obtained with uncollimated detector and broad (collimated) light source. Density profiles are also recorded on the image. The lower pictures are the intensity profiles reconstructed from the counts of transmitted photons when the source and detector were scanned synchronously.

be practical with clinically acceptable scan times.

6.0 CONCLUSIONS

We have shown that tissue of up to several cms. in thickness is sufficiently transparent in the near infra-red to allow detection of transmitted photons. Analytical expressions for the transmitted flux as a function of tissue characteristics and structure are formidable but provide a formalism within which to investigate the degree of information available as we impose different forms of specificity on the measurements.

Spectral specificity provides good sensitivity to changes in oxygenation state, and is likely to provide a useful clinical tool. Spatial specificity appears to be poor, although there is a possibility of resolving structure to a depth of at least one cm. Temporal specificity would provide well- resolved structure provided that noise levels are not too high. A combination of these methods (i.e. a narrow-bandwidth, small diameter, time gated source and collector) would allow analysis mathematically in the same way as CT, NMR etc.

We have presented only some preliminary results. More detailed experimental determinations of tissue absorption and scattering characteristics are necessary. Monte-Carlo models for photon propogation would provide useful predictions about the usefulness of different instrument designs. Analytical techniques are likely to be prohibitive with present methods. Although a great many instrumentational difficulties remain to be solved, we feel that infra-red transillumination provides many exciting possibilities for future work, and we hope to be able to present **in-vivo** images in the near future.

ACKNOWLEDGEMENTS

We would like to thank Professor EOR Reynolds, Dr. P Hope, Dr. P Hamilton, and Dr. J Wyatt, and other members of staff in the Neo-Natal Unit at UCH for their continuing advice, interest and assistance in clinical trials. Also Mr. J Treherene, Mr. G Brown, and other members of UCH Medical Physics workshop for their skill in instrument manufacture.

This work was supported by a Wolfson Foundation grant number Z/81/21, and SERC grant number GR/C/b5582, and by Hamamatsu Photonics K.K.

REFERENCES

1. Pape KE, Wigglesworth JS : Haemorrhage, Ischaemia and the Perinatal Brain. Heinemann, London,1979.

2. Stewart AL, Thorburn RJ, Hope PL, Goldsmith M, Lipscomb AP, Reynolds EOR : Ultrasound Appearance of the Brain in Very Preterm Infants and Neurodevelopmental Outcome at 18 Months of Age. Arch. Dis. Child **58**, 598- 604, 1983

3. Cady EB, Costello AM deL, Dawson MJ, Delpy DT, Hope PL, Reynolds EOR, Tofts PR, Wilkie DR : Non-Invasive Investigation of Cerebral Metabolism in Newborn Infants by Phosphorous Nuclear Magnetic Resonance Spectroscopy. Lancet, **14th May**, 1059-1062, 1983.

4. Wharton DC, Tzagoloff A : Studies on the Electron Transport Chain - LVII: The Near Infrared Absorption band of Cytochrome Oxidase. J. Bio. Chem.**239**(6) 2036-2041, 1963

5. Jobsis FF : Noninvasive, Infrared Monitoring of Cerebral and Myocardial Oxygen Sufficiency and Circulatory Parameters. Science **198** : 1264-1267,1977

6. Mook P, Proctor H, Jobsis F, Wildevuur Ch R : Assessment of Brain Oxygenation: A Comparison between an Oxygen Electrode and Near Infrared Spectrophotometry. Adv. Exp. Med. Biol. **169** : 841-847,1984.

7. Van der Hulst H : Light Scattering by Small Particles . Wiley (New York),1957.

8. Takatani S, Graham MD : Theoretical Analysis of Diffuse Reflectance from a Two-Layer Model. IEEE Bio. Eng. **BME 26(12)** 656-664,1979.

9. Anderson NM, Sekelj P : Light Absorbing and Scattering Properties of Non-Haemolysed Blood. Phys. Med. Biol. **12** 173-184,1966

10. Anderson NM, Sekelj P : Reflection and Transmission of Light by Thin Films of Non-haemolysed Blood. Phys. Med. Biol. **12** 185-192,1966

11. Barbenel JC : Backscattering of Light by Red Cell Suspensions. Med. Biol. Eng. **17** 763-768,1979.

12. Eason G, Veitch A, Nisbet R, Turnbull F : The theory of the Backscattering of Light by Blood. J.Phys D **11**: 1463-1479,1978.

13. Gate LF:The Determination of Light Absorbtion in Diffusing Materials by a Photon Diffusion Model. J. Phys. D : Appl. Phys. **4** 1049-1056,1973.

14. Janssen FJ: A Study of the Absorbtion and Scattering Factors of Light in Whole Blood. Med. Biol. Eng. **10** 231-240,1972.

15. Johnson CC: Optical Diffusion in Blood. IEEE BME **17(2)** 129-133,1970.

16. Longini R, Zdrojkowski R : A Note on the Theory of Backscattering of Light by Blood. IEEE Trans. Bio-Med. Eng. **BME-15** 4-10,1968.

17. Svaasand LO, Doiron DR, Profio AE: Light Distribution In Tissue During Photoradiation Therapy. University of Southern California, Institute for Physics and Imaging Science, Report MISG 900-02,1981.

18. Wilson BC, Jeeves WP, Lowe DM, Adam G : Light Propagation in Animal Tissues in The Wavelength Range 375-825 Nanometers. Report from Ontario Cancer Foundation and McMaster University, Hamilton, Ontario, Canada,1984.

19. Svaasand LO: Dosimetry for Photodynamic Therapy of Malignant Tumours. Report RB/PE 032 Divisions of Radiation Biology and Physical Electronics University of Trondheim, Norway,1984.

20. Maarek JM, Jarry G, De Cosnac B, Bui-Mong-Hung: Simulation of Transillumination Through Blood and Tissues. Proc. World Congress on Medical Physics and Biomedical Engineering, Hamburg,1982.

21. Wilson BC, Adam G : A Monte-Carlo Model for the Absorbtion and Flux Distribution of Light in Tissue. Med. Phys. **10**: 824-830,1983.

22. Kubelka P: New Contributions to the Optics of Intensely Light-

Scattering Materials Part 1. J. Opt. Soc. Am. **38(5)** 448-457,1948.

23. McKelvy JP, Longini RL, Brady TP : Alternative Approach to the Solution of Added Carrier Transport Problems in Semiconductors. Phys. Rev. **123(1)** 51-57,1961.

24. Shockley W: Diffusion and Drift of Minority Carriers in Semiconductors for Comparable Capture and Scattering Mean Free Paths. Phys. Rev. **125(5)** 1570-1576,1962

25. Kaneko M, Goto S, Fukaya T, Isoda H, Hayashi T, Hayakawa T, Yamashita Y : Fundamental Studies of Image Diagnosis by Visual Lights. Proc of Medical Imaging Technology Conference, Tokyo,1984.

26. Jarry G, Ghesquiere S, Maarek JM, Debray S, Bui-Mong-Hung, Laurent D : Imaging Mammalian Tissues and Organs Using Laser Collimated Transillumination. J.Biomed. Eng. 6 70-74,1984

27. Duguay MA, Mattick AT : Ultrahigh Speed Photography of Picosecond Light Pulses and Echoes. Appl. Opt. **10(6)** 2162-2170,1971.

THE USE OF SET THEORY AND CLUSTER ANALYSIS TO INVESTIGATE THE CONSTRAINT PROBLEM IN FACTOR ANALYSIS IN DYNAMIC STRUCTURES (FADS)

A.S. HOUSTON
Department of Nuclear Medicine, Royal Naval Hospital, Haslar, Gosport, Hampshire. PO12 2AA. UK.

1. INTRODUCTION
1.1. Conventional Factor Analysis in Dynamic Studies

In recent years factor analysis has played an increasingly important role in the analysis of nuclear medicine dynamic studies. Schmidlin (1979) demonstrated how the technique could be applied to a time sequence of images where each pixel gives rise to a dynamic curve (sometimes called a dixel). The premise is made that each dixel may be approximated by a linear combination of a few components. These are chosen in such a way that, for a given number of components, the least squares error of the approximation to the population of dixels is a minimum.

Schmidlin pre-processes the data using the normalisation of Benzécri (1973), ie if n_{it} is the count in the ith pixel of the tth frame, and if $n_i = \sum_t n_{it}$ and $n_t = \sum_i n_{it}$, then the processed value is $p_{it} = n_{it}/\sqrt{(n_i n_t)}$. With this normalisation it may be shown that the original counts may be approximated by

$$n_{it} \approx \frac{n_i n_t}{n} \sum_{k=0}^{T-1} \frac{F_{ik} G_{kt}}{\sqrt{\lambda_k}}$$

where $n = \sum_i n_i$, T is the number of components, G_{kt} and λ_k are the factors and eigenvalues calculated by orthogonalisation of the correlation matrix

$$r_{tt'} = \sum_i (n_{it} n_{it'}/(n_i n_t \cdot n_i n_{t'})^{\frac{1}{2}})$$

and F_{ik} are the factor loadings or coefficients which are calculated using

$$F_{ik} = \frac{1}{n_i} \sum_t n_{it} \frac{G_{kt}}{\sqrt{\lambda_k}} \quad k = 0, 1, ---$$

It should be noted that $G_{Ot} = 1$; $f_{iO} = 1$ and $\lambda_0 = 1$ for all values of t and i. This is called the trivial factor. Note also that factors $n_t^{\frac{1}{2}} G_{kt}$ are orthogonal.

The results of applying such an analysis to a gated cardiac study of a patient with a large aneurysm are shown in Fig 1 where the first two non-trivial factors and the corresponding factor loading images are displayed.

Two views (anterior and LAO) were used to create the factors although only one (anterior) is shown.

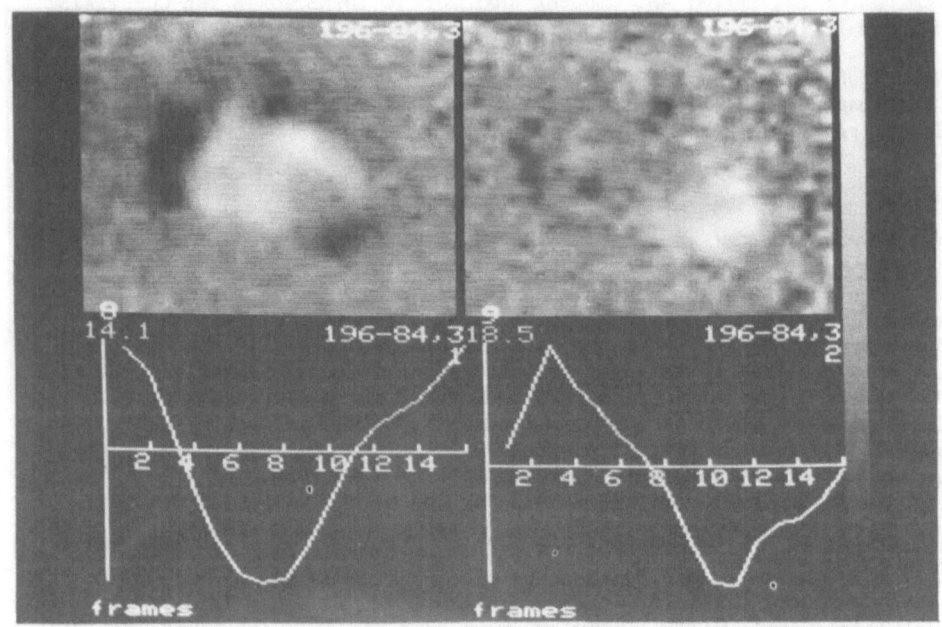

FIGURE 1. First two non-trivial factors and corresponding anterior factor loading images for gated cardiac study of patient with a large aneurysm.

1.2. Factor Analysis in Dynamic Structures

While such a technique is useful in reducing the dimensionality of the problem, it has been criticised as bearing little relationship to physiology. In an attempt to overcome this objection, Bazin et al (1979) and Barber (1980) have attempted to transform the data in such a way that the results are physiologically meaningful. This technique has become known as FADS (Factor Analysis in Dynamic Structures) (Cavailloles et al, 1984).

The criterion adopted is that physiological data in nuclear medicine never contain negative values. Hence if the results of a factor analysis can be transformed in such a way that the factors and factor loadings are non-negative, then this may bear some resemblence to the true physiological situation.

In order to demonstrate how such a transformation is implemented, it is useful to assume that three homogeneous compartments are involved. It may then be shown in the absence of noise that any dixel may be formed using two non-trivial components. In fact, the representative physiological curve for each compartment may also be formed in this way. If the non-trivial factor loadings are plotted against one another, it follows that there will exist three points in the plane corresponding to the physiological curves.

These points will lie within the domain of non-negative factors, ie the domain inside which all reconstructed curves will be non-negative. If the coefficient or contribution images are to be non-negative, it is a necessary

and sufficient condition that all dixel points lie inside or on the
triangle formed with the physiological factor points as its apices.
Barber (1980) used an apex-finding routine to find a close-fitting triangle
around the dixel points with apices inside the domain of non-negative
factors, although, in theory, any triangle inside the domain and including
the dixel points will satisfy the non-negativity criterion. Fig 2 shows
the dixel points (F_{ik}) and domain of non-negative factors for the gated

cardiac study used in Fig 1. Factors formed from points within the domain
will be positive everywhere while points on the domain limits will produce
factors with at least one zero. It is apparent that the scope for choosing
a triangle is great. Since the choice of triangle is crucial, it is clear
that further investigation into the use of the technique is warranted.

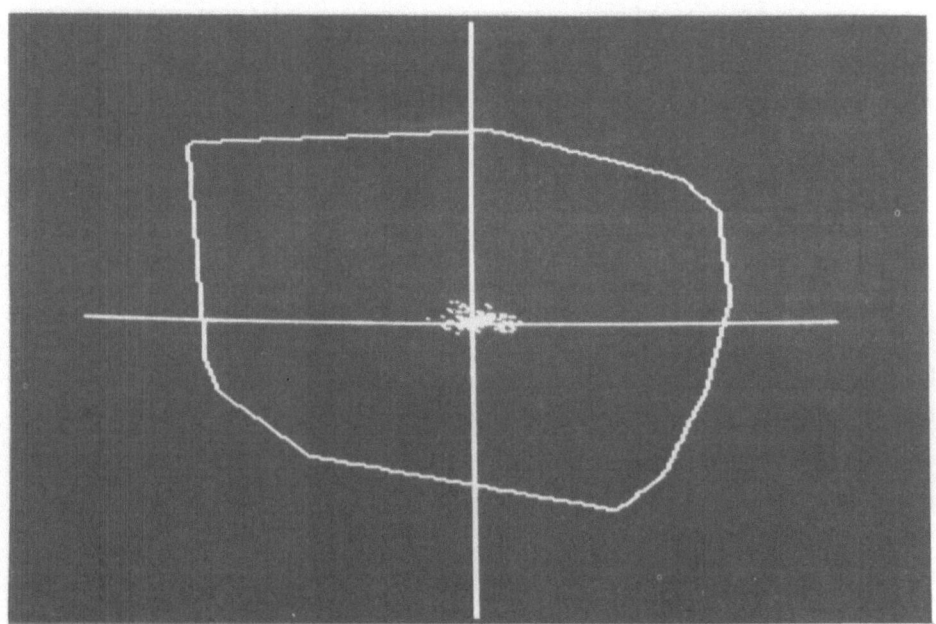

FIGURE 2. Dixel points and domain of non-negative factors for gated
cardiac study.

NB Here and elsewhere in the paper a two dimension situation corresponding
to three compartments is adopted for demonstration purposes. The theory
can be extended to N compartments and N-1 factors using the appropriate
geometrical configurations.

2. RELATIONSHIP BETWEEN APICES AND FACTOR IMAGES
In a recent paper, Houston (1984) examined the effect on the factor images
of errors in the position of an apex. It was concluded that such an error
merely scaled the corresponding factor image but could have quite significant effects on the other images. This rather paradoxical result further
demonstrates the need for controlling how these apices are chosen.
  In the same paper it was shown that the line joining two apices represented
the line of zero contribution of the compartment corresponding to the third

apex. It was also shown that the contribution, α_i, of this compartment to the ith pixel, is given by dividing the perpendicular distance from the ith dixel point to the line by the perpendicular distance from the apex to the line. This result is shown in Fig 3 where

$$\alpha_i = \frac{XE}{AD} = \frac{HD}{AD} = \frac{FB}{AB} = \frac{GC}{AC}$$

If β_i and δ_i are the contributions of the other compartments we have

$$\alpha_i + \beta_i + \delta_i = 1$$

Factor (or contribution) images are formed using $n_i\alpha_i$, $n_i\beta_i$, and $n_i\delta_i$.

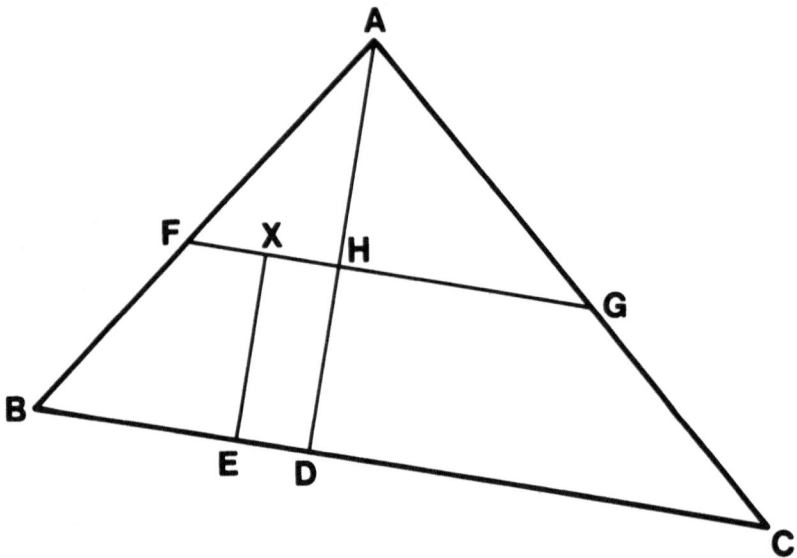

FIGURE 3. Contribution of compartment (A) to dixel (X).

3. USE OF SET THEORY
3.1. Set Theory and Assumptions
Set theory is used to investigate the conditions under which the use of an apex-seeking routine is valid.
 Again, let us assume that there exist three homogeneous compartments, A, B and C. Each dixel will be represented by one of the following sets: $\{A\}$ (defined by $A_\cap B'_\cap C'$; or A present, B and C absent), $\{B\}$, $\{C\}$, $\{A,B\}$, $\{B,C\}$, $\{C,A\}$, $\{A,B,C\}$ (It is assumed that $S_\cap A'_\cap B'_\cap C' = \emptyset$, since such dixels would not be of use).
 Two assumptions are made:
(i) If two or more compartments overlap, it is assumed that they contain sufficient relative contribution variation within the dixels in order to be identified as independent.
(ii) Sufficient prior physiological knowledge is available to say which sets are present in any study. Practically, this may be difficult in

certain pathological situations but is assumed for the present as a means to an end.

Given the validity of these assumptions it is clear that each set will define a geometrical configuration, the dimension of which equals the number of elements in the set. In particular, a one-element set will define an apex and a two-element set a side of the triangle to be used in the transformation (the line of zero contribution of the missing element). The first assumption ensures that a two-element set will not plot onto a single point.

Suppose that sets $\{A,B\}$ and $\{A,C\}$ are present in a study. Then we are able to define lines AB and AC which intersect at point A. This corresponds to an intersection of sets, ie $\{A,B\} \cap \{A,C\} = \{A\}$. Similarly if sets $\{A\}$ and $\{B\}$ are present, then the line joining points A and B is known, corresponding to a union of sets, ie $\{A\} \cup \{B\} = \{A,B\}$. Hence as well as explicitly defined sets, ie sets which are actually present, we also have implicitly defined sets, ie sets that may be formed from explicit sets using union or intersection.

The apex-seeking routine assumes a triangle tight around the dixel points. Hence some points will always lie on each side of the triangle (either between or at both apices). It follows that the routine may be used only when all possible sets are defined either explicitly or implicitly. Note that set $\{A,B,C\}$ corresponds to the plane and will always be defined (from the union of all explicit sets).

3.2. Cardiac Example

Let us now consider an example. Suppose sets $\{A,B\}$, $\{A,C\}$ and $\{A,B,C\}$ are present, as might be the case if A were background. $\{A\}$ may be defined implicitly from $\{A,B\} \cap \{A,C\}$ even if there are no pixels corresponding to pure background. Sets $\{B\}$ and $\{C\}$ remain undefined. However, we know that apex B must lie on line AB and apex C on line AC. Hence we require two one-dimensional constraints.

The domain of non-negative factors may be used to define the limits of the constraint. It may be shown that the line AB will cut the domain at precisely two points, D and E. Hence B must lie between or at one of these points. In general, dixel points from set $\{A,B\}$ will lie to one side of apex A, say towards D. Point B will therefore lie in the interval $]A,D]$.

It is clear from this argument that, if the domain is reasonably tight around the dixel points, errors produced by the apex-seeking routine will be small.

4. APPLICATION TO THE DEPENDENT FACTOR PROBLEM
4.1. Dependent Factor Problem

Figs 1 and 2 showed the results of applying factor analysis to a gated cardiac study of a patient with a large aneurysm. When FADS is applied, the resulting curves correspond to ventricular, atrial, and pathological compartments. It may at first seem logical to go to three-dimensions in order to identify a fourth compartment corresponding to background. However, in the case of cardiac dynamic studies obtained at equilibrium the background curve is almost identical to the mean curve, ie flat. Hence the coefficients of all non-trivial components will be close to zero, ie background will be well described by a point close to the origin on the plane described by the first two orthogonal factors.

The four physiological factors are therefore linearly dependent, ie each may be constructed using a linear combination of the other three.

4.2. Assumptions and General Solution

Four linearly dependent factors will plot in the plane in one of three ways (see Fig 4).

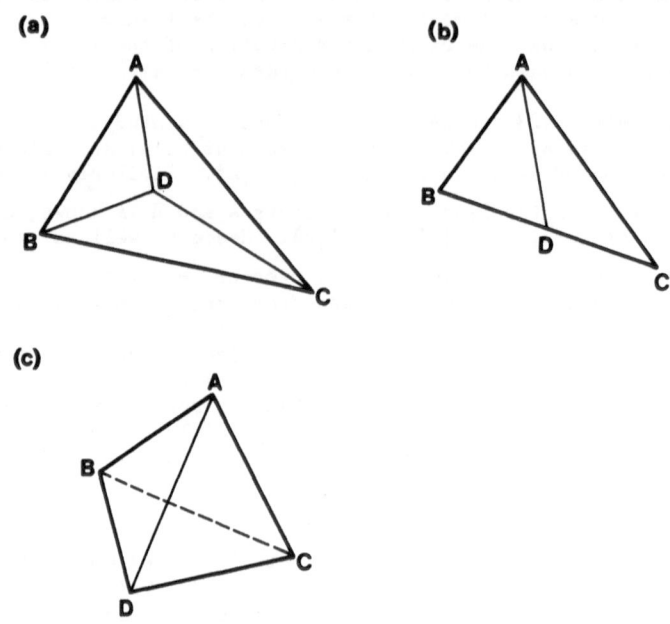

(a)

(b)

(c)

FIGURE 4. Possible configurations for four dependent factors plotting in two dimensions.

Let us consider case (a). In the absence of factor D, we have for the i^{t} dixel

$$f_i(t) = \alpha_i g_A(t) + \beta_i g_B(t) + \gamma_i g_C(t)$$

where f_i is the dixel, and g_A, g_B, g_C are the physiological factors corresponding to A, B and C respectively. If factor D exists, we have

$$g_D(t) = a g_A(t) + b g_B(t) + c g_C(t)$$

Hence, for some δ_i

$$f_i(t) = (\alpha_i - a\delta_i)g_A(t) + (\beta_i - b\delta_i)g_B(t) + (\gamma_i - c\delta_i)g_C(t) + \delta_i g_D(t)$$

Suppose we choose δ_i such that $\min\left\{(\alpha_i - \delta_i a), (\beta_i - \delta_i b), (\gamma_i - \delta_i c)\right\} = 0$

Without loss of generality we may assume that

$$\alpha_i = \delta_i a; \ \beta_i \geqslant \delta_i b; \ \gamma_i \geqslant \delta_i c$$

Then $f_i(t) = (\beta_i - b\delta_i)g_B(t) + (\gamma_i - c\delta_i)g_C(t) + \delta_i g_D(t)$

ie our assumption is equivalent to dixel i having no contribution from one
of the other factors, in this case A.
Let us now assume that $A_\wedge B_\wedge C = \emptyset$. From Fig 5 we have

$$a = \frac{BF}{AB}; \quad b = \frac{CG}{BC}; \quad \alpha_i = \frac{BE}{AB}; \quad \beta_i = \frac{CH}{BC};$$

$$\delta_i = \frac{\alpha_i}{a} = \frac{BE}{AB} \frac{AB}{BF} = \frac{BE}{BF} = \frac{GL}{GD}$$

$$\beta_i - \delta_i b = \frac{CH}{BC} - \frac{GL}{GD} \frac{CG}{BC} = \frac{CH}{BC} - \frac{GL}{BC} \frac{CG}{GD} = \frac{CH}{BC} - \frac{HX}{BC} \frac{HK}{HX}$$

$$= \frac{CH-HK}{BC} = \frac{CK}{BC}$$

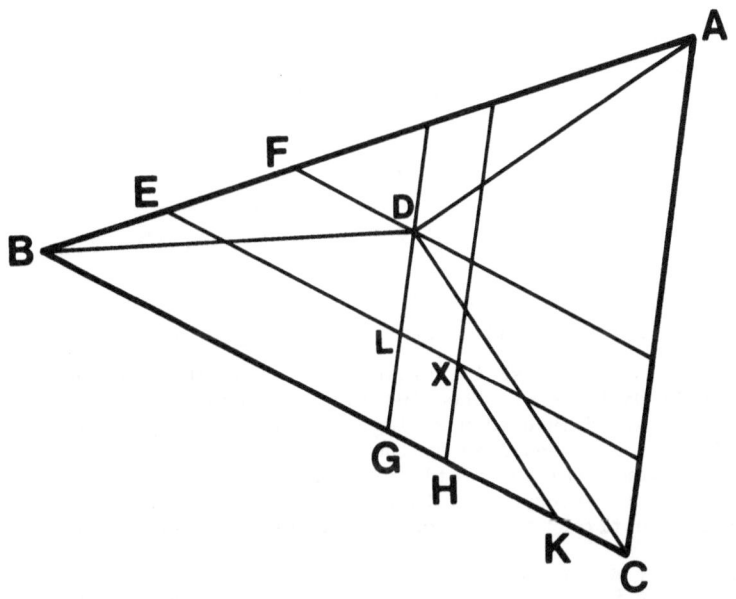

FIGURE 5. Configuration corresponding to case (a).

These are the coefficients of g_D and g_B that would be obtained by applying
the conventional method to ΔBCD. Since a similar result holds for the
coefficient of g_C, it may be concluded that we may apply the method to Δs
BCD, CAD and ABD (and the dixel points therein). Similar results may be
proved for cases (b) and (c), although the assumptions will be different.
In case (b), it must be assumed that $B_\wedge C = \emptyset$ while case (c) needs one of
two assumptions, ie either (i) $B_\wedge C = \emptyset$, where Δs ABD and ACD would be
considered separately, or (ii) $A_\wedge D = \emptyset$, where Δs ABC and BCD would be used.

These assumptions are necessary to ensure the non-ambiguity of contributing compartments to any given dixel. If this is known from physiological considerations then the assumption may be relaxed to $A_\wedge B_\wedge C_\wedge D = \emptyset$ for cases (a) and (c), and $B_\wedge C_\wedge D = \emptyset$ for case (b).

4.3. Cardiac Example
In the case of the cardiac example, let us define compartment A as aneurysm, B as atrium, C as ventricle, and D as background. Sets present will include $\{A,D\}$, $\{B,D\}$, $\{C,D\}$, $\{D\}$; while $\{A,C,D\}$ and $\{B,C,D\}$ will almost certainly be present also. Hence, if this example corresponds to case (a), the assumption that $A_\wedge B_\wedge C = \emptyset$ will hold. However, if case (b) is true (assuming D lies on line BC), the assumption that $B_\wedge C = \emptyset$ will probably not be true. In the unlikely event that case (c) is true (with D opposite A), then neither $B_\wedge C = \emptyset$ nor $A_\wedge D = \emptyset$ will hold.

5. USE OF GRAVITATIONAL CLUSTER ANALYSIS
5.1. Generalised Markovian Model
The problem of identifying sets in both pattern and feature space is tackled using gravitational cluster analysis on the dixel points. An adaptation of the generalised Markovian model (Wright, 1977) is adopted. In this model the gravitational function is

$$g(i,t,dt) = dt^2 \sum_{\substack{j \in N(t) \\ j \neq i}} \frac{m_i^p(t)\, m_j^q(t)}{m_i(t)} \cdot \frac{s_j(t) - s_i(t)}{\left| s_j(t) - s_i(t) \right|^3}$$

where $m_i(t)$ and $m_j(t)$ are the masses of the ith and j^{th} particles, $s_i(t)$ and $s_j(t)$ their positions, and p and q real numbers. In each time interval the length dt of the interval is determined so that the fastest moving particle travels distance δ. When two particles come within distance ϵ of each other, they are joined into a single particle at their centroid. Parameters δ and ϵ are specified by the operator. The Markovian model differs from conventional gravitational clustering in that $g(i,t,dt)$ is independent of past history. In other words, the velocities of the particles are effectively set to zero at the start of each interval.

5.2. Adaptation of Model
In the adopted model, p and q are given zero values. This is known as the unit attraction Markovian model and is less dependent on large clusters. The model is adapted by dividing by $\sqrt{m_i(t)}$ instead of $m_i(t)$ in the formula for the gravitational function. This ensures that, while large clusters do not have a greater attraction due to size (since p=q=0), neither do they move more slowly in direct proportion to their size (Wright, 1977). It should be noted that this adaptation of the model is not centroid-preserving.

5.3. Cardiac Example
Fig 6 shows the results of applying the model to the gated cardiac study previously considered. For demonstration purposes five clusters are shown in both pattern and feature space. These could be said to correspond to sets $\{D\}$, $\{D,B\}$, $\{D,A\}$, $\{D,A,C\}$ and $\{D,C\}$ in order of increasing

brightness. The cluster corresponding to $\{D,A,C\}$ also contains points from $\{D,C\}$ with low ventricular contribution, while set $\{D,B,C\}$ is not identified.

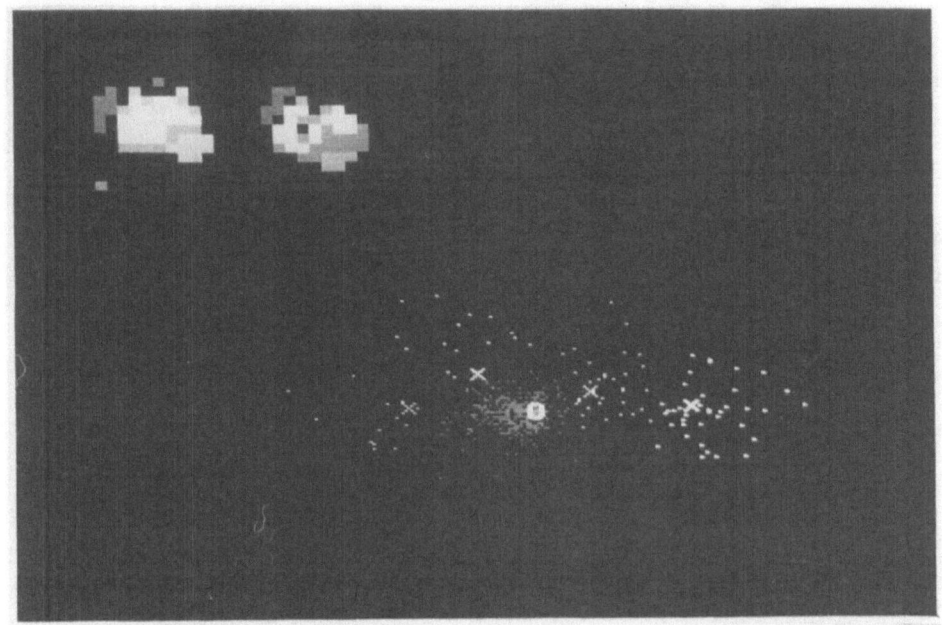

FIGURE 6. Gravitational clustering applied to gated cardiac study. Five clusters are depicted with current positions of centroids shown as crosses.

6. DEFINITION OF TRANSFORMATION ELEMENTS
6.1. Definition of Elements
Given that sets present in a study may be defined using gravitational clustering, the next problem is defining the geometrical configuration corresponding to that set. For instance how does one define the point D from the cluster corresponding to the set $\{D\}$, or the line DC from the cluster corresponding to $\{D,C\}$.

In the one-dimensional case it seems sensible to use the centroid of the cluster. For higher dimensions, a least-squares fit, with or without constraints to pass through points, lines etc., would appear to be fairly realistic. A problem which arises is that conventional least-squares fitting is axis dependent, eg different straight lines may be drawn through a set of points depending on whether errors are assumed in y or x. Since it is felt that errors in F_{ik} will be of the same order for different k, it was decided to use the squares of the perpendicular errors as the criterion for minimisation.

For two non-trivial components this corresponds to
(a) One dimensional set: point (x_c, y_c) is given by

$$x_c = \bar{x} = \frac{\sum x_i}{N}; \; y_c = \bar{y} = \frac{\sum y_i}{N}$$

(b) Two dimensional set (unconstrained); line $y = mx + c$ is given by

$$m = \frac{B \pm \sqrt{B^2 + 4A^2}}{2A} \quad ; \quad c = \frac{-m\Sigma x_i + \Sigma y_i}{N} = -m\bar{x} + \bar{y}$$

where $\quad A = \Sigma x_i y_i - \frac{\Sigma x_i \cdot \Sigma y_i}{N}$

$$B = \frac{(\Sigma x_i)^2}{N} - \frac{(\Sigma y_i)^2}{N} - \Sigma x_i^2 + \Sigma y_i^2$$

(c) Two dimensional set (passing through point (x_o, y_o)): line $y = mx + c$ is given by

$$m = \frac{B \pm \sqrt{B^2 + 4A^2}}{2A} \quad ; \quad c = -mx_o + y_o$$

where $\quad A = \Sigma \left\{ (y_i - y_o)^2 - (x_i - x_o)^2 \right\}$

$$B = \Sigma (x_i - x_o) \cdot (y_i - y_o)$$

In each case the summations are over all relevant values of i.
Clearly the methodology may be extended to deal with situations involving higher dimensions.

6.2. Cardiac Example
Fig 7 shows the results of using clusters to define one apex (D) and three lines corresponding to BD, AD and CD and numbered clockwise starting at $y = -\infty$. An unconstrained line is also defined using the clusters identify-ing $\{C, D\}$ and $\{B, D\}$. Given that fairly large clusters spreads are apparent, the difference between this line and BD and CD as previously defined is very small. It would appear that this case corresponds to case (b) of section 4. In order to proceed we must now assume $B_\wedge C = \emptyset$, an assumption which is

probably invalid. The effects of this will be apparent later.
In practice, it was found that 5 clusters were too few in order to define the transformation. For example, in Figs 6 & 7 several of the points in the background cluster were thought to contain some contribution from the other compartments. A purer solution was found by displaying 15 clusters and defining unconstrained lines AD and BC using combinations of these clusters. Unfortunately, this is impossible to display in black and white.

7. DEFINITION OF CONSTRAINTS
7.1. Examples of Constraints
Although it is not the main purpose of this paper to define the form of the constraints, it might be interesting to discuss constraints which could be applied in certain situations.
Perhaps the simplest situation is where it is known that a physiological factor will have at least one zero. If we also know that the apex lies on a line, then it may be defined to lie at the intersection of the line and the boundary of the domain of non-negative factors.
Nijran and Barber (1983) proposed that a physiological factor could be constrained to lie at the intersection of study space, defined by the

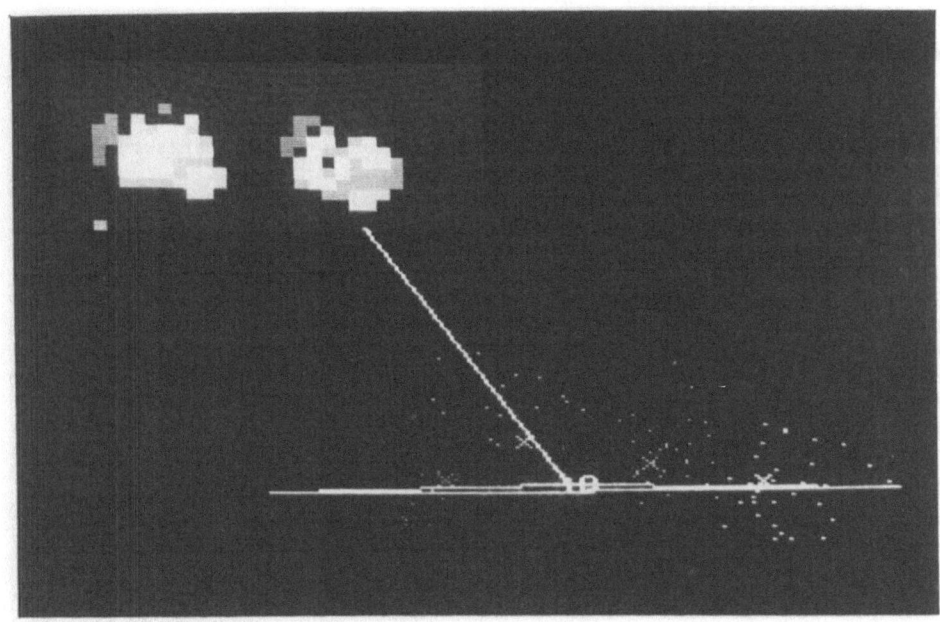

FIGURE 7. Apex (corresponding to D) and three constrained lines (corresponding to BD, AD, CD) defined as in text. Unconstrained line (corresponding to BC) is also shown.

orthogonal factors, and theory space, which is defined from physiological considerations such as a compartmental analysis. In two dimensions, this may be regarded as finding the point in the plane which makes most physiological sense, eg gives the best fit to a family of possible curves. If we know that this point lies on a line, the dimension of the domain of the constraint is reduced. This will be more significant at higher dimensions where, for example, a five dimensional problem might be reduced to a one, two, or three dimensional problem.

7.2. Cardiac Example

Unfortunately, neither of these procedures is applicable to our gated cardiac problem. Ventricular curves never contain zeros, and the line corresponding to ventricle will give rise to a family of ventricular-like curves with different ejection fractions. If the ejection fraction is known, it is possible to use this as a constraint, but this would appear to defeat the object of the entire exercise.

7.2.1. Interpolative Background Subtraction. Goris (1976) has suggested using interpolative background subtraction as a pre-processing routine. A rectangle is chosen surrounding the organ and with the perimeter passing through background alone. If the co-ordinates of top left and lower right corners of the rectangle are (k, m) and (l, n) then the amount of background subtraction at point (i, j) within the rectangle is given by

$$B_{ij} = (B_i + B_j)/2$$

where $B_i = \left\{ (j-m)c_{in} + (n-j)c_{im} \right\}/(n-m)$

and $B_j = \left\{ (i-k)c_{1j} + (1-i)c_{kj} \right\}/(1-k)$

If this is used before factor analysis, two problems arise.
(i) The rectangle must be defined. If this is done by an operator, the method becomes subjective.
(ii) Since a subtraction technique is involved, noise in the image will be increased. This leads to noisier orthogonal factors with a subsequent increase in errors.
7.2.2. <u>Definition of Constraint</u>. It is however possible to use an adaptation of this technique as a constraint. Background pixels may be defined using the appropriate cluster. Values of these pixels may be set from the summed view. The remaining values may be calculated using the Goris formula and the nearest background value in each of four directions (horizontally and vertically). Suitable adaptation of the formula is made if such a value is not found in any direction. In this way a composite background matrix $\left[B_{ij} \right]$ is formed. An attempt is now made to find apices on the three lines previously defined (case (b) of section 4 applies).
It is convenient to transform the axis so that the centroid of the background cluster (x_c, y_c) is the new origin, ie,

$$x'_{ij} = x_{ij} - x_c$$

$$y'_{ij} = y_{ij} - y_c$$

If a dixel point lies in the sector defined by lines 1 and 2, it may be shown that the background contribution image will be B_{ij} ,

where $\hat{B}_{ij} = n_{ij} + n_{ij} \dfrac{(y'_{ij} - m_1 x'_{ij})}{(m_1 - m_2)\, X_2} - n_{ij} \dfrac{(y'_{ij} - m_2 x'_{ij})}{(m_1 - m_2)\, X_1}$

where (x'_{ij}, y'_{ij}) is the position of (i, j)th dixel, n_{ij} is the summed view value, m_1 and m_2 are the slopes of lines 1 and 2, and X_1 and X_2 are the apices required in the transformed co-ordinate system.

Let $Z_1 = 1/X_1$; $Z_2 = 1/X_2$; $Z_3 = 1/X_3$

The co-efficients of Z_1 and Z_2 (a_{ij} and b_{ij}) are then defined by

$$a_{ij} = n_{ij}\,(y'_{ij} - m_1 x'_{ij})/(m_1 - m_2); \quad b_{ij} = -\,n_{ij}(y'_{ij} - m_2 x'_{ij})/(m_1 - m_2)$$

The coefficient of Z_3 (c_{ij}) will be zero in this case. Similar formulae for points between 2 and 3, and between 3 and 1 may be obtained from symmetry.

Hence $\hat{B}_{ij} = n_{ij} + a_{ij}Z_1 + b_{ij}Z_2 + c_{ij}Z_3$

We now require that the least-squares difference between the background estimates be a minimum, ie we require a turning value of

$$Q = \sum \left\{ (n_{ij} - B_{ij}) + a_{ij} Z_1 + b_{ij} Z_2 + c_{ij} Z_3 \right\}^2$$

This yields the equations

$$Z_1 \sum a_{ij}^2 + Z_2 \sum a_{ij} b_{ij} + Z_3 \sum a_{ij} c_{ij} = - \sum a_{ij} (n_{ij} - B_{ij})$$

$$Z_1 \sum a_{ij} b_{ij} + Z_2 \sum b_{ij}^2 + Z_3 \sum b_{ij} c_{ij} = - \sum b_{ij} (n_{ij} - B_{ij})$$

$$Z_1 \sum a_{ij} c_{ij} + Z_2 \sum b_{ij} c_{ij} + Z_3 \sum c_{ij}^2 = - \sum c_{ij} (n_{ij} - B_{ij})$$

where the summations are over all i and j, although, in practice, points from the background cluster are usually omitted.

These equations may be solved for Z_k, k = 1, 2, 3 and hence for X_k.

7.2.3. Problems and Alternatives. An interpolative background subtraction was used estimate B_{ij}. However, as an alternative, it is possible to define B_{ij} by means of an equation and solve for the unknowns, eg.,

$$B_{ij} = p + qi + rj$$

where p, q, r could be found as part of the least-squares procedure. A disadvantage of this method is that, either an unrealistic formula is used (as above), or the computation becomes unmanageable.

Since the apices must lie within the domain of non-negative factors, the solution must satisfy either $0 < X_k \leqslant X_D$ or $0 > X_k \geqslant X_D$ where X_D is the limiting value defined by the domain. It is usually known which of the inequalities applies. Since these inequalities correspond to $Z_k \geqslant Z_D$ and $Z_k \leqslant Z_D$ respectively, it should be possible to use the method of undetermined multipliers for inequality constraints to solve for Z_k subject to this condition. This possibility is currently being investigated.

A problem arising when considering case (b) concerns how to deal with points lying in the 180° sector, ie (see Fig 4) on the side of BC opposite A. These will contain negative elements of one of the factors (A in Fig 4) which in turn will increase the background estimation. In practice it was found better to set such negative contributions to zero.

7.2.4. Results. The apices found using this method are shown in Fig 8. It is apparent that such points would never be chosen by an apex-seeking routine. The factors and anterior contribution images for the three non-background compartments are displayed in Fig 9. These may be compared with the results of the apex-seeking routine (Fig 10). It is the contention of the author that the constrained results are more realistic. Note, however, that, because of the assumption made in case (b), no pixel contains both ventricular and atrial contributions.

8. DISCUSSION AND CONCLUSION

Using set theory, it is shown that the apex-seeking algorithm for determining the oblique transformation used in FADS will be valid only under conditions which are rarely met in nuclear medicine. An alternative

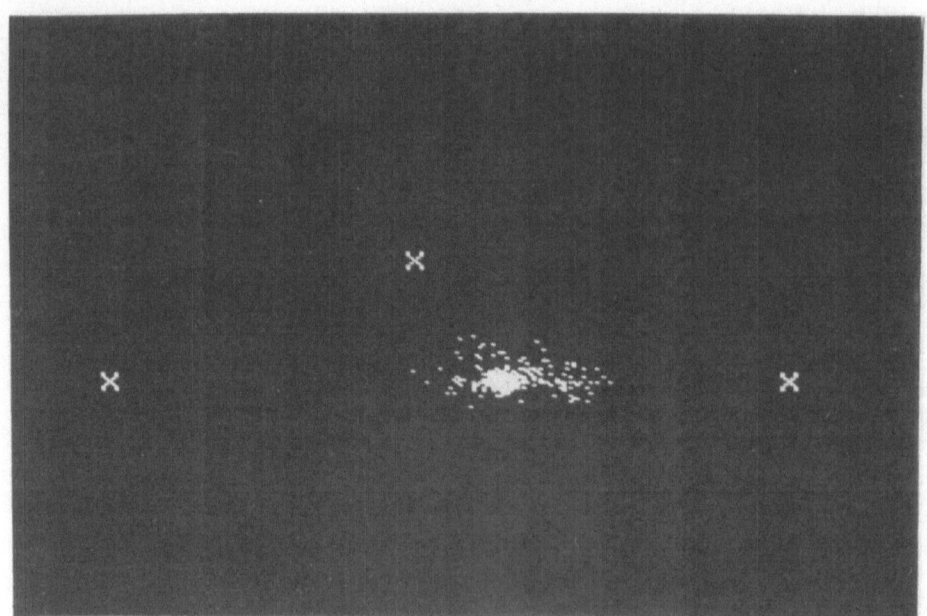

FIGURE 8. Apices for gated cardiac study found using constraints.

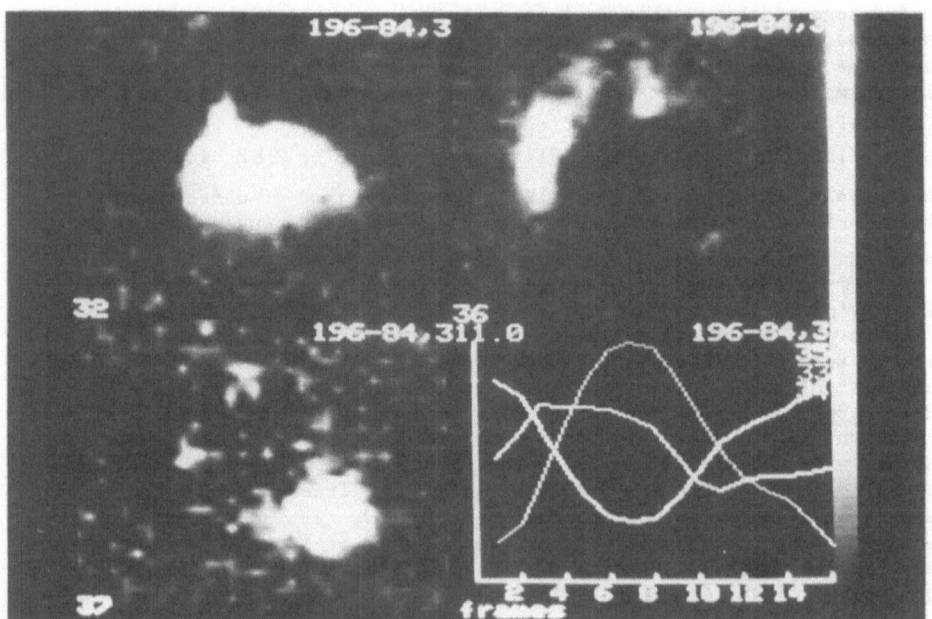

FIGURE 9. Factors and anterior contribution images found using constraints. Ventricular, pathological and atrial curves are shown in decreasing order of brightness and correspond to the upper left, lower left, and upper right images.

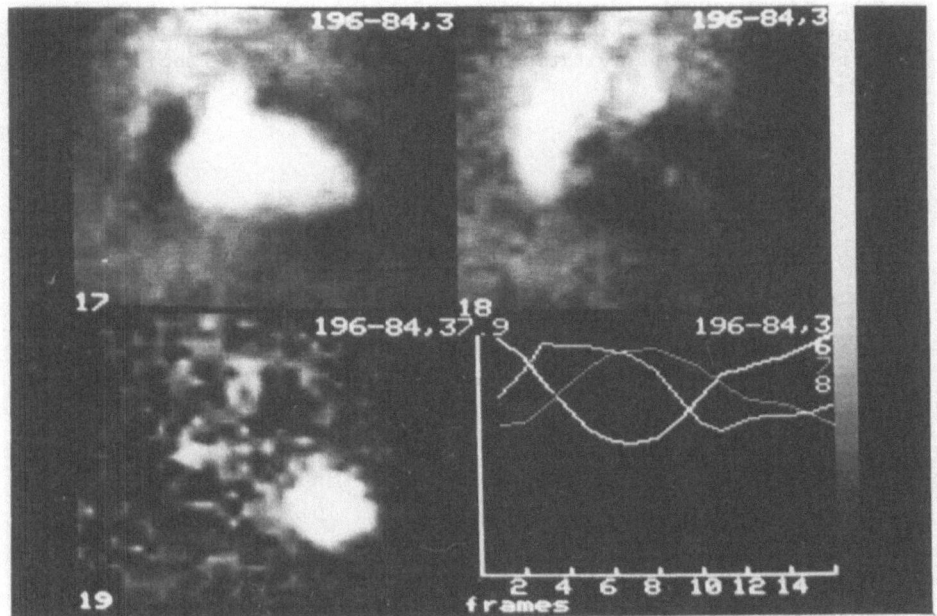

FIGURE 10. Factors and anterior contribution images found using the apex-seeking routine, and depicted as in Fig 9.

approach using cluster analysis is suggested. It is shown using these methods that the problem of dependent factors may be reduced to one of constraint finding.

Using the example of an abnormal gated cardiac study, it is shown that a more realistic solution is found using the new methodology and a background constraint. The problem of non-homogeneity, present in cardiac studies and contrary to the theory of FADS, remains.

REFERENCES

1. Barber DC (1980): The use of principal components in the quantitative analysis of gamma camera dynamic studies. Phys. Med. Biol., 25(2), 283-292.
2. Bazin JP., DiPaola R., Gibaud B., Rougier P., Tubiana M (1979): Factor analysis of dynamic scintigraphic data as a modelling method. An application to the detection of metastases. In: Information Processing in Medical Imaging. Eds. Di Paola and Kahn, Inserm, Paris, 345-366.
3. Benzécri JP (1973): L'analyse des Correspondances. Dunod, Paris.
4. Cavailloles F., Bazin JP., DiPaola R (1984): Factor analysis in gated cardiac studies. J. Nucl. Med., 25, 1067-1079.
5. Goris ML., Daspit SG., McLaughlin P., Kriss JP (1976): Interpolative background subtraction. J. Nucl. Med., 17, 744-747.
6. Houston AS (1984): The effect of apex-finding errors on factor images obtained from factor analysis and oblique transformation. Phys. Med. Biol., 29(9), 1109-1116.
7. Nijran KS., Barber DC (1983): Analysis of dynamic radionuclide studies using factor analysis - a new approach. In: Information Processing in

Medical Imaging. Ed. Deconinck, Martinus Nijhoff, the Hague, 30-44.
8. Schmidlin P (1979): Quantitative evaluation and imaging of functions using pattern recognition methods. Phys. Med. Biol., 24(2), 385-395.
9. Wright WE (1977): Gravitational clustering. Pattern Recognition, 9, 151-166.

FACTOR ANALYSIS: ITS PLACE IN THE EVALUATION OF VENTRICULAR
REGIONAL WALL MOTION ABNORMALITIES.

D.G. Pavel, J. Sychra, E. Olea, C. Kahn, S. Virupannavar, K.
Zolnierczyk, J. Shanes. University of Illinois Medical Center, Chicago, IL.

The detection and evaluation of regional wall motion abnormalities (RWMA) represents clinically relevant information. It
is also increasingly important because the presence and extent of RWMA can guide the therapeutic approach and enable
precise follow-up. As a consequence, there is a need to
refine the methods of detection by improving the topographic
localization of the abnormality as well as the evaluation of
its extent and type (hypokinesia, akinesia, dyskinesia).

The main problem encountered by any two dimensional technique including equilibrium gated study is due to the anatomical superimposition of cardiac structures i.e. ventricular
walls. This in turn leads to functional superimposition,
which limits the sensitivity of RWMA detection especially
when single oblique views are used. The recent advent of
newer algorithms for factor analysis (1, 2, 3, 4) has given
some hope that, at least within limits, this superimposition
can be unraveled and thus the detection of abnormal regional
wall motion improved. In addition, it should be possible to
develop simple means of quantification of the information
obtained.

In order to assess such possibilities, the present study
compares factor analysis results with contrast angiography
and also with phase analysis.   Specifically, the comparison
was performed with the phase image which lends itself easily
to interpretation and quantification and which is presently
used extensively for RWMA evaluation in daily routine.

Material and Method.

Fourteen normal cases were compared to 41 patients who underwent biplane contrast angiography.   In addition, 18/41 had
Tl-201 and/or surgery and/or autopsy.   The worst abnormality
found in each patient by contrast angiography was dyskinesia
in 15, akinesia in 19, hypokinesia in 4 and no evidence of
RWMA in 3. Most patients had multiple segments involved. In
order to standardize the wall motion reading a segmentation
model was agreed upon with the cardiologists for the localization of abnormalities (Fig. 1).   This model included the
RAO view even though no corresponding view was obtained

during the gated study. The information from the RAO view was used only to help explain differences between LAO contrast and radionuclide views in some cases. Every case was completely reviewed by the same team and no use was made of the original reports found in the patient's chart.

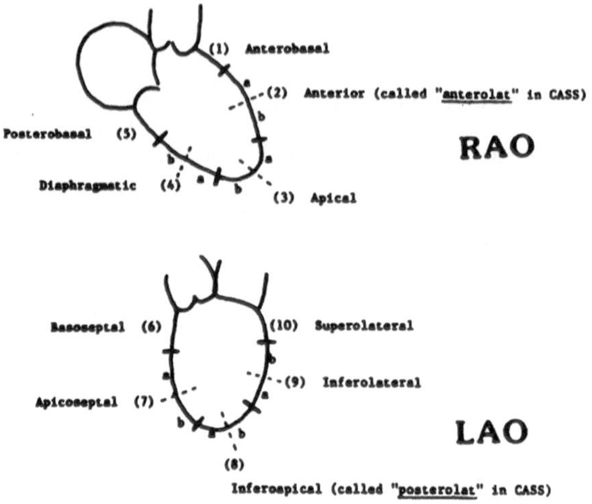

Fig. 1. Segmentation model (see legend of Figures)

Data acquisition: Large field of view camera (LFOV) and optimized LAO view in all cases. In addition, in 21/41 an additional view was obtained but used only as support, not included in correlation. A 64 frame, 32 x 32 acquisition was then obtained on a dedicated computer (SOPHA S-4000). The number of counts was between 200-250 K/frame (up to 16MK total).

Processing: As first step, a preprocessing was performed consisting of late count loss correction (by the R-R histogram method), followed by interpolation and compression to 16, 64 x 64 frames/cardiac cycle. The ventricular regions of interest (ROI) were obtained by the standard method (5) and then used to mask the field. This preprocessing resulted in a final sequence of 16 frames subsequently used as input for final processing and containing solely the ventricular regions, subsequently zoomed by a factor of 2.

Factor analysis was based on the algorithm developed by Bazin and Di Paola (2, 3). A search for two and for three factors was performed in all cases on both ventricular ROI-s taken together, (two ventricle ROI) as well as on the LV ROI alone. The size of the trixel (elemental search unit as described by Di Paola (3)) was 8 x 8 two ventricle ROI and 4 x 4 for LV ROI alone. Briefly, the algorithm follows the following sequence: before the actual analysis starts, the algorithm performs normalization of pixel intensities by dividing each pixel value in each input image by the sum of all 16 intensities of the particular pixel. This operation decreases the dimensionality of the problem by one and the time dependency of pixel values is stressed in the new images.

Principal component analysis of the image data is then performed in order to estimate the minimum number of significant components contained in the dynamic data. In so doing one also diminishes noise considerably. A constrained factor analysis is then performed in the intrinsically 15-D space of pixel intensities of the normalized 16 input images (for details see (4)). The analysis is based on the assumption that the time development of a pixel value can be expressed in the form of a linear combination of factors, where each factor represents an individual, separate physiological process. The method then requires all factor components and the coefficients in the linear combination to be non-negative (2, 3, 4). To satisfy these positivity constraints of the factor analysis, an iterative process is employed in the search for the factor definitions, with the user specifying the convergence criteria. The factor analysis results are then presented in the form of loading curves and factor images for each requested factor.

Over 50% of normal and abnormal cases were processed repeatedly in order to test reproducibility.

Results.

No significant negative images were found in any of the normals or abnormals. The highest values obtained in negative images were below 3% of the corresponding positive image. Repeated processing of the same data did not generate significant differences.

Normals: The two factor display showed a distinct "ventricular" type factor with a loading curve similar to the ventricular time activity curve. The corresponding image was always very similar to the ventricular amplitude image obtained by phase analysis. The second factor had a generally flat loading curve and the corresponding image had a "peninsula" or a "crescent" shape at the base of the left ventricle (Fig.

2). No difference was found between processing both ROI-s together or just the LV ROI.

The three factor display showed that the ventricular factor appearance described above was not affected but that the non-ventricular factor was always split in two images and was thus the main contributor to the third factor image. Generally this third factor image had a scattered irregular appearance spread over the whole ROI and its corresponding loading curve had a "wavy" appearance (Figure 2).

When only the isolated LV ROI was processed, several features occurred which were not apparent when both ventricles were processed together. First, in 4/14 cases the ventricular factor was also split and thus out of the three factor images two had loading curves of "ventricular type". In such cases these curves were only slightly different and their nadir occured very close in time to each other. Second, in 6/14 cases the third factor was associated with a well defined "dyskinetic" loading curve and the corresponding high image intensities concentrated at the base of the LV. This appearance strongly suggested atrial contamination.

In 2 cases, the isolated LV was processed with an 8 x 8 trixel size, besides the standard 4 x 4 size. In such circumstances, no significant difference was found for the two factor search but there were noticeable differences for three factor searches.

Abnormals. The following patterns were observed in the presence of RWMA: The two factor display showed already clearly the presence of abnormality in 33/40 cases with evidence of RWMA and suggested abnormality in the remaining 7. If the LV ROI alone is used the abnormality is clearly seen in 38/40. In the specific case of dyskinezias the ventricular factor image was clearly different from the corresponding amplitude image (Fig. 3).

The three factor display showed the RWMA with greater clarity. In 34/40 cases with evidence of RWMA the abnormality was equally well seen if processing was performed on both ROI-s or on isolated LV ROI. In the remaining 6 the abnormality was clearer in the latter case. The existence of a third factor image allowed the detection of areas of RWMA with different characteristics (Figs. 3, 4). This improvement was made possible by evaluating the images as well as their corresponding loading curves. In particular it enhanced the detection and localization of dyskinetic areas (Fig. 3).
If one considers normality versus abnormality, as sole criteria, there are 7 discordant cases for phase images (6

are false negatives), and only two discordant cases for factor analysis, none being false negative (Table I).

Factor (+)	Factor (−)		Phase (+)	Phase (−)
38	0	Angio (+)	32	6
2	1	Angio (−)	1	2

Table I. Distribution of the 41 abnormal cases, considering as variables only normality, versus abnormality of the respective procedures.

In 2/41 cases there was evidence of abnormality by factor analysis not confirmed by angiography. Those two patients had coronary artery disease, marked LVH with compliance abnormality, and one of them had major aterosclerotic changes, with peripheral amputation and previous coronary bypass.

The specific comparison with phase analysis was done based on two criteria: 1) detection of number of segments involved; 2) evaluation of type of worst abnormality found. For number of segments, factor analysis appeared better than phase image in 82% of cases and for evaluation of type of abnormality in 77% of cases.

Discussion.

The use of factor analysis for ventricular RWMA evaluation has been previously advocated by Cavailloles et al (4). Nevertheless, their conclusions appeared rather pesimistic in light of our preliminary results. One possible explanation was that in 40% of their abnormals, RWMA was compared to ECHO findings only (because no contrast ventriculography was available). In addition, the ECHO and angiography results were just taken from patient charts, while we have found that such data can be at considerable variance with those obtained by a careful subsequent review. While the principles and main steps of the original algorithm used by Cavailloles have not changed, there have been improvements added by their group subsequently. Consequently we had decided to take a new look at our database, using the latest software modifications available and confining the processing strictly to the ventricular ROI-s. This has the theoretical and practical advantage of not "wasting" factors for the detection of atrial function which is of no concern for the study of ventricular RWMA. Also we have tried to explore the effect of further confining the search just to the LV ROI.

Based on past experience we have decided to limit the search to two and three factors. Going to four factors often generates curves which are too noisy and too irregular in shape to allow a clear interpretation.

Concerning the topographic segmentation of the left ventricle a detailed model was agreed upon with the cardiologists (Fig. 1). This made it possible to minimize the errors of localization of a given abnormality, but even so there is still subjectivity in the qualitative evaluation of contrast angiography. One source of error still remaining is the difference in LAO angulation: it is always about 60 in contrast angiography and much less in radionuclide studies. For this reason, we have taken into account the information obtained from the RAO contrast angiography even though no corresponding view was obtained from radionuclide angiography. This enabled us sometimes to solve apparent discrepancies between the two techniques. A typical example is in separating anterior wall from septum lesions. Indeed what is called septum on a 60 LAO is often mostly an anterior wall area.

The acquisitions were of high information density in order to minimize noise and improve the quality of factor images.

Concerning the normal population the following observations can be made. In all normals it is possible to extract 3 factors which satisfy the positivity constraint. This is one major difference between our analysis and the results obtained by others (4). The difference is due to the new improved algorithm as we have been able to demonstrate by running, the old and the new one, on all cases.

Concerning the two factor search we found that the non-ventricular factor generated an image with a significant amount of structure at the base of the LV. It usually has the shape of a peninsula (Fig. 2) or of a more or less accentuated crescent. While this appearance is different enough from the one found in abnormal patients, one cannot disregard the fact that some confusion could arise in cases with only minimal abnormalities.

The fact that the normal ventricular factor image is very similar to the amplitude image turned out to be an important adjunct means of differentiating dyskinezia from other RWMA as will be discussed below.

The two factor display is not influenced by entering both ROI-s or the isolated LV ROI into the search. Neither is it influenced by the trixel size.

Concerning the three factor search, in normals, it appears
more difficult to standardize and thus to evaluate. For
example, there are significant differences when the two
ventricle ROI or the LV ROI alone are processed. It would
appear that the most simple and reliable interpretation is
the one based on the two ROI-s search. The major advantage
there, is that the ventricular factor image and its corresponding loading curve, are carried almost unchanged into the
three factor display. This means that the third factor is
mainly generated as a subset of the non-ventricular factor
originally found by the two factor search. If the LV ROI is
processed independently there are cases in which the ventricular factor is also split and thus the three factor display
winds up with two ventricular factors. At this point the
separation from abnormals can be made only by the fact that
the two corresponding ventricular type curves reach their
nadir at almost the same time. The significance of this
difference is not yet certain but one can speculate that
isolating the left ventricle and going to a smaller trixel
size (4 x 4) elicits additional details from the dymanic of
the structures included in the respective ROI. The same
speculation may also help explain the appearance of falsely
"dyskinetic" areas at the base of the ventricle when processing the isolated left ROI. Whether this can be looked at as
processing artifact or "additional detail" indicating atrial
contamination in that area, remains to be seen.

In the abnormal population 38/41 were confirmed by contrast
angiography as having RWMA and in these the presence of
abnormality can be detected very efficiently even by the two
factor display: in 87% of cases, if two ventricle ROI is
used, and in 100% if LV ROI alone is used. Nevertheless, the
latter finding has to be viewed with some caution in light of
the fact that processing left ventricular ROI alone may
possibly generate false positive results, as discussed above.

Of interest is the possibility to establish the presence of
diskinezia in most cases by detecting dissimilarities between
the amplitude image obtained from phase analysis and the
ventricular factor image obtained from two factor search.

This is not surprising in view of the fact that: 1) the
theory of phase analysis requires that any amplitude of the
first harmonic be represented on the same image irrespective
of its phase shift, 2) the stated goal of factor analysis of
a dynamic structure is to place areas containing different
dynamics on different images.

In general the three factor search and display confers additional precision to the evaluation of RWMA by giving topogra-

phic details on the image and dynamic characteristics. This improvement was particularly striking when processing was done on the isolated LV alone.

In the two cases where factor analysis suggested abnormality not confirmed by angiography it is noteworthy to consider that both had LVH in addition to coronary artery disease. The latter was responsible for the symptoms which lead the patients to contrast angiography and thus to the inclusion in our patient population. Both LVH and coronary artery disease affect significantly the left ventricular compliance and thus early filling rate. It is thus possible to raise the hypothesis, which remains to be proven, of subtle dynamic changes, detected by factor analysis, in cases with such combined pathology.

The comparison with phase analysis was chosen because it is commonly used and easy to quantify. It is of course agreed that no phase image should be evaluated without considering the amplitude image as well. Nevertheless the latter, being modulated by anatomy is only amenable to qualitative evaluation and can thus add subjectivity to the evaluation. Factor analysis images, while also modulated by anatomy, are not presenting the same difficulty because each factor is displayed separately in a different quadrant in association with its respective loading curve.

By using factor analysis the improvement obtained both for number of segments as well as for type of maximum abnormality found is very significant when compared to the respective phase images: in 83% and 78% of cases respectively. If one considers the number of cases where phase images were normal (8 cases) in 6 of them factor analysis and contrast angiography were abnormal (Table I). Of the remaining two one has definite coronary artery disease and abnormal factor image (as discussed above) and the last one had no evidence of RWMA by either contrast angiography nor factor analysis.

The intra and inter observer variability of the processing has been insignificant. This was not surprising, in view of the high degree of automation of the algorithm in which the only operator dependent variable was the placement of the zoom cursor. This has not generated significant differences in the final results, provided both ventricles were clearly included in the zoomed area. In one case with akinezia/dyskinesia there were two LAO views available (acquired during the same session) but only with a five degree difference in position. The processing of both views yielded very similar results. This fact strengthens the confidence in the underlying principles of the method and in the algorithm itself. Indeed this was not just a repeat processing as done in other cases, but a processing of two different acquisitions which, because they differ by only five degrees, have no theoretical or practical reason to show significantly different information. The existence of differences in shape of ROI-s, of slight location shifts of the projected lesions, of count rates, etc. did not change the results. This is indeed of great practical importance and tends to prove that the assumptions and the model are adequate but does not necessarily prove that the algorithm is also optimal.

In conclusion, factor analysis enables the evaluation of RWMA with significantly increased accuracy by using an algorithm which is essentially automatic. At this stage the concept appearing as a valid and useful one, the remaining task is to improve the algorithm in such a way as to enhance further the differences between normal and abnormal population. Consequently the detection, localization and characterization of regional wall motion abnormalities on an individual basis could become even clearer and simpler.

References.

1. Barber DC.: The use of principal components in the quantitative analysis of gamma-camera dynamic studies. Phys. Med. Biol. Vol. 25: 283-292, 1980.

2. Bazin JP, Di Paola R.: Advances in factor analysis applications in dynamic function studies. Proceedings of the Third World Congress of Nuclear Medicine and Biology, Edit. C. Raymond, Pergamon Press, Paris, 1982, p. 35-38.

3. Di Paola R., Bazin JP, Aubry F., et al: Handling of dynamic sequences in nuclear medicine. IEEE Transactions of Nuclear Science, Vol. NS-29, 1982, p. 1310-1321.

4. Cavailloles F., Bazin JP., Di Paola R.: Factor analysis in gated cardiac studies. J. Nucl. Med. 25: 1067-1079, 1984.

5. Pavel D, Byrom E, et al: Detection and quantification of regional wall motion abnormalities using phase analysis of equilibrium gated cardiac studies. Clin. Nucl. Med. 8: 315, 1983.

Legend of Figures

Figure 1: Segmentation model used for topographic location of RWMA. In order to better reflect the reality of wall notion evaluation on contrast angiography and on radionuclide studies, subdivisions were used for all segments except the ones located at the base of the ventricle.

Figure 2: Normal Case (case M.M.) (A) represents the standard display of ED, ES, amplitude and phase images. (B) normalized phase image with frequency distribution histogram. Note great similarity of amplitude image in (A) and ventricular factor in (C). The second factor in (C) shows a "peninsula" structure (which proved to be a frequent normal variant). The three factor display (C) shows that 2 of the 3 factors are very similar in appearance to the two factor display. In right upper quadrant of (D) the new factor generated, shows noninterpretable loading factor curve and image. Such features are found in the normal population.

Figure 3: Hypokinesia (case V. H.) Contrast angiography showed: Hypokinesia at apex and lower septum and akinesia of upper septum.
Amplitude image in (A) and ventricular factor in (C) are similar. There is a distinct abnormal appearance of second factor image in the two factor display (C). The three factor display (D) indicates very clearly a large area of hypokinesia at apex and inferior septum and the akinetic area in the upper septum.
In contradistinction, the LV phase image in (B) although abnormal shows only minor abnormality and only in the inferior septum. This is often the case for RWMA of the septum.

Figure 4: Akinesia/Dyskinesia (case A.J.) Contrast Angiography: Apical akinesia/dyskinesia and large extension of akinesia to part of septum, anterior and diaphragmetic walls.
Apical discrepancy between amplitude image in (A) and ventricular factor in (C) (this is a first indication of a dyskinetic component). The second image in (C) is extensively abnormal. The three factor images and curves (D-E) confirm apical dyskinetic component (in right upper quadrant)

extension of RWMA to inferior septum. It also
suggests extension in the 3-D dimension (anterior
and diaphragmatic walls). The third factor (left
lower quadrant) confirms the extension of abnormality to upper septum and anterior wall.
In contradistinction LV phase analysis in (B) only
shows apical akinesia, and localized surrounding
abnormality, extending to inferior septum.

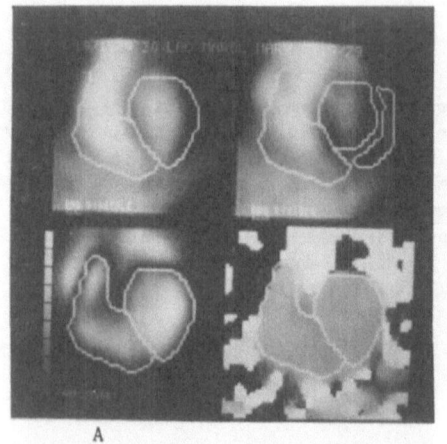

A

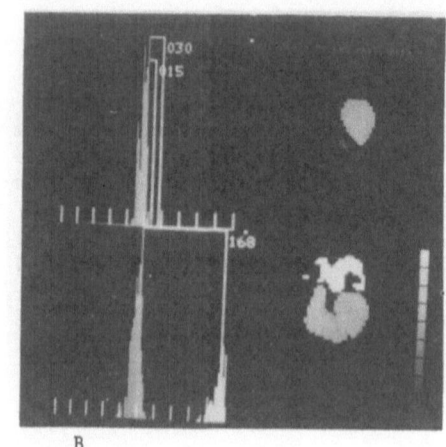

B

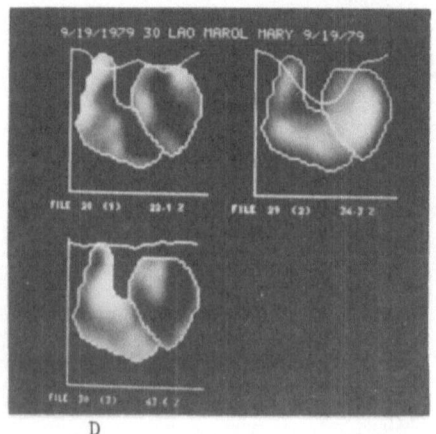

C

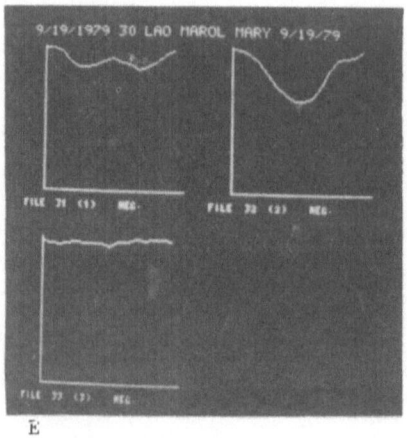

D

E

FIG 2

NORMAL CASE

(see legend of figures)

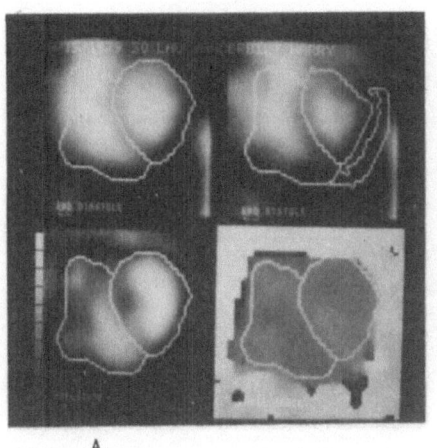

A

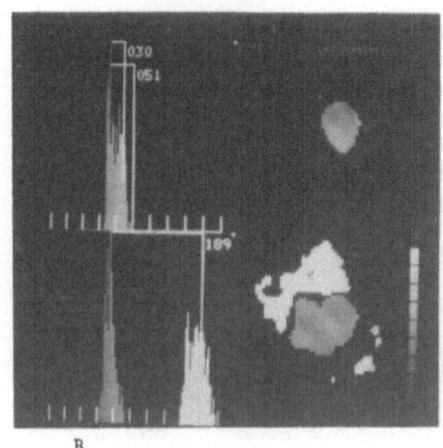

B

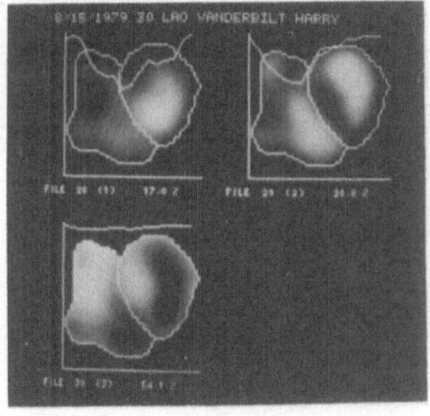

C

FIG 3

HYPOKINESIA

(see legend of figures)

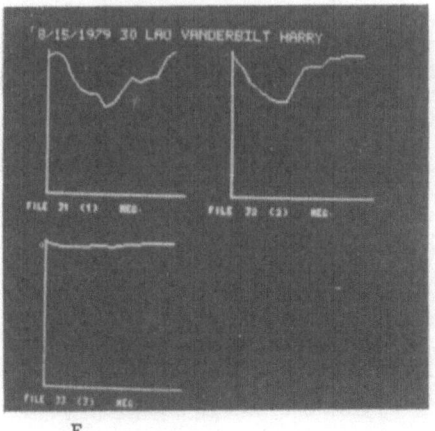

D

E

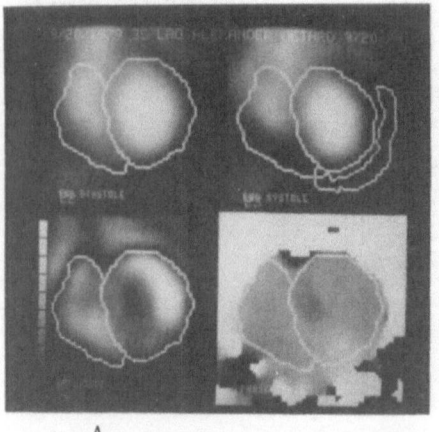

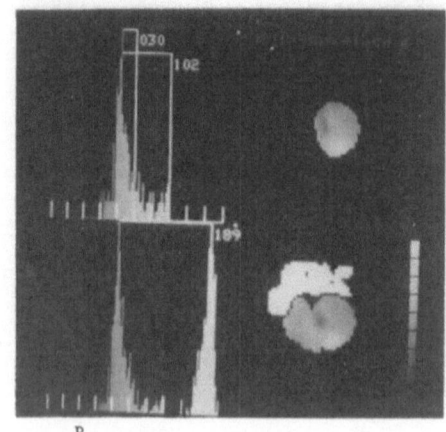

A B

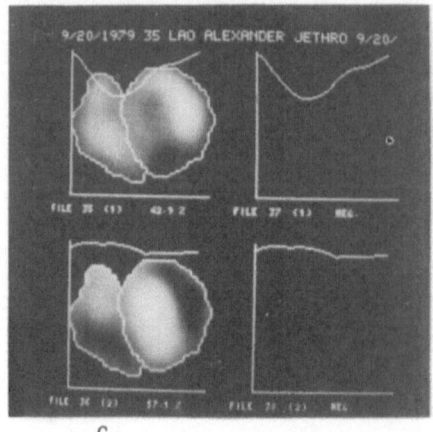

C

FIG 4

AKINESIA / DISKINESIA

(see legend of figures)

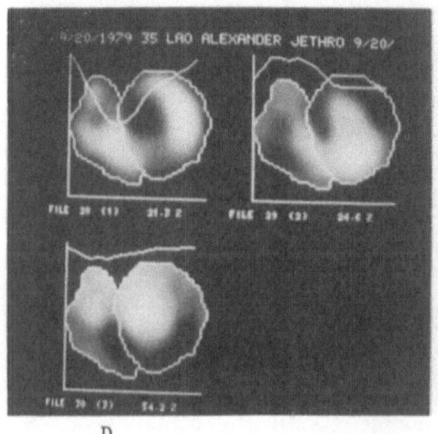

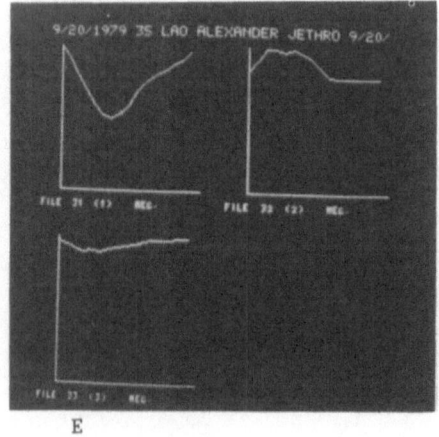

D E

ADAPTIVE FREQUENCY-DOMAIN FILTERING OF DYNAMIC SCINTIGRAPHIES

A. BOSSUYT, R. LUYPAERT, J. VAN CRAEN, F.DECONINCK, A.B. BRILL

1. INTRODUCTION

The predominant role of amplitude/phase analysis in parametric imaging of radionuclide ventriculographies has emphasised the importance of including both time and motion variables in the description of cardiac pump dysfunction. The accuracy of phase analysis for the visualisation of time patterns is hampered by the fact that a first harmonic model for the temporal behaviour of a pixels' activity changes is assumed. We therefore have proposed a framework of alternative data extraction procedures which do include the information of the higher harmonics as well (1).

When the visual perception of time patterns in a dynamic image series is limited due to low temporal contrast, strong temporal contrast enhancement can be achieved by substracting for each pixel its minimum value from the whole image series. By further normalising each pixels' value for its magnitude, an image series is obtained which only displays the fractional variation of the blood volume changes reached at each part of the cardiac cycle taken separately. As regional evaluation of time patterns is performed by a counting process on a pixel by pixel basis, a major drawback of these procedures is that they are distorted by large fluctuations induced by statistical noise. In terms of a temporal Fourier analysis the contrast enhanced series of images contains all the Fourier frequencies except the zero frequency component. In order to retain only those harmonics that contain relevant information we have developped a low frequency filtering technique of the original cardiac cycle data in which the cut-off value varies spatially in function of pixel noise. In a first stage it was therefore necessary to characterise the way noise is passed on into the frequency domain.

2. NOISE BEHAVIOUR IN THE TEMPORAL FREQUENCY DOMAIN

2.1. Computer simulation

In order to simulate the behaviour of noise in widely varying circumstances, use was made of computer generated data of equilibrium gated cardiac blood pool studies. The time evolution of single pixels was described by 16 frames per cycle time activity curves (TAC), $s(t)$, constructed on the basis of a truncated Fourier representation, $f(t)$, of the noise free data and additive, gaussian noise, $n(t)$:

$$s(t) = f(t) + n(t) \tag{1}$$

$$f(t) = a_0 + \Sigma\, c_m \cos\,(\, m\omega t + F_m\,) \tag{2}$$

$$n(t) = \text{rand}\,\{\,N\,(\,\text{mean=0}\,,\,\text{s.d.}=\sqrt{f(t)}\,\} \tag{3}$$

The resulting discrete, noisy TACs gave rise to 8 Fourier components calculated as follows:

$$c_m = \sqrt{(a_m^2 + b_m^2)} \tag{4}$$

$$F_m = -\text{arctg}\ b_m/a_m \tag{5}$$

where

$$a_m = \Sigma_t\ s(t) \cos m\, 2\pi/16\,t \tag{6}$$

$$b_m = \Sigma_t\ s(t) \sin m\, 2\pi/16\,t \tag{7}$$

The whole process was repeated 50 times yielding average values and standard deviations for each frequency component.

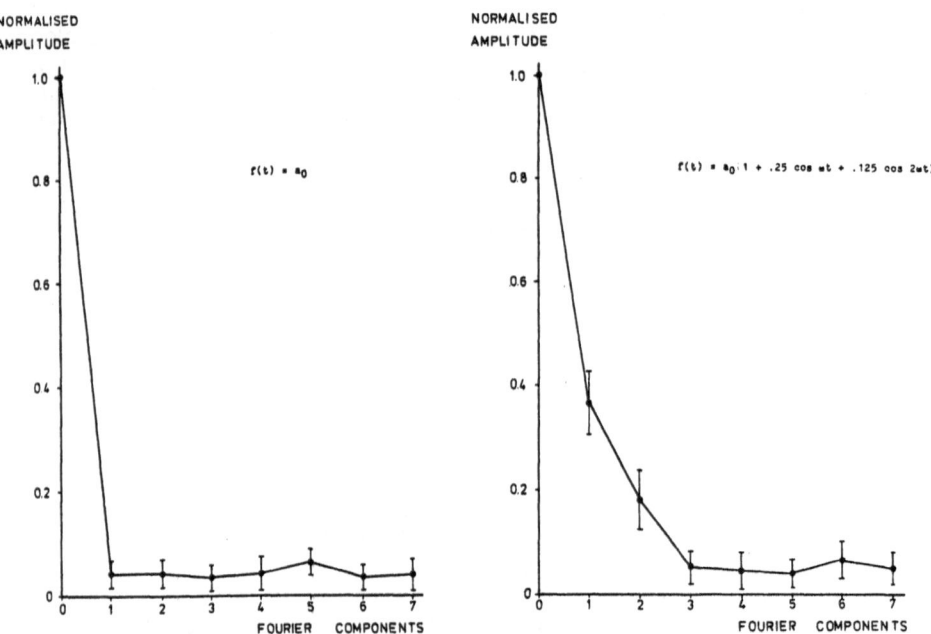

FIGURE 1. Fourier components of $f_1(t)$ and $f_2(t)$.

In Fig. 1 the way in which noise is transferred from the time domain into the frequency domain is compared for two different functions f(t)

$f_1(t) = a_0$ and $f_2(t) = a_0 (1 + .25 \cos \omega t + .125 \cos 2\omega t)$.

It was found that noise-only components have very similar amplitudes, independent of the exact form of the underlying time behaviour: the only factor which influences the noise level is the background value a_0.

In Fig. 2 the plots show the evolution of mean and standard deviation of an arbitrary noise-only component as a function of a_0. A linear regression analysis indicates that, to a very good approximation, both parameters have a linear dependence on $\sqrt{a_0}$: mean $= .20 + .39 \sqrt{a_0}$ ($r = .99$) and
s.d. $= .12 \pm .29 \sqrt{a_0}$ ($r = 1.00$)

Finally, Fig. 3 shows the results of a detailed study of the Fourier amplitude distributions behind these expressions. Histograms of noise only components corresponding to reasonable values for a_0 (~100) and a wide range of values for a_0/c_1 (.2, ... , .8) in (2) were obtained. Comparison of the shapes, means and s.d. characterising these distributions confirms our previous conclusion: the behaviour of noise in the frequency domain is, to a good approximation, determined by the magnitude of the constant background signal.

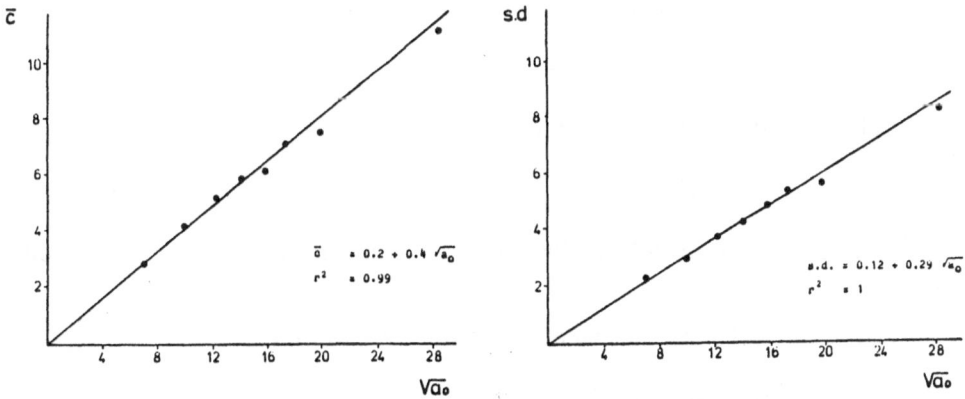

FIGURE 2. Parametrisation of noise only components as a function of $\sqrt{a_0}$.

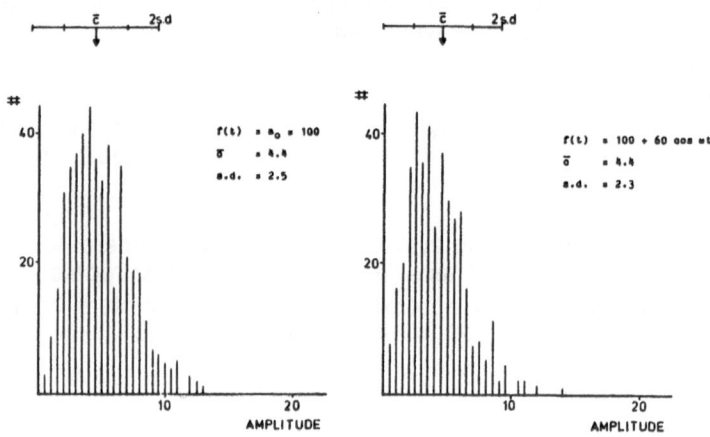

FIGURE 3. Distribution of the amplitudes of noise only components in the Fourier spectrum (450 simulations).

2.2. Generalised noise behaviour

The results obtained by the computer simulations provide a quantitative description of the noise behaviour in the frequency domain specific to the case where the heart cycle is sampled at 16 points in time. In order to generalise these results, an attempt was made to derive analytical expressions for both mean ($< N_m >$) and s.d. (v_m) of the noise only frequency components. Introducing the complex Fourier components of the noise contribution to the signal,

$$N_m = 1/N \ \Sigma \ n(t) \ e^{im\omega t} \qquad (8)$$

use could be made of th following relationship

$$v_m = 2 \, | N_m | \qquad (9)$$

in order to obtain the noise level Fourier amplitudes that are usually encountered in nuclear medicine.

Conserving our earlier hypothesis of gaussian noise, we have:

$$< |N_m| > = \int |N_m| \ P(|N_m|) \ d|N_m| \qquad (10)$$

with

$$P(|N_m|) \, d|N_m| = \frac{1}{(\sqrt{2\pi}\sigma)^N} \int e^{-\Sigma n(t)^2/2\sigma^2} \, \Pi_t \, dn(t)$$

(11)

where σ represents the standard deviation governing the noise distribution in the time domain. (In accordance with the findings of the simulation study we have assumed the noise to be determined by the stationnary background value: $\sigma \sim \sqrt{a_0}$).

Inserting (8) and (11) in (10) and evaluating the resulting integrations leads to the following expression:

$$<|N_m|> = \frac{\sqrt{2\pi}}{N.2^{(N/2-1)}} \cdot \frac{1.3....(N-1)}{[(N-2)/2]!} \cdot \frac{7N+18}{8N+16} \, \sigma$$

(12)

On the other hand

$$<|N_m|> = 1/N^2 \; \Sigma_t \; <n(t)\,n(t')> e^{\,i(t-t')m\omega}$$

$$= 1/N^2 \; \Sigma_t \; <n(t)^2>$$

$$= \sigma^2/N$$

(13)

On the basis of expressions (9) (12) (13) following results are obtained for the mean and standard deviation of the n_m:

$$<v_m> = \frac{4\sqrt{2\pi}}{N.2^{(N/2-1)}} \cdot \frac{1.3....(N-1)}{[(N-2)/2]!} \cdot \frac{7N+18}{8N+16} \cdot \sigma$$

(14)

and

$$s.d.(v_m) = 2\left[<|N_m|^2> - <|N_m|>^2 \right]^{1/2}$$

(15)

The results are found to be independent of m. In table 1 we have listed means and standard deviations obtained for a number of values of N.

Table 1.   Mean and standard deviation of noise only components as a function of sampling frequency.

N	$<v_m>$	$sd(v_m)$
4	.901	.434
8	.634	.313
16	.444	.230
32	.312	.166
64	.220	.119

2.3. Phantom studies

In a first study using a Tc filled flood phantom, 6 image series of 16 frames each, and containing respectively 100, 200, 400, 800, 1600 or 3200 kcts/frame, were acquired. In a second study using the same flood phantom a 16 frame image series was created in which the countrate varied as follows: 700, 680, 640, 580, 500, 420, 360, 320, 300, 320, 360, 420, 500, 580, 640, 680 kcts /frame; thus corresponding to $f(t) = 1 + .40 \cos \omega t$. For each of these image series 1st, ... , 7th harmonic amplitude parametric images were calculated. Within a constant ROI of 840 pixels in the center of the image, the distribution, mean and standard deviation of the pixel's amplitudes was measured.

The distribution of the pixel's amplitudes for a given Fourier component within the ROI was slightly oblique as might be expected from the computer simulations. As well in the study with stationnary signals, as in the study with a 1st harmonic signal, the noise contribution was distributed uniformly over all "higher" Fourier components (fig 4). In all studies, the magnitude c^* of those Fourier components that contained only noise was related to the time independent part a_0 of the signal by: $c^* = (.44 + .23) \sqrt{a_0}$ (fig 5).

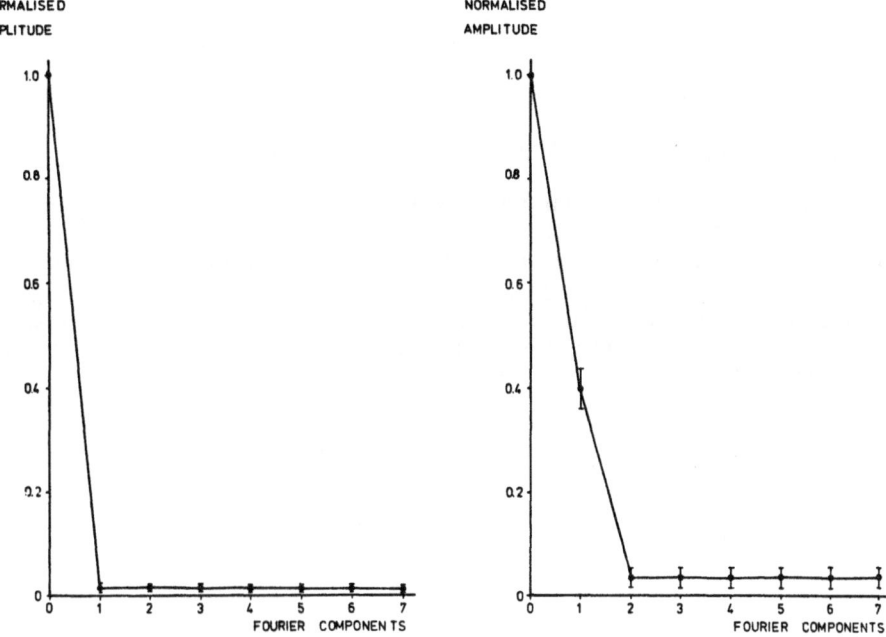

FIGURE 4. Fourier components in a phantom study with a stationnary signal (left) and with a 1st harmonic signal (right).

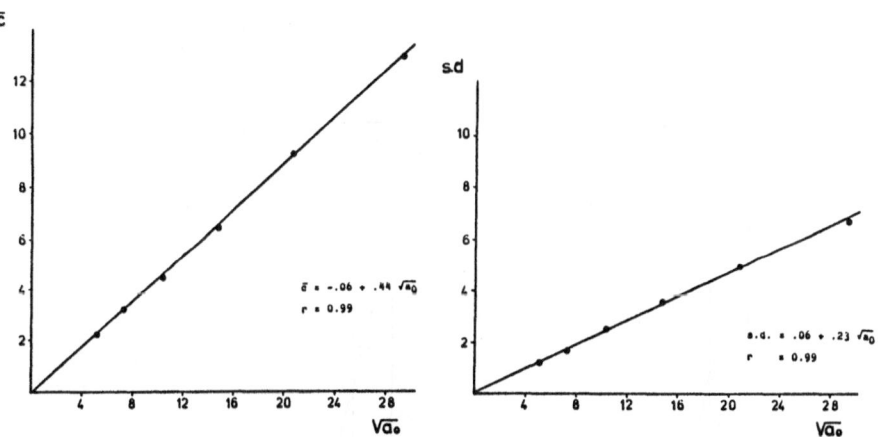

FIGURE 5. Parametrisation of noise only components as a function of $\sqrt{a_0}$.

3. CLINICAL APPLICATION

3.1. Noise propagation in equilibrium gated cardiac blood pool studies

      4 consecutive equilibrium gated cardiac blood pool studies were performed in the same patient without changing his position. The data aquisition periods were so that respectively 1, 4, 8 and 15 * 10^6 counts were obtained in the total field of view. For each of these image series 1st, ... , 7th harmonic amplitude images were calculated. Fig. 6 shows for each study the mean and standard deviation of the pixel amplitudes of the successive Fourier components within a left ventricular ROI.

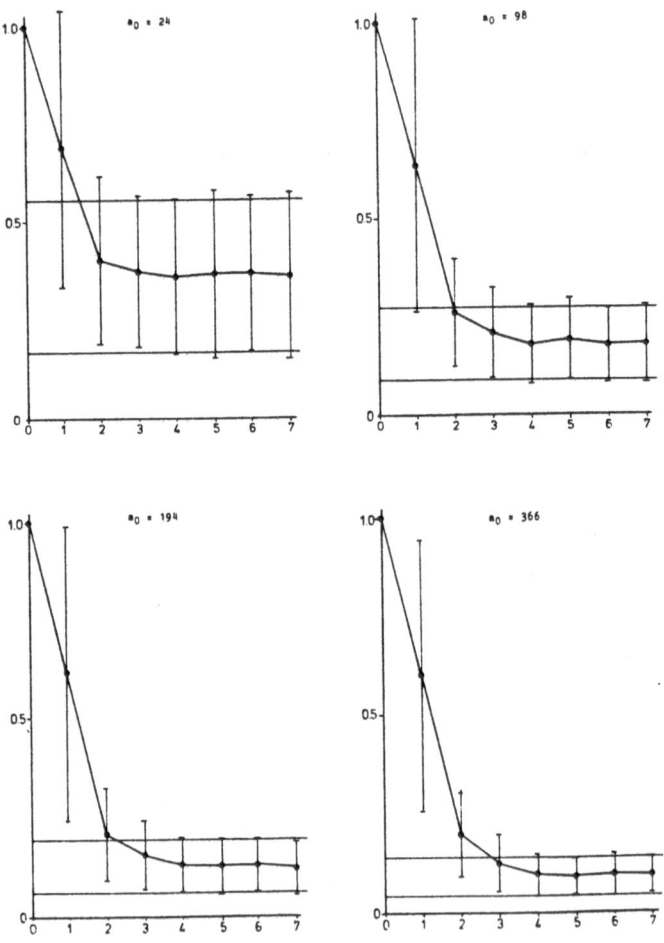

FIGURE 6. Fourier components within a left ventricular ROI of 4 consecutive EGNA studies with increasing counting statistics. (indicated range corresponds to $.44 \pm .23 \sqrt{a_0}$).

3.2. Adaptive frequency domain filtering

These consistent observations on the behaviour of noise in the temporal frequency domain, provide a basis for a filter technique operating in the frequency domain and adaptive in function of the noise present in different anatomical structures. In the version used here, significant Fourier components of each pixels' TAC are required to exceed a 2 standard deviations upper limit of c'_m. Components that do not satisfy this criterion are judged to be indistinguishable from the noise and put equal to zero. Assuming that non-clustered, isolated pixels cannot have a physiological meaning, it seems also reasonable to remove isolated pixels from the amplitude images resulting from the sifting process. This was actually performed by spatial median filtering (2) of the tresholded amplitude images in a second step. The use of weighted contributions of the Fourier components and a suitable cluster filtter will be further evaluated. In a third and final step, reconstruction of the TACs on the basis of the residual Fourier components yields the filtered version of the dynamic scintigraphies.

The proposed filtering technique conserves the statistically relevant information in higher harmonics, and does not induce spatial blurring. It was therefore applied as a basic tool for a multiharmonic analysis of right ventricular performance by means of steady state Krypton 81-m infusion. The important displacements of the right heart during an averaged cardiac cycle necessitate the use of different ED and ES ROIs for the calculation of RVEF, and make it difficult to evaluate regional wall motion from simple first harmonic amplitude and phase functional images. During the filtering procedure, background, evaluated by use of a Tc-99m   MAA lung perfusion scintigraphy, is substracted from the time independent Fourier component. After the filtering procedure, the magnitude and synchronicity of regional blood pool movements is further investigated by means of temporal contrast enhancement and fractional variation imaging.

REFERENCES

1. Bossuyt A, Deconinck F: Amplitude/phase patterns in dynamic scintigraphic imaging. Martinus Nijhoff Publishers, 1984.

2. Luypaert R, Deconinck F: Design and evaluation of median filters for scintigraphic image filtering. IEEE Computer Soc. 82 CH 1804-4, 20-23, 1982.

APPLICATION OF THE FOURIER DESCRIPTORS METHOD FOR PLANE CLOSED CURVES TO THE ANALYSIS OF SEQUENCES OF LEFT VENTRICULAR CONTOURS IN CARDIAC RADIONUCLIDE ANGIOGRAPHIES.

DUVERNOY J., JOUAN A., Laboratoire d'Optique C.N.R.S.
CARDOT J.C., BAUD M., VERDENET J., BIDET R., Service de Biophysique
FAIVRE R., BERTHOUT P., BASSAND J.P., MAURAT J.P., Service de Cardiologie.
Université de Besançon, FRANCE

1 - INTRODUCTION

A general solution to the problem of automatic determination of cardiac cavities contours has not yet been found. As an obvious consequence, the quantitative characterization and exploitation of the contours has not been proposed. The Fourier Descriptors (FDs) method for plane closed curves offers original solutions to this problem. Especially it allows the quantitative characterization and reconstruction of the shape of the successive contours of the acquisition sequence. This method initiates a new approach to problems such as the automatic detection of abnormal contours, the assessment of the isotropy of the contraction and the analysis of the temporal evolution of the shape of the cardiac cavities. This paper presents the principle of the method, and describes the computational procedure for extracting the successive left ventricular contours from the acquisition sequence, and their corresponding FDs. The respective influences of the sampling noise, the reconstruction bandwidth, and the related smoothing effects are discussed. The above mentionned topical applications to cardiac analysis are illustrated.

2 - PRINCIPLE AND METHODOLOGY

2.1 - Principle

A plane closed curve is usually described by a 2-D function, $K(u,v)$. However it can be characterized by a mere 1-D angular function, $\varphi(l)$, which accounts for the variations of the angle defined by the tangent to the curve $K(u,v)$ (at point of curvilinear abscissa l); and a fixed reference axis (fig. 1). This angular function of period 2 is expanded into a Fourier serie :

$$\varphi(l) = \mu_0 + \sum_{n=1}^{\infty} a_n \cos\left(2\pi n \frac{l}{L}\right) + b_n \sin\left(2\pi n \frac{l}{L}\right)$$

where L denotes the total contour length. The knowledge of the Fourier coefficients μ_0, a_n, b_n allows an exact reconstruction of φ. The Fourier Descriptors of the curve are conventionally defined by the moduli A_n and phases α_n of the Fourier coefficients :

$$A_n = \sqrt{a_n^2 + b_n^2}$$

$$\alpha_n = \tan^{-1}\left(\frac{b_n}{a_n}\right)$$

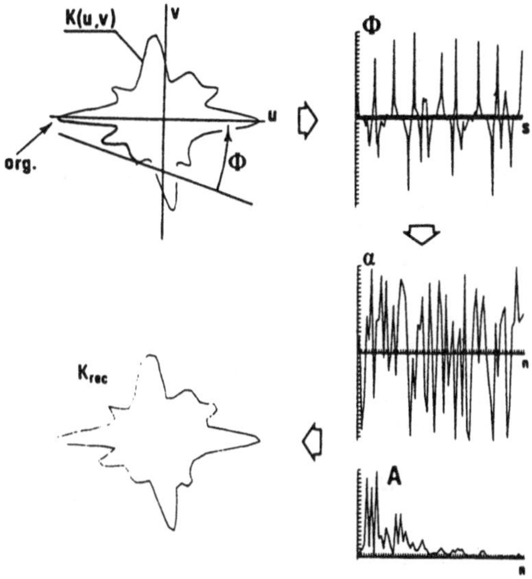

Figure 1

It has been shown (1) that the moduli A_n are **invariant** by **rotation** of the curve, and by **change of scale**. The phases α_n carry relevant information about these changes. In the following the set of A_n of a contour will be referred to as FDs spectrum ; notice that the spectrum is invariant by rotation and change of scale of the contour. Obviously the classical properties of Fourier analysis hold, the FDs being nothing else but the spectrum of the angular function. For example the information relative to the contour details is located in the high frequencies, as the low frequencies account for the general shape of the contour.

This powerfull method of shape analysis offers the cardiac scintigraphy a tool for the quantitative study of the contours of the cardiac cavities. It will be applied here to the case of the left ventricle. The first step is the extraction of the 16 successive contours from the sequence of 16 frames delivred by a gamma camera performing a classical LAO (left anterioroblique) investigation.

2.2 - <u>Preprocessing : extracting the rough contours from the sequence</u>

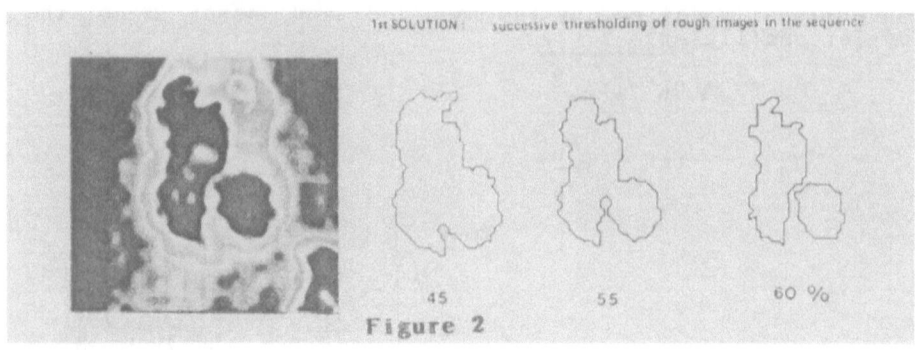

Figure 2

The contours to be quantified must be extracted from distributions of energy displayed in each frame of the sequence. An obvious solution consists of thresholding (2) each frame at a given level; in order to obtain a closed curve representative of the left ventricle (figure 2). The sequence of contours extracted according to this procedure need not be very accurate, because the whole temporal story of the modifications of the ventricle shape can be assessed from the corresponding sequence of FDs. The differences between any ideal contour and that obtained by thresholding behave as an uncorrelated spectral noise when looking at the structure of successive FDs spectra.

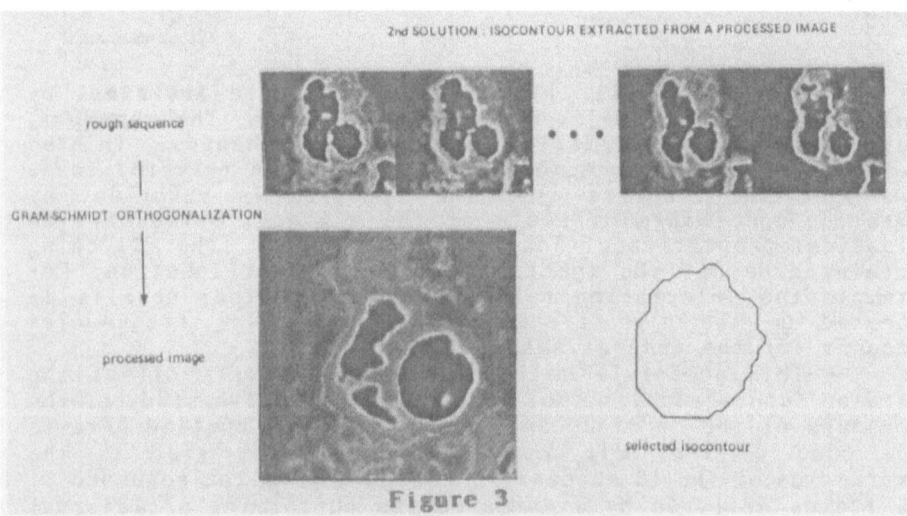

Figure 3

A second solution consists of starting from a single processed image which summarizes the information scattered in the 16 frames of the sequence. It has been shown (3) that the Gram Schmidt orthogonalization procedure gives the best results as to the representation of the left ventricle contour. This optimal contour (figure 3) plays the role of a reference with respect to the successive rough contours above defined, which can be synthetized from it by a quantitative geometric transformation.

2.3 - Quantitative characterization of the shape of the contours

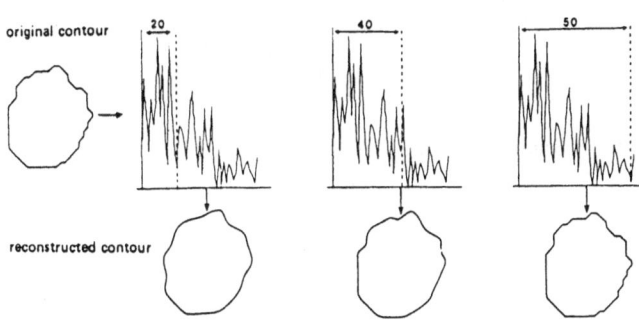

Figure 4 INFLUENCE OF THE NUMBER OF DESCRIPTORS

The contours of the left ventricle extracted from each frame are sampled at a given number of points where (1) is measured. After an expansion into a Fourier series, the FDs of each contour are available. These descriptors allow the reconstruction of the corresponding contours (figure 4). The wider the spectral band, the more detailled the reconstructed contour shape. Two consequences are noticed :

- 1st : it is possible to determine characteristic frequency bands in the FDs spectrum ;
- 2nd : smoothing effects are expected from a low-pass filtering of the spectrum, inducing a reduction of the noise that impairs rough contours.

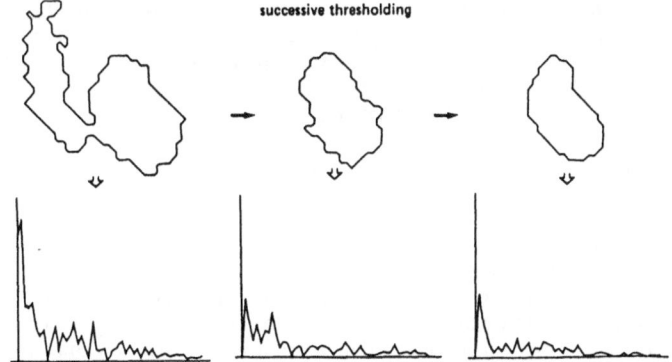

Figure 5 INFLUENCE OF THE CONTOUR EXTRACTION PROCEDURE

With a contour sampled at 100 points, 40 FDs were found sufficient for a satisfactory reconstruction.

The influence of the thresholding level on the content of the FDs spectrum is depicted in figure 5. The high frequency noise decreases, and the relative medium frequency content increases, as the threshold increases. This effect is consistent with the fact that a higher threshold selects regions of the left ventricle with a higher counting rate. Because of the counting statistics, the S/N ratio is higher and the contours are smooth (i.e. rich in medium angular frequencies).

2.4 - Sampling noise assessment

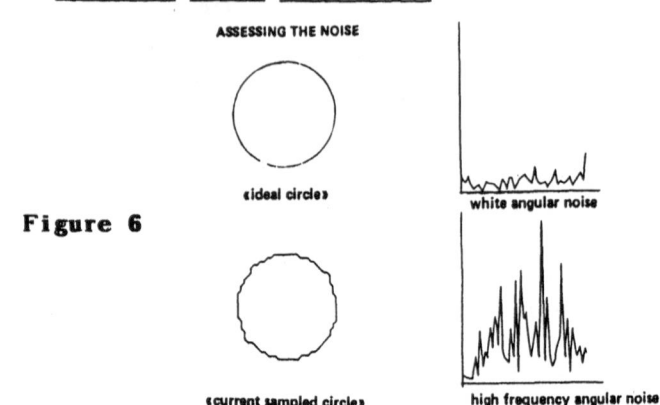

Figure 6

The total number of points sampled along a contour determines the accuracy of the description of the left ventricle. With a small number of points the sampled contour exhibits a staircase structure with wide rectilinear segments. The right angles introduce high frequencies in the FDs spectrum ; the segments are described by medium angular frequencies. These effects are shown in figure 6. The ideal FDs spectrum of a circle contains a single fundamental harmonic. The FDs spectra of the two actual sampled circles contain noise : the best sampling rate is characterized by a white angular noise of small amplitude, the worst sampling rate results in medium and high frequencies angular noise.

2.5 - Detection of abnormal contours in a sequence

The FDs spectrum of a contour displays the angular frequency content of the shape. Morever it represents the result of an information procedure, since 40 FDs are sufficient to reconstruct a contour sampled at 100 points. Shape modifications along a sequence of contours can be read in the corresponding sequence of FDs spectra. The example shown in figure 7 illustrates the detection of a burst of medium and high frequencies in the FDs spectrum of the 11th frame. The associated contour may represent either a wrong manual contour, or a kinetic trouble. An automatic detection algorithm can be designed from the measurement of the ratio of medium to high angular frequencies.

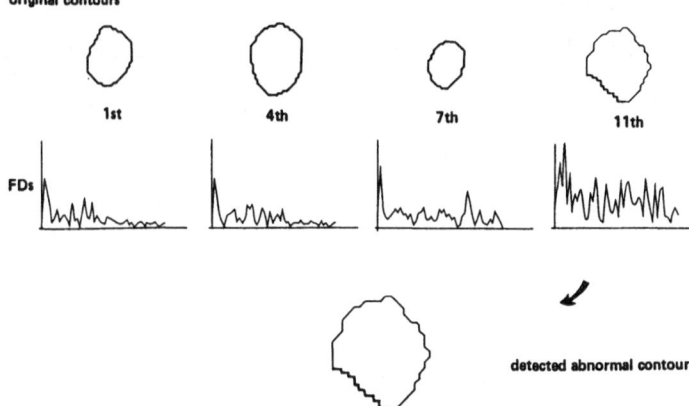

Figure 7

2.6 - Temporal evolution of the contours in a sequence

A quantitative analysis of shape modifications along a sequence is made possible by comparing the successive FDs spectra. The integrated square differences between the FDs spectra gives an estimation of their degree of resemblance. The example in figure 8 presents 5 contours on both sides of the systolic one. An euclidian distance between successive FDs spectra is obtained by normalization of their integrated square differences. This index is minimum at the systolic time. This result agrees with the fact that the volume variations of the left ventricle are minimum around this time.

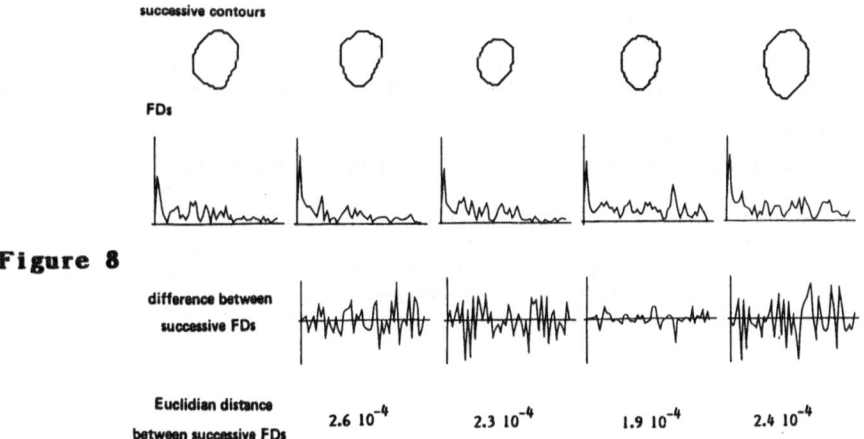

Figure 8

The temporal evolution of the sequence of contours will be determined in a further work by the Karhunen Loeve

transform. This information compression technique is expected
to extract the dominant temporal behaviour for the
modifications of the shape of the left ventricle.

3 - CONCLUSION

This "work in progress paper" illustrates some basic
properties of a new tool for a quantitative analysis of the
shape of cardiac cavities. The clinical validation has not
yet been undertaken.
The main results are :

- FDs account for the quantitative description of the shape
  of ventricular contours ;
- FDs introduce smoothing effects on rough contours ;
- FDs allow the detection of abnormal contours in a
  sequence.

Current problems are under investigation :

- The analysis of the isotropy of the contraction of the
  left ventricle, by using the scale invariance of the FDs
  spectra ;
- The extraction of the dominant behaviour of the cardiac
  contraction ;
- The automatic recognition and drawing of the contours.
- In a further study we will investigate the properties of
  the phase of the FDs, which may offer the possibility of
  locating abnormal parts along each contour.

4 - REFERENCES

1) Zahn C.t., Roskies R.Z., Fourier Descriptors for plane
   closed curves,
   I.E.E.E. Trans. on Computers ; vol. C-21, n° 3 (1972),
   269-281

2) Duvernoy J., Optical-digital processing of directional
   terrain textures, invariant under translation, rotation
and
   change of scale.
   Applied Optics, vol. 23, n° 6 (1984), 828-837

3) Duvernoy J., Cardot J.C., Baud M., VerdenetJ. Xia Y.,
   Berthout P., Faivre R., Bassand J.P., Bidet R.,
   Maurat J.P., Application of linear classifiers to the
   recognition of the temporal behaviour of the heart.
   Proc. IPMI VIII Conf. Bruxelles (1983), 202-222.

THYROID TOMOGRAPHY USING A SEVEN PINHOLE COLLIMATOR

John W. van Giessen[*], Max A. Viergever[*], Wouke H. Lam[*],
Cornelis N. de Graaf[**] and Peter J. van Noorden[**]

* Delft University of Technology, The Netherlands
** University Hospital Utrecht, The Netherlands

ABSTRACT
    In this paper we discuss a new application of the seven pinhole (7-P)
collimator: tomographic imaging of the thyroid. The collimator has been re-
optimized for this purpose by diminishing the distance from the aperture
plate to the crystal and by choosing a smaller diameter for the pinholes.
The reconstruction technique employed is the same as introduced by us for
7-P tomography of the heart [1]. This combination of imaging system and reconstruction method produces images of good quality and high resolution.
Therefore, it seems to offer a promising alternative to conventional planar
imaging (using a single pinhole or a parallel-hole collimator).

1. INTRODUCTION
    Applying a seven pinhole collimator for tomographic imaging of the heart
(using Tl-201 or Tc-99m) is a simple and cheap way of obtaining information
about possible ischaemic or infarcted areas of the heart muscle.
    The device has, however, a few restrictions which is why the 7-P colli-
mator has not gained wide appreciation. One of the restrictions is the
limited angle of view. Although this in itself does not prevent a proper
reconstruction of the projection data, the fact that gamma radiation follows
Poisson statistics and also is scattered and attenuated, produces so much
noise in the data that well known reconstruction techniques (such as the
class of convolution methods) cannot be used. Another restriction is the
fact that background activity accumulated from surrounding tissue structures
will produce artefacts. Therefore the quality of the reconstructions depends
greatly upon the way in which the background is subtracted.
    Nevertheless, reconstructions of a reasonable quality can be obtained
by using a suitable iterative algorithm [1].
    If the 7-P collimator is applied to perform thyroid tomography, the
above mentioned restrictions will not apply to the same extent:
- By re-optimizing the 7-P collimator design such that the thyroid can be
  brought nearer to the aperture plate, the angle of view can be enlarged.
  This advantage will be slightly undone by the fact that gamma rays emitted
  by source points very near the collimator can have a large angle of incidence upon the NaI crystal. In practice, this results in less accurate xy
  position detection of the incoming gamma quanta.
- The thyroid is a relatively small organ lying close beneath the surface of
  the skin. We therefore expect that the influence of scatter and absorption
  will be less than in the heart configuration. Of course, this will strongly depend upon the chosen isotope. If Tc-99m is used, the above mentioned
  expectation will probably come true, but if I-123 is used the expectation
  may well prove wrong.
- We expect, furthermore, that the amount of background activity from surrounding tissue structures will be smaller than in the heart configuration,

and, therefore, will have less influence upon the quality of the reconstructions. Especially, if I-123 is used, which is more specific for the
thyroid than Tc-99m, we expect very little background radiation.

In this paper we will discuss some preliminary experiments performed
with three different isotopes: Co-57, I-123 and Tc-99m.

2. COLLIMATOR DESIGN AND HARDWARE PERIPHERALS

The commercial 7-P heart collimator (as first proposed by Vogel et al.
[2]) can, in principle, be used for imaging the thyroid. The reconstructions,
however, will not be very satisfying because the system configuration has
been optimized for the heart geometry.

We modified the geometrical design in such a way that the organ under
investigation can be positioned closer to the collimator which, together
with choosing a smaller diameter for the pinholes, will result in improved
resolution throughout the Simultaneous-Field-Of-View (SFOV) of the system.
Accordingly, we diminished the distance between collimator and detector to
get a proper magnification factor for the projection of the thyroid upon
the crystal surface. In order to make positioning in the directions parallel
to the collimator non-critical we did not change the spacing between the one
central and the six peripheral pinholes. The differences between the heart
collimator and the thyroid collimator are demonstrated schematically in
Fig. 1.

The SFOV is divided into 8 slices of 7.5 mm thickness beginning at
41.25 mm from the collimator midplane, that is 35.50 mm from the outer surface of the collimator plate (see Fig. 2). Normally, the deterioration of
the resolution with increasing distance to the collimator is taken into
account by using variable slice thicknesses. In clinical practice, however,
this variability makes the quantitative evaluation of the reconstruction
more difficult because physicians are not used to non-equidistant slices
(cf. CT and MRI images).

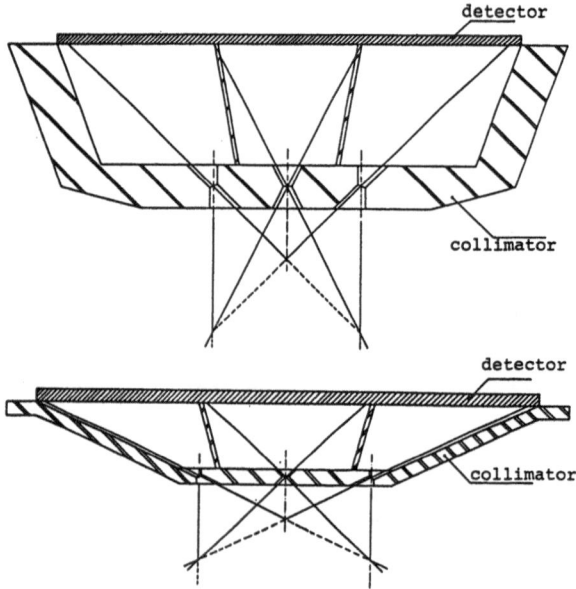

FIGURE 1. The heart collimator (top) and the thyroid collimator (bottom).

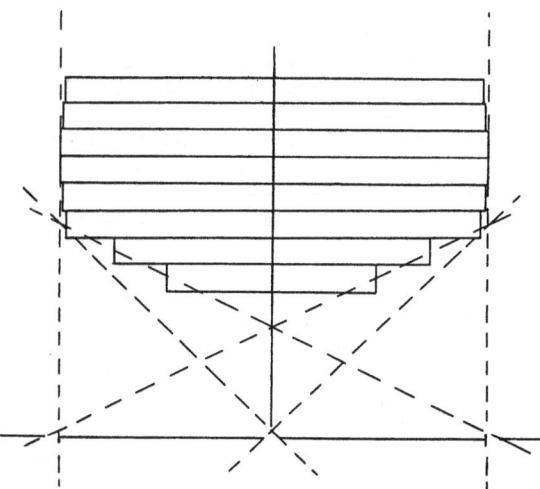

FIGURE 2. The eight reconstruction slices in the simultaneous field of view (SFOV). The dashed lines are the boundaries of three projection cones (one central, two peripheral).

The projection matrix, which gives the relation between pixels and corresponding voxels, has been built up under the assumption that each pixel "sees" nine voxels in each reconstruction plane. This results in voxels with small dimensions in the x- and y-directions, which is necessary to make good in-plane resolution possible.

The in-plane voxel size varies from 3.1 mm in the first slice (nearest to the collimator) to 6.1 mm in the last slice. These sizes are approximately a factor 2 smaller than the corresponding ones in the heart configuration [1,3]. This reflects the fact that we expect a better resolution of the present device.

The 7-P collimator is mounted on a large field of view gamma camera with an intrinsic resolution of 4.0 mm. The processing software is implemented on a HP1000F minicomputer. Both the input data and the reconstructed tomograms can be displayed on a video image processor linked to the minicomputer.

3. DATA PROCESSING

Before reconstruction, the raw projection data should be preprocessed in two ways:

- the 7-P projection of a reference point source is used to spatially transform raw projection data such that they will fit the geometry expected by the reconstruction software.
- the image of a sheet source is used to correct for spatial non-uniformities and to compensate for gamma camera inhomogeneities.

After reconstruction, the tomograms should be postprocessed individually to correct for voxel size, distance to the collimator and, if appropriate, attenuation. These corrections could be performed on-the-fly (that is, during reconstruction) involving a certain amount of extra CPU-time. The accuracy of the reconstruction, however, will not improve significantly by on-the-fly correction [1].

The reconstruction algorithm is a modified version of Herman's ART3 [4]. We gave our algorithm the acronym ART3H, in which the H stands for histogram and is added because we introduced a dependence of one of the parameters on the mode of the histogram of the input data. This reconstruction technique has been thoroughly discussed in one of our previous papers [1], so we here confine ourselves to discussing its most important characteristics. The algorithm is a row action method which means that in each iteration one raysum is adjusted by correcting all voxels contributing to the relevant pixel. In one iteration cycle all pixels are accessed once. By accessing the rays in a random sequence the speed of convergence can be increased. The number of manipulations needed to correct the voxel intensities is small and therefore the algorithm is fast. Furthermore, the algorithm consumes relatively little computer memory space. Best results were achieved with a zero initial distribution, a relaxation factor of .4 for the correction feedback to the voxel intensities, and constraining negative reconstruction values to zero after each iteration cycle. The optimum number of iteration cycles depends, among other things, on the noise in the data and may be different for each class of objects.

An extra step in the reconstruction consists of processing the resulting tomograms by an operator which we gave the acronym FIZEVO (FInd ZEro VOxels). This operator searches for all voxels seen by zero-valued pixels: for each zero-valued pixel the voxels in the corresponding ray are set equal to zero (that is, if they are not zero already) except for the voxel with the highest intensity in the ray, the value of which is left unchanged. Although it would seem more logical to assign the value zero to all voxels seen by zero-valued pixels, the operator described here has a decidedly better effect upon the reconstruction. Apparently, the highest intensity voxel in a zero-pixel ray often has a non-negligible value. The fact that this occurs may be attributed to the Poisson statistical nature of gamma emission or to scattering processes. Since removing non-zero voxels from the reconstruction process (resulting in ragged object boundaries) clearly does more damage to the image than taking zero-valued voxels into account, the procedure as described above was followed.

We introduce this operator, because it had a very good influence upon the quality of the reconstructions acquired with the 7-P heart collimator [1].

4. EXPERIMENTS

In order to evaluate the performance of the imaging system in combination with the reconstruction algorithm, a number of experiments have been performed:
- Phantom studies. We used four real objects to evaluate the performance of the system: a point source positioned on the axis of the imaging system, an F-shaped phantom, an array of narrow spaced point sources (all of the same intensity), and a thyroid phantom with three cold spots and one hot spot. After reconstruction of the objects the quality of the results can be judged on the basis of likeness to the original object, (visual) resolution and presence or absence of artefacts.
- FWHM and linearity studies. We can determine point source FWHM (Full Width at Half Maximum) resolution in the xy-plane (parallel to the detector) as well as in the z-direction (along the system axis) by calculating least-squares fits of point source reconstructions to 3D gaussoids. Furthermore, the displacements due to reconstruction of the point sources both in-plane (dxy) and in the z-direction (dz) can be computed using the gaussoids to determine the source centre locations.
- Depth homogeneity studies. One of the objectives of tomographic reconstruction is to produce quantitative images which requires that depth homogeneity should be preserved. This can be investigated on the basis of the

reconstruction of the array of point sources.

The source which was used in the single point source measurements and in the point source array measurement (which in fact is built up by adding single point source images) was a small Co-57 emitter (diameter smaller than .5 mm). The F-phantom consists of a combination of Co-57 line sources (about 1 mm thick) in the shape of an F, of which width and height are approximately 50 mm (the line sources are enclosed by two perspex plates). The thyroid phantom, which has a rather complicated design, is shown in Fig. 3.

All of the thyroid phantom measurements were performed twice: once using Tc-99m and once using I-123.

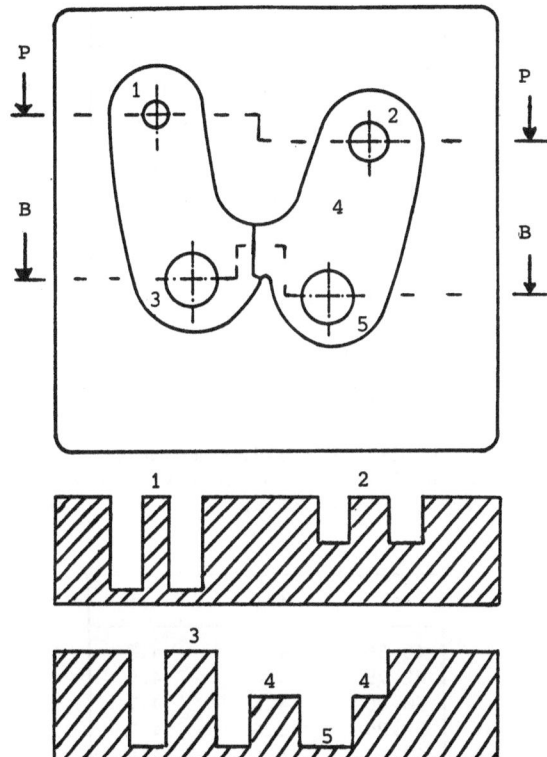

FIGURE 3. The thyroid phantom. Top: frontal view of the phantom. Middle: cross-section PP. Bottom: cross-section BB. The following features can be distinguished:
- Three cold spots indicated (1), (2) and (3) having diameters of 6, 9 and 12 mm, respectively.
- A 'cold block' of perspex (4).
- A local hot spot (5) of 12 mm diameter, consisting of a cylindrical hole in the perspex block and having the same activity as the rest of the phantom.

5. RESULTS

In this section the results of the experimental studies are discussed.

In Table 1 the results of the linearity studies are shown: the calculated displacements are almost uniformly distributed throughout the SFOV with an average of 0.8 mm (standard deviation = 0.5 mm) in the xy-direction and 0.7 mm (s.d. = 0.4 mm) in the z-direction. Hence, the reconstruction will not be seriously affected by non-linearities.

z	dxy	d̄z
49.50	1.1	0.2
52.75	1.5	0.5
56.00	1.4	1.0
59.25	1.4	0.5
62.50	1.4	0.5
69.00	0.9	0.3
72.25	0.6	0.6
75.50	0.4	0.5
78.75	0.5	0.9
82.00	0.4	0.7
85.25	0.5	0.2
88.50	0.3	1.4
95.00	0.3	1.7

TABLE 1. Displacements of on-axis point sources by the reconstruction procedure. z = distance from the point source to the pinhole plane; dxy = displacement parallel to the detector plane; dz = displacement parallel to the system axis, all in mm's.

Table 2 shows the results of the resolution measurements for point sources in air (no surrounding scattering medium).

The average of the in-plane resolution fxy is 4.9 mm with a standard deviation of 0.3 mm. The z-resolution fz averages 5.5 mm (s.d. = 0.9 mm).

z	fxy	fz
49.50	4.6	4.2
52.75	4.4	4.9
56.00	4.6	4.7
59.25	4.6	4.7
62.50	4.6	4.6
69.00	4.8	5.2
72.25	4.9	5.5
75.50	5.0	5.9
78.75	5.1	5.5
82.00	5.1	6.5
85.25	5.2	6.5
88.50	5.3	7.1
95.00	5.5	6.3

TABLE 2. FWHM resolution values for on-axis point sources in air. z as in Table 1; fxy = FWHM resolution parallel to the detector plane; fz = FWHM resolution parallel to the system axis, all in mm's.

Hence, in-plane resolution and depth resolution are almost equal. Moreover, these calculations indicate that, as expected, fxy and fz figures are correlated with the distance from the point source to the collimator: the nearer to the aperture plate the better the resolution.

The depth homogeneity of the system can be derived from Fig. 4. Depth homogeneity is certainly not uniform along the axis of the system, especially because there is an unexpected jump in intensity from the second to the third plane. A possible explanation for this strange phenomenon may be the fact that for the lower slices the angle of incidence of a gamma quantum on the camera can be large, resulting in a large uncertainty as to where the quantum will be detected. Moreover, the depth homogeneity profile is rather sensitive to changes in the parameters of the reconstruction algorithm.

All of the above results were obtained without the FIZEVO operator. FIZEVO is a non-linear operator and therefore can diminish depth homogeneity. This is especially true in the cases that the reconstructed object is very small in the xy-direction (like the line source). Also, in the case of single point source reconstructions, FIZEVO will sharpen up the point source, resulting in better, but somewhat flattered, FWHM figures.

Figure 5 shows the raw projection data of the (calibration) point source, the array of point sources, the F-phantom and the thyroid phantom (filled with a Tc-99m solution). No extra perspex plates were placed around any of these objects.

Figure 6 shows reconstructions (without FIZEVO) of the above mentioned raw projection data. The point source reconstruction confirms that the resolution of the system is very good (considering the fact that the intrinsic resolution of the Anger camera is 4.0 mm an average resolution of 5.2 mm in the object space is very good indeed). The reconstruction of the point source array has been discussed before, see Fig. 4. The reconstruction of

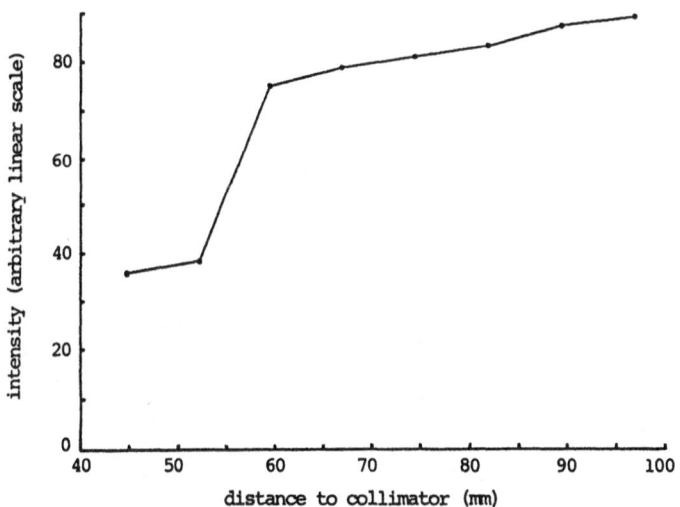

FIGURE 4. Depth homogeneity of the imaging device (including reconstruction). The plotted intensities are the sums of counts within the reconstructed point source regions.

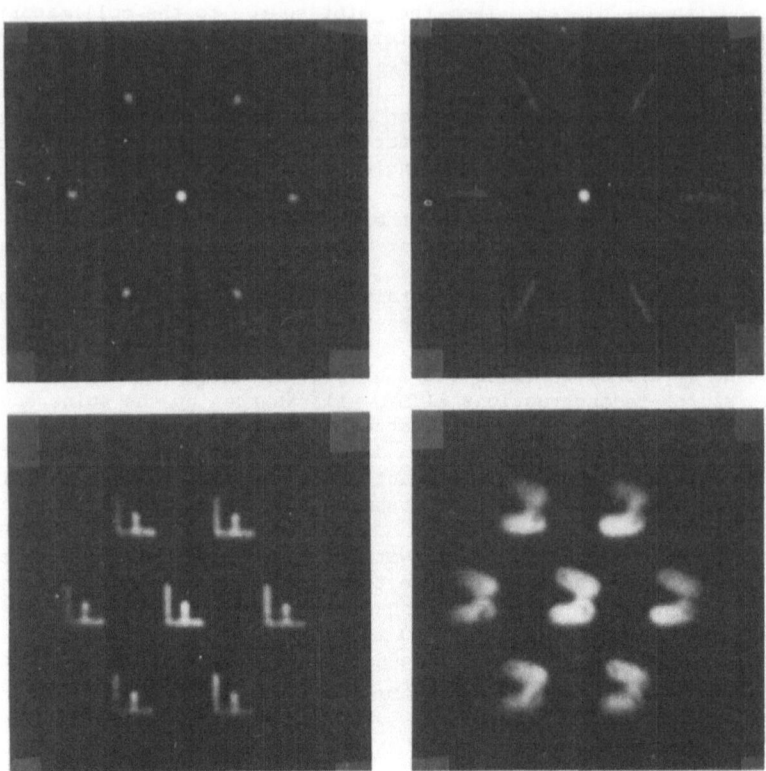

FIGURE 5. Raw projection data acquired with the 7-P collimator. Top left: point source on the axis of the imaging system at 60 mm from the collimator midplane. Top right: the array of point sources (narrow spaced, on-axis). Bottom left: F-shaped phantom, parallel to the detector. Bottom right: thyroid phantom.

the F-shaped phantom is sharp and clear and contains only a few artefacts. The reconstruction of the thyroid phantom is quite good. Two cold spots can be clearly distinguished, the third one, however, is too small (6 mm in diameter) to be detected. This is a good example of the fact that point source resolution is only an indication of the overall (extended source) resolution of the device. Furthermore, one can clearly observe the local hot spot (i.e., the cylindrical hole in the perspex block) in the fifth slice.

Figure 7 shows the same reconstructions as Fig. 6 but now with application of the FIZEVO operator. For the point source, the F-shaped phantom and the thyroid phantom the effect of using this operator is that it deletes some of the artefacts without influencing the object itself. The effect of the operator on the reconstruction of the array of point sources is, on the contrary, quite large and not at all positive.

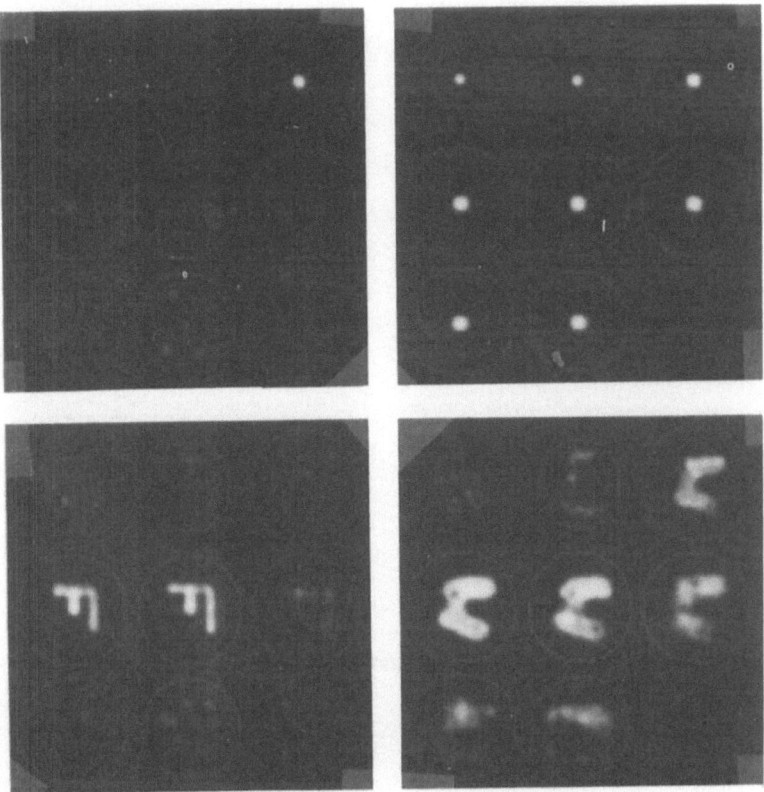

FIGURE 6. Reconstructions without FIZEVO of the projection data presented in Fig. 5. The reconstructed tomograms are stored from left to right and from top to bottom (the upper left slice is nearest to the collimator). Each of the slices is encompassed by a circle to indicate its boundary.

Figure 8 shows thyroid phantom reconstructions for the case that I-123 is used instead of Tc-99m. The reconstructions are not as good as those presented in Fig. 6 & 7. Although I-123 may be a more interesting radiofarmacon from a clinical point of view, it seems to induce more scatter than Tc-99m, resulting in poorer reconstructions. A definitive conclusion about the most suitable radionuclide will have to await the evaluation of patient studies, however.

6. CONCLUSIONS
In this paper we have discussed the application of a seven pinhole collimator to thyroid tomography. The design of the original 7-P collimator, which was developed for imaging of the heart, has been adapted to fit the needs of thyroid tomography.

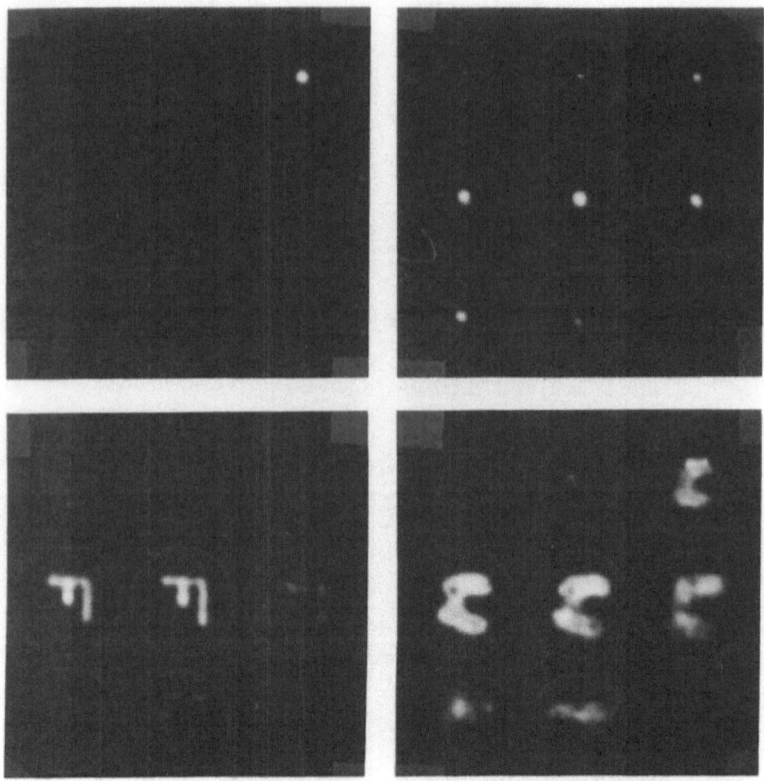

FIGURE 7. Reconstructions with FIZEVO of the raw projection data presented in Fig. 5.

For the reconstruction of the 7-P projection data we use a variant of Herman's ART3 algorithm. A special operator (FIZEVO), which resets to zero all but one of the non-zero voxel intensities corresponding with a zero projection pixel, can be added to the reconstruction process.

The present combination of imaging device and reconstruction technique produces images of good quality. The average in-plane FWHM resolution for point sources in air is 4.9 mm, the corresponding axial resolution is 5.5 mm. Reconstructions of a thyroid phantom show that a cold spot of 6 mm diameter cannot be detected, but 9 mm and 12 mm cold spots and a 12 mm hot spot are clearly visible in the tomograms. Based on these results, we expect that the 7-P device is suitable for tomographic imaging of the thyroid.

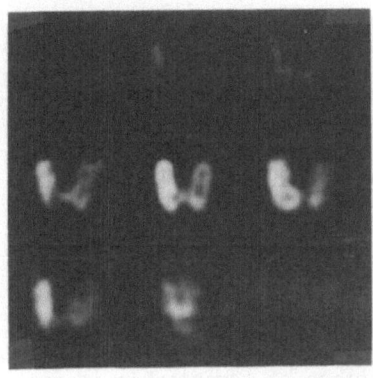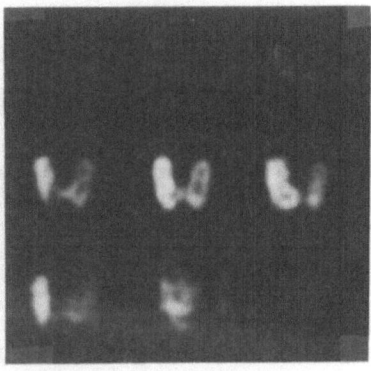

FIGURE 8. Reconstructions of the thyroid phantom filled with a I-123 solution. Left: without FIZEVO. Right: with FIZEVO.

REFERENCES

1. Van Giessen, J.W., Viergever, M.A. and de Graaf, C.N. (1985). Improved tomographic reconstruction in seven-pinhole imaging, IEEE Trans. Med. Im. 4, 91-103.
2. Vogel, R.A., Kirch, D.L., LeFree, M.T. and Steele, P.P. (1978). A new method of multiplanar emission tomography using a seven pinhole collimator and an Anger scintillation camera, J. Nucl. Med. 19, 648-654.
3. LeFree, M.T., Vogel, R.A., Kirch, D.L. and Steele, P.P. (1981). Seven pin-hole tomography - A technical description, J. Nucl. Med. 22, 48-54.
4. Herman, G.T. (1975). A relaxation method for reconstructing objects from noisy X-rays, Math. Programming 8, 1-19.

STRATEGIES FOR INFORMATIVE DISPLAYS OF BLOOD VESSELS USING MAGNETIC
RESONANCE IMAGING DATA

JD Hale, PE Valk, L Kaufman, LE Crooks, CB Higgins and JC Watts,
UCSF Radiologic Imaging Laboratory, 400 Grandview Drive,
South San Francisco, CA 94080

INTRODUCTION
   Magnetic resonance imaging (MRI) generates a series of cross-sections,
or slices, of the human body. The advantage of tomographic images over
planar images such as those of standard x-rays is that overlap is avoided.
The disadvantage is that the planar view is unfamiliar to most people, and
to make use of the information in the images it is often necessary to
study many slices and to visualize mentally features in three dimensions.
   Algorithms which aid three-dimensional visualization of particular
structures have been developed for MRI and x-ray CT (1-5). This involves
identifying regions of interest, placing them in a three-dimensional
context, and displaying projections onto a two-dimensional monitor. The
projections have the more familiar appearance of, say, standard x-rays but
without the overlapping of unwanted tissue. The images can be displayed
from various perspectives, contrast-enhanced, or encoded by color or gray
scale to show relationships other than signal intensity to differentiate
tissues.
   In order to be useful, the new images must provide more information or
facilitate some other even more tedious procedure. In the case of
three-dimensional skeletal images now being made from x-ray CT data, not
only the diagnosis but also the surgical planning and the manufacture of
prosthetic templates are aided by the computer. The MRI vessel
reconstructions, in addition to the improved anatomic visualization,
display information about flow and patent area which is difficult to
determine by looking at the original slices.

Spin echo MRI and flow
   The potential use of spin echo, dual echo MRI to diagnose diseases of
the cardiovascular system has been described (6-7). Both the anatomic
structure and the flow dynamics of blood vessels can be derived from the
data. Using this information, we are making reconstructed projections of
vessels which help to assess patency, to demonstrate pathology, and to
contribute to the understanding of the effect of flow on signal intensity.
   The intensity of a pixel is described by:

$$I = N(H)\ f(v)\ e(-TE/T2)\ [1 - e(-TR/T1)] \qquad (1)$$

N(H) is the number of hydrogen nuclei in the volume of the pixel; TE and
TR are computer-controlled timing parameters; T1 and T2 are time-dependent
properties of the tissue; and f(v) is the flow function, which is a
combination of motion effects we have been studying for some time. With a
TR of 2 seconds and a TE of 28 msec, we find an inverse relationship

between velocity of blood flow at a pixel and the intensity of that pixel.
Fast flowing blood has low intensity because the hydrogen nuclei, the
source of the signal, move through the slice plane too fast to be
detected. We call this the outflow effect. As flow decreases, blood
begins to give a detectable signal, but it is still somewhat
attenuated by its motion. Some of the attenuation is a result of the
dephasing of neighboring nuclei moving across magnetic gradients. In spin
echo, dual echo acquisition, first and second echo images are collected at
slightly different times. For stationary tissue, the second echo shows
signal decay relative to the first echo. The decay is determined by the
T2 value of the tissue, which we calculate from the equation:

$$T2 = TE/\ln(I1/I2) \qquad\qquad (2)$$

where I1 is the first echo intensity and I2 is the second. Where there is
nonuniform motion, there is attenuation of I1 from dephasing but little or
no attenuation of I2. This results in an increase in the calculated T2
value wherever: 1) flow velocity within a pixel is variable enough to
cause dephasing; and, 2) absolute mean flow velocity is slow enough to
produce detectable signal in both echoes.

Singer (8) described dephasing in terms of isochromats, groups of spins
moving at the same velocity. All spins traveling across magnetic
gradients experience a shift in phase (relative to the phase of stationary
tissue) proportional to their velocities. Axel (9) notes that if within a
pixel there is a significant range of velocities (i.e., many isochromats)
there will be different phase shifts and the intensity of that pixel will
be reduced (Fig. 1). Singer illustrated this by graphing the phase
changes of five isochromats through the spin echo pulse sequence. The
graph showed that for the second echo and all even echoes the isochromats
are brought back to zero phase and no loss of intensity is predicted.

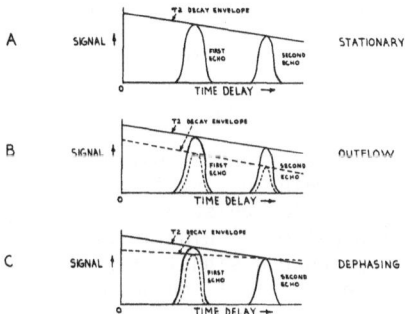

FIGURE 1. Dotted lines show effects of outflow and dephasing on intensity. The net effect is a combination of the two.

There are two mechanisms which cause variations in velocity across a
pixel and thus induce dephasing. In the laminar flow model, the velocity
profile across a vessel is parabolic, with greatest velocity in the center
and lowest velocity near the wall. Variation within a pixel is
proportional to the slope of the parabola, which is zero in the center and
greatest at the wall. Thus, dephasing is greatest at the wall, where flow
is slowest (Fig. 2).

236

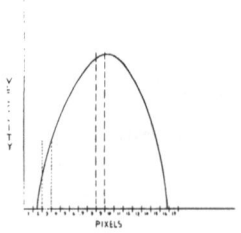

FIGURE 2. Laminar flow has a parabolic velocity profile, flat in the center (pixel 9) and steep near the wall (pixel 3). Pixel 3 will experience much more first echo dephasing.

The other cause of dephasing is turbulence, by which we mean rapid fluctuations in the velocity profile. In laminar flow, turbulence occurs at velocities above a certain threshold determined by the diameter of the vessel and the viscosity of blood. Turbulence can also result from the acceleration and deceleration of pulsatile flow, from obstructions within the vessel, or from sudden changes in vessel diameter. Whatever the cause of turbulence, it can only be detected in MRI images where the mean flow velocity is low enough to allow signal to be acquired from the moving blood.

Dephasing and outflow both reduce signal. If the signal intensity is low enough to provide contrast with surrounding tissue, we can detect it with an intensity threshold. Gas in lung and bowel also has low intensity, so that a region of interest (ROI) must be drawn to eliminate these nonvascular features. More slowly flowing blood whose signal is as high as its surroundings can be found by calculating its T2 value pixel by pixel and selecting pixels with a T2 longer than any stationary tissue in the ROI. We have determined that blood flowing faster than 17 cm/sec will produce a signal less than 15% of image maximum in our spin echo data. We have also found that blood producing signal greater than 15% maximum tends to have a T2 longer than 100 msec. In the abdomen, a two-tiered threshold routine which first selects pixels lower than 15% of maximum, then selects pixels with a T2 longer than 100 msec according to equation (2), is successful in finding vessel flow channels.

Another flow effect can increase intraluminal signal. During the spin echo sequence most spins in a sample will remain in a state of partial saturation from the repeated 90 degree excitation pulses. Nuclei of blood without previous exposure to an excitation pulse, flowing into a slice, will not be partially saturated and will produce a signal greater than nuclei of stationary blood. We call this paradoxical enhancement (6). This is a potential problem when we are counting on signal attenuation to reveal flow, because enhancement will counteract attenuation. The multi-slice technique confines the problem to the first few slices encountered by the unirradiated blood, since the deeper the "fresh" blood travels into the sample, the greater the probability that it will receive its first 90 degree pulse. Furthermore, by using a TR of 2 seconds, we give all the spins in the sample 2 seconds to recover magnetization. Since most tissue, and certainly blood, will reach full remagnetization in less than 2 seconds, there will, in effect, be no partial saturation state.

Both stationary and flowing spins will always be fully magnetized at the beginning of each 90 degree pulse.

METHODS
Pixel classification

The detection of flowing blood in MR images is accomplished by a combination of two threshold operations. The first is an intensity threshold which finds pixels less than or equal to 15% of image maximum. The second finds pixels with a T2 value greater than or equal to 100 msec. The operator draws an ROI to eliminate lung and bowel from the search.

Pixels chosen by the intensity threshold are classified as fast flowing blood and those found by the T2 threshold are classified as slowly flowing blood. The flow pixels are highlighted to show the operator the result of the search and to permit editing. Optional subroutines fill in pixels which were not selected but which are surrounded by those that were, or delete pixels that were selected but have no orthogonal neighbors that were. Such isolated pixels are often caused by image noise. If these "smoothing" routines are used, the order in which they run is important. Suppose that as a result of thresholding, part of a vessel cross-section contains a checkerboard pattern of chosen pixels. The checkerboard indicates that there are several pixels within a vessel that do not meet the flow criteria. This might be a lesion, turbulence, or a region of very slow flow. If the filling routine runs first, the checkerboard will be completely filled in, but if the deleting routine runs first, it will be erased. Filling before erasing tends to make the outlines of vessel highlights smoother. Erasing before filling brings out potential intra-luminal lesions. The operator may decide whether to aim for a smooth vessel image or one that emphasizes lesions by choosing the order of "smoothing." Alternatively, "smoothing" may be disabled completely, leaving a rougher but statistically more rigorous vessel highlight.

Segmentation

Assuming that there is not a profusion of vessel segments in a slice, it is relatively easy to automate the detection of connected groups of pixels. In a single pass, the computer can scan a line at a time, determine contiguous pieces of highlighted pixels in a line, and connect the pieces into two-dimensional regions representing vessel cross-sections.

For each line, the algorithm keeps track of the starting and ending points of each uninterrupted piece of highlighted pixels. The previous line is checked for pieces which touch. The operator may decide in advance whether pieces which touch only diagonally at the end points should be connected. Touching pieces merge together into ever-expanding regions until the entire image has been scanned.

To facilitate the reconstruction process, the algorithm creates a record of data describing each region with the following values: 1) the coordinates of the smallest rectangle (parallel to the x an y axes) that surrounds the region; 2) left, right, top, and bottom projection outlines; 3) the number of pixels in the region (cross-sectional area); and 4) the number of pixels found by the T2 threshold (low velocity area).

Connecting the region

Once vessel cross-sections have been outlined it would be possible to create longitudinal views immediately. We could display the regions edge-on, stacked vertically, and thick enough either to touch each other or to reflect the original slice thickness. The resulting image has jagged contours. Any color or gray scale coding showing depth would have abrupt changes between slice boundaries. Our approach is to determine connections between the vessel segments in adjacent slices and then to interpolate along the vessels within the individual contours of connecting segments.

Connecting two-dimensional regions from slice to slice is more difficult than joining pieces of lines into two-dimensional regions, primarily because the slice thickness and center-to-center offset are substantially greater than the x-y pixel size. A vessel running obliquely through the slice plane can be offset more than its whole diameter from one slice to the next, so that the planar cross-sections do not appear connected in three-space. Also, a pair of oblique vessels running parallel to each other may create a situation where the cross-section of one vessel in one slice appears connected to the cross-section of the other vessel in the next slice.

The algorithm works sequentially through the slices in a direction away from the heart. In the following discussion of connections, the term "region" refers to a vessel cross-section in a arbitrary slice and "candidate" denotes a cross-section in the next (more distal) slice that is a potential continuation of a given region.

We employ a combination of size, shape, and location clues to decide connections of vessels between slices. The rectangle in the record for each region is projected onto the next slice to determine the search space for potential connections. The operator has the option to expand the rectangle several pixels in x and y. By default, the expansion in pixels is the ratio of the resolution in z (center-to-center slice distance) and the resolution in x and y, typically 5 to 1, or 5 pixels. This allows for a certain amount of relative x-y offset between slices. Any region which touches this rectangle becomes a connection candidate for the original region. For each candidate, a connection probability is calculated, as well as the amount of x-y overlap between the region and its candidate. These two values are stored in a table for further processing. Each region in a slice has a table of candidates in the next slice.

The connection probability is based on the relative sizes and shapes of the regions. Size probability is the ratio of the area of the smaller region to that of the larger region. Shape is compared in the same way, the lower shape value being divided by the higher value. To compute the "shape value" of a region we again consider the region's rectangle. The first clue to the shape of a region is the ratio of the rectangle's width to its length. Round regions have square rectangles. As a region is flattened along its x or y axis, the rectangle gets longer and thinner, so that the width/length ratio decreases. If, however, the region is flattened along an axis 45 degrees from the x and y axes, the rectangle remains square. In this case, another ratio can reveal that the region is out of round, namely the ratio of the region's area to the area of the rectangle. All of these ratios are computed with the smaller value in the numerator so that they fall in the (0-1) range. Thus they can be treated as probabilities - multiplied or weighted and added with the results still in (0-1). The two shape ratios (rectangle width/rectangle length and region area/rectangle area) are multiplied to give the shape value. The more nearly round the region, the higher the value. The shape probability and the size probability are averaged to give the connection probability.

The algorithm uses the connection probability and the amount of overlap between a region and its candidates to decide which of them connect. All candidates which have no overlap and whose probability is below a threshold entered by the operator are eliminated. The best candidate is labeled as connected, the rest remain tentative. To find the best candidate, it is necessary to combine the connection probability and the overlap into a single value to be compared to values of other candidates. Two new ratios are calculated: overlap/region area and overlap/candidate area. The ratios are then added to the connection probability. The highest scoring connection (best candidate) is chosen as the continuation for the region.

If a candidate is chosen by more than one region as a continuation, there is a potential merging of vessels, something that is rare but possible when working distally. The algorithm avoids merges if other connection configurations are available. Just as regions can have best candidates, candidates can have favorite regions among those that have chosen them as continuations. The algorithm finds the best connection from the candidate's point of view (its favorite region) and seeks other unconnected candidates for the other regions. Any region-candidate pair found is connected, and the connection from that region to the original candidate is eliminated. If the original candidate still has multiple connections after this, another unconnected candidate is sought for the favorite region as well. Then if there are still multiple connections to the original candidate, they are allowed to stand (i.e., the vessels are allowed to merge).

Any candidates that have not been connected are potential bifurcations of vessels that are already connected. These candidates are connected to their favorite regions. The operator may prevent some or all bifurcations by specifying a range of slices within which they are allowed. Outside this range, the only bifurcations permitted are branches, connections in which one of the candidates is much smaller than the bifurcating region. The operator also specifies how much smaller these branches must be.

Drawing vessels

Once all the connections are established, the algorithm can work directly from the projection outlines of the regions to make a two-dimensional reconstructed vessel image. From the longitudinal view, the outlines are one-dimensional arrays of pixels which are displayed horizontally. Outlines from different slices are separated vertically according to the center-to-center distance between slices, which, as explained above, is typically 5 pixels. The four image lines between the slice projection are filled in by interpolating from each region to its continuation 5 lines away. Regions with no connections are not displayed, a kind of "smoothing" along the original z axis.

The pixel values of the projection outlines contain depth information, the pixels nearer the front of the reconstructed image being brighter than those deeper in the image. Starting with the left-most pixel of each pair of connecting regions, the algorithm performs a linear interpolation along the straightest possible path from one pixel to the other. The same is done with the right-most pixels. Following parallel paths, the algorithm works from the edges to the center until the entire vessel is filled in. This interpolates not only depth but also width. The width of a vessel as seen on the display will be equal to the size of the region outline at the slice level of the region and will gradually change to the size of the continuation's outline at the next level (Fig. 3). For overlapping vessels, the highest value only is retained for each pixel. This way the vessels are clearly delineated, and the order in which they are filled in is irrelevant.

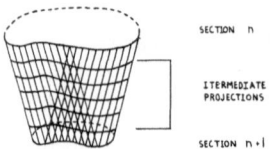

FIGURE 3. Standard interpolation is done starting with straight lines between the outer edges of the projections and working towards the center.

There are other ways to fill in vessels. One method connects a vessel to a branch, a bifurcation in which one region is much smaller than the other. Here only one edge is used as a starting point, the shorter of the two paths between left-most pixels or right-most pixels of the two projection outlines. Filling in is done along parallel paths starting at the chosen edge and stopping at the other side of the smaller region. The displayed width of such a vessel will be constant and equal to that of the smaller region (Fig. 4).

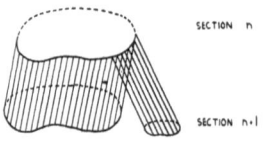

FIGURE 4. Small branching segments connect along the shortest straight path to the main vessel in the previous section.

So far we have assumed that the vessel regions are cross-sections, and that the vessels are moving perpendicular to the slice plane. In fact, we prefer this situation and choose our imaging orientation (e.g., transaxial slices of the abdomen) so that all or most of the large vessels are as near as possible to intersecting the image plane at 90 degrees. Even so, we often encounter vessels parallel to the plane and must deal with regions that are length-wise cuts rather than cross-sections of vessels. The algorithm recognizes these regions using operator-entered thresholds on the shape values. Recall that the shape value is proportional to the roundness of the region. Regions are divided into three categories: ROUND for high values, SNAKE for low values, and EITHER for intermediate values. The filling-in schemes described above apply only when neither region is a SNAKE, and the displayed vessel width depends on the size of one or both of the projection outlines. For a SNAKE, the outline is a projection of its length, not its width. We must find the diameter of the vessel and connect one end of the SNAKE to the other region.

To find the diameter of a region we use the rectangle much the same way we use it to find shape. The width (shorter dimension) of the rectangle is an approximation of the vessel diameter. To correct for SNAKEs not parallel to the x or y axis, we multiply the rectangle width by the ratio of region area to rectangle area. The connection is made from the end of

the SNAKE nearest to the region to which it is connecting (if it is also a
SNAKE, then to the nearest endpoint of it). If both are SNAKEs and they
overlap, the connection takes a straight path through the overlap. Any
part of a SNAKE not involved in a connection is filled out to the proper
diameter and centered around its own slice projection (FIG 5).

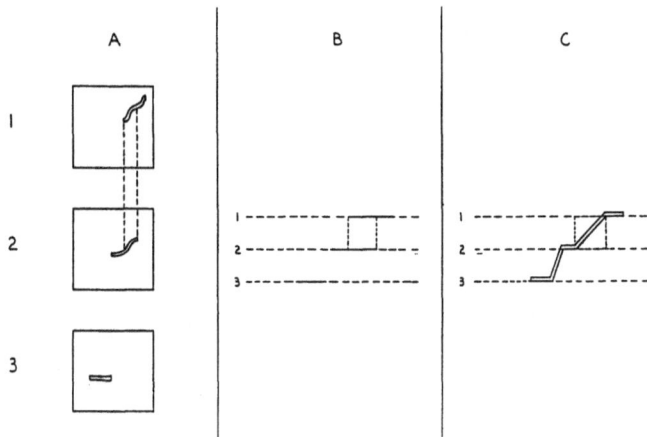

FIGURE 5. Connecting SNAKES. Column A shows three sequential sections
containing a vessel running almost parallel to the slice planes. Vertical
dotted lines indicate the overlap of two of the vessel segments. Column B
shows the sections rotated 90 degrees toward the reader with projections
of each vessel segment in solid lines. Column C shows the result of the
drawing routine. The connection path between sections 1 and 2 takes an
angle through the area of overlap. The path between 2 and 3 simply
connects the nearest endpoints of the two segments. At each section
level, the nonoverlapping parts of the vessels (all of segment 3 and
portions of segments 1 and 2) are "thickened" to their original diameters
and drawn along the slice planes (horizontal dotted lines).

If an intermediate shaped region (EITHER) connects to a SNAKE, it is
treated as a SNAKE. Otherwise, it is treated as ROUND.

Display options
The standard output of the algorithm consists of depth-encoded vessel
reconstructions. Anterior, posterior, and lateral views can be displayed,
as well as images of individual vessels. A vessel map containing the
region records and the table of connections is stored on the disk.
Vessels are numbered as they are being reconstructed, and the numbers are
stored in the low-order bits of the pixel values in the depth images.
This provides a pixel-by-pixel cross-reference between the image and the
map.

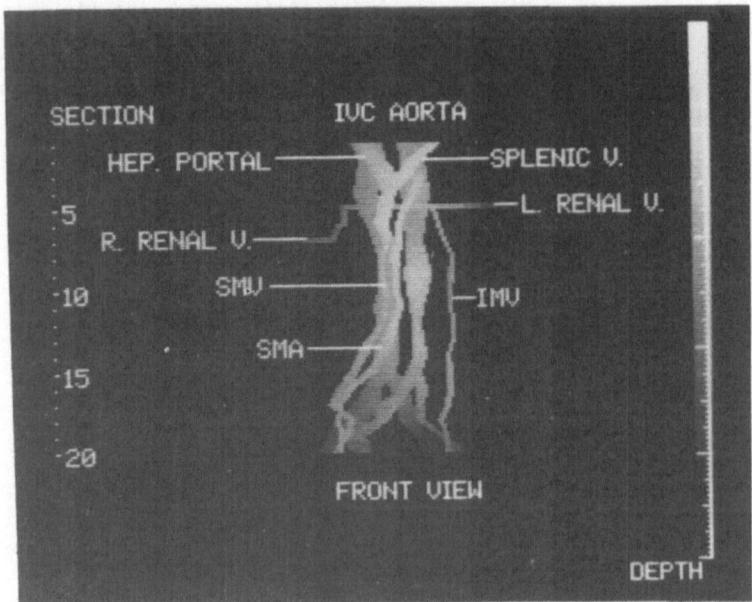

FIGURE 6. Depth-encoded reconstruction; original section levels are marked on reader's left.

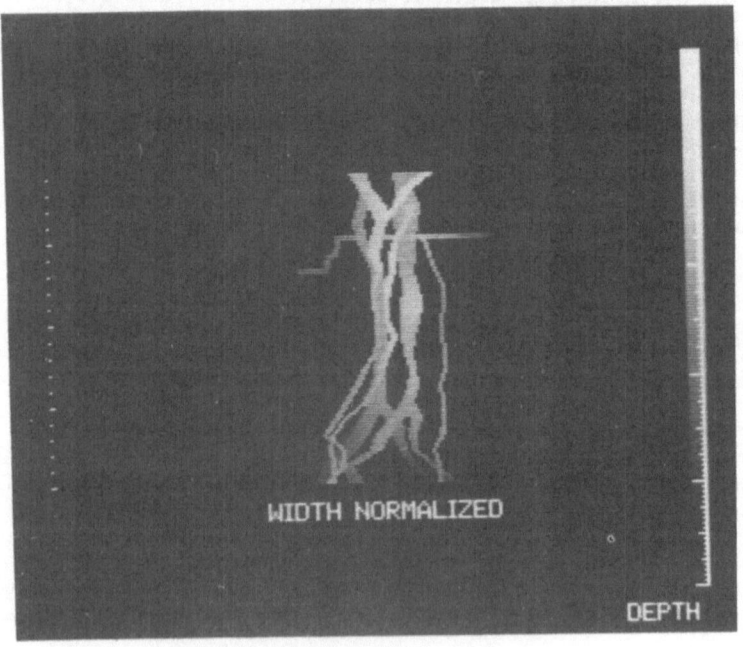

FIGURE 7. Width-normalized verstion of FIGURE 6.

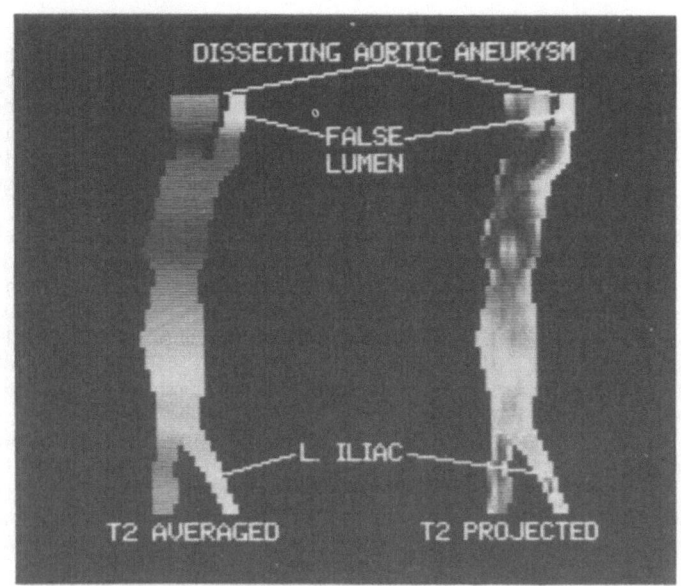

FIGURE 8. Higher intensity means more T2 pixels (slower flow).

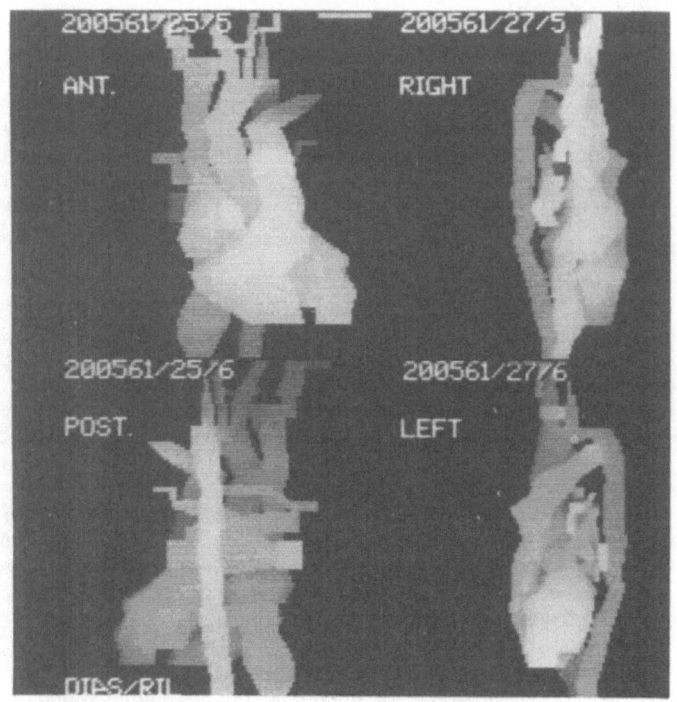

FIGURE 9. Chambers and major vessels of a normal human heart.

As noted above, depth encoding resolves overlapping vessels when we retain only the highest-valued pixel for each vessel occupying the same position on the reconstructed image. Deeper vessels are hidden by those in front of them. Other encoding options we wish to use cannot do this, so we let the depth image decides which pixels of a vessel are visible in a particular projection, and we make new images by replacing visible pixels with values containing information other than depth. We get these other values from the map.

The map keeps track of the number of pixels in each vessel which were detected by each of the two thresholds, intensity (fast flow) and T2 (slow flow). The ratio of these pixels is an indication of flow velocity within the vessel - the more T2 pixels, the lower the mean velocity. We display relative mean flow velocity by mapping the percentage of T2 pixels either to a gray scale or to a color sequence (red for 0%, violet for 100%). To show this percentage as a cross-sectional average, we replace the depth-encoded projection outline in a slice with the appropriate gray scale or color for that region in that slice and interpolate between slices. Only one interpolated value is computed for each vessel in each line, since all the pixels in that line for that vessel will be in the same cross-section and thus will represent the same cross-sectional percentage of T2 pixels. We can show flow patterns in finer detail by finding the T2 pixel percentage within a single line or column of a vessel cross-section. Here we replace the depth projections with T2 projections and interpolate pixel by pixel from edge to center just as we did with the original depth image.

If all vessels had round cross-sections, the displayed width in the reconstructed image would reflect the true patent area of each vessel, but vessels can be distorted by surrounding muscle or asymmetrically narrowed by disease, so that the projected width can vary with the viewing angle. Instead of providing many viewing angles, we have found two faster and simpler ways to depict patent area. One is to convert cross-sectional area region by region into a gray scale or color value and then to interpolate between slices in the same manner as for the cross-sectional T2 average image. The other is to redraw the depth image itself. The size of each projected outline is stretched or shrunk to conform to the "true" diameter, which is calculated from the cross-sectional area, and another depth image is created. We call this width normalization. The patency of any vessel at any level can be measured directly, regardless of view angle. Furthermore, we can convert the width normalized depth image to a width normalized, average T2-encoded image, combining these two important data sets into one picture. This single display provides information about anatomic structure, mean flow velocity, and patent area.

RESULTS

Figures 6 and 7 are vessel projections of a patient with an aortic aneurysm. A narrowing of the aortic flow channel is seen near the center of the images in an area corresponding to the aneurysm, indicating that the bulk of the tissue there (not seen in the projections) is stationary. The width normalized version (Figure 7) provides a better representation of the true cross-sectional areas of the flow channels.

Figure 8 is a projection of a dissecting aortic aneurysm with two different modes of T2 encoding. T2 encoding corresponds roughly to flow velocity. The fact that patterns in these images agree with hemodynamic models gives evidence of the validity of the T2-flow relationship and the accuracy of the reconstruction technique.

The heart in Figure 9 was reconstructed with the same algorithm, although more post-highlight editing was required in determining segment outlines. The anterior and posterior views were created simultaneously, as were the right and left lateral views.

DISCUSSION

We have compared our reconstructed vessel images with angiograms of the same patients and found good anatomic correlation (10-11). Angiograms have better two-dimensional spatial resolution. Volume resolution (three-dimensional) of the MRI reconstructions is better than angiograms, and consequently the reconstructions have better contrast and display overlapping structures more clearly. Patient risk and procedure time factors heavily favor the reconstruction technique. A scan takes half an hour and the reconstruction takes about 45 minutes.

The potential of MRI to show smaller vessels has probably not yet been fully developed. Reconstructed projections should play an important role in the non-invasive imaging of coronary and cranial arterial pathology.

Although radiologists may in general be able to get most of the necessary information directly from the original images, the reconstructed displays bring out less visible data such as flow in a manner easy to interpret, and give radiologists a communication tool for consultations with physicians less familiar with MRI and tomography. Since the T2 encoded reconstructions conform to expected flow patterns in normal and diseased vessels, they serve to corroborate the validity of using T2 to discriminate flow in MRI data and should assist further investigations in this area.

REFERENCES

1. Herman, GT: Three-dimensional Computer Graphics Display in Medicine. Proc. Fifth Ann. Conf. National Computer Graphics Assoc., Vol I, 1984, pp. 131-147.
2. Chen GTY, Pitluck S, Richards T: Three-dimensional Graphics in Radiation Therapy. Proc. Fifth Ann. Conf. National Computer Graphics Assoc., Vol II, 1984, pp.61-65.
3. Farrell EJ, Zappulla R, Yang WC: Color 3-D Imaging of Normal and Pathologic Intracranial Structures. Comp. Graphics and Applications, Vol. 4, September 1984, pp. 5-17.
4. Vannier MW, Marsh JL, Stevens, WG, Dye, DW, Warren JO: Surface Reconstruction and Computer-aided Design of Craniofacial Surgical Procedures Based on CT Scans. Proc. Fifth Ann. Conf. National Computer Graphics Assoc., Vol II, 1984, pp. 116-130.
5. Meagher DT: Interactive Solids Processing for Medical Analysis and Planning. Proc. Fifth Ann. Conf. National Computer Graphics Assoc., Vol II, 1984, pp. 96-106.
6. Kaufman L, Crooks LE, Sheldon PE, Rowan W, Miller T: Evaluation of NMR Imaging for Detection and Quantification of Obstructions in Vessels. Invest. Radiol., Vol. 17, Nov./Dec. 1982, pp. 554-560.
7. Kaufman L, Crooks LE, Sheldon PE, Hricak H, Herfkens R, Bank W: The Potential Impact of Nuclear Magnetic Resonance Imaging on Cardiovascualar Diagnosis. Circulation, Vol. 67, No. 2, 1983, pp. 251-257.
8. Singer J: NMR Diffusion and Flow Measurements, and an Introduction to Spin Phase Graphing. J. Phys. E., Vol II, 1978, pp. 281-291.

9. Axel L: Blood Flow Effects in Magnetic Resonance Imaging. AJR, 1984, pp. 1157-1166.
10. Valk PE, Hale JD et al: Magnetic Resonance Imaging With 3D Vessel Reconstruction I: Imaging of Aortic Aneurysms. Twenty-third Ann. Meeting, Assoc. of Univ. Radiologists, 1985.
11. Valk PE, Hale JD et al: Magnetic Resonance Imaging With 3D Vessel Reconstruction II: Imaging of Aorto-Iliac Atherosclerosis. Twenty-third Ann. Meeting, Assoc. of Univ. Radiologists, 1985.

PULSATILE BLOOD FLOW MEASUREMENTS WITH THE AID OF 3-D RECONSTRUCTIONS FROM DYNAMIC ANGIOGRAPHIC RECORDINGS

A.C.F. COLCHESTER, Department of Neurology, Atkinson Morley's and St. George's Hospital, London, SW20 ONE; D.J. HAWKES, Department of Medical Physics, St. George's Hospital, London, SW17; J.N.H. BRUNT, Department of Medical Biophysics, Manchester University Medical School, Oxford Road, Manchester; G.H. du BOULAY and A. WALLIS, Institute of Neurology, Queen Square, London, WC1.

1. INTRODUCTION

Flow measurements in individual vessels may be of value in a variety of circumstances. 1.) Total organ flow can be derived from flow in a vessel when there is a single inflow artery or outflow vein in an organ. 2.) The commonest type of vascular disease is atherosclerosis, which tends to affect larger vessels. It may be advantageous to measure flow or change in flow in the diseased vessel(s), rather than attempt to measure tissue flow in its region of supply of the vessel, which may be spatially irregular and hard to define when using tissue flow measurement techniques. Furthermore, several arteries may potentially supply one territory and vessel flow measurement may allow estimation of the relative contribution of particular vessels. 3.) Similarly, measurement of flow in bypass grafts or natural anastomoses can be of particular clinical importance. 4.) Along an unbranched vessel (where volume flow must remain constant) velocity flow is inversely proportional to vessel cross sectional area. Moreover, blood flow velocity normally changes little at branches and large velocity changes often indicate abnormal haemodynamics. Thus, velocity flow (e.g. as provided semi-quantitatively by Doppler methods) may give valuable indirect information about vessel geometry.

5.) Studies of rapid changes in flow or pulsatile flow are usually dependent on vessel flow measurement techniques as most tissue flow methods provide insufficient temporal resolution. 6.) There is still much to be learnt about the physics, physiology and pathology of blood flow and vascular resistance in individual vessels. Flow measurements in individual vessels, especially with methods allowing quantitative or qualitative study of the distribution across the vessel lumen, are a central part of this research. 7.) Finally, combination of vessel flow estimation with multiple measurements of calibre and with path length makes possible calculation of approximate pressure gradients. This allows assessment of the contribution of a vessel to total or segmental resistance (Colchester 1985) and of the haemodynamic significance of stenoses.

Unfortunately, many of the potential applications are difficult or impossible to realise in clinical practice because of methodological deficiencies which are reflected in the large number of different techniques which are available for vessel flow measurement. As is so often the case, the more accurate techniques tend to be more invasive which limits their clinical use. Volumetric measurement of haemorrhage from a vessel is the most accurate method for estimating absolute mean volume flow but prohibitively invasive. EM flowmeters have very good temporal resolution and are used for experimental studies of pulsatile flow, but they require direct exposure of a vessel and can only be used clinically during surgery. Non-invasive Doppler ultrasound techniques also have good temporal resolution but are inaccurate and usually limited to vessels close to the body surface. Magnetic resonance techniques are in their infancy but present methods are time consuming and have poor spatial resolution.

Indicator techniques are of intermediate invasiveness. Two classes can be distinguished: firstly, where knowledge of the quantity of injected indicator is used (known constant rate of injection or known total indicator dose), and secondly, where flow is derived from bolus transport time (BTT), vessel path length and cross-sectional area (CSA). The amount of indicator in the vessel after injection has traditionally been estimated by direct blood sampling but more than 25 years ago researchers were exploring the possibility of doing this by X-ray densitometry using radio-opaque contrast medium (CM) as an indicator (see review by Heintzen, 1978). BTT : path length : CSA methods, while still requiring catheterisation and CM injection, potentially allow flow to be estimated in numerous vessels a long way downstream of the injection, and in this sense are less invasive than the the known-injection-quantity methods.

Mainly because of technical difficulties, development of these angiographic blood flow measurement techniques has only been pursued in a few research centres. They have remained too time consuming and too inaccurate to be used clinically, despite their potential use for many of the applications listed above. We have examined separately the methods and limitations of angiographic measurement of BTT, vessel path length and calibre.

1.1. Estimation of Bolus Transport Time

The earliest angiographic velocity flow estimates were made in the superior vena cava following intravenous injections of iodine oil drop by drop into a neck vein (Bohme 1936). With insoluble contrast media the individual droplets are clearly defined in their position and can usually be tracked over time. Inaccuracies in transit time measurement are related to: (a) the inherent time-sampling limitations of the recording (Crepeau and Silverman 1973), (b) the location of particles within the trans-axial flow distribution, and (c) the phase(s) of the cardiac cycle being sampled during transit of the droplet(s).

Unfortunately, insoluble contrast media are not likely to be suitable for use in human subjects and, in the animal experiments described, only very small quantities of oil could be used without causing major problems from embolism and intravascular coagulation.

With soluble contrast media, the basic concept of transport time measurement is the same, but the passing stream of the bolus has to be treated as a population of individual particles which cannot be identified separately. The inability to identify the individual particles leads to an uncertainly both in distance down the vessel and in trans-axial position in a blood vessel image. When analysing the passage of a radio-opaque bolus with very sharp leading or trailing edges, it may be possible to define the locus of part of the bolus with little difficulty, and one study analysing aortograms recorded at 60 frames/second was able to show the trans-axial distribution of velocities at certain stages of the cardiac cycle (Kedem et al 1978). In the present paper we will regard the aim of measurements as providing an estimate of transport time which represents a mean across the lumen and also across the cardiac cycle. With most techniques, densities across the image of a blood vessel (background having been subtracted) are integrated, and density : time curves are constructed depicting the passage of the bolus by plotting the mean density within a window over time (Rutishauser et al 1974; Bursch et al 1974; Yerushalmi 1976). The density : time curves from two windows (a known distance apart) are compared to establish the mean transport time. Various different methods for comparing the curves have been used and are discussed below. Most have been shown empirically to make possible approximate measures of blood flow.

1.1.1. BTT Estimation Using Part of the Density : Time Curve. The time separation of the peak of the two curves has been used as the mean transport time (e.g. Hohne et al 1978), while Silverman and Rosen (1977), Kedem et al 1978 and Bursch (1979) have estimated transport times from the time separation of the half-peak height densities. Hohne et al (1978) also measured transport times from the difference between the points of maximum slope on the density : time curve. Others have attempted to define the passage of the bolus from the arrival moment i.e. the time at which the density : time curve exceeds a certain threshold value (e.g. Heuck and Vanselow 1969; Silverman and Rosen 1977). When the curves have a similar amplitude, the time separation of isodensity parts of the two curves has been used to estimate transport time (Silverman et al 1973). This is the one approach which potentially makes possible multiple transport time estimations from the passage of a single bolus.

A successful method for estimating mean transport time from the initial portion of a density: time curve was described by Bursch et al (1979,1981). The peak of the curve is identified, and area of the initial curve up to the peak divided by its height, subtracted from the time of the peak, is taken as the arrival amount for each curve. This method has the advantage of utilising and averaging all the data from the first part of the curve. Where the curve has a rather flat top, even though the time of peak density may be poorly defined, small errors in the localisation of the peak have no significant effect on the calculated time-parameter.

1.1.2. BTT Estimation Using the Whole Density : Time Curve. Theoretically, the mean transport time of the population of particles represented by the bolus of soluble contrast medium can be measured accurately by comparing the centres of gravity of the two density : time curves. This method has been used by many authors, for example Smith et al (1973), Rutishauser et al (1974), and Hamby et al (1977). Another method is a cross-correlation procedure which is less sensitive to variations in the shape of the curve (Silverman and Rosen 1977; Bursch et al 1979). The latter group found the cross-correlation method the most consistent of the methods they compared, but it was felt that the small improvement offered by the cross-correlation method when compared to the pre-peak area divided by height did not justify the extra computation time.

Simple concentration : time curves have been satisfactorily modelled as gamma variate curves (Thompson et al 1964) which are completely specified by four parameters. This prompted Kruger et al (1983) to attempt to improve the calculation of time parameter(s) from angiographic contrast medium dilution curves by finding the best-fit gamma-variate of the type used by Thompson et al. Forbes et al (1982) and others have used this technique with modern digital radiography systems.

1.1.3. The Problem of Pulsatile Flow. Very few of the existing techniques used for angiographic flow measurement have addressed the central problem of inaccuracies in mean flow estimation caused by pulsatile flow. Typical density : time curves last for one half to two seconds and transport times are derived from an uncontrolled and asymmetrically-weighted sample of the cardiac cycle.

The most successful previous measurement of pulsatile flow by an angiographic technique was probably that described by Korbuly (1973) who injected CM at a known constant rate, but his technique is a simple development of the indicator dilution method which measures flow only at the site of injection. This restricts the usefulness of angiographic flow measurements, which have the potential for estimating flow in a large number of vessels which are opacified following an angiographic injection. Also, direct disturbance of normal flow by the introduction of the indicator fluid is maximal at the site of injection and, together with the artefactual effects of the presence of the catheter, effectively limits the dye dilution method to the aorta and large arteries. The same limitation applies to the method developed by Lantz (1975).

There are potential ways with the BTT technique of coping with the difficulties caused by pulsatile flow. One possibility is to introduce a long bolus lasting several cardiac cycles. However, accurate estimation of the very small time difference between curves is difficult with a long bolus. This problem is seen in an extreme form following intravenous injections of contrast medium. The other factor which makes long injections unacceptable even with arterial injection is the fact that data collection continues for so long that the artefactual effects of contrast medium on small vessels (producing vasodilatation and increased flow) may have begun to take effect.

A more acceptable possibility is to average several flow estimates which are discrete in time and at specific phases of the cardiac cycle. One approach to this is to deliver a series of injections at different stages of the cardiac cycle. Kedem et al (1978) proposed injecting multiple small boluses within one cardiac cycle, a tactic which undoubtedly confines pulsatile flow estimation to points near the injection site because the very short boluses will soon intermix. Busch and Piroth (1980) gave about four small injections whose onset was timed to occur at progressively later stages of consecutive cardiac cycles. A second approach is to process the curves obtained from a single bolus so as to derive more than one velocity estimate from the passage of a single bolus. In the present paper, we explore this approach and treat a bolus as a series of iso-concentration sub-boluses arranged contiguously along the leading and trailing edges of the parent bolus.

When flow is markedly pulsatile and short boluses are injected, the form of density : time curves can be very complex, with gross qualitative differences in shape. Establishing when to begin or end computation of time parameters can then be very difficult. Busch and Piroth (1980) discussed this, but were unable to solve the curve matching problem with a systematic algorithm. For simple curves, they calculated the centre-of-gravity, but in difficult cases they presented the two density : time curves on the same axes to the observer who was required to shift one with respect to the other over time until he judged that the curves were correctly matched. The criterion the authors recommended in the case of these difficult curves was to align appropriate peaks.

We propose that the most helpful way of analysing bolus transport, especially with pulsatile flow, is to regard distance down the vessel as a continuum and to construct a three-dimensional surface where the X-axis is time, the Y-axis is vascular path length, and the Z-axis or grey scale is mean CM concentration averaged across the lumen. Each horizontal line represents a concentration : time curve recorded at a particular point down the vessel. The conventional pair of windows used for construction of two density:time curves would be represented by a pair of lines, one at the top and one at the bottom of the graph.

An example using this data structure shows very clearly why density : time curves may assume a complex shape when flow is pulsatile (Figs. 1 and

2). The bolus is shown as very short and discrete, and it is assumed there is some back flow during diastole. Depending on the sites of recording of a pair of concentration : time curves, simple matching may be impossible. Furthermore, a gamma variate is not an appropriate general model for describing the range of possible curves.

·We have previously given a brief description of this approach and shown an example of in vivo flow measurement in a small intracranial artery 1 mm

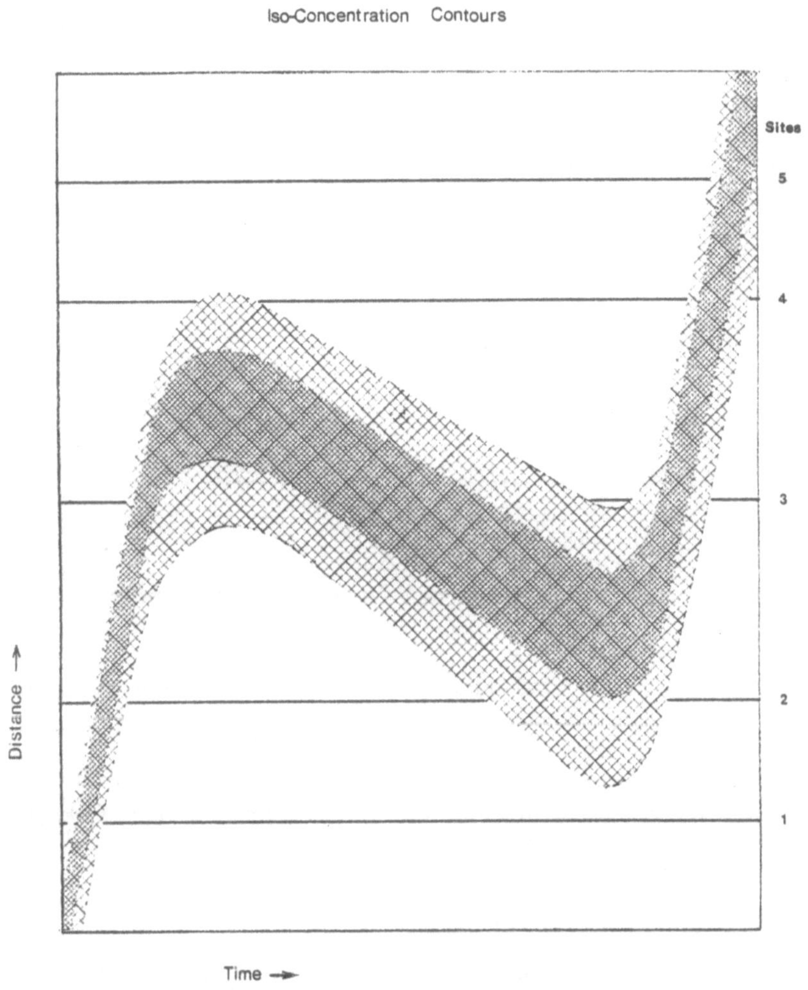

Iso-Concentration Contours

FIGURE 1. Simplified example of a concentration : distance : time surface with iso-concentration contours representing passage of a bolus of indicator down a vessel during one cardiac cycle. Y axis = distance down vessel; X axis = time; Z axis or grey scale = mean concentration of CM across the vessel lumen.

252

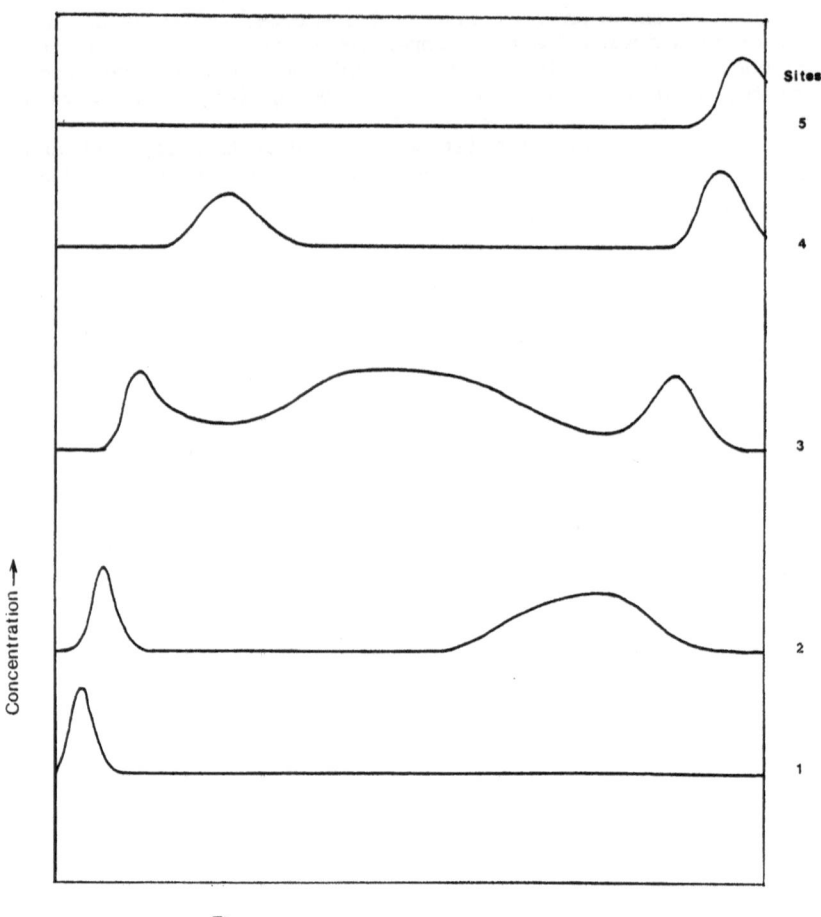

Sites

5

4

3

2

1

Concentration →

Time →

FIGURE 2. Concentration : time curves based on Fig. 1 at the sites indicated

in diameter (Colchester & Brunt 1983). In the present paper we present phantom data where we have obtained simultaneous angiographic and EM flow-meter measurements in a tube about 4 mm diameter.

1.2. Estimation of Vessel Path Length

In the past angiographic measurements of blood flow have usually been restricted to vessels which are assumed to be straight and running perpendicular to the X-ray beam. This assumption may be justified by prior anatomical knowledge (e.g. anterior cerebral/pericallosal artery in a lateral view : Colchester & Brunt 1983),or may be validated by inspection of a second view in another plane, but is frequently a source of error. However, the recent development of methods to reconstruct the 3-D course of vessel centre-line from biplane angiograms (Mackay et al 1982; Hawkes et al

1985) deserves further evalutation as a source of path-length information
in flow computation, and should improve accuracy and allow flow measurements to be made in a much wider range of vessels than at present.

1.3. Estimation of Vessel Cross-Sectional Area (CSA)

Inaccuracy of vessel CSA estimation from angiograms has been a major
source of error in calculation of volume blood flow. Two basic approaches
to calibre measurement have been used (Brown et al 1982). Firstly, the
width of the vessel image may be obtained by estimating the location of the
edges.   Accurate edge location is difficult and dynamic angiographic
recordings used for flow measurements (especially video) do not provide
optimum radiographic spatial resolution. The lumen normally has to be
assumed circular and the CSA calculated from the squares of the width
estimate, thus exaggerating any error. An advantage of the edge location
methods is that they are relatively insensitive to the density calibration
factor. Also it has usually been assumed that width estimates are not
affected by concentration of contrast medium (CM). However, a recent
phantom study has shown that the CM concentration does have a significant
effect (Spears et al 1983), offsetting this apparent advantage of edge
location versus densitometric methods.

Secondly, vessel calibre may be estimated by densitometric methods, i.e.
methods which make use of the idealised relationship derived from Lambert-
Beers Law between the density of an angiographic image after background
subtraction and the concentration x depth of CM:

$$\log B2 - \log B1 = N.C.Z$$

where $B1$ = brightness (grey scale value) of background or mask image at a
point before opacification with contrast medium (CM),
$B2$ = brightness of image at that point after opacification with CM,
N = densitometric calibration factor (related to the mass
absorption coefficient of the CM),
C = concentration of CM, and
Z = depth, i.e distance in a direction parallel to the x-ray beam,
of the CM-containing compartment at that point on the image.

In practice, polychromatic X-rays, beam hardening, scatter and multiple
non-linearities in the contrast transfer functions of the imaging chain
tend to make this relationship imperfect i.e. N does not remain constant
(Hilal 1966; Reiber et al 1983) and special precautions are necessary to
minimise the difficulties. Vessel CSA is estimated from the area under the
transverse density profile (TDP) i.e. the graph of image brightness, after
log transformation and background subtraction, along a track perpendicular
to the vessel long axis. The most important advantage of this densitometric
method is that CSA measurements are valid regardless of lumen shape and for
this reason we have adopted it.

2. METHODS

In all the experiments 35 mm cine recordings at 50 frames per second
were obtained using a 17 cm or 25 cm image intensifier field of view. The
nominal x-ray tube focal spot size was 0.3 mm for calibre measurement work
(filtered with 0.17 mm copper) and 0.6 mm for experiments evaluating the
3-D calibration and blood flow methods. Radiographic magnification was
approximately 2.

2.1. 3-D Centre-Line Reconstruction

In collaboration with Dr. Chris Mol of the IBM UK Scientific Centre, Winchester (Hawkes et al 1985) we have developed a 3-D calibration method based on that described by Mackay et al (1982). A paper giving further details of our technique has been submitted for publication (Mol et al 1985). A perspex cube containing small steel balls at each corner and the centre of each face was constructed. The distances between balls were known accurately. After biplane cine angiography, the x-ray tubes and intensifiers were not moved but the perspex cube was substituted in the field-of-view in place of the patient. Radiographs of the cube were then obtained in both planes. This procedure was easily accomplished for clinical as well as phantom studies. Cine frames were digitised to 1024 x 1024 pixels using a slow-scan plumbicon system to give an approximate magnification of 5.5 pixels per mm in the mid-subject plane and processed in an IBM 4341 computer. Spatial distortion produced by the image intensifier was corrected by a rubber-sheeting procedure. Images of the calibration cube were used to solve the matrix which describes the 3-D relationship between the x-ray foci and the image planes and which maps the 3-D location of a point on to a specified 2-D image. The 3-D course of a vessel centre-line was then reconstructed by identifying a sequence of corresponding points on the two views. Identification was assisted by a computer generated 'auxiliary line' which was the projection onto the image in the second plane of the back-projection line of a selected point on the image in the first plane. The course of the vessel was coded as a list of 3-D vectors arranged hierarchically under the location of 'nodes' which represented the origin of a branch from a parent vessel.

From the 3-D location of points on the vessel centre-line, the precise magnification factor relating the vessel of interest to the computer image (Mi), the angle between vessel long axis and x-ray beam (ϕ), and the true vascular path length between selected points (L) were calculated. These data were then used in the further measurements of vessel calibre and velocity blood flow: Mi for measurements of width of the vessel silhouette, Mi and ϕ for densitometric calibre and CM concentration measurements, and L for velocity flow measurements.

2.2. Cross Sectional Area-Measurements

A special phantom was constructed for evaluation of calibre measurement methods (Colchester 1985). Dummy vessels ranging from 0.1 mm to 3.2 mm diameter were made by pouring a liquid epoxy mixture into a mould across which wires or rods of precisely measured external diameter were stretched. When the epoxy had hardened the wires were withdrawn leaving a smooth-walled hole of known internal diameter. The epoxy was in fact a complex mixture consisting of phenolic microspheres, polyethylene powder and calcium carbonate powder which was added to a low exotherm epoxy base and mixed thoroughly under a vacuum. This epoxy mixture had very similar properties of radiation absorption and scatter to water or soft tissue. The dummy vessels were filled with contrast medium of accurately measured concentration and sealed. The block of dummy vessels was introduced into the centre of a head phantom made of a baboon skull surrounded by a tough plastic shell and filled with water.

Cine angiograms of dummy vessels containing six different concentrations of Urografin 290, ranging from approximately 10 to 60 gm diatrizoate salt per 100 ml solution (assayed as 49.4, 98.9, 148, 199, 253 and 299 mg iodine/ml), were obtained.

Transverse density profiles (TDPs) perpendicular to the centre-line of dummy vessel images on successive cine frames were digitised to a 9-bit grey scale with a magnification of approximately 35 pixels/mm in the mid-subject plane. Each transverse profile represented integrated data from 1.5 mm length of vessel. Profiles were processed in a Hewlett-Packard 9845B computer. TDPs were re-registered with each other by searching for the relative position which gave the least variance of the difference between them. Four to twelve frames were then averaged, according to the signal-to-noise ratio judged by the user. Background density was subtracted by extrapolating a straight baseline (horizontal or sloping) under the TDP from the mean level either side of the vessel image. This produced a TDP with zero baseline.

Vessel CSA (A) was derived from TDP area according to the equation:

$$A = \frac{S}{M.N.C.\sin\phi}$$

where ϕ = the angle between x-ray beam and vessel long axis,
    M = the magnification calibration factor,
    N = densitometric calibration factor,
    C = CM concentration,
and S = TDP area.

During peak opacification of an 'in vivo' angiogram there is usually a period of uniform filling when CM concentration is constant down the length of vessel as well as across the vessel lumen. If uniform filling is achieved, $S/(M.\sin\phi)$ should be directly proportional to vessel CSA. This relationship was evaluated empirically for vessels perpendicular to the x-ray beam using the phantom images.

In vivo criteria that we use to establish uniform filling are that the mass : time curves for all TDPs in the length of vessel being studied (see below) are at their maxima and remain so for several frames, and also that the edges of the vessel silhouette on the original image do not change between frames. M & ϕ are both derived from the 3-D calibration procedure. This allows calculation of relative vessel CSA. For absolute CSA measurements, the product of N and C is calculated from TDP parameters of vessel segments which are identified as having circular cross-section using biplane images and a model-fitting procedure. This method has been used previously by our group (Duffield et al 1983) and a detailed description will be presented elsewhere.

2.3. Pulsatile Flow Experiments

Pulsatile flow of tap water was generated in a 4.15 mm diameter tube by a peristaltic pump used for cardiac bypass (Fig. 3). Mean volume flow was about 40 ml/min. Contrast medium was injected via a 'T' piece 12 cm upstream from the region imaged. The flow tube was connected in series with an EM flowmeter. Mean flow readings from the flowmeter were calibrated by measuring the outflow volume in a timed period. Approximately 1 ml of CM was injected during 'diastole'. The region of interest was digitised to 256 x 256 pixels x 8 bits using a chalnicon TV camera and transferred to a CVAS-3000 computer (Computer Vision Analysis System, made by Visual Machines, Manchester, England). Sixteen video images of each cine frame were averaged to reduce noise. The magnification was 3.7 pixels/mm on the subject plane. After a densitometric correction procedure, log transformation and automatic re-registration, an unopacified frame from the

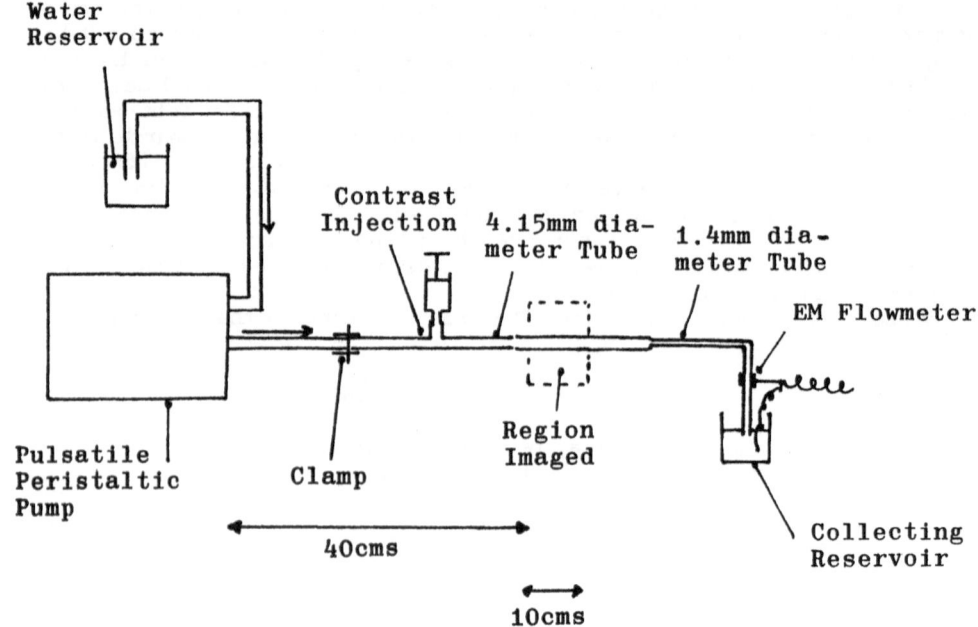

FIGURE 3. Pulsatile flow phantom.

beginning of the run was subtracted from each opacified frame. TDP's were constructed at one-pixel intervals along a 6.5 cm length of vessel and any residual background density subtracted by interpolation between the TDP edges. The area under each TDP was calculated and the values were used to construct a single vertical column of a parametric image where each grey value was proportional to [CM concentration x vessel CSA] at a particular point and time, the vertical axis was distance down the vessel, and the horizontal axis was time. Frames showing uniform filling (see above) were used to calculate relative vessel CSA at each point and each grey value of the parametric image was divided by the appropriate CSA to convert the parametric image to a concentration : distance : time surface.

Blood flow velocity was calculated from the movement of iso-concentration portions of the bolus over time. This movement was represented by the slope (distance/time) of iso-concentration contours on the concentration : distance : time surface. Each contour was divided into a series of segments, to each of which a straight line was fitted. With our present software the number of segments and positions of inflection points are decided interactively by the user. The slope of each segment of each contour provided a mean velocity estimate for the time period and distance down the vessel covered by the length of the contour segment. It can be seen that multiple estimates from different positions down the vessel at a particular time, and at different times for particular position down the vessel, are generated by these calculations.

Flow during the angiograms was measured simultaneously by the EM flow-meter. The output was recorded on a paper chart. Time marks from a pulse generator were shown on the chart and a photodiode in the cinecamera was

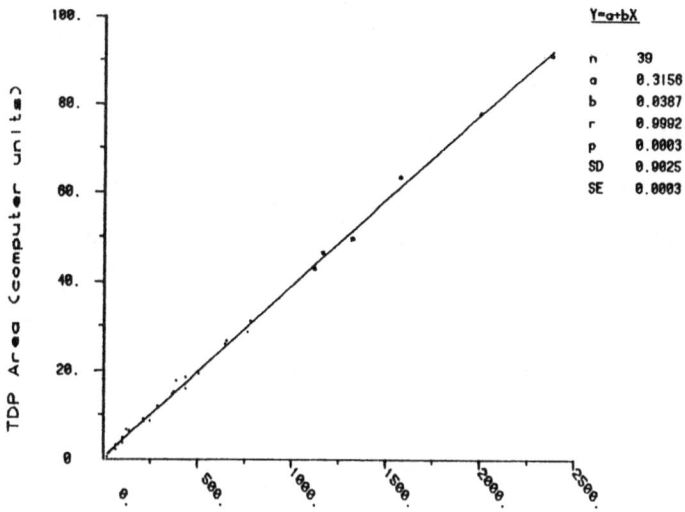

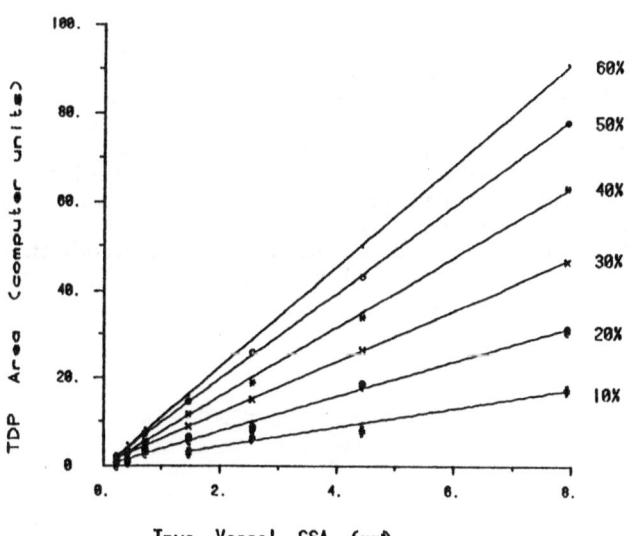

FIGURES 4 (top) and 5 (bottom). Scatter plots of area under the Transverse Density Profile (TDP) of phantom vessels from 0.5 to 3.2 mm diameter containing Contrast Medium (CM) strengths from 10% to 60% (50 to 300 mg iodine/ml) versus: a) true CM concentration x vessel cross-sectional area (CSA) for all vessels and concentrations (Fig. 4), and b) true vessel CSA for each concentration separately (Fig. 5).

simultaneously illuminated, exposing a small spot in the corner of a cine frame, to allow accurate synchronisation of the flow measurements.

3. RESULTS

3.1 Evaluation of 3-D Calibration

Images of the same perspex cube used for 3-D calibration were analysed to assess the accuracy of the technique. Steel balls near the edge of the field of view were chosen because errors due to the rubber-sheeting procedure were likely to be greater at the periphery. For biplane views at 90° to each other, points which are unambiguously identified in both views can be located in 3-D with an accuracy of 0.7 mm (one standard deviation).

3.2 Evaluation of Cross-Sectional Area (CSA) Measurement

The results of quantitative processing of dummy vessels between 0.5 and 3.2 mm diameter are presented. Smaller vessels than this could be identified visually; for example the diameter of the smallest vessel containing 30 gm diatrizoate salt/100 ml (145 mg iodine/ml) which could be confidently detected was 0.38 mm. However, quantitative processing became unreliable with smaller vessels and measurements on vessels less than 0.5 mm diameter were excluded. With the most dilute Urografin solution (49 mg iodine/ml), the three vessel sizes between 0.5 and 1 mm diameter were also excluded.

Overall TDP area was very highly correlated with the known contrast medium mass per unit length of vessel, i.e. true vessel cross-sectional area x CM concentration (Fig. 4). The correlation coefficient was 0.999 and the residual deviation was equivalent to 23 ug/mm length of vessel. The slope of this plot is equal to the product of the densitometric and magnification calibration factors. A plot of the overall TDP area versus the known vessel cross-sectional area for each CM dilution separately is shown in Fig. 5. The residual deviations of the figures from vessels containing more than 140 mg/ml of iodine were all less than 0.09 mm^2. The slope of each plot on Fig. 5 is equal to the product of (a) the densitometric calibration factor, (b) the geometric calibration factor and also (c) the CM concentration.

FIGURE 6. Parametric image with 6-bit grey scale representing a concentration : distance : time surface (axes as Fig. 1).

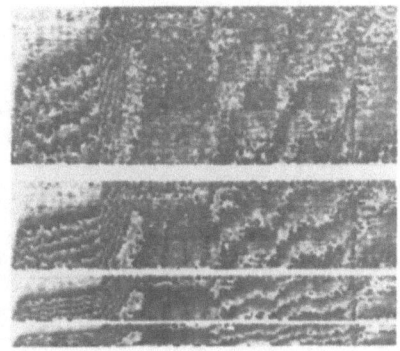

FIGURE 7 (left). As Fig. 6 with compression of the vertical (distance) axis by factors of 2, 4, 8 and 16.
FIGURE 8 (right).   Display of the three most significant bit-planes of Fig. 7 to clarify iso-concentration contours.

3.3. Evaluation of Blood Flow Measurement

The concentration : distance : time surface generated by a single 1 ml injection of contrast medium is shown as a 6-bit grey image in Fig. 6. The parametric image was smoothed with a 9-point Hanning filter and the distance axis was compressed by factors of 2,4,8 and 16 to simplify estimation of the slope of different concentration contours (Fig. 7). Iso-concentration contours were clarified by displaying only the three least significant bits of the 6-bit image (Fig. 8).   Flow velocities for

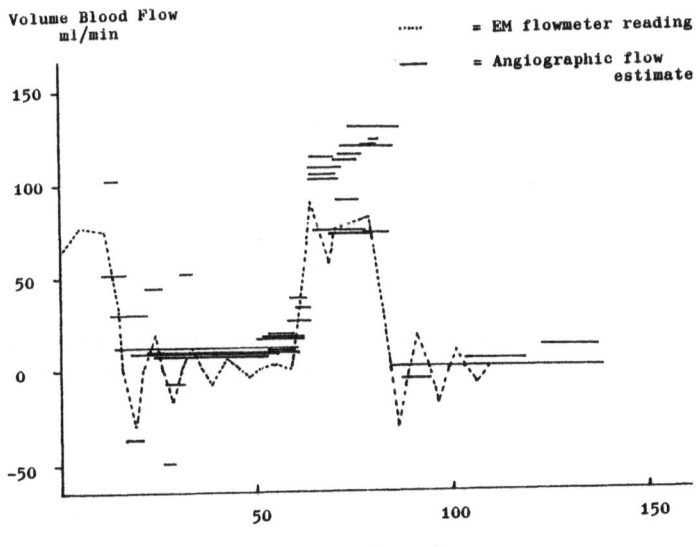

FIGURE 9. Plot of flow measurements against time. Angiographic estimates (solid lines) are calculated from the slopes of straight line fits to segments of the iso-concentration contours of Fig. 8. EM flow meter estimates are shown dotted.

different portions of the bolus were estimated for every contour on this image. The estimated velocities (slopes of each straight line subdivision) were multiplied by the known cross sectional area of the tube to produce volume flow values. These values were plotted against time (Fig. 9). The angiographic flow estimate from a single portion of an iso-concentration contour is shown as a horizontal line to indicate the time period covered.

On the same graph (Fig. 9), EM flowmeter readings are also shown. These were taken from the continuous paper trace, and spaced so that all the major fluctuations in flow were represented. Thus, for example, during 'diastole', when there were small fluctuations in flow due to the mechanics of the pump, EM flowmeter readings at the peaks and troughs of these fluctuations were transferred to the graph of Fig. 9.

In general, the angiographic estimates agreed well with each other and with the known true flow. Flow tended to be over estimated, especially during 'systole'.

Angiographic estimates were then averaged for each point in time and replotted (Fig. 10). Overall the agreement was very good, and readings were obtained for the whole 'cardiac' cycle. However, during the peak flow period the angiographic method overestimated true flow by about 15%.

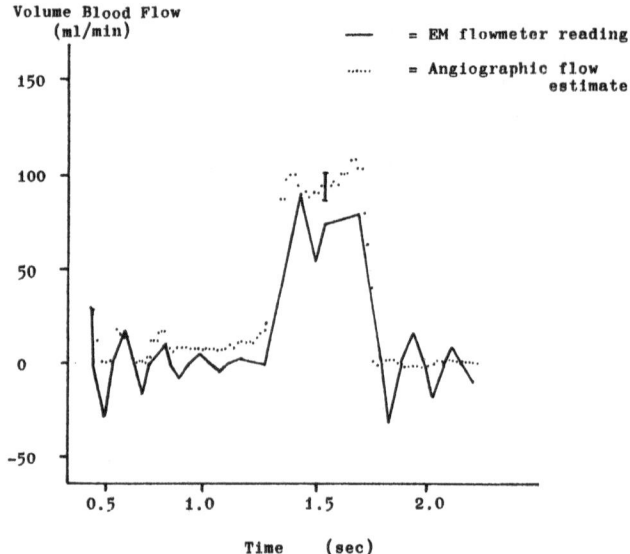

FIGURE 10. Plot of flow measurements against time. Angiographic estimates (dotted) at each point in time on Fig. 9 were averaged. The error bar at 1.5 secs (± 1 S.D. of the angiographic estimates) is shown as an example. EM flow measurements are shown as a solid line.

4. DISCUSSION

We have attempted to improve the methodology of angiographic blood flow measurement by identifying causes of inaccuracies and tackling each separately. We have not yet evaluated the combined new methodology with tortuous vessels in phantoms or in vivo, but we feel that we have demonstrated significant advances in accurate measurement of calibre, vessel path length, and blood flow velocity which are the factors necessary for improved accuracy and wider applicability in vivo.

We are in the process of implementing the 3-D vascular tree reconstruction technique on our new computer, the Visual Machines CVAS 3000. At present, 3-D calibration data derived on the IBM mainframe in Winchester have to be entered into the Visual Machines system at St. George's by hand when running the flow program.

Our adaptation of the 3-D calibration method of Mackay et al (1982) allows satisfactory reconstruction of the 3-D course of the vessel centre-line in vivo as well as in phantom studies. The 3-D locations are an important source of data (radiographic magnification, angle between X-ray beam and vessel long axis, and vessel path length) which are needed for calculation of vessel calibre and flow velocity, and are otherwise difficult to obtain accurately. This is especially true for curved or tortuous vessels. We also use the 3-D data, in combination with calibre measurements, to generate high quality graphical displays of a solid model of the vascular tree with full surface shading from any chosen viewpoint (Hawkes et al 1985; Mol et al 1985). This model does not reproduce any irregularities of the shape of the luminal cross section; regardless of the actual shape, the luminal shape at any point is represented by a circle of the same cross-sectional area as the true lumen.

The very good correlation between TDP area and vessel CSA in the vessel calibre experiments shows that the densitometric calibration factor remained constant across the field of view in the baboon skull vault containing the vessels as well as for the different quantities of iodine across the TDP's. Across a field of view containing greater changes in bone thickness, for example where the carotid artery shadow crosses the cervical vertebrae in the neck, and where there are much larger changes in iodine mass, for example across the aorta, correlations would be less good. Never-theless, we believe that considerable improvements over existing techniques for densitometric calibration in these more difficult circumstances are possible and are likely to confirm the general preferability of densito-metric over edge detection methods in estimation of vessel CSA.

While the present experiments used phantom vessels with a circular cross-section, we do not believe that this contributed to the accuracy of the radiographic measurements. Estimation of vessel CSA from the TDP area can be regarded as integration of the chord length information coded by the amplitude of the TDP at each point across the lumen, and no information about luminal shape is retained in the TDP area value.

We have found that the problems of analysing bolus transit have been greatly clarified by our method of constructing a concentration : distance : time surface. We display this as a parametric image, on which each vertical line represents the profile of changing CM concentration down the length of the vessel. This is the key to the data structure. Most previous analyses of bolus transport have ignored this vital dimension. It makes possible confident analysis of bolus behaviour regardless of the type of flow profile. Velocity can only be detected when there is a significant longitudinal concentration gradient down the vessel. Either when there is no CM present, or during the plateau stage of bolus passage when concentration does not alter down the stretch of vessel under study, there is no way of detecting motion; the bolus could be stationary or moving quickly without any change in signal. On the other hand, the steeper the bolus edge, the more reliable becomes any velocity estimate. Zero, positive, or negative velocities can then be measured with confidence.

In the present phantom study the calibre of the vessel did not change down its length, and the transformation of the parametric image from a mass

: distance : time surface into a concentration : distance : time surface had no effect on velocity flow calculation. However, when vessel calibre alters down its length, the transformation is essential. For example, a local stenosis in a vessel or a change in calibre after a side branch would produce horizontal contours in the mass: distance : time surface which would not, of course, indicate stationary flow. The transformation removes this potential artefact and allows valid measurement of velocity.

Data from the analysis of the parametric image can easily be combined in different ways. Our method of fitting a straight line to selected sub-divisions of the iso-concentration contours averages velocity information from a certain part of the bolus. On Fig 10 we have averaged data from each vertical column on the image, assuming that there are no significant changes in flow velocity down the length of the vessel. On the other hand, we have carefully preserved the time-variant data in order to record the pulsatile flow changes.

The extent to which velocity estimates can be obtained for all parts of the cardiac cycle from the passage of a single bolus is very variable in practice and we are exploring different injection tactics to optimise this. More than one small injection may be required in some instances.

Our aim for mean flow calculation is to construct a curve of velocity against phase of the cardiac cycle by fitting a smooth curve of appropriate shape to the points obtained, and then to divide area under this curve by the cardiac cycle time (Colchester & Brunt 1983). This should make the measurement much less dependent on achieving an even distribution of velocity estimates.

The reason for the overestimation of flow by our angiographic method in the example presented remains to be analysed. The explanation is likely to be due to the fact that most of the flow estimates through the single cardiac cycle chosen were derived from the leading edge of the bolus, where indicator is being carried by the central fastest-flowing streamlines. We expect to find a comparable underestimate of mean flow across the lumen if we analyse the trailing edge of the bolus.

One factor limiting the applicability of our method in vivo is the framing rate of the imaging system. Accurate measurement of the peak velocities in large vessels may require rates as high as 100 frames/sec or more. However, this limitation will to some extent be offset by our ability to analyse longer lengths of vessel with the aid of the 3-D centre-line reconstruction technique. These and other factors which impose basic physical limits on the accuracy of the velocity calculation require systematic evaluation.

As with all techniques, artefactual effects as well as the physics of the data collection system combine to limit the validity of measurements. The effects of the process of introducing a catheter into a blood vessel, the continuing presence of the catheter, the disturbing influence of the injection, the volumetric, viscous and inertial consequences of having introduced a foreign fluid, and the pharmacological effects of contrast media must all be considered as possible sources of artefact (Colchester 1985). Despite the potential problems, the data quoted in the literature comparing angiographic and independent flow measurement methods show that the artefacts can be kept to acceptable proportions when small volume injections are used.

The fact that angiography remains an important and frequent clinical procedure, despite improvement in other less invasive techniques such as ultrasonography and computerised tomography, underlines the value of the structural information it provides even without quantitative processing. Considering the risks of angiography, every effort should be made to extract all the potentially useful quantitative information from the procedure, especially if further investigations might thereby be avoided. Furthermore, as has been shown by the commercially available digital subtraction angiography systems, computer processing makes possible the use of smaller volumes and/or less selective contrast medium injections to produce clinically acceptable images, thus decreasing the risks as well as potentially increasing the usefulness of the procedure.

5. SUMMARY AND CONCLUSIONS

1. Flow measurements in individual vessels have a number of important clinical and research applications but all the more widely used methods have serious clinical limitations such as prohibitive invasiveness, limitation to very few anatomical sites, or inaccuracy.

2. Angiographic blood flow measurement is a technique of intermediate invasiveness and accuracy. Despite a large literature showing its feasibility it is not widely used. This has been partly due to the time-consuming data reduction but modern computer techniques are greatly improving this. We now use a small but powerful image analysis computer which could be used in a clinical environment.

3. We have analysed the causes of inaccuracy in measurement of volume blood flow from vessel path length, cross-sectional area (CSA), and bolus transport time (BTT), and tackled each separately.

4. We have implemented a technique for locating the 3-D course of the centre-line of a blood vessel from biplane angiograms. This makes possible accurate path length measurement even with tortuous vessels. The precise radiographic magnification, and the angle between vessel centre-line and X-ray beam at each point down the vessel, are also derived. These figures are used in the estimation of vessel calibre.

5. We use a densitometric method for cross-sectional area estimation and have obtained very favourable figures for its accuracy ($\pm$ 0.1mm^2 = 1 S.D.) in small phantom vessels 0.5 to 3 mm diameter containing at least 140 mg/ml of iodine.

6. We regard the problems caused by pulsatile blood flow as the major cause of inaccuracy in mean bolus transport time calculation using existing angiographic techniques. We have therefore developed a method which allows discrete flow measurements at many stages of the cardiac cycle and treats distance down the vessel as a continuum. This method uses a 3-D data structure which we display as a parametric image with distance down the vessel as the Y-axis, time as the X-axis, and mean contrast medium concentration across the vessel lumen as the Z-axis or grey scale (Colchester & Brunt 1983). Blood flow velocity is calculated from the slope (distance/time) of iso-concentration contours on the parametric image.

7. In an experiment using a pulsatile flow phantom, flow measurements across the whole cardiac cycle were obtained by analysing the leading edge of a single 1 ml bolus injected into a 4 mm diameter vessel. The angiographic measurements followed the true flow fluctuations extremely closely, as shown by a simultaneous EM flowmeter recording. However, the angiographic measurements consistently overestimated flow in the example presented. We believe this is due to the fact that the leading edge of the bolus is formed by the faster-flowing components at the centre of the vessel and expect to be able to improve accuracy by including velocities calculated from the trailing edge of the bolus which is formed by the slower-moving components at the periphery of the stream.

REFERENCES

BOHME, W. Uber den activen anteil des herzens an der forderung des venenblutes. **Ergebn Physiol 38:** 251-338. Translation. eds. COLCHESTER, A. & PALMER, J. 1980. Available from the RAF Library, Q4 Building, RAF Farnborough, Hants.

BROWN, B.G., BOLSON, E.L. & DODGE H.T. (1982). Arteriographic assessment of coronary atherosclerosis. **Arteriosclerosis 2:** 2-15.

BURSCH J.H., RITMAN E.L., WOOD, E.H. & STURM, R.E. (1974). Roentgen videodensitometry. In **Dye curves: The theory and practice of indicator dilution.** Ed. BLOOMFIELD, D.A. Univ Park Press pp 313-333.

BURSCH, J.H., HAHNE H.J., BRENNECKE R., HETZER, R. & HEINTZEN, P.H. (1979). Functional-angiograms derived from densitometric analysis of digitized x-ray picture series. **Biomedical Engineering (Berlin) 24 (suppl),** 189-90. (In German).

BURSCH J.H., HAHNE, H.J., BRENNECKE, R., GRONEMEIER, D. & HEINTZEN P.H. (1981). Assessment of arterial blood flow, measurements by digital angiography. **Radiology 141:** 39-47.

BUSCH, H.P. & PIROTH, H.D. (1980). Clinical flow measurements with an automated general purpose video-densitometry system (unpublished).

COLCHESTER, A.C.F. & BRUNT J.N.H. (1983). Measurement of vessel calibre and volume blood flow by dynamic quantitative digital angiography: an initial application showing variation of cerebral artery diameter with $PaCO_2$. **J Cereb B Flow Matabol 3:** S640-641.

COLCHESTER, A.C.F. (1985). **The Effect of Changing $PaCO_2$ on Cerebral Artery Calibre Estimated by a New Technique of Dynamic Quantitative Digital Angiography.** PhD Thesis, University of London.

CREPEAU, R.L. & SILVERMAN, N.R. (1973). Videodensitometric vascular flow rate measurement: some error considerations. **Med Biol Engin 11:** 319.

DUFFIELD, R.G.M., LEWIS, B., MILLER, N.E., JAMIESON, C.W., BRUNT J.N.H., & COLCHESTER, A.C.F. (1983). Treatment of hyperlipidaemia retards progression of symptomatic femoral atherosclerosis. **Lancet, I.** 639-642.

FORBES, G.S., EARNEST, F., KISPERT, D.B., FOLGER, W.N., 7 SUNDT, T.M. (1982). "Digital angiography": introducing digital techniques to clinical cerebral angiography practice. **Mayo Clin Proc 57:** 673-693.

HAMBY, R.I., AINTABLIAN, A., WISOFF, B.G. & HARTSTEIN, M.L. (1977). Comparative study of the post-operative flow in the saphenous vein and internal mammary artery bypass grafts. **Amer Heart J 93:** 306-315.

HAWKES, D.J., COLCHESTER, A.C.F., & MOL, C. (1985). The accurate 3-D reconstruction of the geometric configuration of vascular trees from x-ray recordings. In **Physics & Engineering of Medical Imaging.** Ed. Guzzardi, R. The Hague: Martinus Nijhoff. (In press).

HEINTZEN, P.H. (1978). Review of research into and some aspects of the modern development of densitometry, particularly roentgen-video-computer techniques. **Ann Radiol (Paris) 21,** 343-348.

HILAL, S.K. (1966). The determination of the blood flow by a radiographic technique. **Amer J Roentgenol 96:** 896-906.

HOHNE, K.H., BOHM, M., ERBE, W., NICOLAE, G.C., & PFEIFFERSONNE, B. (1978). Computer angiography: A new tool for x-ray functional diagnostics. **Med Prog Technol 6:** 23-28.

KEDEM, D., KEDEM, D., SMITH, C.W., DENAN, R.H., & BRILL, A.B. (1978). Velocity distribution and blood flow measurements using videodensitometric methods. **Invest Radiol 13:** 46-56.

KORBULY, D.E. (1973). Determination of the pulsatile blood flow by a radiographic method. **Invest Radiol 8:** 255.

KRUGER, R.A., BATEMAN, W., LIU, P.Y. & NELSON, J.A. (1983). Blood flow determination using recursive processing: a digital radiographic method. **Radiology 149:** 293-298.

LANTZ, B.M.T. (1975). Relative flow measured by Roentgen videodensitometry in hydrodynamic model. **Acta Radiol Diagnosis 16:** 503-519.

MACKAY, S.A., POTEL, M.J., & RUBIN, J.M. (1982). Graphics methods for tracking three-dimensional heart wall motion. **Comput Biomed Res 15:** 455-473.

MOL, C., COLCHESTER, A.C.F., & HAWKES, D.J. (1985). Three dimensional reconstructions of vascular configurations from biplane angiography. Submitted to Brit J Radiol.

REIBER, J.H.C., SLAGER, C.J., SCHUURBIERS, J.C.H., den BOER, A., GERBRANDS, J.J., TROOST, G.J., SCHOLTS, B., KOOIJMAN, & SERRUYS, P.W. (1983). Transfer functions of the x-ray-cine-video chain applied to digital processing of coronary cineangiograms. In **Digital Imaging in Cardiovascular Radiology.** Eds. HEINTZEN, P.H., & BRENNECKE, R.

RUTISHAUSER, W., STEIGER, U., SIMON, R., HARLANDER, W. & WELLAUER, J. (1974). Roentgendensitometry: an indicator-dilution technique for blood flow measurement after contrast medium injection. **Biomed Engin 9:** 472.

SILVERMAN, N.R., INTAGLIETTA, M., & TOMKINS, W.R. (1973). Television densitometer for blood flow measurement. **Brit J Radiol 46:** 594-598.

SILVERMAN, N.R. & ROSEN, L. (1977). Arterial blood flow measurement: assessment of velocity estimation methods. **Invest Radiol 12:** 319-324.

SMITH, H.C., STURM, R.E. & WOOD, E.H. (1973). Videodensitometric system for measurement of vessel blood flow, particularly the coronary arteries in man. **Amer J Cardiol 32:** 144.

SPEARS, J.R., SANDOR, T., ALS, A.V., MALAGOLD, M., MARKIS, J.E., GROSSMAN, W., SERUR, J.R. & PAULIN, S. (1983). Computerised image analysis for quantitative measurement of vessel diameter from cineangiograms. **Circulation 68:** 453.

THOMPSON, H.K., STARMER, C.F., WHALEN, R.E. & MCINTOSH, H.D. (1964). Indicator transit time considered as a gamma variate. **Circ Res 14:** 502-515.

YERUSHALMI, S. & ITZCHAK, Y. (1976). Angiographic methods for blood flow measurements. **Med Prog Technol 4:** 107-15.

CORRELATION METHODS FOR TOMOGRAPHIC
IMAGES USING TWO AND THREE
DIMENSIONAL TECHNIQUES

GERALD Q. MAGUIRE JR.[*+], MARILYN E. NOZ[+], EVAN M. LEE[+] AND JAMES H. SCHIMPF[$]

1. INTRODUCTION

The aim of any project which involves the use of radionuclides, is to determine whether or not an organ is functioning correctly. Two areas of great concern at present, are the evaluation of cardiac function and of brain function. Tomographic methods have proved to be very valuable in both cases. The problems encountered have many things in common as well as many differences.

It is usual to use Single Photon Emission Computer Tomography (SPECT) as well as Positron Emission Tomography (PET) to evaluate myocardial function under conditions of both rest and stress. In this case, small differences in activity are being sought and the eye is often not accurate enough to detect them. By registering the images so that the rest image lies directly over the stress image, subtraction can be performed. The differences in activity will then become more pronounced. Additionally, a cardiac patient might be followed with successive PET or SPECT studies to determine the effect of treatment. In this case also, small differences might be missed, if the two images could not be analytically compared.

The brain on the other hand is a very complex structure composed of many organs which vary in position and size from person to person. In studying a particular function of the brain, therefore, it is essential to have the ability to overlay images which show good anatomic resolution such as computer tomography (CT) or magnetic resonance imaging (MRI) images onto images such as those obtained from PET or SPECT which show physiologic function. This is especially important with the present generation of tagged amino acids and monoclonal antibodies which are being used to determine very specific and very small focal areas of brain function. Hence, it is important to have an objective and reproducible means for identifying brain structures, [1] since the aim of any neurological project is to accurately determine brain function.

[*]Department of Computer Science, Columbia University New York, NY 10027

[+]Department of Radiology, New York University New York, NY 10016

[$]Department of Computer Science, University of Utah Salt Lake City, UT 84112

This research was supported in part by the Defense Advanced Research Projects Agency under contract N00039-84-C-0165 and an IBM Faculty Development Award.

Once a patient is removed from the imaging apparatus of any sort, it is very difficult, in fact impossible to reposition this patient in exactly the same manner again. In the case of brain studies, even though head holders and a common reference point such as the canthomeatal line are used, it is virtually impossible to position a patient precisely twice. Indeed, "scout" images performed with the CT scanner before and after a study often reveal slight position shifts. Patient movement, even when a head holder is used, is a commonly reported problem in PET studies. With respect to heart studies where a scintillation camera is used, it is very difficult to get the camera head exactly the same distance from the chest wall even though the skin is used as a reference point.

In this study, we have concentrated on the correlation or registration of tomographic images of the brain. The method of correlation described below, was originally developed for cardiac studies.

2. BRAIN TOMOGRAPHY

The use of positron emitting radionuclides tagged to a suitable pharmaceutical as well as the development of rotating scintillation cameras, has allowed tomographic reconstruction of brain activity. However, the specific functional centers can only be mapped out by having an absolutely accurate anatomical blueprint. One method of accomplishing this is to construct an anatomic atlas of the brain. [9, 4] This atlas can be then be deformed elastically [3] and fit to images such as those obtained from CT where edge detection is at least possible. Once the anatomic structures are well defined, then it should be possible to overlay the CT image onto the PET image. However, even the calculation of the atlas to CT transformation cannot be accomplished without some difficulties. If the CT slices do not exactly match those of the atlas, then some compromise must be made or three dimensional techniques must be employed. When a computerized atlas is used, and elastic deformation methods are employed, it must be possible to form curved surfaces which are then stretched or shrunk until a minimum of the potential energy function is found. This implies being able to find the edge of the structure. Unfortunately, for metabolic images such as PET or SPECT, this is not easily possible. Most edge finding techniques fail due to the nature of the statistics governing the quanta in the image. Hence, for analysis of radionuclide images, the structures must first be located unambiguously on the CT (or similarly on an MRI) image and then this must be correlated with the radionuclide image. This implies possibly two oblique reconstructions.

On the other hand, there is also a great deal of interest in correlating image data obtained from such sources as Landstat images. [2] Unlike graphics data, for which geometric transformation means a mathematical calculation to move the data (a vector or a surface), image data should be manipulated by resampling the original spatial continuum. Such a method, employing a polynomial technique was proposed by Frei [20] and is now implemented in hardware in at least one image processor (International Imaging Systems, Model 75). Alternatively, there is a image rotation controller chip whose functions include image resampling (rotation, scaling) and two dimensional convolution (image filtering), again developed primarily for the geometric correction of satellite digital image data [21]. Since, in medical images, we have bandlimited continuous images, a perfect reconstruction is possible, provided the digital image was obtained by sampling at least at the Nyquist sampling rate. However, even here, while two-dimensional transformations such as translate, rotate and scale are relatively easy, skew remains a difficult problem. The software we have developed to do the image transformation could and really should be replaced by hardware such as the chip mentioned above (developed by Stroll, et al.). New and improved hardware is also being developed by I^2S.

This paper will describe the methods developed by the authors for correlating tomographic images obtained from different modalities, namely, positron emission tomography (PET), computer tomography (CT) and magnetic resonance imaging (MRI).

3. METHODS

For this analysis, two PET images of the same patient, taken at different times, and a CT image of the same patient were used. The PET images had a pixel resolution of 128x128 and the CT of 256x256. The PET images were obtained using the PET camera developed by and presently in operation at the Karolinska Institute/Hospital. [13, 8] The CT was obtained using a GE8800 scanner. In each case, a head holder specifically molded to the patient's head [7] was used. In spite of these precautions, the PET images are quite different. (See figure 1.)

A 512x512 Grinnel 270 frame buffer used as a raster display was employed for viewing the images simultaneously and thus aiding in characterizing their geometric relationship. This is done by comparing the relative positions of features on each image and measuring their respective coordinates. These features are referred to in our terminology as "landmarks", and are features that appear to be similar on each image. Visual acuity is somewhat limited in nuclear medicine type images because of photon difficiency. The skull as seen on the CT image and the edge of the picture in the PET image, as well as the ventricles, make suitable landmarks. When comparing two PET images, both the image edge and the ventricles can be used. Usually between seven and ten such pairs of landmarks are chosen. (We have found that five landmarks are too few and that fifteen are not any better than ten, but we have not tried large numbers like fifty.) [12] Figure 2 shows a typical screen for choosing landmarks.

Landmarks are chosen on the reference image and on the image to be moved (i.e., rotated, scaled, skewed and/or translated. Although we included skew, we feel that it is better accomplished using the tilt algorithm described below).

Each landmark from the reference image is then cross-correlated with the corresponding landmark from the other image. A search window (smaller) on the reference image is moved through an area (larger) in the image to be moved. The best matched pair (using the original coordinates from the reference image) is chosen (the coordinates on the image to be moved are updated). It is at this point that careful attention to matching data size and meaning must be made. For example, if the reference image is a CT with a pixel size of 256x256 and the image to be moved is a PET image with a pixel size of 128x128, one or the other must be changed. Additionally, CT numbers are usually assigned with the opposite meaning of activity numbers, i.e., where there is a lot of attenuation (skull) there is little activity from the metabolism point of view. Letting $a_{i,j}$ and $b_{i+k,j+1}$ designate the pixels of the window and the search areas respectively, the cross-correlation coefficient function is defined as:

$$R(k,l) = \frac{\sum\limits_{i=1}^{n}\sum\limits_{j=1}^{n} a_{ij}\, b_{i+k,j+l}}{(\sum\limits_{i=1}^{n}\sum\limits_{j=1}^{n} a^2_{ij} \cdot \sum\limits_{i=1}^{n}\sum\limits_{j=1}^{n} b^2_{i+k,j+l})^{1/2}}$$

At the end of this procedure, we have sets of coordinate pairs $(x_i,\ y_i;\ u_i,\ v_i)$ which relate the respective locations of the anatomical landmarks in the two images.

Following Frei's algorithm [20], we form two-dimensional polynomials

$$x = a_0 + a_1 u + a_2 v + a_3 uv + a_4 u^2 + \ldots \tag{1}$$

$$y = b_0 + b_1 u + b_2 v + b_3 uv + b_4 u^2 + \ldots \tag{2}$$

The coefficients a_i, b_i are determined using a linear regression technique which employs a least squares fit on the set of landmarks already obtained. [10, 15] We used only the first three terms of each polynomial which corrects for translation, rotation, scale and skew. The Gauss-Jordan formalism is then employed to obtain the eigenvalues of the matrix of coefficients. [16] These eigenvalues are then used together with an averaging technique for partial pixels, to determine the new coordinates for each pixel in the image to be moved.

This averaging technique deserves some comment. We used a four pixel area to estimate what fraction of each of the original pixels should be moved to the new pixel. Contributions to a moved pixel, from one or more original pixels are simply summed to give a total activity in that pixel. Currently, we just divide proportional to the "area" of the pixel to be included. It might be worthwhile to try a gaussian point spread function, where the distance is proportional to the weighted distance. The assumption however, would still be that only the nearest four pixels are affected. Figure 3 shows how pixels in this four pixel array could match. Figure 4 demonstrates a worst case match where the two images are mismatched by $\pi/4$. Figures 5 and 6 show two different ways in which pixels could be mismatched.

4. RESULTS

This method has been used with success to register two dimensional images [20] of the heart (obtained via standard nuclear medicine techniques using Thallium-201) and for two dimensional data from three dimensional PET and CT images obtained at the Karolinska Institute. [14] Figure 7 shows two PET images aligned and Figure 8 shows the PET image aligned with the CT image.

In addition, it was suggested to the authors by Stephen M. Pizer of the University of North Carolina, that the correlation of three dimensional images might be better accomplished by choosing the landmarks using a three-dimensional viewer such as that developed by Pizer [11, 17] or by Brent Baxter [5, 6] at the University of Utah, as opposed to reconstructing an oblique slice of one modality to correspond to the exact planar location of the slice associated with the second modality. In an effort to examine this, we chose landmarks on three contiguous slices and extended the polynomial equations to three dimensions:

$$x = a_0 + a_1u + a_2v + a_3t + a_4uv + a_5ut + a_6vt + \dots \qquad (3)$$

$$y = b_0 + b_1u + b_2v + b_3t + b_4uv + b_5ut + b_6vt + \dots \qquad (4)$$

$$z = c_0 + c_1u + c_2v + c_3t + c_4uv + c_5ut + c_6vt + \dots \qquad (5)$$

The coefficients a_i, b_i, c_i are again determined using a linear regression technique which employs a least squares fit on the set of landmarks already obtained. [10, 15] We used only the first four terms of each polynomial which corrects for translation, rotation, scale and skew. We then examined the coefficient of z that was produced. If the coefficient was close to one, we felt confident that the two dimensional planar transformation was sufficient. If the coeficient of z was not close to one, we expect that it can be resolved in a such a manner that the inputs necessary for the oblique reconstruction could be obtained.

Thus the actual manner in which the original landmarks are chosen becomes a matter of which techniques make the the the user of the program feel more confident. Ideally, the choosing of the landmarks should be automated, but this is somewhat in the future for radionuclide type images. Once a number of landmarks are chosen, the program can then be continued. The effect of the number of landmarks chosen on the values of the coefficients obtained was studied by using the same PET image and varying the number of landmarks used in the calculation of the coefficients.

In the present work, we first determined the eigenvalue coefficients for the two PET images and then for the CT image. These eigenvalues are then used together with the averaging technique described above to determine the new coordinates for each pixel in the image to be moved.

Figure 9 shows a PET image in the upper left corner, its shifted image (x + 5, y + 3) in the upper left hand corner, it registered (x - 5, y - 3) with itself in the lower right hand corner and it registered with itself again (x - 10, y - 6) in the lower left corner.

5. OBLIQUE SLICE RECONSTRUCTION

As an alternative to the three-dimensional viewer mentioned above, one can employ a tilt algorithm to obtain an oblique slice of the PET and/or MRI image which most closely aligns with the CT image. [18, 19]

In our development of the method, a transaxial (usually centrally located) slice is displayed in the upper left quadrant of the video screen. The levels for sagittal and coronal reconstruction are chosen by separately moving an automatically displayed set of crosshairs. The x and y position of the crosshairs is written in the text area of the screen and is updated as the crosshairs are re-positioned. When the levels have been chosen, the sagittal and coronal views are reconstructed and displayed in two additional separate quadrants. At the bottom of the sagittal view, a cursor (along with its coordinates) is displayed. This is moved through the sagittal view for the purpose of obtaining the z coordinate of the pixel which will be the pivot point for the oblique slice. After this point has been chosen, a line appears on the sagittal view and the user is asked to choose the incremental angle in degrees through which the line should be rotated each time a numerical key is struck. The line is rotated (either clockwise or counter-clockwise) until the desired tilt is obtained in the x-z plane. A line then appears on the coronal view at the correct z height, the rotation increment is again specified (it may be different from that specified above) and the tilt in the y-z plane is selected. In both cases, the numerical value of the angle through which the line is tilted is continuously updated in the text area. The construction of the oblique slice follows if the user agrees. The slice is stored in a file for future use and is displayed in the remaining quadrant of the screen as it is produced. Figure 10 shows a typical screen at the end of this procedure.

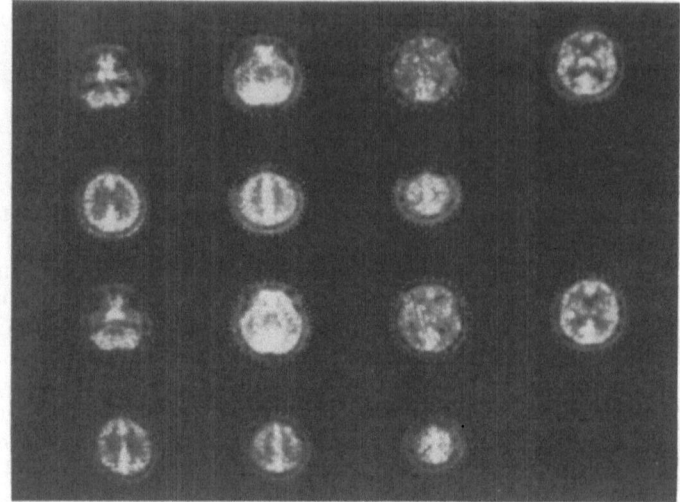

Figure 1: Original PET images. Those on the top were taken before those on the bottom

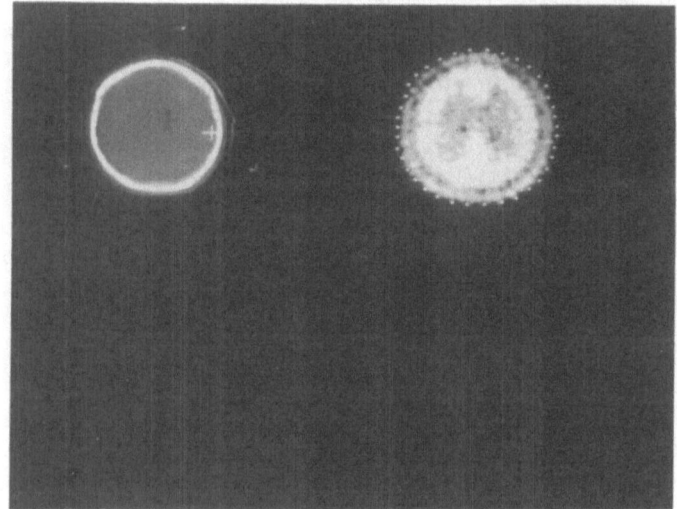

Figure 2: Typical Screen for Choosing Landmarks

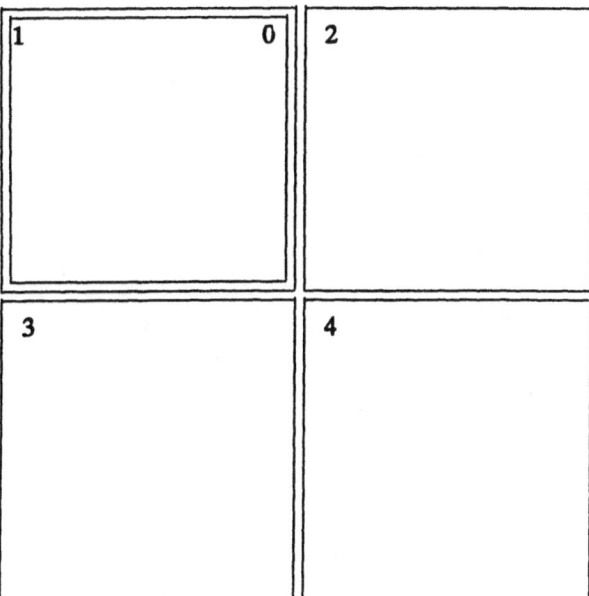

Figure 3: In this case, the pixel is moved exactly onto the upper left hand pixel

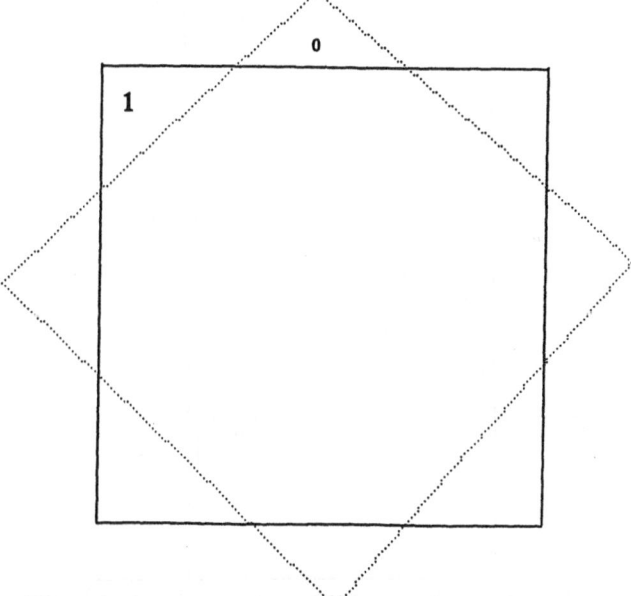

Figure 4: The pixel to be moved is exactly $\pi/4$ out of phase

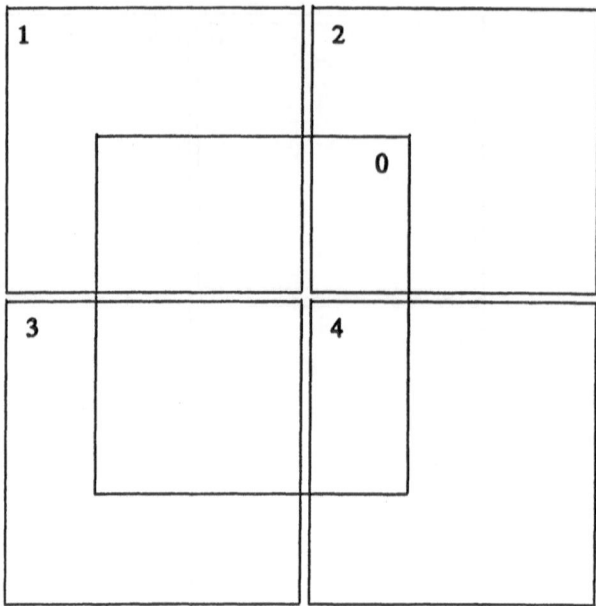

Figure 5: Pixels mismatched, but not rotated

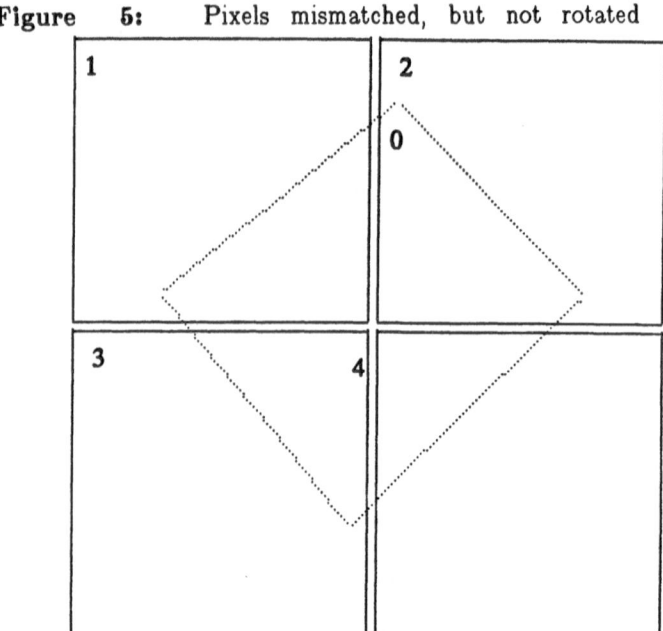

Figure 6: Pixels mismatched and also rotated

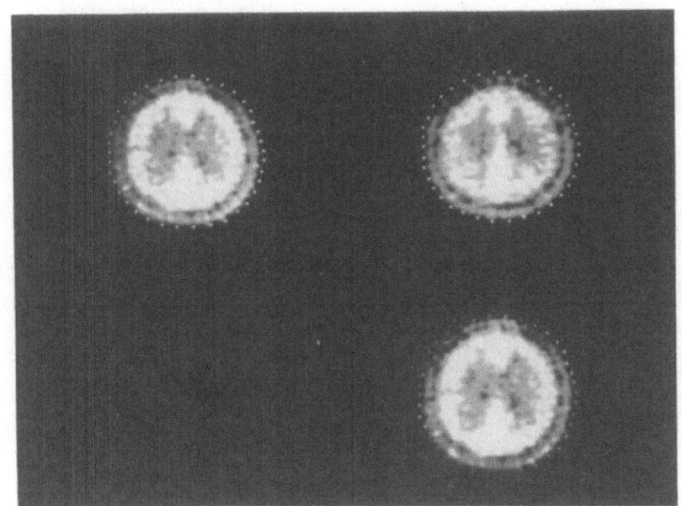

Figure 7:   Two PET images aligned

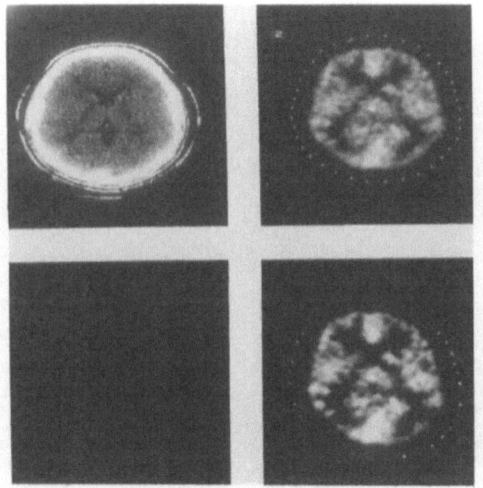

Figure 8:   Alignment of a PET and CT image

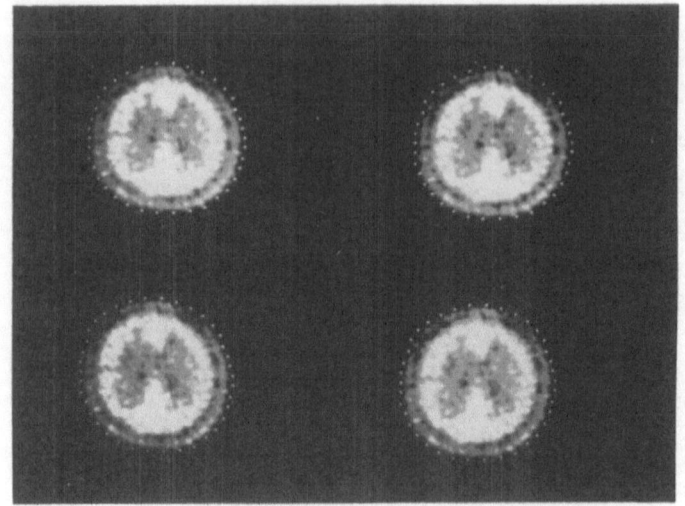

Figure   9:   PET image shifted and registered
with itself

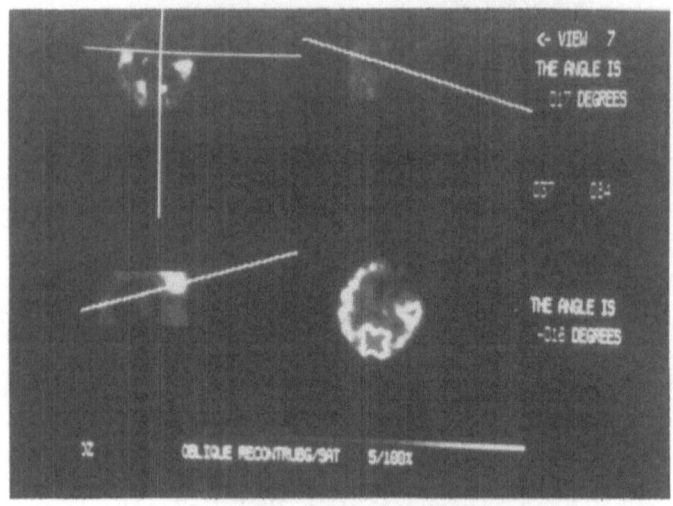

Figure   10:   Detailed Result of Graphically
Oriented Oblique Reconstruction

REFERENCES

[1] Adair, T., Karp, P., Stein, A., Bajcsy, R. and Reivich, M.
Computer Assisted Analysis of Tomographic Images of the Brain.
Journal of Computer Assisted Tomography 5:929-932, December, 1981.

[2] Adams, J., Patton, C., Reader, C. and Zamora, D.
Hardware for Geometric Warping.
Electronic Imaging 3:50-55, April, 1984.

[3] Bajcsy, R., and Broit, C.
Matching of Deformed Images.
In *Proceedings of the Sixth International Conference on Pattern Recognition*, pages 351-353. Institute of Electrical and Electronics Engineers, October, 1982.

[4] Bajcsy, R., Lieberson, R. and Reivich, M.
A Computerized System for the Elastic Matching of Deformed Radiographic Images to Idealized Atlas Images.
Journal of Computer Assisted Tomography 7:618-625, August, 1983.

[5] Baxter, B.S.
A Three-Dimensional Display Viewing Device for Examining Internal Structure.
In *Proceedings of the Conference on Technical Issues in Focal Plane Development*, pages 111-115. Society of Photo-Optical Engineers, December, 1981.

[6] Baxter, B.S. and Hitchner, L.E.
Applications of a Three Dimensional Display in Diagnostic Imaging.
Nuclear Medicine and Biology, Vol. 2.
Pergamon Press, Paris, 1982, pages 2173-2176.

[7] Bergström M., Böethius, J. Eriksson L., Greitz, T., Ribbe, T. and Widèn, L.
Head Fixation Device for Reproducible Position Alignment in Transmission CT and Positron Emission Tomography.
Journal of Computer Assisted Tomography 5:136-141, February, 1981.

[8] Bergström, M., Eriksson, L. Bohm, C. Blomqvist, G. and Litton, J.E.
Correction ofr Scattered Radiation in Ring Detector Positron Camera by integral Transformation of Projections.
Journal of Computer Assisted Tomography 7:42-50, February, 1983.

[9] Bohm, C., Greitz, T., Kingsley, D., Berggren, B.M. and Olsson, L.
Adjustable Computerized Stereotaxic Brain Atlas for Transmission and Emission Tomography.
Am. J. Neuroradiology 4:731-733, March, 1983.

278

[10]   Eadie, W.T., Drijard, D., James, F.E., Roos, M. and Sadoulet, B.
Statistical Methods in Experimental Physics.
North Holland Publishing Company, New York, NY, 1971.
pp. 121-124.

[11]   Fuchs, H., Pizer, S.H., Cohen, J.S. and Brooks Jr., F.P.
A Three Dimensional Display for Medical Images from Slices.
Information Processing in Medical Imaging.
INSERM 88, Paris, 1979, pages 581-602.

[12]   Hall, E.L.
Computer Image Processing and Recognition.
Academic Press, New York, NY, 1979.
pp. 186-189 & pp. 468-554.

[13]   Litton, J.E., Bergström, M., Eriksson, L. Bohm, C. Blomqvist,
G. and Kesselberg, M.
Performance Study of PC-384 Positron Camera System for Emission
    Tomography of the Brain.
Journal of Computer Assisted Tomography 8:74-87, February, 1984.

[14]   Noz, M. E.; Maguire Jr., G. Q.; Lee, E.; Schimpf, J. H.; and
Horii, S. C.
Computerized Correlation of Tomographic Images.
In *Proceedings of the 1984 International Joint Alpine Symposium*,
    pages 85-88. IEEE, February, 1984.

[15]   Ostle, B. and Mensing R.W.
Statistics in Research.
The Iowa State University Press, Ames, Iowa, 1975.
pp. 165-236.

[16]   Pizer, S.H. with Wallace V.L.
To Compute Numerically.
Little, Brown & Company, Boston, MA, 1983.
pp. 182-204.

[17]   Pizer, S.H., Fuchs, H., Heinz, E.R., Bloomberg, S.H. and Tsai, L.C.
Varifocal Mirror Display of Organ Surfaces from CT Scans.
Nuclear Medicine and Biology, Vol. 2.
Pergamon Press, Paris, 1982, pages 2177-2180.

[18]   Rhodes, M.L.
Interactive Object Isolation from Parallel Image Planes.
PhD Thesis, University of California at Los Angeles :200pp,
    1978.

[19]   Rhodes, M.L., Glenn, W.V. and Azzawi, Y.M.
Extracting Oblique Planes from Serial CT Sections.
Journal of Computer Assisted Tomography 4:649-657, October, 1980.

[20]   Singh, M., Frei, W., Shibita, T., Huth, G.H. and Telfer, N.E.
A Digital Technique for Accurate Change Detection in Nuclear
Medicine Images - with Application to Myocardial Perfussion
Studies Using Thallium 201 .
IEEE Transactions on Nuclear Science NS-26:565-575, February,
1979.

[21]   Stroll, Z.Z., Swartalander Jr., E.E., Eldon, J. and Ashburn, J.L.
Image Rotation Controller Chip.
In *Proceedings of the International Conference on Computer Design
(ICCD84)*, pages 274-279.   Institute of Electrical and Electronics
Engineers, October, 1984.

A NEW APPROACH TO DOUBLE TRACER STUDIES.

JC LIEHN, A VENOT and JF LEBRUCHEC.

Institut Jean Godinot and Faculté de Médecine BP 171 F51056 Reims FRANCE.

FR Synthèse et Analyse d'images médicales and Service d'Explorations
fonctionnelles par les radioisotopes, Hopital Cochin. Paris.
INSERM U194. Pitié-Salpétrière. Paris.

1.INTRODUCTION
1.1) The problems of Double Tracer Studies processing and their classical
solutions.
Many scintigraphic studies are based on the comparison of two images
recorded using different tracers. The processing of these Double Tracer
Studies (DTS) combines the difficulties of any image comparison and those
arising from the fact that the images are obtained with different tracers.
This is the reason why DTS are usually analysed visually. In this case, any
number of views can be used and the acquisitions can take place at
different times. However, when the construction of a parametric image, such
as the difference or the ratio image is planned, constraints are imposed on
the acquisition protocol. One of the most serious constraints is the
absence of patient motion which limits the number of views, and also
imposes, in most cases, the use of radionuclides with different energies.
Even if these constraints are fulfilled, difficulties still remain, such as
the differences in crosstalk (or background), in absorption and in the
Point Source Responses of the detector (1). In this text we present a new
method of DTS processing which is based on an original and rigorous
approach to the problem.
1.2) A generalized definition of DTS.
In fact, the difficulties arising from the differences in energies are
only one part of the problem. Registration and Normalization are necessary
prior to subtraction of any couple of scintigraphic images. This is the
reason why the method we propose is applicable to a wide range of
scintigraphic tests which can be included in a generalized definition of
DTS. In this text, a DTS is defined as study involving the comparison of
images recorded with tracers having different metabolisms. These two
tracers can be :
1) Different radio-isotopes (e.g. : Tl-Tc Parthyroid study) (case 1).
2) Different molecules labelled with the same radio-isotope (e.g.:Micro-
sphere-Aerosol Lung Study) (case 2).
3) The same radio-isotope used under different physiological conditions
(e.g. : Tl Stress-Rest Myocardial study) (case 3).
1.3) Origin of the new approach.
In previous works, we have developed (2,3,4,5) and tested (6) new methods
for simultaneous Geometric and Grey-Level image Registration and for the
statistical comparison of registered images. These methods can be used to
solve some of the problems of DTS processing and to free the acquisition
protocol of the above mentioned constraints.

2) METHODOLOGY.
2.1) The basic concept.
  2.1.1) The double origin of the differences between the two images.

Using the proposed method, we can analyse DTS which lead to couples of images recorded on the same view. These images are only partly similar. Several processes contribute to the differences between the two images :
1) The different metabolisms of the tracers within the organ of interest.
2) The different metabolisms of the tracers outside the organ of interest.
3) The patient motions.
4) The different acquisition times and activities.
5) The different Point Source Responses of the detector. (case 1 only).
6) The different absorption of the rays. (case 1 only).
7) The contribution of one ray in the window of the other.(cased 1 only).
8) The noise in each image.
Amongst these processes, process 1 can be considered as the process of interest, while the other processes have disturbing effects.
2.1.2) The modelling approach.
Although numerous and complex, processes 2 to 7 can be analysed and a transformation can possibly be found which transforms one of the images into the other. For example, a geometric transformation can correct patient motions, a normalization can correct the differences in acquisition times and activities and the addition of a constant can correct differences in the crosstalks, at least within a certain ROI. We call this transformation THE REGISTRATION MODEL. It transforms one of the images into the other (except for the statistical fluctuations) within the region where no differences are due to process 1, i.e. in normal regions. In the abnormal regions, the differences are due to process 1 and cannot be explained by the Registration Model, which is built in order to describe the differences due to other processes. The pixels of these regions can be considered as OUTLIERS according to the terminology of data modelling techniques. Therefore the interpretation of a DTS is based on the detection of outliers with respect to the Registration Model. This approach differs from the general method of data modelling where outliers are generally discarded.
2.1.3) The robustness problem.
The identification of the Registration Model consists of different steps
1) Selection of the structure of the model.
2) Selection of a criterion.
3) Selection of an optimization method.
Each model chosen at step 1 is characterized by the MODEL PARAMETERS whose values are determined by optimizing the criterion. The main problem is, that in this identification process, only the normal regions have to be taken into account, since the outlier pixels of the abnormal regions disturb the identification. Therefore the criterion must be insensitive to the presence of outliers. An estimation procedure based on such a criterion is called a ROBUST estimation. Robustness is thus the main quality of the criterion we use for this particular model identification problem.
2.1.4) The statistical comparison.
The Registration Model explains the differences between the two images in the normal regions. Since the two original images are noisy, a further statistical test is necessary to select the outlier pixels where the residuals (the differences between the observed images and what the model predicts) are significantly different from zero. Each test depends on the structure of the model.
2.2) THE REGISTRATION MODEL.
  2.2.1) The different models.
  2.2.1.1.) Notations :
Let F1 be one of the two images to be compared,F2 be the other image.
F3 be the registered version of F2 : F3 = T (F2)

where T is the transformation which defines the Registration Model.
T is the product of simpler transformations :

$$T = G \times L$$

G is Geometric Registration Model.
L is the Grey-Level Registration Model.

2.2.1.2) Geometric Registration Models

G models a geometric transformation between two images. The two simple transformations we use are the translation in the plane of the image characterized by two parameters Dx and Dy and the rotation in the plane characterized by one parameter. When applying these transformations, no interpolation is performed in order to maintain the statistical properties of noise.

2.2.1.3) Grey-Level Registration Models.

The normalization of two scintigraphic images is very often considered as a multiplicative process, we call the corresponding model the 1 PARAMETER LINEAR GREY LEVEL REGISTRATION MODEL. This single parameter is noted as NF (for Normalization Factor). But very often, in the special case of DTS processing , the multiplication by a constant does not lead to a Good Grey-Level Registration. The differences in Tissue Crosstalks require a more sophisticated model. The addition of a constant BG (for Background), is the simplest way to model these differences. The Grey-Level Registration Model is therefore the 2 PARAMETER GREY LEVEL REGISTRATION MODEL with parameters NF and BG. For example, a 4 parameter model which includes a translation and a 2 Parameter Linear model is :

F3 (x,y) = NF (F2(x + Dx, y + Dy) + BG)

The hypothesis supporting this model is generally too simple to explain the differences in the whole image, but is suitable for modelling procedures applied to limited ROI

2.2.1.4) Other models.

This modelling approach allows us to envisage more sophisticated models. For example, the convolution by a blurring filter could model differences in the Point Source responses of the detector. Differences in the absorption of the rays could be modelled by a non-linear transformation.

2.2.2) Model Selection.

2.2.2.1) Prior information.

As in any model selection problem, prior information and empirical data are useful in the selection of a model structure. Prior information can help in the selection of a Geometric Registration Model if, for example,it is known that the images are recorded at different times.

2.2.2) Empirical information.

But most of the useful information for the selection of a model is provided by the analysis of actual images.

2.2.2.2.1) Selection of the Geometric Registration Model. The visual analysis of several cases, with the help of ROI drawing facilities generally shows whether patient motions can occur between the two acquisitions.

2.2.2.2.2) Selection of the Grey Level Registration Model : the Scatter Diagram : Selecting a Grey Level Registration Model is more difficult. The first reason is that this point can only be studied once the geometric registration problem has been solved. In practice, we have to carry out this analysis on manually registered images. The second reason is that a difference in grey levels is not easily analysed visually. In order to make the choice of a Grey Level Registration Model more practical, we use SCATTER DIAGRAMS. These graphs display the pixel values of one image versus the values of the corresponding pixels on the second image. Figure 1A shows

such a graph for Thallium-Pertechnetate Thyroid-Parathyroid images. The Thallium image pixel values are plotted versus Pertechnetate image pixel values. This scatter diagram clearly demonstrates that a 1 parameter normalization cannot model the differences between the two images ; a 2 Parameter Linear Model seems more suitable. Figure 1B shows the values of a Thallium Redistribution myocardium images versus the stress image values. In this case, a 1 Parameter Linear model seems adequate. On both scatter diagrams, the regression line obtained by the non-parametric procedure described in section 2.3 is plotted.

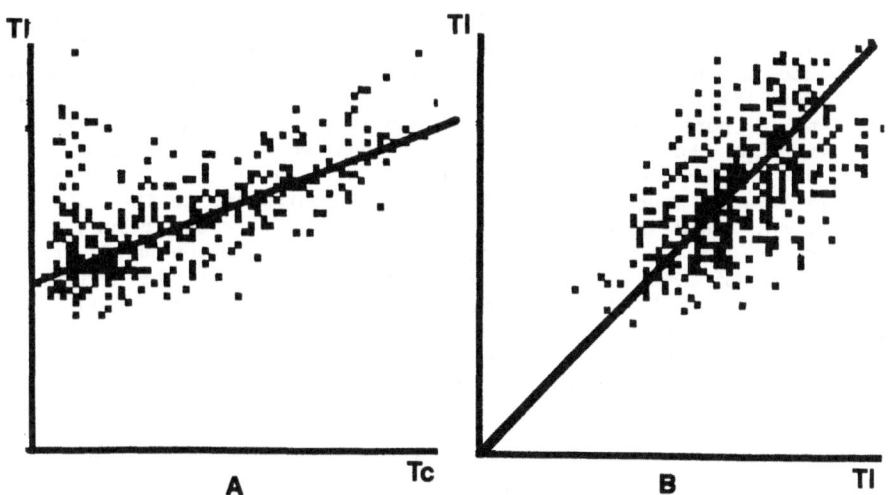

Figure 1 : Scatter Diagrams used in the selection of Grey-Level Registration models   A : Parathyroid-Thyroid   Tl-Tc   scintigraphy .B : Myocardium Stress-Rest Tl scintigraphy.

2.2.2.3) The method based on the value of the criteria.

The above-described methods do not lead to a rigorous choice of a model structure. An alternative approach is based on the value of the criterion used to identify the parameters of the model. This method is quantitative. If the statistic of the criterion value is known in the case of similarity of the two images, two tests can be carried out. Firstly, the suitability of a chosen model can be tested if similar images are available. Secondly, the degree of significance of the improvement of fit obtained by adding more parameters to the model can be tested. Hierarchical or Nested models can be selected by performing a statistical test between the values of the criterion obtained with two models of increasing complexity, (e.g. : 2 Parameter Linear Grey-Level Registration Model versus a 1 Parameter Linear model).

2.2.3) The effect of noise.

As in any data modelling process, the residual F1 - F3 is the sum of two terms. The first term is a statistical term whose value depends on the noise in the original images F1 and F2. The second term depends on the goodness of fit. If the noise in the original images is low, the residuals are mainly determined by the second term. Therefore, it is more difficult to find a good model for high count images. For example, a good model for 128 x 128 images may be unable to model images packed to the 64 x 64 format. Nevertheless, as seen in the next section, images with high pixel values are more sensitive in the detection of outliers.

2.3) The robust criterion.

As pointed out in section 2.1.3. the use of a robust criterion is an essential step in the modelling process. In fact, the development of this methodology has its origin in the introduction of a new class of similarity measures (3) which have been proven to be efficient distribution-free criteria for robust estimation problems (5,6). In order to compare noisy images, we have to use the STOCHASTIC SIGN CHANGE criterion (SSC) which is calculated in the following way : Given two observed images F1 and F2, a Registration Model T and the transformed F3 = T (F2) of F2, we calculate the residual image D = F1-F3. We scan this image line by line within a defined window and count the number of changes of the residual sign. In the regions where the model is adequate, the probability for the difference D (i,j,) to be positive equals the probability to be negative and the density of sign changes is high. In regions where the model is not adequate, the differences are either all positive or all negative and no sign change occurs. Thus, these regions do not contribute to the value of the criterion. This property makes the SSC criterion robust. The distribution of SSC is closely related to the distribution used in the non-parametric RUN TEST. If N is the number of pixels in the window in which SSC is calculated, SSC is normally distributed with mean (N-1)/2 and variance N/4. This can be used in order to perform the tests described in section 2.2.2.3. Furthermore an image of the Sign Changes (SC), made of 0 and 1, is generated. It can be analysed visually in order to evaluate the goodness of fit and to identify the regions where the fit is good and where it is not. Up to now,no automatic segmentation of this image has been performed. As an example, figure 2 shows the result of a Tl-Tc parathyroid study. A parathyroid adenoma is visible on the Thallium image (Figure 2A) The image of the Sign Changes shows a random distribution everywhere except in the region of the adenoma (Figure 2C).

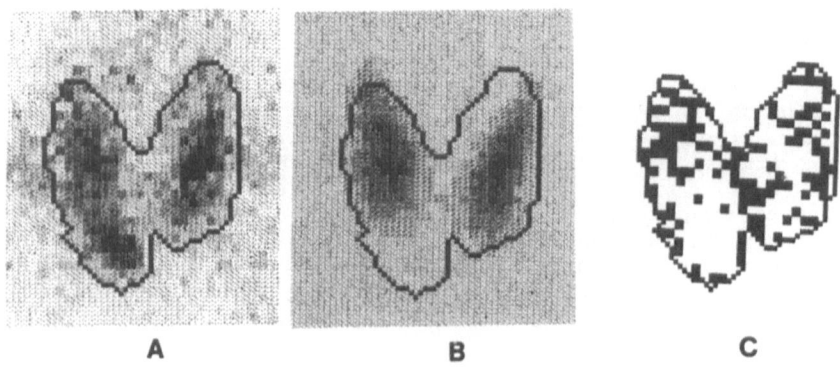

Figure 2 : The Sign Change image. A : Tl Parathyroid Thyroid image. B : Tc Thyroid images. C : The Sign Change image.

2.4. The estimation of the parameters.

2.4.1 The necessity of derivative-free algorithms.

Given two images F1 and F2 and a window, SSC is a function of the

registration model parameter values. The estimation of the value of these parameters requires the maximization of SSC with respect to these parameters. The problem has the following characteristics :
1) The number of parameters ranges generally from 1 to 5, but can be higher.
2) The function to optimize is not a linear function of the parameters (7).
3) The problem is not constrained.
4) Some parameters take only integer values (the translation shifts), while others are real numbers (the normalization factors).
5) The function to optimize is not differentiable, small variations of the parameters may have no effect on SSC.
6) The function to optimize can be multimodal.
7) The calculation of the function value can be time consuming, especially if the window is large.
All these characteristics make this optimization problem a non-classical one. As a consequence, trajectory-description methods, such as those derived from the Newton method are unusable.

2.4.2) The Adaptative Random Search (ARS) method (8).

In such difficult cases, probabilistic methods are appropriate. The basic step of these methods is the calculation of the criterion for a randomly chosen parameter vector and the replacement of the old optimal parameter vector by the new one if the criterion value is better. In our implementation of the ARS strategy, two phases are repeated alternatively. During the first phase, the variances of the normal distributions in which the further parameter values are randomly chosen are selected. During the second phase, the selected variances are used for a fixed number of iterations. A characteristic of this implementation is that it spends more time in looking for the subspace where it has to search for the optimal values (phase one) than in searching for the exact location of these values (phase two).

2.4.3) Other algorithms.

2.4.3.1) Optimization.

The main advantage of the ARS method is its versatility. We found it very efficient in identifying 5 parameter models. But such an optimization requires typically 2000 function evaluations. This can be too time consuming for implementations made on slow systems. Therefore, we developed a less versatile but faster algorithm. It is based on a relaxation method which combines two optimization procedures. At each step of the Geometric Registration procedure, the parameter values of the Grey Level Registration Model are estimated by the Fibonnaci (or Golden section) search if a 1 Parameter Linear model is used, or by the Simplex (also called flexible polyhedron) (9) method if a 2 Parameter Linear model is used. The latter method requires initial estimates of the parameters. For Geometric Registration, a method applicable only for a Translation Model was developed. It is an integer version of the Steepest Descent Method which consists of different trials made around a starting initial estimate and a step by step progression toward the high values of SSC. The search is completed when a maximum is found. This simple method is reasonably fast and reliable if the initial estimate is not located too far from the solution.

2.4.3.2) The initial estimate.

As mentioned, both the Geometric Registration and the Grey-Level Registration methods require accurate initial estimates. These estimates can be obtained by using less robust criteria, but which can be computed more quickly. For Geometric Registration, we found the Correlation

Coefficient to be a good criterion. The optimal value of the registration parameters are estimated by means of the same integer version of the Steepest Descent method. At this early stage, the estimates are given manually after visual inspection of the images. The optimization is fast because no Grey Level Registration has to be performed at each step of the Geometric Registration. The Grey Level Registration is performed once the Geometric Registration is completed. The parameters of the Linear Grey Level Registration model are obtained by using the Weighted Least Squares method. In order to fulfil the requirements of this method (no variance on X), we have to use the pixel values of the image with the better count density as the explicative variable and the more noisy image as the dependant variable.

2.5) <u>Pixelwise comparison of the registered images</u>.

Once the model is identified, a further test is performed in order to find the location of the abnormal pixels i.e. those where the residuals are significantly different from zero. Basically, the Sign Change Image contains this information, but its analysis faces the following problems :

1) The limits of the regions with no Sign Change are difficult to determine.

2) Generally, only the regions where the residuals have a certain sign are of clinical interest. The Sign Change Image does not provide the sign of the residuals.

3) The magnitude of the residuals are of clinical interest. The Sign Change Image does not provide this magnitude.

4) Small regions with no Sign Change or regions with slightly less than 50 % Sign Changes are not easily identified.

On the contrary, the images of the Significant Differences (SD) (or residuals) provide the sign and the magnitude of the differences. They can also identify small abnormal regions. Two SD images are generated, one for the positive differences, one for the negative differences. They are obtained by applying a suitable test to each pixel of the original couple of images. Where the residuals are not significantly different from zero the SD image is set to zero, elsewhere, the value of the residual is used.

The test takes into account the estimated values of the model parameters, therefore they can only be applied within the window used at the model identification step.

2.5.1) <u>Tests for the 1 Parameter Linear Grey-Level Registration model.</u>

Two tests have already been proposed for the 1 Parameter Linear Grey-Level Registration model (4). The first one is the Maximum Likelihood Test and is called C1. The second one is an approximation of the UMP test and is called C2. They are performed in the following way :

Given two observed values X1 and X2 and an estimate of the single parameter of the model NF :

1) The null hypothesis Ho is : X1 and X2 come from two Poisson distributions with means M1 and M2 such that : M1 = NF M2.

2) The alternative hypothesis is : M1 = NF M2.

3) C1 and C2 are calculated as :

$$C1 = 2\ (X1LogX1 + X2LogX2 - (X1 + X2)\ Log\ \frac{X1 + X2}{NF + 1} - X1LogNF)$$

$$C2 = (X1 - X2)^2\ /\ (NF\ (X1 + X2)$$

Under Ho, C1 and C2 follow CHI-SQUARE distribution with one degree of freedom. C2 is valid only when the observed counts are larger than 30.

2.5.2) <u>Tests for the 2 Parameter Linear Grey-Level Registration model.</u>

Since the 2 Parameter Linear Grey-Level Registration model is very useful for DTS processing, we have developed tests for this more complicated model. In this case the null hypothesis is : M1 = NF (M2 + BG). Where NF and BG are the estimated values of the two model parameters. Two approaches were used. Firstly, we attempted to use modified versions C1* and C2* of C1 and C2. They are calculated as C1 and C2, except that X2 is replaced by X2 + BG. Secondly, we developed the Maximum Likelihood Ration Test called C3. Under Ho, the Likelihood Lo of the two mesures X1 ad X2 is :

$$P(X1,X2|Ho) = e^{-NF(M2 + BG)} \frac{(NF \ (M2 + BG))^{X1}}{X1 \ !} \ e^{- M2} \frac{M2^{X2}}{X2 \ !}$$

Then,

Log (Lo)= -NF(M2 + BG) + X1LogNF + X1Log (M2 + BG) -M2 + X2LogM2 - Log X1 ! - Log X2 !

The Maximum Likelihood estimator $\hat{M2}$ of M2 is given by :

$$\frac{d(LogLo)}{dM2} = 0 \ or \ -NF + \frac{X1}{\hat{M2} + BG} - 1 + \frac{X2}{\hat{M2}} = 0$$

M2 is a solution of the second order equation :

$$(NF + 1) \ \hat{M2}^2 + ((NF + 1) \ BG - (X1 + X2)) \ \hat{M2} - BG \ X2 = 0$$

M2 is the positive solution if the two original images are chosen such that BG 0.Log (Lo) is calculated by using this estimation of M2.
Under the alternative Hypothesis H1, the likelihood of the two measures X1 and X2 is :

$$P(X1, X2 \ |H1) = e^{-X1} \frac{X1^{X1}}{X1 \ !} \ e^{-X2} \frac{X2^{X2}}{X2 \ !}$$

Then.

Log (L1) = -X1 + X1Log X1 - X2 + X2logX2 - LogX1 ! -Log X2 !

The C3 test is :
$$C3 = -2Log \ (Lo/L1) = -2(-NF(\hat{M2}+BG)+X1LogNF+X1Log(\hat{M2}+BG)-\hat{M2}+ X2Log\hat{M2}$$
$$+X1-X1LogX1-X2LogX2)$$

Under Ho, C3 follows CHI SQUARE distribution with 1 degree of freedom.

2.5.3) <u>The power of the C1*, C2* and C3 tests</u> :

Since C3 requires more calculations than the C1* and C2*, we compared by simulation the power of these tests in different circumstances. Firstly, these powers depend on the value of BG, for example C1* and C3* have the same power when BG = 0. Secondly, these powers depend on the numbers of counts X1 and X2. Therefore we proceeded in the following way :
1) Given two numbers S and BG, we generate two series of 10,000 Poisson variables with means M1 and M2 such as : M1 + M2 = S and M1 = NF (M2 + BG) with NF = 1 for the first series and Nf = 1.1 for the second series.
Then, NF = 1 is considered as the null Hypothesis and this value is used in the calculation of the tests. The Type I Error (alpha) is the proportion of the test values greater than a certain Threshold in the first series. The Power of the test (1 - beta = 1 - Type II Error) is the same proportion in the second series. Thus, for each Threshold value, a couple (alpha,1 - beta) is obtained. This analysis is identical to ROC analysis. The results

of this simulation study are :
1) As expected, C1* and C3 have the same Power when BG = 0.
2) As expected, the Type I Error of the C3 test is determined by the CHI-SQUARE distribution e.g. it is .05 for a threshold value of 3.84.
3) The couples (alpha, 1 - beta) are on the same curves for the C1 and C3 tests. (Figure 3).
4) The type I Error of the C1 test is NOT determined by the CHI-SQUARE distribution. Given a certain threshold value, alpha is smaller for the C1* test than for the C3 test which follows the CHI-SQUARE distribution. But the power of C1 is also smaller.
5) For S 30 C1* and C2* are equivalent.
6) For BG = 0 and S 30 C2* differs from C1* in the same way that C1* differs from C3, i.e. the C2* Type I Error does not follow CHI-SQUARE distribution. but the couples (alpha, 1 - beta) are on the same curve.
7) The power of C3 increases with S.
Figure 3 shows such a curve for S = 1000 and BG = 100.

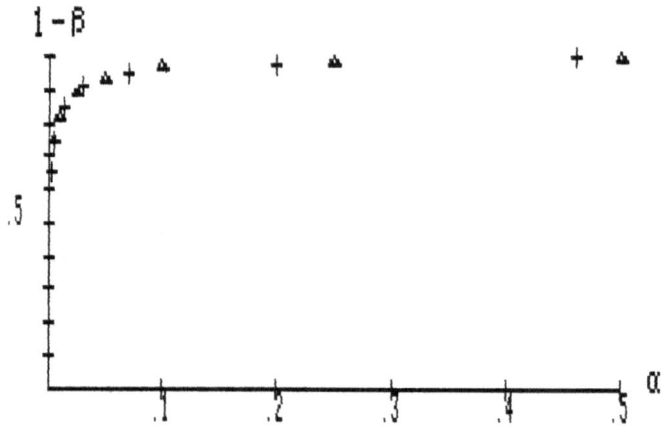

Figure 3 : The power of the C1* and the C3 test evaluated by simulation. The power is plotted versus the Type I Error. Crosses are for the C3 test, triangles for the C1* test.

For DTS processing, the important point is that C1* is not by itself less powerful than C3. However it does not allow the choice of the Threshold value and of the Type I Error. Therefore, the use of the C3 test for the 2 Parameter Linear Grey-Level Registration Model is mandatory.

   2.5.4) Increasing the power of the test.
The power of the test largely depends on the number of counts in the two original images. Therefore, it is possible to increase the power of the test by packing the original images to a lower format. This is made at the expense of the spatial resolution, but is helpful, in the search for slightly abnormal regions.

3) IMPLEMENTATIONS.
Two implementations of the method, one on a fast system, the other on a classical one are described.
   3.1) The first implementation.

This implementation is made on a CGR-IMAC 7300 system (French version of the ADAC system 1) connected to an AP 120B Floating Point System Array Processor. This powerful tool allowed the development of a complete implementation of the method. It is written in FORTRAN with some subroutines in the Assembly Language of the Array Processor. It is interfaced with the other programs of the system so that all the display, ROI, and other facilities of the system are used for analysing the obtained images. The entire modelling procedure is carried out using the SSC criterion and the ARS optimization strategy.

The characteristics of the programme are :

1) It processes 128 x 128, 64 x 64 or 32 x 32 images.

2) It requires the choice by operator of the window in which the criterion is calculated.

3) It requires the choice by the operator of a search domain for each parameter of the model. A 5 parameter model is proposed (Translation + Rotation + 2 Parameter Linear Grey-Level Registration model). Nested models are simply chosen by selected a null domain for the parameter to be excluded.

4) The results include the registered version (F3) of the second image (F2) and the images of the significant differences, either positive or negative or both. The value of Type I Error (initially set to 5 %), as well as the format of the SD image may be chosen. The registration of 128 x 128 images and the generation of SD images, using a window of 8K pixels and a 5 Parameter model is performed in 30 seconds.

3.2) The second implementation.

This implementation is made on a SOPHA-INFORMATEK SIMIS IV system. Since this system is slow compared with the previous one, the optimization technique described in section 2.4.2 is used. Furthermore, only 64 x 64 images can be used and rotation is not taken into account in the Geometric Registration model. This implementation is more operator dependant : in order to speed up the optimization process, if the initial estimate of the Geometric Registration is visually correct, no Geometric Registration using the SSC criterion is performed. Nevertheless, a Grey-Level Registration is always carried out using this criterion. The Grey-Level Registration is either a 1 or a 2.

Parameter Linear model. When 128 x 128 images have to be processed, either the images are packed in to the 64 x 64 format, or 64 x 64 windows are extracted from the images. This procedure is possible when the ROI is a small portion of the original image as in Parathyroid scanning. The registration of 64 x 64 images, using a window of 2 K pixels and a 4 parameter model is generally performed within 3 minutes if the Geometric Registration is correctly performed using the Correlation Coefficient. When all the registration is performed using the SSC criterion, 10 to 20 minutes are required. Notwithstanding these limitations, this interactivie implementation was found very useful in practice. Most of the applications presented in this text were carried out on this system. But, it seems that the versatility of the method can only be appreciated using a fast system.

4) APPLICATIONS.

In this section our experience in the application of the method is presented. Up to now, the method has been mainly used for Parathyroid scanning and Immunoscintigraphy, but some other examples are also given.

4.1) Parathyroid scintigraphy.

Parathyroid scintigraphy is used for localizing parathyroid adenoma or hyperplasic glands in the presence of Hyperparathyroidism. It is based on the comparison of Thallium and Pertechnetate images. There is an uptake of Thallium in both the Thyroid and Parathyroid tissues,while only the Thyroid concentrates Pertechnetate. Regions with Thallium uptake and no or lower Pertechnetate uptake are considered as abnormal Parathyroid glands. The visual inspection of the two images can only demonstrate large abnormalities. Many authors process the images by subtracting the Pertechnetate image from the Thallium image (10). In this process they face the problems of spatial registration and normalization. What we call a 1 Parameter Linear Grey-Level Registration Model is generally used, the normalization factor being often chosen as the ratio of the maxima of the images.

4.1.1) The scintigraphic technique.

The acquisition of the images presented in this study is made in the following way :

1) 2 mCi of 201 Tl are injected IV.

2) 15 minutes later the patient is placed supine under a gamma camera. His head is placed in a Head-Holder. A static image is obtained with a pinhole collimator within 15 minutes. The frame format is 64 x 64 or 128 x 128.

3) Then, 3 mCi of Pertechnetate are injected IV.

4) 15 minutes later an image is recorded during 5 minutes.

4.1.2) Selection of a model.

In order to select a Registration Model, the methods described in the preceding sections were used on many studies. The visual inspection of the images with a ROI drawn around the Thyroid gland shows that patient motions are very common, even with a Head Holder. This was already noticed by others (10). The scatter diagram was used to choose the Grey-Level Registration Model. All the Scatter Diagrams look like figure 1A. This demonstrates the necessity of a 2 Parameter Model which takes into account the Tissue Crosstalk which is higher for the Tl image than for the Tc image. The scatter diagram shows also that a linear model is able to describe the relation between the two images. Although the energies of the tracer are different (80 and 140 KeV), this simple model is adequate, probably since the investigated organs are superficial. The application of the method to 30 studies gave the following results :

1) A translation of 1 or more pixel units is very common.

2) It is not necessary to take rotation into account.

3) Typical values of NF and BG are .1 and 500 (The maximum values of the Tl and the Tc images are, typically 200 and 1500, for a 64 x 64 image).

4) Even for visual inspection, the Grey-Level Registration is very useful because it makes the Grey-Scale similar in the two images, while the use of standard display softwares makes the Tl and Tc normal images look very different.

4.1.3) Quantitative analysis of the Significant Difference image. In order to assess the diagnostic value of this method, an attempt was made to quantify the Significant Difference image. Once this image is built, the operator chooses a point located at the top of the Thyroid Isthmus. The Thyroid-Parathyroid ROI is then divided into four quadrants. Each of them is characterized by the sum of the Significant Residuals, expressed as a percentage of the Thallium image in this portion of the ROI.

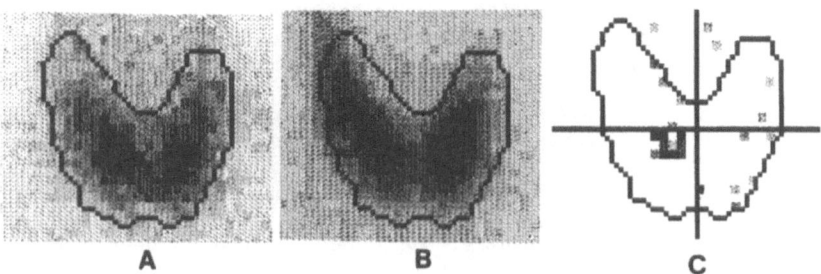

Figure 4 : Parathyroid-Thyroid Tl-Tc scintigraphy. A : Tl image. B : TcO4 image. C : Significant Difference image. A Parathyroid adenoma is seen in the left inferior quadrant.

In 14 patients who were operated on after the scintigraphic examination, the diagnostic value of this numerical test was evaluated using the ROC technique. The Golden Standard is the result of the histological examination when a biopsy of the parathyroid gland was performed, but glands considered as normal and not biopsied by the surgeon were classified as normal.Figure 5 shows the corresponding ROC curve.

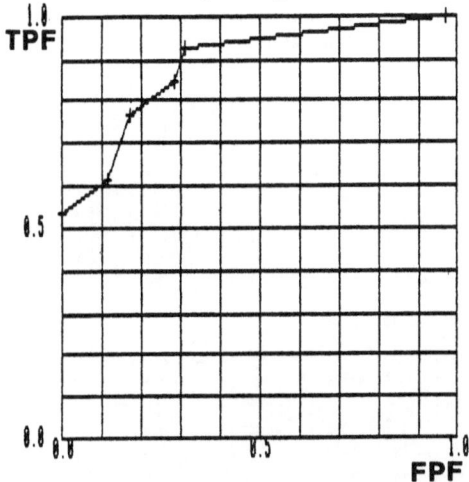

Figure 5 : The ROC curve for the diagnosis of Parathyroid adenoma using the quantitative description of the Significant Difference image as a test and Histology findings as the Golden Standard.

4.2.) Immunoscintigraphy.

Labelled Monoclonal Antibody (MA) scintigraphy is a promising technique for locating primary or secondary tumors. But this method suffers from a lack of specificity. Diffuse uptake in many tissues, such as the liver, the stomach or the large intestine makes the analysis of the images sometimes difficult. In order to help the image interpretation, the comparison of MA images with images obtained using other tracers is widely used. Most of the time, images obtained with tracers such as bone or kidney agents are only used as landmarks. In this case 99 m Tc agents are adequate, assuming the Antibodies are labelled with 131 I. But when a true image comparison is

performed, tracers with high energy, such as 113m In, are required. Different types of image comparison can be performed :
1) First type of comparison : MA images and a liver scan.
2) Second type of comparison : Initial (purely vascular) MA images and late (48 or 72 h) MA images.
3) Third type of comparison : 48 h (or earlier) images and 72 h (or later) images. These image comparisons encounter the problems of Spatial and/or Grey-Level registration. In this context, the availability of an efficient image registration method improves the method in the following way :
1) The images on which a type I comparison is performed have not to be recorded the same day. Consequently, the liver scan can be performed before MA injection and not contaminated by Iodine rays.
2) Types 2 and 3 comparisons which require a registration step become possible.
3) Many views can be obtained and processed.
Figures 6,7 and 8 show examples of types 1,2 and 3 comparisons. All the MA images were obtained with I 131 labelled anti CEA and anti CA 19-9 MA (provided by ORIS FRANCE) in patients with proven secondary lesions of rectal or colic carcinomas. Figure 6C shows a liver metastasis (upper left) and an abdominal metastasis (center).
Figure 7C shows two bone metastases (arrows) and diffuse intestine uptake.
Figure 8C is useful for identifying the uptake located near the left lobe of the liver (arrow) as colon activity. The comparison of 48 h with 72 h images shows that this uptake takes place at the same time as the colon uptake. The patient was colostomized.

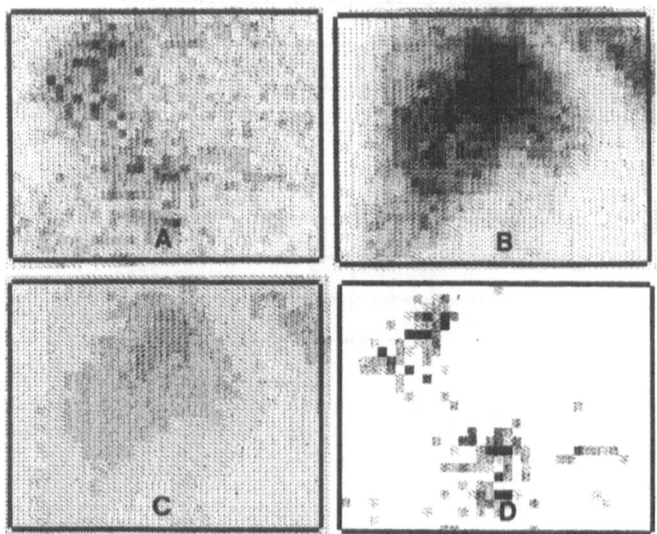

Figure 6 : Immunoscintigraphy, comparison of the 48 h MA image with a 113m In liver scan. A : MA image. B : Liver image. C : Registered version of B. D : Significant Difference Image.

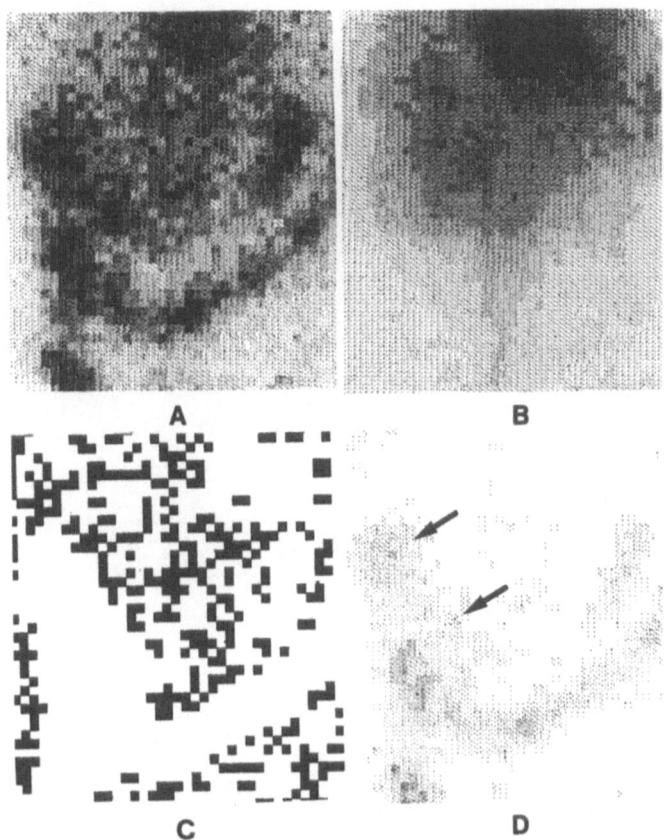

Figure 7 : Immunoscintigraphy, comparison of the 72 h MA image with the vascular image. A : 72 h MA image. B : Registered version of the vascular image. C : Sign Change image. D : Significant Difference image.

294

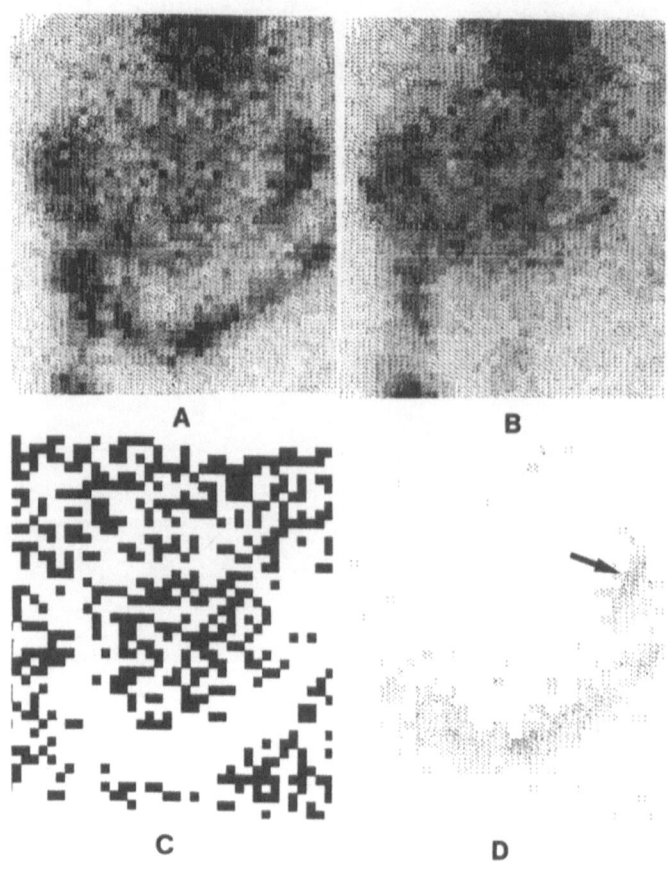

Figure 8 : Immunoscintigraphy, comparison of the 48 h MA image with the 72 h MA image. A : 72 h MA image. B : 48 h MA image. C : Sign Change image. D : Significant difference image.

4.3) Kr-Tc Lung scan.

Ventilation-Perfusion mismatch demonstrated by Lung scanning is a common application of DTS. The use of 81m Kr makes possible the recording of ventilation images which can be compared to 99m Tc microspheres Perfusion images. In order to generate a Ventilation to Perfusion ratio image, Geometric Registration is necessary. Another possibility is the use of the Significant Difference image. In this study, we do not test the clinical value of these images but we investigate the robustness of the Geometric Registration procedure. In the case of Pulmonary Embolism, the images to be registered can be strongly different and the problem of robustness is

essential. A simulation study was therefore performed in the following
way :
1) Actual 128 x 128 Kr and Tc microspheres images are used.
2) Two normal Kr-Tc images are registered using a 5 Parameter model.
3) On the perfusion image, defects of increasing size are generated via
software.
4) The Ventilation and each simulated Perfusion image are registered.
On a normal couple of anterior views, defects with area corresponding to
20,30 and 40 % of the total lung area and to 9,12 and 20 % of the total
number of counts were generated. The parameter values of the Geometric
registration performed on the initial normal image were Dx = -1 and
Dy = 14. The values obtained for the images with increasing defects were Dx
= -1, -1, -1 and Dy = 13,13,14. The rotation was always less than 1 degree.
These results illustrate the Robustness of the method, even for large
defects. Figure 9,10 and 11 show the original images, a simulated image and
the result of registration.

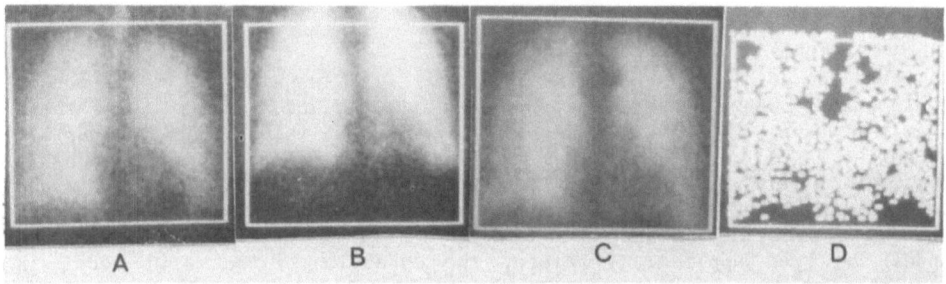

Figure 9 : Ventilation-Perfusion Kr-Tc Lung scan. A : Ventilation image. B.
Original Perfusion image. C : Registered version of the Perfusion image.
D : Sign Change image.

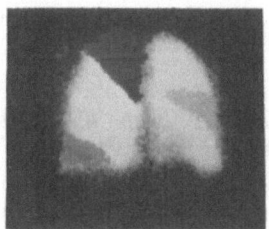

Figure 10 : Perfusion image with simulated defects.

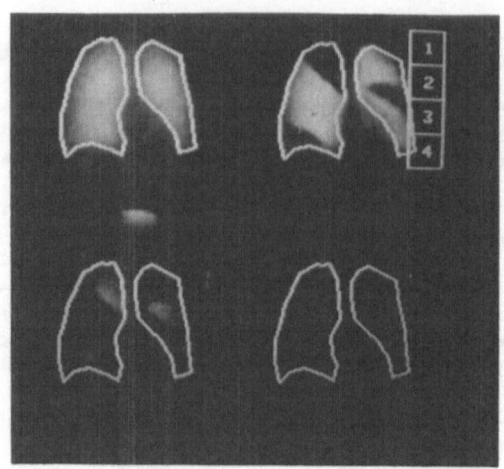

Figure 11 : Registration of a simulated Perfusion image and the Ventilation image.

5) CONCLUSION.
In this paper, a new methodology for DTS processing is proposed, implementations are described and some examples of application given. These examples have illustrated the efficiency of this image comparison technique. Applications in other fields of Nuclear Medecine will probably be found. Nevertheless, it must be emphasized that only comparable images can be compared. The SSC criterion allows robust registration, but requires that some part of the images are similar, once the proper registration model has been applied. Therefore, the selection of a valid model is crucial. But the validity of a model is largely dependant of the noise level. High count images can be found difficult to process. Large image formats are recommended.
The proposed methodology is based on a statistical approach of DTS processing which is considered as a robust estimation problem in the presence of outliers. It offers a theoretical frame which contrasts with the empirical techniques commonly used in Nuclear Medicine.

6) ACKNOWLEDGMENT.
We would like to thank Dr JM ROCCHISANI and Dr MJ DELISLE for providing some of the images, Dr JY DEVAUX, Mr M VALTON and Ms A FORTIER for their help in the implementation of the software, Caroline EVANS for correcting the manuscript, Ms M OUDIN for typing the manuscript and ORIS FRANCE for providing the Labelled Monoclonal Antibodies.

7) REFERENCES.
1) SOUSSALINE F, TODD-POKROPEK AE, DI PAOLA R, BAZIN JP : Techniques for combining isotopic images obtained at different energies. INFORMATION PROCESSING IN SCINTIGRAPHY. ORSAY 1975.
2) VENOT A, LEBRUCHEC JF, GOLMARD JL, ROUCAYROL JC. An automated method for the normalization of scintigraphic images. J Nucl Med 24, 1983, 529-531.
3) VENOT A, LEBRUCHEC JF, ROUCAYROL JC, A new class of similarity measures for robust image registration, Computer Vision, Graphics and Image Processing, 28, 1984, 176-184.
4) VENOT A, GOLMARD JL, LEBRUCHEC JF, PRONZATO L, WALTER E, FRIJA G,

ROUCAYROL JC. Digital methods for change detection in medical images. In DECONINCK F. (Ed) Information Processing in Medical Imaging. Martinus Nijhof, The Hague, 1984, 1-16

5) VENOT A and LECLERC V. Automated correction of patient motion and gray values prior to subtraction in digitized angiography. IEEE Trans. Med.Imag. MI-3, 4, 1984, 179-186.

6) LIEHN JC, VENOT A, VALTON M, VALEYRE J. Registration of scintigraphic images : a comparison of four methods on Thallium simulated images. In HAE SCHMIDT and DE VAURANO (Ed). Nuclear Medicine in Research and Practice. Proceedings of the 25 th Congress of the Society of Nuclear Medicine 1984 SCHATTAUER VERLAG, 36-39.

7) HIMMELBLAU DM, Applied Nonlinear Programming. 1972 McGRAW-HILL.

8) PRONZATO L, WALTER E, VENOT A, LEBRUCHEC JF. A general purpose global optimizer : implementation and applications. Math Comp Simul, 26, 1984, 412-422.

9) NELDER JA, MEAD R, A simplex method for function minimization. Computer J, 7, 1964, 308-313.

10) BASARAB RM, MANNI A, HARRISON TS, Dual Isotope Subtraction Parathyroid Scintigraphy in the Preoperative Evaluation of Suspected Hyperparathyroidism, Clin Nucl Med, 10, 1985, 300-314.

SOME MAXIMUM LIKELIHOOD METHODS USEFUL FOR THE REGIONAL ANALYSIS OF DYNAMIC PET DATA ON BRAIN GLUCOSE METABOLISM

G. PAWLIK, K. HERHOLZ, K. WIENHARD, C. BEIL, and W. D. HEISS

1. INTRODUCTION

Impairment of regional energy metabolism in morphologically intact areas of the brain beyond the bounds of focal lesions has been of considerable interest to neurologists, since v. Monakow (1914) introduced the term "diaschisis" to denote the transient phenomenon of transneural depression of CNS function. However, despite decades of anatomical and physiological work, due to the complexity of neuronal interaction, the relationship between major topographical and functional characteristics of a focal pathology on the one side and the extent and severity of remote deactivation on the other remained largely obscure. It was only after the introduction of positron emission tomography (PET) as a diagnostic instrument in clinical neurology (PHELPS et al., 1979; REIVICH et al., 1979) that diaschisis could be noninvasively studied in three dimensions. Because of the close coupling between neuronal activity and local glucose consumption the 2(F-18)-fluoro-2-deoxy-D-glucose (FDG) method soon served as sort of a gold standard for the assessment of functional brain anatomy. But it did not take long until problems of quantitation became apparent - some unique to PET, some common the all nuclear medicine imaging techniques, others related to any diagnostic test.

2. RATIONALE

Given sufficient training in neuroanatomy and physiology, reasonable interpretation of the metabolic brain maps obtained by FDG-PET is readily achieved even by readers with little specific experience.
For example, in Fig. 1 showing seven tomographic images of a patient with left temporoparietal infarction, the metabolic "black hole" corresponding with the defect on CT is quite conspicuous. But is the overall level of glucose consumption still normal?

FIGURE 1. FDG-PET images
of a stroke patient

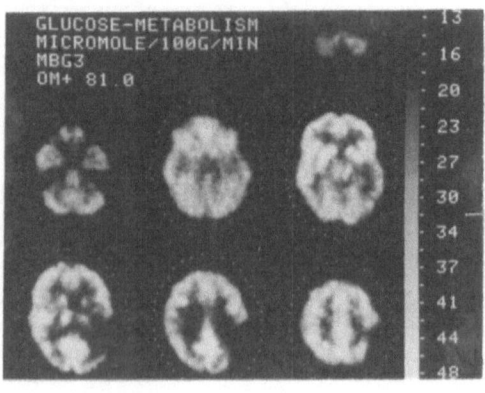

A closer look may reveal some metabolic depression of the ipsilateral cerebral cortex and deeper gray matter as well as hypometabolism in the contralateral cerebellum. But where is the anatomical boundary between normal and abnormal tissue? Apparently, the visual information encoded in those images is dense enough as to allow rather rapid formation of fairly congruent individual standards of normal that are then applied to define localized metabolic abnormalities. But does the physiological model really hold - even in severely altered tissue; or do the calculated local metabolic rates need some correction? Decision problems get still worse when data reduction, from the complex pixel-by-pixel to the more convenient regional level of topography, is attempted for statistical comparisons and communication of numerical results. Because of the large variety of brain shapes and sizes, and the numerous arbitrary choices that must be made in the process of defining regions of interest, no universal standard scheme of topography-related analysis has been generally agreed upon to date. For all of these reasons published reference values of regional brain glucose metabolism are quite scattered, both within and among laboratories (HEISS et al., 1984). Statistical hypothesis testing is further rendered inefficient by legal and ethical restrictions on the group size of healthy controls that may be exposed to nuclear radiation for scientific purposes. Fortunately though, experience from hundreds of dynamic FDG patient studies carried out and analyzed in the same standardized manner in this laboratory, indicates that part of those problems can be overcome by stepwise optimization and by the application of computerized maximum likelihood methodology as outlined in the following.

3. METHODS & RESULTS
3.1. Data collection
   Optimization necessarily starts with the physical, physiological, and psychological conditions during measurement that should be as stable and reproducible as possible. Appropriate standard procedures are elsewhere described in detail (HEISS et al., 1984). Briefly, from the time of FDG injection, seven equally spaced, 11-mm-thick slices centered from the canthomeatal line to 82 mm above are simultaneously scanned for 40 min at consecutive intervals gradually increasing from 1 to 5 min, using a four-ring positron camera (Scanditronix PC 384) (ERIKSSON et al., 1982). A continuous write-out of the instantaneous whole-head coincidence counting rate is obtained on paper chart for the monitoring of the stability of head positioning. Data from the tomographic device, the radioactivities of arterialized venous plasma samples measured in a cross-calibrated well counter, and plasma glucose values are stored in the memory of a VAX 11/780 (DEC) computer. The spatial activity distribution in the image planes is reconstructed using an edge-finding algorithm to determine the skull contour for attenuation correction (BERGSTRÖM et al., 1982), a deconvolution for subtraction of scattered radiation (BERGSTRÖM et al., 1983), and a filtered backprojection algorithm resulting in a 128 x 128 matrix to be displayed by means of a Ramtek 9050 system as an interpolated 256 x 256 pixel image. All measured radioactivities are corrected for decay before entering into any model equation.

3.2. Metabolic quantitation
3.2.1. Static methods. In the course of time, the deoxyglucose model (SOKOLOFF et al., 1977) and its FDG modifications frequently have been shown to be remarkably insensitive to violations of the underlying

assumptions concerning the various rate constants and the lumped constant.
While the inclusion of a dephosphorylation parameter is not a crucial
point in measurements taken during the first hour after FDG injection,
spurious metabolic results, though, are obtained in severely altered
tissue when standard constants determined in healthy resting subjects
are employed to calculate glucose consumption rates from single activity
measurements (HAWKINS et al., 1981; WIENHARD et al., 1985; GJEDDE et al.,
1985). A recent comparison of the various proposed correction methods
(WIENHARD et al., 1985) indicated that an adjustment of the rate constants
k1 and k3, according to the ratio of the measured tissue activity Ci* to
the one expected from solving for Ci* the original Sokoloff equation
with standard parameters, is best-suited to compensate for such a bias.
Therefore, this adjustment should be made in the pixel-by-pixel reconstruction of metabolic maps for visual interpretation. The practical significance of an appropriate rate constant correction is illustrated in
Figs. 2 and 3 showing the same infarcted brain slice, at the same window
setting, before and after k1,3-adjustment. Only on the latter image the
considerable residual metabolism of the right frontal temporal region can
be detected.

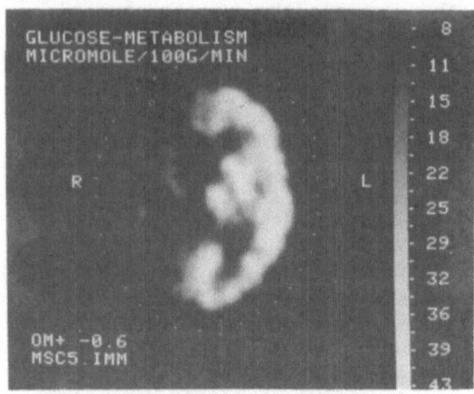

FIGURE 2. Standard metabolic map

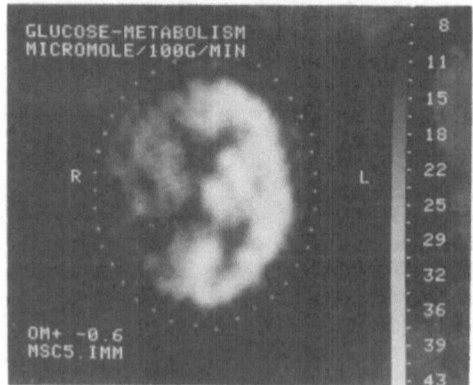

FIGURE 3. Metabolic map after
          k1,3-adjustment

3.2.2. Dynamic method.

Clearly the most accurate metabolic results and other, more detailed information on the actual physiological state of the brain tissue are obtained from full-length sequential recordings of regional radioactivities, characterizing the net tracer uptake in the brain, from the time of injection until a steady state is reached. A least-squares fit to those time-activity data then yields the parameters of the rearranged Sokoloff equation. In order to avoid uncontrolled bias, the data accumulated during the first 5 min should be excluded from curve-fitting because during that initial period, when plasma activity is comparatively high, poorly defined experimental errors due to differences in regional blood volume or in the tracer appearance time in the brain and at the peripheral blood sampling site, respectively, still are quite large, while at later times they are of little effect. Numerical results can be stabilized further by secondary reduction of the number of fit parameters: From the Sokoloff equation it follows that the ratio of regional tissue activity and the plasma activity-time integral converges to the rate constant $k1$, as time tends to zero. Even 6 min after injection, the regional $k1$ estimate still is a linear function of Ci^* and, therefore, after fixing all $k1$ values on that straight line, only $k2$ and $k3$ remain to be estimated (WIENHARD et al., 1985). The regional cerebral metabolic rate for glucose (rCMRGlc) is then calculated according to rCMRGlc = ((plasma glucose concentration)/0.42) x $k1$ $k3$/($k2$ + $k3$) (PHELPS et al., 1979).

3.3. Region mapping

For topography-related analyses of the physiological PET data, a comprehensive set of regions of interest is marked on all functional images by means of an interactive FORTRAN program in connection with the computer's image display system, providing fast and largely user-independent mapping with excellent reproducibility and flexible adaptation to individual anatomical variations (HERHOLZ et al., 1985). After determining the outer brain contour on a tomographic image by edge finding, generous region raw contours (Fig. 4) are placed relative to that outer contour one after the other according to geometrical standard parameters (representing sector segments, circles, and rectangles) specified in a permanent file. For the cerebral cortex the program proceeds in angular steps of 20 degrees measured from the center of the brain contour.

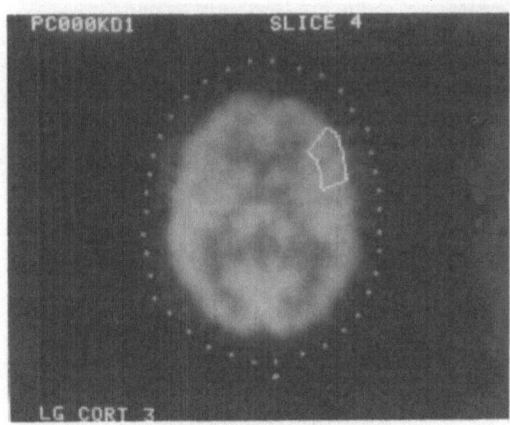

FIGURE 4. Cortical raw region contour (adjusted sector segment)

Within each gray-matter raw region, the final subregion of interest is marked so that it covers all pixels with a metabolic activity above a pre-defined proportionate level (Fig. 5, note the frequency histogram of relative activities within raw region in lower right-hand corner).

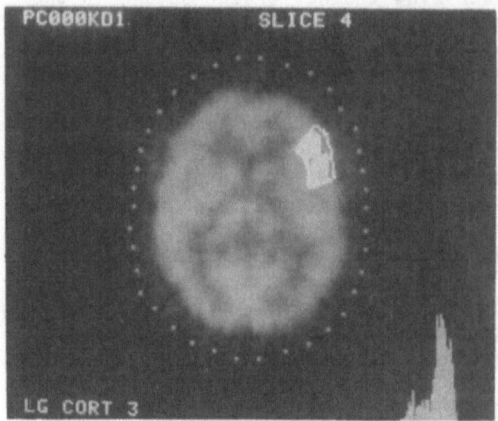

FIGURE 5. Final cortical region of interest (shaded area within raw region contour)

A more compex definition including lower and upper thresholds as well as a distance condition applied to white matter, where regions are placed after all gray-matter regions are finished. If present, the contours of morphological lesions as demonstrated by CT or MRI are manually copied on the PET images by joystick input prior to the automated procedure which then spares those areas. Fig. 6 shows a fully regionalized tomographic image of a patient with left striatal infarction.

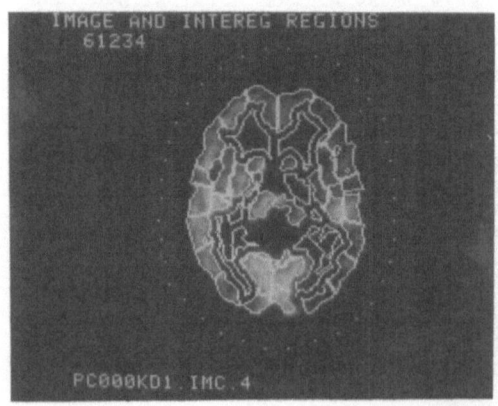

FIGURE 6. All final region contours on a brain slice across basal ganglia

That way, a whole set of seven slices is represented by approx.150 regions with different mnemonic names, for each of which the individual set of rate constants and, hence, the mean metabolic rate is computed by curve-fitting as described above, utilizing an advanced system for fast function minimization (JONES and ROOS, 1976), including a Monte Carlo search routine, a reasonably fast simplex method, and an extremely fast gradient search procedure.

3.4. Morphological matching

The comparability of topography-related functional data is substantially improved, when the intersubject variation in brain shape and size is accounted for. This is most readily achieved by adjustment of those aspects of the individual anatomy that are least-suited for transaxial tomographic representation - i.e., most of all any deviation from the standard occipitofrontal and craniocaudal axes. Therefore, at first the average set of region names characteristic of each brain level was established in 30 FDG-PET studies of healthy human subjects, and was divided into an anterior, middle, and posterior subset. The same subsetting is performed on each patient's regions. Each stack of regions then is separately shifted upward and downward by 13.7 mm (= center-to-center distance between contiguous slices). At each step, the correspondence between the region names of the patient's and the reference subsets is determined by the TANIMOTO coefficient as the most appropriate measure of similarity, which is defined as the number or regions common to both subsets, divided by the sum of common regions and regions unique to either subset. Fig. 7 illustrates the region stacks and the respective slice levels in a lateral standard skull projection.

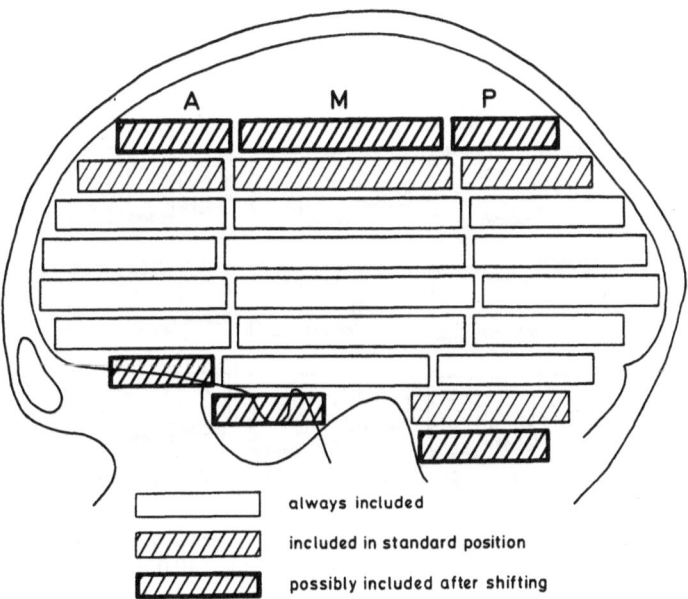

always included

included in standard position

possibly included after shifting

FIGURE 7.
Stacks of slice segments for
TANIMOTO matching

The matching position with the highest similarity coefficients out of all 27 possible combinations (Fig. 8) then forms the topographical basis of further statistical comparisons.

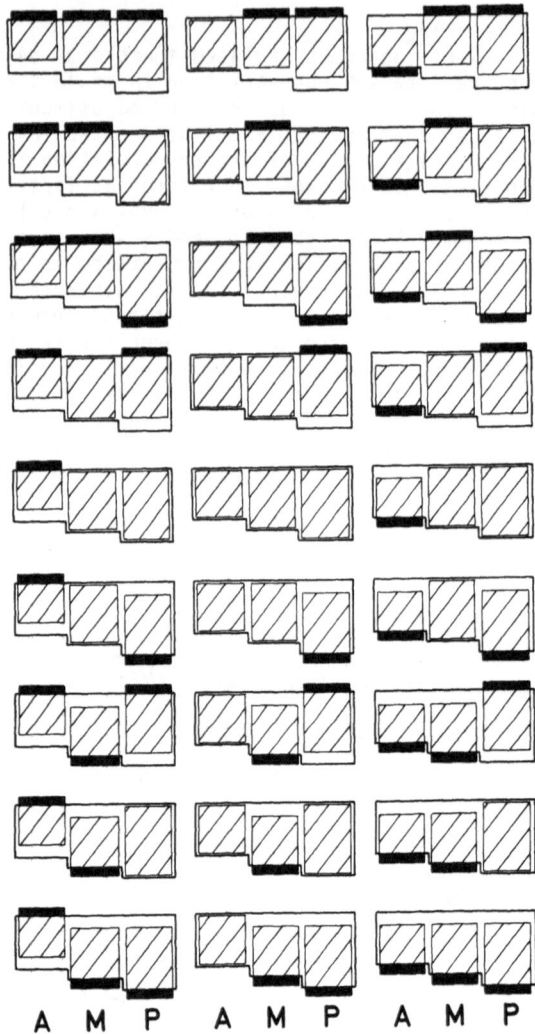

A M P   A M P   A M P

FIGURE 8. Schematic of all the topographical variations in comparison with reference standard, accounted for by TANIMOTO matching

3.5. Diagnostic classification

3.5.1. <u>Significance probability mapping.</u> As a diagnostic instrument pro-
viding large matrices of regional metabolic data, in principle, PET requires multivariate analytical strategies, where each patient represents a point in metabolic region space, and a very large sample of normal control subjects serves to define the reference space. However, as reference groups of a sufficient size are nowhere available, rather inefficient uni-

variate techniques must be resorted to - at least as a first step. For example, the mean metabolic rate and prediction limits for comparing a single case with a sample, can be calculated for all standard regions according to well-known t-test principles. The result of this procedure, a set of regionally distributed P values, is demonstrated in Fig. 9 showing a top lateral view of the cortical regions of a stroke patient's left hemisphere, with the respective significance probabilities appearing in different shades of gray. In this particular case, midfrontal hypometabolism is prominent.

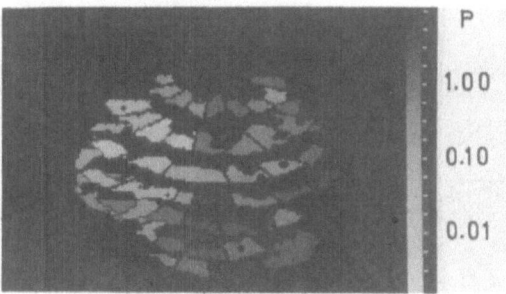

P

1.00

0.10

0.01

FIGURE 9. Left lateral view of significance probability map

3.5.2. Cluster analysis. Although quite useful to designate gross metabolic abnormalities, the above significance probability procedure usually is not powerful enough to indicate the more subtle changes occurring in diaschisis. A more detailed representation of the physiological state of the tissue may be expected from the regionally fitted rate constants, k_1, k_2, and k_3, because this set of parameters fully (except for a scaling factor) describes regional glucose metabolism. Furthermore, the behavior of the rate constants is basically the same in morphologically altered and functionally deactivated regions remote from the primary lesion site. This is illustrated in Fig. 10 comparing the relationship between the ratios of the various rate constants in pathologic and homotopic regions of the other hemisphere, and the respective ratios of rCMRGlc, in both cerebrum and cerebellum of 64 patients with supratentorial infarction.

Starting from the original m x 3 data matrix representing all of a patient's regions in rate constant space, at first a MAHALANOBIS transformation is performed to remove the apparent correlations among rate constants, and to shift all aspects of similarity toward the regions. Next, according to the previous significance probability test, regions are classified (Fig. 11, upper graph, reduced exemplary sample) as belonging either to the inactive (= abnormal, full circles), the active (= normal, open circles), or an uncertain (dotted circles) group. This is followed by iterative partitioning of the whole region sample into an active and an inactive/uncertain cluster by successive assignment of uncertain regions to the active class and, at each step, computation of the product of the generalized variances of the two submatrices, each raised to the n-th power (n= cluster size). The grouping that minimizes this test statistic is the final maximum likelihood solution (MARDIA et al., 1979) within the pre-defined constraints (Fig. 11, middle and lower graph).

Ratio of rate constants $K_1, K_2, K_3,$ and CMRGlc

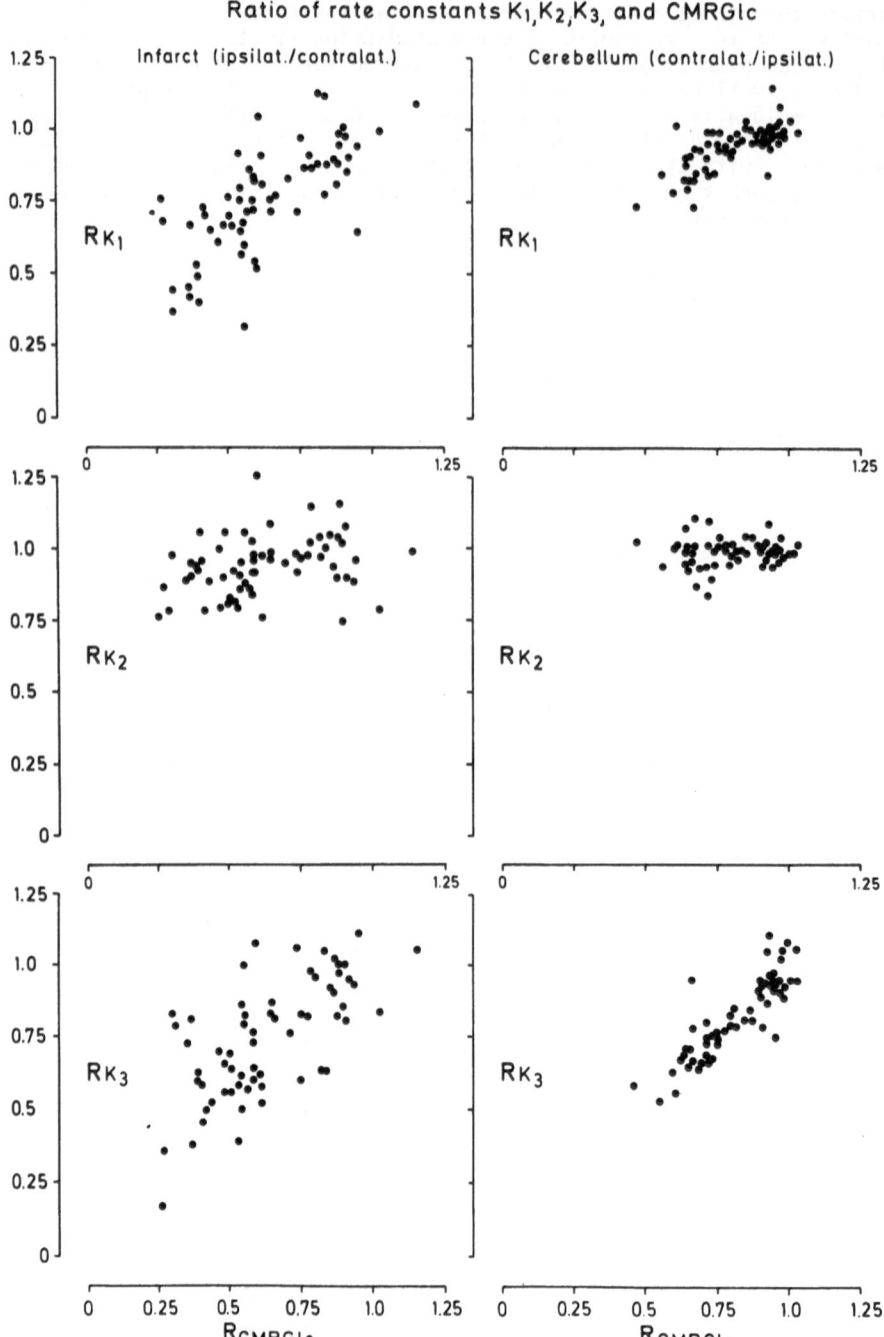

FIGURE 10. Relationship between rate constants and metabolic rates in injured and deactivated tissue

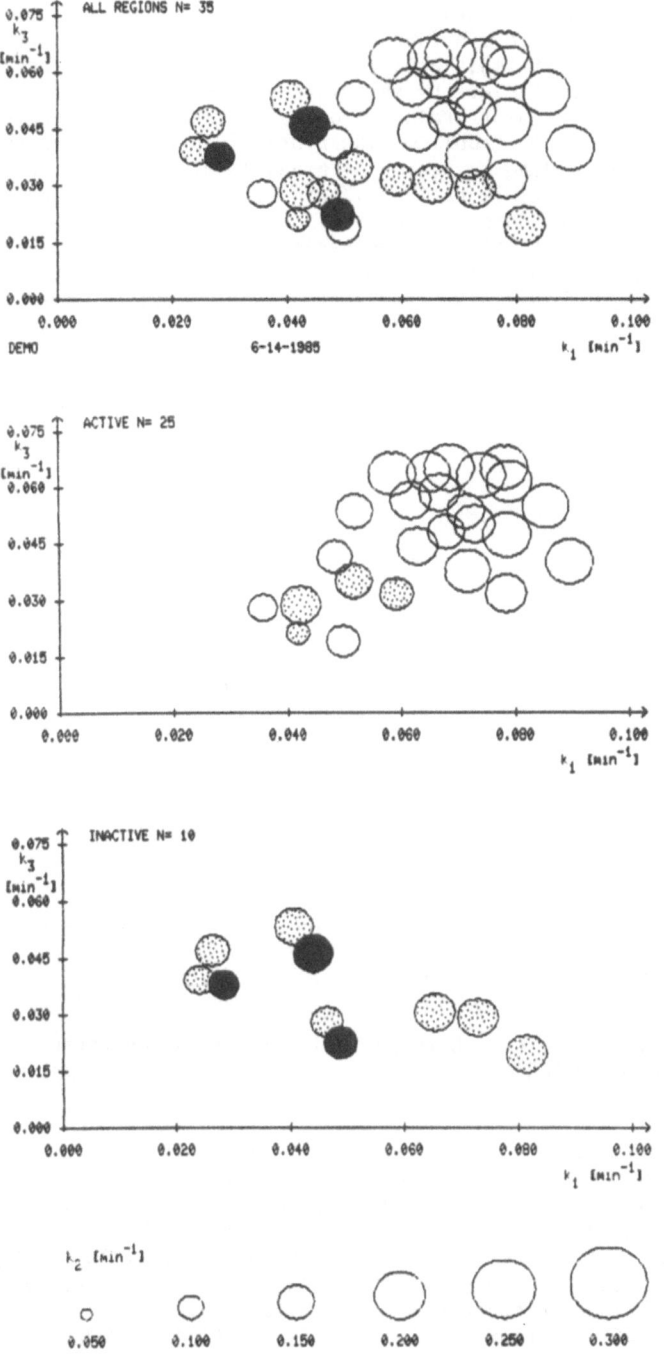

FIGURE 11. Principle of constrained maximum likelihood cluster analysis

3.6. ROC analysis

All the methods outlined so far were aimed at the most precise partitioning of a patient's brain into regions with normal or abnormal energy
metabolism. How well this is achieved is best described by the relative
operating characteristic of the entire procedure (SWETS, 1979), considering the whole spectrum of brain lesions and diaschistic phenomena, from
minimal to severe hypometabolism. Therefore, 10 patients were chosen from
a large series according to lesion size and focal metabolic rate to reflect the largest possible variety. Their full sets of k1,3-adjusted metabolic brain maps were interpreted by six PET experts, whose classification
of active and inactive regions then served as the standard against which
the results of the computerized procedure were tested. The corresponding
ROC curve (Fig. 12) indicates excellent diagnostic performance, with an
overall accuracy index Az of 0.87.

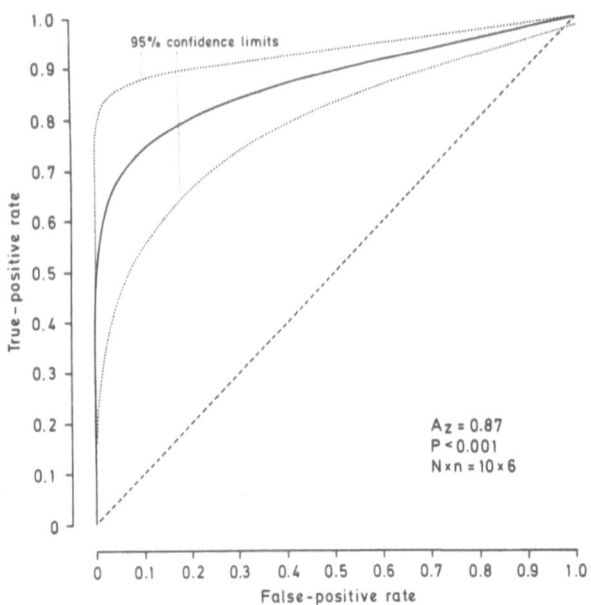

FIGURE 12. ROC analysis of computerized classification versus expert
interpretation

4. Conclusion

The described combination of metabolic quantitation by regional curve-
fitting, computer assisted brain mapping, topographical maximum likelihood matching, significance probability mapping, and iterative partitioning cluster analysis based on the trivariate kinetics of FDG, unlike exclusively metabolic-rate-oriented conventional univariate statistical
procedures, matches the diagnostic accuracy of expert interpretation as to
regional functional disturbances of detailed metabolic PET images, but
concurrently affords reproducible data reduction in a reader-independent
form.

5. References

Bergström M, Litton J, Eriksson L, Bohm C, Blomqvist G (1982) Determination of object contour from projections for attenuation correction in cranial positron emission tomography. J Comput Assist Tomogr 6: 365-372

Bergström M, Eriksson L, Bohm C, Blomqvist G, Litton J (1983) Correction for scattered radiation in a ring detector positron camera by integral transformation of the projections. J Comput Assist Tomogr 7: 42-50

Eriksson L, Bohm C, Kesselberg M, Blomqvist G, Litton J, Widen L, Bergström M, Ericson K, Greitz T (1982) A four ring positron camera system for emission tomography of the brain. IEEE Trans Nucl Sci 29: 539-543

Gjedde A, Wienhard K, Heiss W-D, Kloster G, Diemer NH, Herholz K, Pawlik G (1985) Comparative regional analysis of 2-Fluorodeoxyglucose and methylglucose uptake in brain of four stroke patients. With special reference to the regional estimation of the lumped constant. J Cereb Blood Flow Metabol 5: 163-178

Hawkins RA, Phelps ME, Huang SC, Kuhl DE (1981) Effect of ischemia on quantification of local cerebral glucose metabolic rate in man. J Cereb Blood Flow Metabol 1: 37-52

Heiss W-D, Pawlik G, Herholz K, Wagner R, Göldner H, Wienhard K (1984) Regional kinetic constants and cerebral metabolic rate for glucose in normal human volunteers determined by dynamic positron emission tomography of (18F)-2-fluoro-2-deoxy-D-glucose. J Cereb Blood Flow Metabol 4: 212-223

Herholz K, Pawlik G, Wienhard K, Heiss W-D (1985) Computer assisted mapping in quantitative analysis of cerebral positron emission tomograms. J Comput Assist Tomogr. 9: 154-161

James F, Roos M (1976) MINUIT - a system for function minimization and analysis of the parameter errors and correlations. Comput Ph 10: 343-376

Mardia KV, Kent JT, Bibby JM (1979) Multivariate analysis. Academic Press, London, New York

Phelps ME, Huang SC, Hoffman EJ, Selin CJ, Sokoloff L, Kuhl DE (1979) Tomographic measurement of local cerebral glucose metabolic rate in humans with (F-18)2-fluoro-2-deoxy-D-glucose: Validation of method. Ann Neurol 6: 371-388

Reivich M, Kuhl D, Wolf A, Greenberg J, Phelps ME, Ido T, Casella V, Fowler J, Hoffman E, Alavi A, Som P, Sokoloff L (1979) The (18F)-fluorodeoxyglucose method for the measurement of local cerebral glucose utilization in man. Circ Res 44: 127-137

Sokoloff L, Reivich M, Kennedy C, Des Rosiers MH, Patlak CS, Pettigrew KD, Sakurada O, Shinohara M (1977) The (14C)deoxyglucose method for the measurement of local cerebral glucose utilization: theory, procedure, and normal values in the conscious and anesthetized albino rat. J Neurochem 28: 897-916

Swets JA (1979) ROC analysis applied to the evaluation of medical imaging techniques. Invest Radiol 13: 109-121

von Monakow C (1914) Die Lokalisation im Großhirn und der Abbau der Funktion durch kortikale Herde. Bergmann, Wiesbaden

Wienhard K, Pawlik G, Herholz K, Wagner R, Heiss W-D (1985) Estimation of local cerebral glucose utilization by positron emission tomography of (18F)2-fluoro-2-deoxy-D-glucose: A critical appraisal of optimization procedures. J Cereb Blood Flow Metabol 5: 115-125

THE DEVELOPMENT AND ASSESSMENT OF A COMPUTER AID
FOR USE IN THE DIAGNOSIS OF CEREBRAL DISEASE

D L Plummer
Department of Medical Physics, University College London, UK

D Teather, B A Morton, K Wills
School of Mathematics, Computing and Statistics,
Leicester Polytechnic, UK

G H du Boulay
National Hospital for Nervous Diseases, London, UK

1. INTRODUCTION

This paper describes the design and development of a computer aid for use in the diagnosis of cerebral disease from CT images. The reasons for the choice of this particular application domain are first discussed, followed by a brief analysis of the techniques available for implementing such a diagnostic computer aid. A description of the system itself is then presented followed by our proposed evaluation procedures.

2. APPLICATION OVERVIEW

Computer aids have been developed for a wide range of diagnostic tasks and with a variety of objectives [1]. So far no systems have achieved impact comparable to that of other technological innovations such as new imaging modalities. Indeed very few systems have escaped the confines of their sites of development. Notable exceptions to this [2,3,4] have been restricted to relatively well delimited areas and have not attempted to provide a general solution to the problem of clinical diagnosis.

Neuro-radiology is a domain that lends itself well to the scrutiny required for the development of a computer aid. The number of diagnostic techniques in use is limited and these are often applied in a very standard manner. Histological or other confirmation of a major proportion of diagnoses is available since many patients undergo surgery. This makes accurate calibration of a system possible. The precision of the methods used to confirm the diagnosis often exceeds that needed to determine subsequent patient management. Thus, for the purposes of clinical diagnosis, the number of disease classes can be quite small (20-30), even though the WHO index lists over 200 types of cerebral disease. This simplifies the requirement on a diagnostic system [5].

In most radiology departments the methodology used for neuro-radiological examination is standardized, with most patients receiving an initial CT scan. Large numbers of these examinations can be analysed to provide basic information. An idealised representation of this diagnostic methodology is as follows: A patient is examined usually by CT initially and the images viewed by a radiologist who reaches a provisional diagnosis. The patient is then referred for either further examination or treatment. At some later stage a confirmed diagnosis is obtained and this may act to reinforce or modify the clinician's diagnostic activity in the future. A complication of this simplistic model is the use of X-ray contrast enhancement. Some pathologies are much more clearly delineated in enhanced scans but the procedure can cause discomfort and is not without risk. The radiologist may choose to wait for the results of a plain scan before proceeding with enhancement.

This system appears to us to be an attractive target for modelling by a computer aid. However this in itself is not a sufficient justification for the attempt and the next section presents our analysis of the possible utility of a computer-based, neuro-radiological advisor.

3. UTILITY OF A DIAGNOSTIC AID

To hope to use a computer aid as a replacement for the critical faculties of a clinician is arrogant nonsense [6]. In all but the most trivial domains, machine intelligence is at best a misnomer and if this is not recognized all attempts are doomed to failure. Rather, an aid must be just that, a device to enhance the powers of the user.

By incorporating knowledge gleaned from several experienced radiologists, a computer-based aid can make available information that no individual clinician could acquire. Further, it may be possible to mechanically elucidate relationships between information that are too complex for a human, however experienced, to manipulate. Such a system might suggest rare diseases that a typical user might not have considered because of their low frequency of occurrence. It might also cause the user to give greater, and more accurate, weight to less likely alternative diagnoses.

We hope this ability will be of particular benefit to less experienced radiologists who may have worked in only a limited range of environments and thus who may have seen only a narrow part of the spectrum of disease. The increasing presense of scanners in smaller hospitals, where staff receive limited specialist training, is producing a need for such a device.

A number of specific positive aspects of diagnostic aids have been identified beyond the ability to simply suggest a diagnosis. It has been established that the very action of eliciting information in a formal manner can enhance the diagnostician's performance [7]. This may be due to the imposition of a more structured mode of working, which aids in the recognition of typical symptoms. It may also be that there is a tendency to diagnose on the basis of the most obvious symptoms without giving due consideration to the less obvious ones, and that this is countered by a formal description process.

A well constructed diagnostic aid embodies a substantial part of the knowledge of at least one human expert. This can potentially be tapped to function as a teaching aid. Diagnostic aids contain several components that may be of benefit in this area. The formal process of eliciting information can form the basis for the development of an understanding of anatomy and its terminology. The process of obtaining advice from a set of typical and atypical cases can build up an understanding of the relationship between symptoms and disease, which would otherwise take many years of experience to acquire. Hence such a device can either implicitly or explicitly embody a computer-aided learning tool of great breadth and scope.

4. FEASIBLE APPROACHES

Having chosen to construct a computer aid for the diagnosis of cerebral disease in neuro-radiology a number of practical aspects were considered in order to limit the project to a realistic scale.

1. Diagnostic techniques to be accommodated
2. Methods of feature extraction from images
3. Methods of representing clinical knowledge
4. Practical limitations on the implementation

We followed the path of moderation with respect to most of these rather than attempting to address every problem at once.

4.1 Sources of information

Although many patients undergo plain X-ray, angiography, etc, the principle neuro-radiological examination in current use in western centres is the CT scan. We thus felt it reasonable to restrict an initial project to this technique. Inclusion of other sources of information would have required an impractical effort in knowledge and data acquisition.

Clearly, in arriving at a diagnosis the physician takes into account a wide range of information, some from diagnostic tests, some from direct observation and some from the case history and verbal reports of the patient. It is important to distinguish between the final diagnosis and that which is suggested by any one test. There is significant evidence that the provision of background information can introduce noise into individual tests. For example, a clinician is more likely to report an equivocal scan as metastasis if it is known that the patient has a primary tumour [8]. If the referring physician unintentionally transmits opinions to the radiologist who then unintentionally uses them to weight the radiological diagnosis, the final result may falsely corroborate the initial suspicions.

For these reasons we chose to restrict our sources of information to radiological ones and indeed to a single modality. In doing this we recognize that the diagnosis arrived at is not definitive but rather the result of a one of several tests. As the technology advances it may become practical to submit the detailed results of several diverse tests to an overall diagnostic system.

4.2 Means of information extraction

Direct feature extraction from CT images is not yet practical. Much work has been done on the mapping of normal and abnormal brain images onto some standard representations. However the computational requirements of this operation are immense and the ability to recognize the more subtle pathological signs remains elusive.

Fortunately we are not aiming to build a 'driverless' system and it is thus possible for the trained radiologist on hand to view images and report their content according to a formal scheme. The radiologist can thus function as a pre-processor, extracting features from the images and presenting them to the computer in a standardized and reduced form. The task of eliciting clinical information is relatively easy compared to that of weighting observations to obtain discriminators between diagnoses [9].

4.3 Possible techniques for knowledge representation

No global solution has been developed for the construction of knowledge-based systems. Two major classes have been proposed. One approach is based on the statistical analysis of past data, the other on sets of 'rules' obtained from a human expert, although this distinction is now becoming blurred with the use of inductive knowledge acquisition [10]. Both these approaches have limitations in specific applications and a new system can rarely use an 'off the shelf' package for knowledge representation. A third approach, that which we have chosen, is to adopt a hybrid of these two classes. The following sections briefly compare the available methods.

4.3.1 <u>Statistical discrimination.</u> It has long been recognized [11] that statistical analysis of a large number of case histories can provide a basis for suggesting diagnoses. Such systems use a finite set to symptoms or 'signs', which are often binary, and tabulate the probability of a particular combination of symptoms occurring in each of a finite set of diseases. The standard discrimination technique used is the application of Bayes' Theorem. Such systems have enjoyed some success but suffer from two main limitations. Firstly, for practical numbers of symptoms, the number of probabilities that must be stored becomes excessive. Secondly, as the 'knowledge' is derived purely from empirical relationships between measurements, there is no scope for introducing basic physiological data that might aid substantially in reaching a diagnosis and have a significant smoothing effect on the statistical noise.

A common solution to the problem of exponential growth in number of probabilities with number of symptoms is to assume independence. This works if the symptoms used are carefully chosen and yields the so called 'Independence Bayes' method. However the assumption of independence is a zero order approximation to a problem that is at least first order and the technique has been criticised widely [12,13,14].

4.3.2 <u>Rule-based systems.</u> More recently great hopes have been pinned on rule-based techniques. The availability of logic programming languages capable of inferring relationships between entities given initial statements about them has led to a widespread belief that a substantial part of human behaviour can be modelled in this manner. Great success has been achieved in those areas where human behaviour is itself based on formal rules eg. advising on rights to benefits, running a nuclear power plant or diagnosing a fault in a car engine. Such systems tend, however, to be less successful when the rules are not readily apparent. Even in the last example a rule such as "if the engine sounds strange, check the timing" may prove unreliable in the absence of a precise definition of 'strange'.

Underlying the construction of such systems is the assumption that the experts have a conscious understanding of how they reach decisions. Although this is clearly the case to a substantial extent, after a little introspection most experts will admit that a degree of 'intuition' or 'inclination towards a particular opinion' is often involved for which no conscious mechanism is apparent. The discipline of 'Knowledge engineering', which devises techniques for obtaining such knowledge in explicit form, has no simple task.

Textbooks may appear to provide a substantial knowledge base on which to build. But when a number of texts are studied in detail it is often found that inconsistencies exist and that what is actually presented is the subjective manifestation of a subconscious process.

4.3.3 <u>Hybrid systems.</u> Several expert systems [2] are based on rules that are not regarded as incontrovertible and instead carry experts' estimates of their degree of certainty. Such systems appear to incorporate the concepts of fuzzy logic that seem to apply in the real world, but they remain at the mercy of the estimated certainties of the rules, and these estimates by experts may be much more suspect than the rules themselves. We have found that radiologists can be quite surprised when presented with simple statistics of the relative frequencies of different disease symptoms. Had these experts been asked for estimates of the figures they would have been substantially in error. The procedure for handling the uncertainties to produce rule-based diagnoses are also questionable [15].

A hybrid system may alternatively be constructed from a statistical database as described above to which a certain amount of expert opinion has been added. Here the expert opinion takes the form of known relationships between symptoms or about the organic similarities of diseases. The addition of this information can lead to a dramatically improved performance over 'Independence Bayes' without the need for the acquisition of a complex rule set. This expert knowledge may be used to refine iteratively a simple statistical model of the association between symptoms and disease [16]. Provided this type of system can explain its basis for a particular diagnosis, it can be relatively easy to 'teach' it new skills.

4.4 Implementation

In selecting the approaches to adopt in designing the various components of our diagnostic aid we kept in mind the hardware and software environments that might be available. We viewed the system as one which might be readily installed in any department of radiology. It should thus be of relatively low cost and have no major requirements for computer hardware. The computational requirements are in fact compatible with the capabilities of a modest micro-computer and a prototype was built on this basis [17]. However the convenience of having image display facilities and substantial disk storage led us to investigate the use of the scanner computer itself or, alternatively, an independent viewing console. This enabled us to envisage a software option that might be supplied by a scanner manufacturer at minimal cost, but also restricted our choice of software and user interface peripherals.

5. A PRACTICAL SYSTEM DESIGN

The system that has been jointly developed at Leicester Polytechnic, The National Hospital, and UCL is the result of lengthy consideration of the above factors. A radiologist views CT scans and is prompted by a scan description program to report which of a specified list of binary signs are visible in the patient images [18]. The scan description is analysed, using a hybrid constrained statistical approach, to produce probabilities for each of 28 disease classes. The three most probable of these are presented to the user along with an indication of the significance of the contribution of the signs specified. Finally, after describing an unenhanced scan, the user can request a computation of the probability that the system would produce a different diagnosis given an enhanced scan.

All scan descriptions are stored indefinitely by the system. If at some time a confirmed diagnosis becomes available, this can be added to the description which then becomes part of the systems' database which currently contains almost 1000 descriptions. In this way the system can progressively refine its statistical precision and can adapt to local variations in disease characteristics. The system includes routines to monitor the reliability of the diagnosis of each disease. This provides a check that new data being accumulated in the database does not degrade the overall performance.

5.1 Scan description dialogue

The signs represent conceptually simple features and fall into the broad classes of: lesion position, lesion appearance and 'other signs', the last relating to signs that are not specific to any lesion. The appearance description includes simple statements about relative attenuation. A typical scan description might contain the signs shown in figure 1.

Position
- One lesion is visible in the scan
- It is located in the left hemisphere in the frontal part of the parasagittal strip

Appearance
- The lesion has a heterogeneous appearance with an irregular surround of relatively low attenuation.
  Some attenuation values within the lesion fall in each of the following classes:
    - Lower than bone but less than 20 units above brain
    - Lower than bone but more than 20 units above brain
    - Lower than brain but greater than CSF
- The lesion has no characteristic shape

Other signs
The following features which are not specific to any lesion are visible in the scan:
- Mass effect

FIGURE 1. Example of signs describing a scan.

The dialogue uses a tree structured approach to minimise the number of responses required to describe a scan. This tree structure takes into account the fact that, depending on the observation of those signs determined earlier in the dialogue, certain signs will not be relevant in the current description. The above example description requires a minimum of twelve responses. If the user asks for help or makes errors the number will of course be larger.

There are a number of specific requirements on the dialogue for scan description. It must be efficient in the sense of allowing the experienced clinician to input the data rapidly and it must minimize the variability introduced by different users of the system. Though the sign definitions have, as much as possible, been made unambiguous there is an inevitable degree of variation between users reporting the same scan. Such variation tends to reduce diagnostic accuracy as a degree of noise has effectively been added to the measurements.

The problem of operator variability can be reduced both by training and by providing a high degree of online help. The former enables users to adapt their behaviour to be consistent with examples presented by the system. The latter is intended to provide highly detailed descriptions of what criteria must be met before a sign is described as present. The need for both training facilities and extensive online help has been a major factor in the system design, particularly of the user interface which is described in more detail below.

5.2 Analysis

By introducing the clinical knowledge that many of the signs are related and by using the dependent Bayes terms selectively, the limitations of the independence assumption have been circumnavigated. In this way medical, anatomical or physiological information can be introduced and used to constrain the purely empirical observations of the standard Bayes' technique.

The relevant set of binary signs describing a particular scan is known as its 'profile'. If a particular profile of signs p is observed and the probability of that profile occurring with disease D_i is $P(p/D_i)$, then the probability of D_i being correct for that profile is:

$$P(D_i/p) = P(p/D_i) \, P(D_i) \, /c$$

where $P(D_i)$ is the prior probability of observing D_i. The normalization constant c is the probability of observing profile p over all n diseases:

$$c = P(p/D_1)P(D_1)+\ldots+P(p/D_n)P(D_n)$$

The standard Bayes' discriminant assumes each profile to be made up of m independent signs s so that $P(p/D_i)$ is replaced with:

$$P(s_1/D_i)*\ldots*P(s_m/D_i)$$

where each term is the probability of a sign having its observed state (TRUE/FALSE) in D_i.

By decomposing the equation in this manner we not only reduce the number of probabilities that must be stored but also introduce the possibility of omitting the probability associated with 'missing' signs. This is useful for cases where information is genuinely unavailable. It also suggests a means of introducing expert knowledge on the correlation of signs in certain diseases. If two signs s_a and s_b are known to be correlated in D_i we can replace the two independent terms with an estimated or measured probability for their combination. Such relationships, which include rules and certain logical dependences, are introduced into the system via text files which are readily modified to permit tuning.

By using the clinical knowledge that certain diseases have features in common, poor statistics for rarer diseases can be improved by exploiting their similarities and pooling probabilities for selected signs. Again, such relations are explicit rather than embedded in the code and can be turned off when sufficient cases for a particular disease have been acquired.

To improve performance for some of the rarer diseases, subjective estimates of probabilities have been combined with the measures from the database. A weighted combination of the measured and estimated probabilities is used in such a manner that, as more measured data becomes available, the probability will tend towards its measured value [19].

5.3 Presentation of diagnoses

The Bayes computation results in a probability that each of the recognized disease categories is the actual disease. To simply present this list without further comment would be unsatisfactory. The approach adopted is to present with each probable disease those signs that have made significant contributions or that are particularly improbable. These are ranked in order of significance. A typical output for one of the three suggested diseases is shown in figure 2.

This information gives an effective explanation of the diagnosis which may make the result more helpful to the user. For example if a sign that is only marginally detectable gives great weight to the diagnosis, the radiologist may choose to reconsider the results.

Computer Aid for Cerebral Disease   V1.0

                    Obtaining advice for patient XX5555
                    from an unenhanced scan.

_____

                    The following signs have been important in
                    reaching the suggested diagnosis.

     69.6%   Extradural haematoma

     Shape: Mantle shaped
     Appearance: Homogeneous
     Attenuation: Lower than bone, >20H units above brain

                    The following signs greatly conflicted
                    with the suggested diagnosis

                    None

                    Press [RETURN] to continue:

                    (Press [HELP] for help)

FIGURE 2. Presentation of one of the three suggested diseases.

6.   INTERFACE REQUIREMENTS
     The user interface is a crucial aspect of the design of any software
system [20]. A significant part of the design effort was thus expended on
this aspect of the system.
     There are a number of important considerations in the design of the
interface. The type of user envisaged is the primary factor and in some
cases, as where multiple types of user are present, the interface may be
required to be adaptable or possibly adaptive.
     Ease of use is the first objective for any interface. Achieving this
involves not only displaying clear instructions to the user, but also
considerations such as avoiding the display of lengthy descriptive text
which the more experienced user will never read.
     Our system is intended for use in an environment such as a large
teaching hospital. It is thus expected to be used by people with a wide
range of experience. There will be a significant number of students and
short term visitors, who may not have time to gain full proficiency, whilst
the resident clinicians will, through daily use, become highly able.
     Several strategies are available to accommodate such a spectrum of
ability. One approach is to provide two or more modes giving the user
different degrees of prompting. The user is then free to switch mode at
any time depending on the degree of familiarity with the particular section
of code being used. This approach can be effective but tends to force
unwanted and often unexpected mode change options on users [21]. Many
workers have advocated adaptive systems [22] which attempt to assess the
user's proficiency and modify the level of prompting accordingly. This can
be most effective if: a) the user can be assessed correctly, and b) there
is a near continuum of degrees of help, so that changes are largely

imperceptible. Sudden modifications in dialogue behaviour can be very disruptive to user confidence and quite counter productive.

We chose to adopt a third and simpler approach, that of always providing minimal information in a clear and concise manner, but making a substantial base of help available on demand. By choosing a standard format for all dialogue screens and always reminding the user that help is available at the touch of a key, a wide range of abilities is accommodated easily. The application requires that even experienced users refer to ancillary information from time to time, for viewing new patient images, changing viewing formats etc. Incorporating these functions with help and other supportive information within a single help mode available at a keystroke, provides a useful degree of uniformity. It is also possible that there is a stigma associated with asking for help which is reduced in this way.

Although the help mode sections of the system are quite distinct from the main description entry sections, they still retain a high degree of homogeneity with the main programs and indeed help on help is available recursively. This type of structure ensures that the user need never feel lost even when in unexplored parts of the program, and this leads to a fast learning curve for the system. The structure also meets the requirement of minimal verbosity, as lengthy dialogue can be replaced by a single easy-to-learn convention: 'If in doubt press HELP'. By providing such a large degree of help on the use of the system, the programs can be substantially self teaching.

In designing the system we took the view that the programmers were also users. They were thus presented with well defined module interfaces. This aspect is of particular importance in a project involving multiple programmers. If the interfaces between the software components are not well defined, the reliability and maintainability will be severely compromised. We accomplished this partly by defining the I/O interfaces before writing any code and partly by using a common file structure that individual modules could access, to effect inter-module communication.

7.   PROGRAM STRUCTURE

Although the object of this particular project was to implement an advisor to run on a particular machine (the GE 9800 Independent Console), transportability was a major consideration. The possibility of adapting the system for alternative environments motivated us to build in a high degree of flexibility with respect to:

1.   Natural language
2.   Operating environment
3.   Medical terminology
4.   Dialogue structure

The need for an efficient means of data entry led us to select a simple menu presentation. Though numerous methods are now available for selection one of a small number of options from a list on a VDU screen (mouse, light-pen, touch-screen etc.) none of these has, in our opinion, demonstrated a clear advantage over menu selection of numeric options. This requires only limited typing skills, which are required anyway for such purposes as entering user and patient identifications. To some extent the example images and diagrams could have been used in the manner of icons for indicating locations and features, but this would have substantially impeded the knowledgeable user, for a questionable gain to the novice.

The system is constructed as a number of modules, each having well defined functions, eg: Log-on and function selection, unenhanced scan description, diagnosis and presentation of advice. Additional modules elicit descriptions for contrast enhanced scans and provide various support functions. The terminal I/O support system, the 'menu driver', is a suite of utility routines that provide a structured and uniform interface between the terminal user and the applications software [23,24]. This module incorporates the interface to the help system which is thus accessible in a uniform manner from every question. A number of databases are accessed by the system to build the screen displays and provide the various types of help. These are used to provide the following features:

    Basic dialogue support
        Standard screen formats, with multiple windows
    Help at question level
        What does this question mean?
        Why are you asking me this?
    Help at feature level
        What do you mean by this term?
        Show me a diagram of this feature
        Show me a typical image of this feature
        Show me an atypical image of this feature
    Image display interface
        Show me the next slice from this patient set

To gain a large measure of system independence, all file structures are accessed via interface routines. All files are modified in 'atomic' operations so reducing the possibility of corruption following software or hardware failure. The dialogue is segmented and each segment journaled. This permits rapid recovery from sessions aborted intentionally or unintentionally, and has also proved useful in fault location.

It was decided to impose simple access control by requesting a user identification at the start of each session. This provides the useful facility of allowing data to be personalized so that, for example, only the scans described by the more experienced users might be incorporated in the system database. Also, operations such as adding a confirmed diagnosis, can be restricted to a senior user. A bonus of identifying the user is that, in evaluating the system, knowing who is doing what provides much information on styles of interaction by more and less experienced users.

8. ASSESSMENT PROCEDURES
    The medical profession can be profoundly conservative in matters of diagnostic methodology. Skepticism of new techniques is justified when the management of patients and the consumption of time, money and other resources is involved and this places the onus on the implementer of a new system to provide a satisfactory justification for its introduction. Unfortunately this can result in a 'catch 22' in which no one wishes to volunteer to take part in an evaluation until the system has been successfully evaluated. By contrast, other areas such as new imaging modalities may exhibit the opposite phenomenon in which everyone wishes to be the first to apply the new technology to their area of interest.

    We have not yet attempted to introduce our system to a site other than The National Hospital. At this stage we recognize that the most hospitable environment possible is required in which an assessment of its capabilities and limitations can be conducted. From this, obviously subjective assessment we hope to go on to a more objective one at another site. Even for an in-house assessment, the problems of devising an appropriate evaluation methodology are severe.

The primary question that must be addressed in assessing a diagnostic aid is: Does the clinician working in conjunction with the program perform better than when unaided? This immediately begs the question of what we mean by 'better performance'. Should we compare the performance of a diagnostic program with a clinician given the same data or with the final confirmed diagnosis?

Our system has the latter type of comparison inbuilt in the procedure of cross validation. Each entry in the internal database of scan descriptions can be diagnosed using the remainder of the database, and the result compared with the confirmed diagnosis. This procedure yields 66% correct first choice diagnosis and 88% first second or third choice.

Unfortunately case notes rarely record, in a useful manner, the radiologist's diagnosis after viewing the scans. Thus to compare the system with an unaided clinician requires an experiment involving several users and a significant number of patient images.

9. EVALUATION METHODS

At the time of writing, the system is installed and in use on a regular basis. The next stage of the project is to conduct a formal evaluation to attempt to measure the performance in meaningful terms and to assess user reaction. It is expected that the results of this evaluation will prompt some changes, particularly in the dialogue. The flexibility of the user interface will permit these to be introduced easily.

The initial evaluation is planned to take 26 weeks and require the involvement of several clinicians and others as test users. The evaluation will consist of two related 'experiments'. The first experiment will consist of training sessions in which the users will gain experience with the system. This will also give information on ease of use and rate of learning. The second, involving the description of more difficult cases, will give information on the performance in the hands of trained users. It is anticipated that at least twelve users will take part in the study. These will be:

> Two experienced users of the system
> Four senior registrars
> Four radiographers
> Two others

The experiments will be conducted in sessions during each of which the user will view and describe five scans. It is expected that sessions will not last more than an hour each and users will be encouraged to complete each session at a single sitting. As the system has the ability to save an interrupted session and resume at a later date, subjects will be permitted to use this if necessary. To reduce the number of variables, the study will be restricted to unenhanced scans at this stage. A further experiment could be performed later to look at the characteristics of enhanced scan description.

Since being made available the system has compiled a log of all activity. This will be used to provide data on learning curves and help usage and will also permit studies of the relationship between speed and performance.

9.1 Training sessions

The training sessions will be based on a set of 10 scans selected to be reasonably easy to describe, but for which the diagnosis is not obvious.

This will combine training with examples of the utility of the system.

The first training scan viewed will be available fully described on the system. This will permit users to step through the description seeing exactly which signs were identified. A detailed document will lead the user through this initial description. The user will then be able to describe this scan and continue with the nine remaining scans over two sessions. The written guide for this experiment will stress the availability of the various forms of help as a means of resolving problems during use.

At the end of the two sessions each user will be asked to complete a short questionnaire on the performance of the system with respect to ease of use and will be encouraged to add additional comments on any aspects.

9.2 System performance measurement

This experiment will be based on two sets of 10 scans each. The first set will be selected to be relatively easy to describe. The scans in the second set will be chosen to have more difficult appearance or other sign descriptions. The scans will be viewed in four sessions of five scans each, each group of five being a random selection of 2/3 scans from the easy set and 3/2 from the hard set.

During the experiment each user will complete a questionnaire giving the following information:

1. User's initial opinion of the diagnosis on seeing the images but not using the system.
2. After describing the scan but before obtaining advice is there a change in that diagnosis and if so to what?
3. Would the user choose to perform an enhanced scan?
4. The system will itself record the sign description, the diagnosis, and its own enhancement advice.

After completing all four sessions the user will be asked to complete a further questionnaire on the performance of the system and given an opportunity to add any general comments.

9.3 Analysis of results

The training experiment will be used to examine patterns of performance in users who are new to the system. This will be derived from the logging data produced by the system. The qualitative responses from the users on the system performance will also be used to make general observations. Learning will be measured by time to complete sections of the program and frequency of help requests. Help system usage will also indicate those areas in which the dialogue requires more clarification.

The main experiment will provide a variety of information:

1. A comparison of unaided radiologist's diagnosis with that of the system.
2. A comparison of the unaided radiologist's opinion on enhancement with that of the system.
3. A measure of the consistency of sign description over a variety of users.
4. A comparison of the performance of users with varying degrees of radiological experience.

10. OTHER USES OF THE DIAGNOSTIC AID

Although the principle reason for developing this system was for use as a diagnostic advisor, several additional facilities have been recognized as being of use. Direct access to statistical database has caused great interest among radiologists and several long held beliefs on the interrelation of certain signs and diseases have been weakened. This is particularly interesting in the case of infrequent occurrences which tend to be forgotten. For example, at first presentation at the National Hospital, the absence of a ring, or indeed any enhancement, in cases later confirmed as cerebral abscess is surprisingly frequent (Only 21% exhibited the 'classic' uniform ring enhancement).

The help databases contain a wealth of information for the less experienced radiologist. The system thus has the potential to be used as a teaching aid. It was originally thought that this would require a quite separate programming effort, possibly offering a variety of computer-aided learning methodologies. In practice, however, the scan description dialogue offers a useful formalism within which students can explore both the anatomy of the brain and many of its pathologies. By studying the statistics and describing hypothetical scans the student can gain a useful insight into the relationship between disease and radiological abnormality. Finally, the base of example images, all annotated by an expert radiologist, is available for study and can be a useful addition to the usual radiological atlas.

11. CONCLUSIONS

It has been demonstrated that the system is capable of aiding a radiologist in reaching a diagnosis. Early experiments [18] suggest that the performance with most diseases is not worse than that of an unaided radiologist. As these studies were performed using a simple system with no online help, a substantially smaller database, and a much simpler statistical advisor, we are optimistic of the performance of this full implementation.

The success so far achieved is, we believe, a justification of the particular hybrid approach we have adopted for discrimination. It is doubtful that a conventional 'expert system' approach would have performed as well in this application.

We stress the point that reaching even this rather early stage in the development of the technique has absorbed a substantial effort (several person years). Whilst some of this effort has gone into producing transportable components, the major part was in data acquisition (over 220 hours has been spent examining case notes) and preliminary analysis. The development of a useful advisor system for medicine can be very time consuming.

Our experience is that this major effort has born fruits beyond the creation of a diagnostic aid. The facility to interrogate a statistical database of CT features, the formalism of the scan description, and the database of example images and text can contribute to an improved performance within the department.

ACKNOWLEDGEMENTS

This work has been supported by:
International General Electric
UK Department of Health and Social Security
Leicestershire Local Education Authority

REFERENCES

1. Wagner G, Tauta P, Wolber U. Problems of Medical Diagnosis: a bibliography. Meth. Inf. Medicine 17:55-74 (1978).
2. Shortliffe EH. Computer-based medical consultations: MYCIN. New York: Elsevier (1976).
3. De Dombal FT, Horrocks JG, Walmsley G, Wilson PD. Computer aided diagnosis and decision-making in the acute abdomen. J. Royal Coll. Physicians, 9:211-218 (1975).
4. Spiegelhalter DJ. Evaluation of clinical decision aids, with an application to a system for dyspepsia. Statistics in Medicine, 2:207-215 (1983).
5. Szolovits P, Pauker SG. Categorical and probabilistic reasoning in medical diagnosis. Artificial Intelligence, 11:115-144 (1978).
6. De Dombal FT. Towards a more objective evaluation of computer aided decision support systems. In: Van Bemmel JH, Ball MJ, Wigertz O, Eds: Medinfo 83, Amsterdam, North Holland 436-439 (1983).
7. De Dombal FT, Leaper DJ, Horrocks JC, Staniland JR, McCann AP. Human and computer aided diagnosis of abdominal pain: further report with emphasis on performance of clinicians, Brit. Med. J. 1:376-380 (1974).
8. Du Boulay GH, Teather D, Morton BA, Wills KM, Plummer DL. BRAINS - A computer advisor to aid in CT scan interpretation and cerebral disease diagnosis. Submitted to Neuroradiology (1985).
9. Leaper DJ, Horrocks JC, Staniland JR, de Dombal FT. Computer assisted diagnosis of abdominal pain using "estimates" provided by clinicians. Brit. Med. J. 4:350-354 (1972).
10. Hart AE. Experience in the use of an inductive system in knowledge engineering. In: Research and development in Expert systems. Ed. M Bramer, CUP 117-126 (1985).
11. Ledley RS, Lusted LB. Reasoning foundations in medical diagnosis, Science 130:9-21 (1959).
12. Teather D. Diagnosis - Methods and analysis. Bull. Inst. Math. Appl. 10:37-41 (1974).
13. Teather D, Hilder W. The analysis of diagnostic data. J. Royal Coll. Physicians, 9:219-225 (1975).
14. Feinstein AR. The haze of Bayes, the aerial palaces of decision analysis, and the computerized Ouija board. Clin. Pharmacol. Ther. 21:482-496 (1977).
15. Spiegelhalter DJ, Knill-Jones RP. Statistical and Knowledge-based Approaches to Clinical Decision-Support systems, with an Application in Gastroenterology. J. Royal Statist. Soc. 147:35-58 (1984).
16. Morton BA, Teather D, du Boulay GH. Statistical Modeling and Diagnostic Aids, Med. Dec. Making 4,3 (1984).
17. Du Boulay GH, Innocent PR, Teather D, Wills K. Programming a PET for computer aided diagnosis with CT scans. Conference proceedings of the 2nd Symposium on Computers in Diagnostic Radiology, Amsterdam, June (1980).
18. Wills K, du Boulay GH, Teather D. Initial findings in the computer-aided diagnosis of cerebral tumours using CT scan results. Brit. J. Radiology 54:948-952 (1981).
19. Du Boulay GH, Teather D, Harling D, Clarke G. Improvements in the computer assisted diagnosis of cerebral tumours. Brit. J. Radiology 50:849-854 (1977).
20. Collard P, Plummer D. Operating system requirements and user interfaces, IEEE transactions on Nuclear Science, 29,4:1291-1298 (1982).

21. Maskery HS. Adaptive interfaces for naive users - An experimental study, Proc.IFIP Conf. on Human Computer Interaction, London, 1:314-320 (1984).

22. Edmonds EA, Adaptive man-computing interfaces. In Alty JL & Coombs MJ, Eds. Computer Skills and adaptive systems, 389-426 London: Academic Press (1981).

23. Todd-Pokropek A, Plummer D, Pizer SM. Modularity and Command Languages in Medical Computing. In: Information Processing in Medical Imaging, Proc. Vth International Conference, 426-455, Biomedical Computing Information Center, Oak Ridge National Lab. TN. (1978).

24. Innocent PR, Plummer D, Teather D, Morton BA, Wills KM, du Boulay GH. The design of flexible interfaces: A Case study of an operational system for assisting in the diagnosis of cerebral disease. Proc. IFIP Conf. on Human-Computer Interaction, London, 1:214-218 (1984).

An Editor for the Acquisition of Medical Expert Knowledge:
Function and Use shown by an Automatic Knowledge-based
System for the Analysis of Heart Scintigrams.

I. Hofmann, H. Niemann, G. Sagerer
Lehrstuhl fuer Informatik 5 (Mustererkennung)
Universitaet Erlangen-Nuernberg
Martensstr. 3
D - 8520 Erlangen (FRG)

1. INTRODUCTION.

The last 20 years have shown a rapid development in building
expert or knowledge-based systems. Those systems are one of the
major objectives in research concerning artificial
intelligence. The areas of application vary from theorem
proving, industry automation, control and, especially,
medicine. Expert systems like MYCIN [BUC84], INTERNIST [MIL82
], CASNET [WEI81] or PATREC [MIT84] are well-known from
literature. Perhaps in near future, they will do their work in
laboratories and clinical environment in everyday use, that is
they will guide a physician interactively to a decision
concerning the special application problem. Another aspect is
to develop knowledge-based systems solving difficult problems
without any user interactions required. This method is
favourable if input data are produced by a camera, for
instance, which could store them in the computer automatically.
Applications would be in ultrasound, radiology, CT, MRI and,
especially, nuclear medicine involving a lot of medical imaging
tasks. Up to now, interpretation of the resulting images is
usually performed by visual inspection. This method is rather
limited in many respects (e.g. estimation of greyscale
thresholds, dependence on image displaying devices etc. affect
a practical interpretation of those data) and necessitates the
repetitive recording of identical phenomena from different
points of view. The experience of the observer and the
knowledge about the problem space are the basis of reliable
decisions. However, representing that knowledge in a computer
and offering the possibility to supplement and modify stored
information might free a physician from routine tasks saving
time for other difficult problems.
The following paper gives an overview of an automatic system
for the analysis of heart scintigrams which has been developped
at the University of Erlangen (FRG) by the Lehrstuhl fuer
Informatik 5 and the Institut und Poliklinik fuer
Nuklearmedizin. Designing such a system demands a large
knowledge base which always has to be modified whenever new
facts or methods occur. Tools are presented to support this
proceeding.

2. System overview.

Defects in the motility of the heart or dilatation could be detected by an analysis of heart scintigrams. Technetium 99m-gated blood pool studies triggered by the ECG result in image sequences showing one cycle of the beating heart. A knowledge-based system has been developped able to analyse those sequences automatically and to derive medical evidence without any user interactions required. Each sequence consists of n images, $12 < n < 32$, with a spatial resolution of 64x64 pixel and an intensity resolution of 8 bit. The images are taken in LaO 45 (Fig. 1).

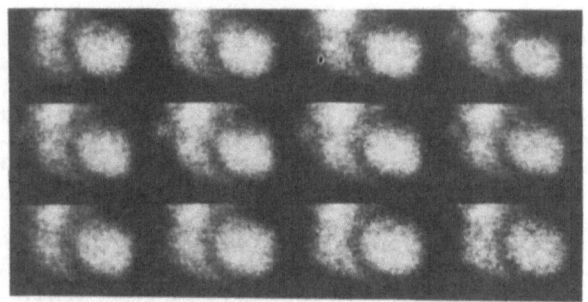

Fig. 1 Input image sequence

The principal architecture of the system is shown in Fig. 2. It is based on the approach proposed in [NIE81]. The system itself consists of three major modules, each of which is concerned with a particular task which is to be described in the following section.

2.1 Module MODEL.

An automatic analysis is guided by stored knowledge. In our case that problem specific knowledge is represented by means of an associative network. The declarative part describes how different types of objects, like the left ventricle and its four segments (see later in this section), motion and medical diagnoses are related with one another. The nodes (concepts) of the network are simply data structures describing terms by a name, attributes and attribute constraints. The latter form the

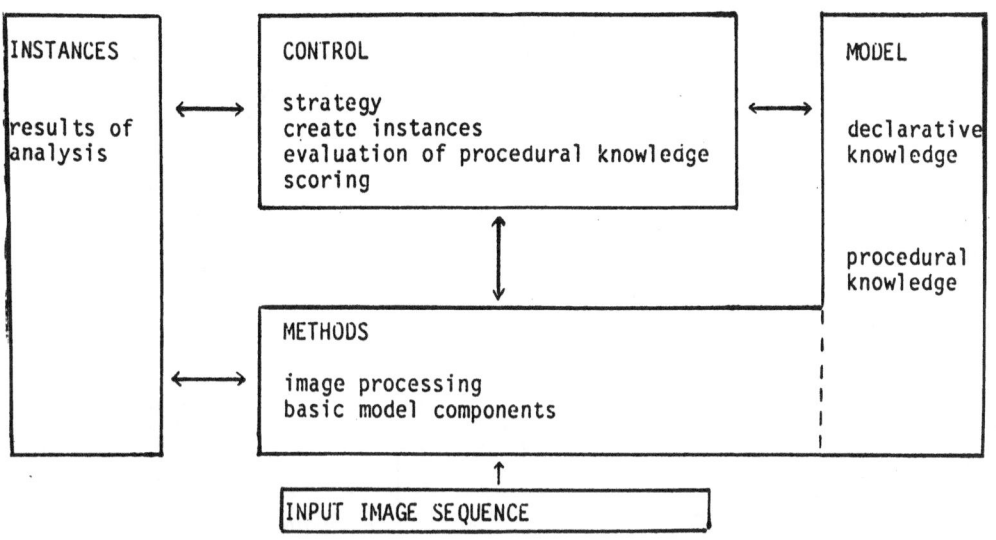

Fig. 2 System overview

relation to the procedural part of the knowledge base. The
edges between the nodes are restricted to three types:
`necessary-parts` which are needed for describing hierarchies
and structuring the knowledge base, `semantic parts` which give
a physical partioning, and `specializations`. Those edges are
represented as links between data structures. The principal
structure of the knowledge base is shown in Fig. 3 [HOF85]. A
more detailed description of contents is given in [SAG85]. A
description of syntactical aspects is given in section `The
Editor`.
The procedures attached to the nodes are straight forward, in
most of the cases. One part is doing image processing. Since
the quality of the given input image sequences is very poor a
smoothing operation (median filtering) is performed followed by
contour detection based on a polar coordinate transform and

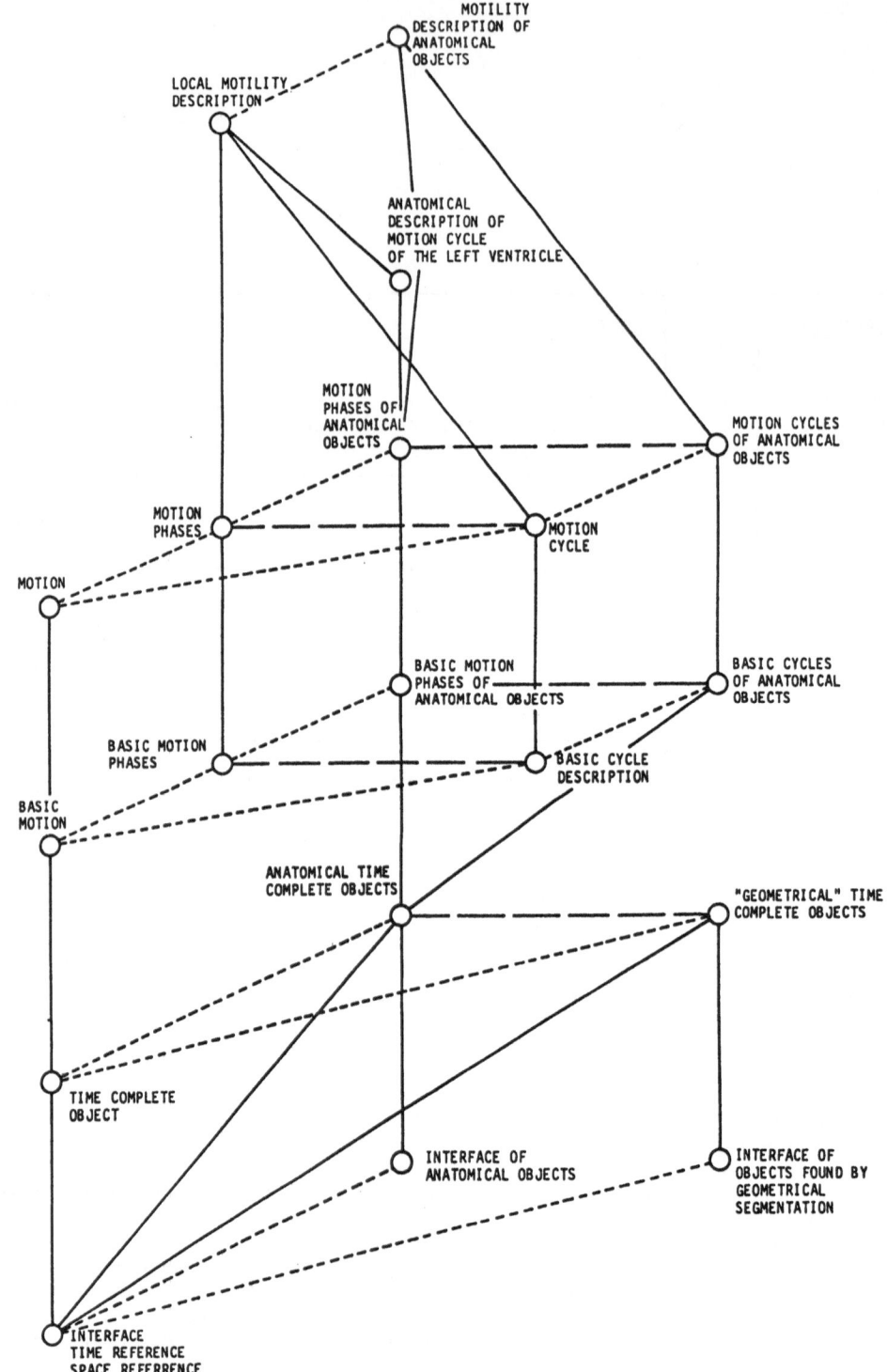

dynamic programming. The contours of the heart, and the left and right ventricle are determined. Additionally, the left ventricle is segmented into four segments guided by medical criteria, and sectors guided by geometric criteria, that is each sector is given by an angle based upon the center of gravity of the left ventricle. Fig. 4 and Fig. 5 show the resulting contours. The algorithms used are described in [BUN82].

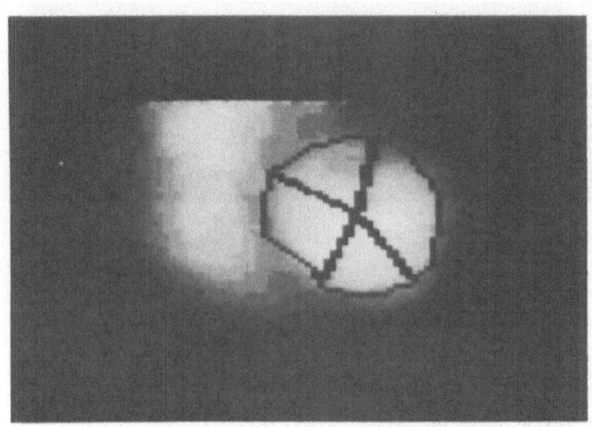

Fig. 4 Medical segmentation

The contours are the basis of further processing steps (determination of areas). Besides calculating angles, areas or lengths of contours, time parameters and testing relations between structures, there are two classes of procedures, which utilise more sophisticated algorithms. Describing the heart cycle by terms like contraction, expansion and stagnation phases is done by means of syntactical pattern recognition (dynamic programming procedure) [BUN84a], where up to nine different prototype heart cycles are matched against actual input data.

Diagnoses are inferred by a rule-based system attached to the associative network as attributes. The automatic system knows about 40 different medical interpretations based on about 120 different rules describing normal, hypokinetic, akinetic or dyskinetic behaviour of the left ventricle and of its segments [BUN84b].

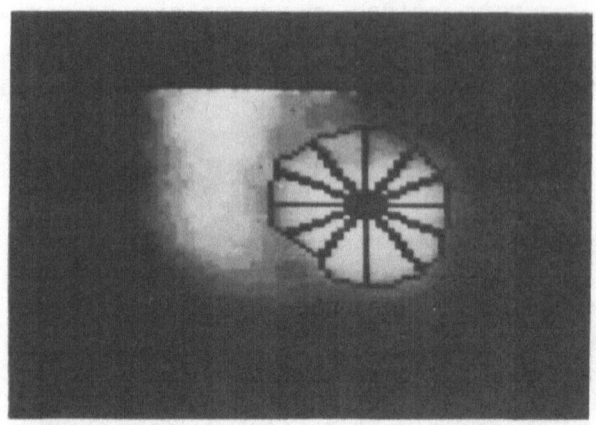

Fig. 5 Geometric segmentation

2.2 Module INSTANCES.

The structure of the module INSTANCES is identical to that of
the module MODEL with the exception that attributes contain the
values computed from actual input data by activating the
corresponding procedures. All results obtained during an
analysis are also represented as an associative network,
offering the possibility to check the way of the automatic
analysis of an actual input image sequence.

2.3 Module CONTROL.

The knowledge base described above is used to guide the
analysis. The user starts analysis by labelling a node (goal
concept) of the knowledge base which is interpreted as a
request to verify this node. Now, the task of this module is
[HOF85]

- to evaluate declarative knowledge by tracing the edges
  `necessary-parts` and `semantic-parts`

- to create an `empty` instance

- to activate procedural knowledge and store actually
  computed values in the instance(s).

A special production rule may be given to instantiate model
concepts. This rule implies a top-down evaluation of the
knowledge base.

On various levels of abstraction competing instances can be

created, each of which is assessed in relation to the goal hypothesis. Therefore, a search space results containing all possible paths to an instance which is the best verification of the goal concept. The strategy is to find this instance on the shortest possible way. In our case a heuristic graph search procedure (A -algorithm) is used.

First results are available concerning a test phase with actual input data. Since contours are the basis of the automatic analysis a validation has been performed. A comparison between manually and automatically outlined contours showed a correlation of about r=0.93 whereas a comparison between different physicians often shows a correlation of r=0.7 [BUN84c, NIE85]. Further tests compared medical diagnoses derived by a physician to interpretations derived by the system. In about 80% of the cases the interpretations had been identical or the system gave even more details, in about 20% the system rejected the input [SAG85].

3. The Editor.

Based on the encouraging results mentioned above further research will accent the expansion of the knowledge base, the development of an utility to list the contents of the knowledge base (which protocol will give the goal concepts of an analysis) and the design of a comfortable interface to the user to extract the results, explain and justify the actions and reactions of the system. Since the memory for the results (module INSTANCES) is structured like the knowledge base, the solution to both of the mentioned problems will be a special tool working like an editor.
The accuracy, performance and, therefore, usefulness of an automatic system is dependent on the completeness of the knowledge base. It should be possible to integrate new terms, experiences, even new technologies when they appear and if they should come to everyday use.
Another aspect is the evaluation of the computed results. A minimal request is the possibility of extracting those values. A more comfortable interface will offer the possibility to trace the history of the analysis and, thereby, explain the reasons for getting a special interpretation of input data.

Fig. 6 outlines the architecture of a human interface surrounding an automatic system. The boxes describe modules dealing with special groups of data, the arrows show access paths of the modules. The kernel of an analysis of results is the module EXPLANATION which guides an extraction of values from the module INSTANCES and traces the way from an input image sequence to the complete description by using the protocol of the history of the analysis. Knowledge acquisition is done by the system designer in cooperation with an expert of the problem space. The process of extracting knowledge from an expert or a source of expertise and transferring it to a

332

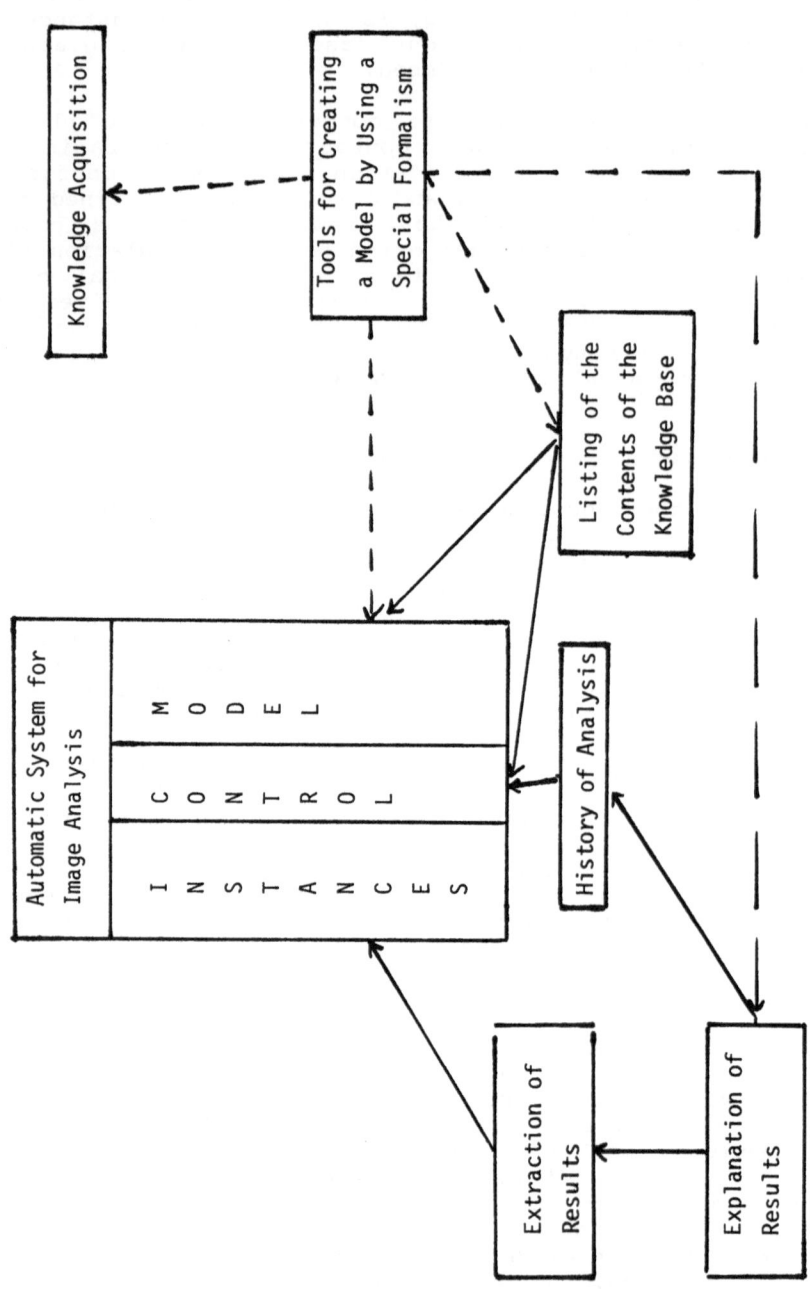

Fig. 6 Human interface of the automatic system

program (knowledge base) is an important and difficult problem. It can reduce the costs of knowledge reproduction and exploitation and it can make private knowledge available for public test and evaluation, but first it involves problem definition and refinement, as well as representing facts and relations acquired from an expert. Up to now, the dialog between the expert and the program is done by the system designer because no automatic facilities for knowledge acquisition are available.

A difficult problem is to structure the knowledge which should be represented in a reasonable way. This has to be done by the expert, but there should be tools which allow for transferring structures to the automatic system, and allow for modifying them, respectively.

Different formalisms for knowledge representation offer different tools

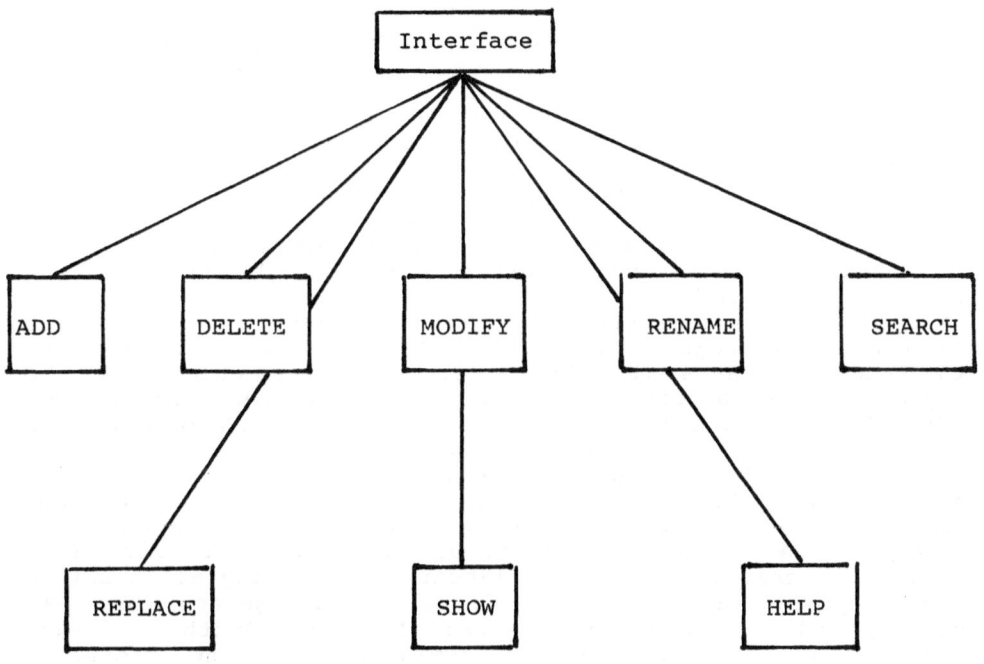

Fig. 7 Functions of the editor

adjusted to a special structure, like query languages concerning relational databases, tools like EMYCIN or TEIRESIAS (containing interpreters) concerning rule based systems, or ARGON [PAT85] concerning frame-based knowledge representation systems. In the following section such a tool will be called an 'editor' having the functions

- to list the contents of the knowledge base by enumerating the names of referenced structures and giving a short user-defined comment on the part of knowledge described by those structures

- to add further knowledge components

- to delete knowledge components contradicting new results in research

- to replace knowledge components by updated ones

- to modify existing knowledge components

- to rename existing knowledge structures

- to search for knowledge components (queries to the database)

- to trace the history of knowledge components and show the kontext of a special component, and

- to help the user applying the editor

moreover never hurting the existing structure (syntax) of a given knowledge base and supporting efforts in being consistent (semantics) (Fig. 7).

Applied to an associative network those functions will operate on nodes and edges. The user will have to structure the knowledge he wants to add getting entities which will be represented as a node in the network. The syntax of a node (Fig. 8a,b) should be given by the editor which prompts for actual input values (The '?' has to be replaced by actual parameters). The coding of such a complex data structure is done automatically by the system, whereas the system designer or an experienced user should be able to easily modify the syntax by adding new components or deleting other ones. This results in creating a 'syntax library' containing all possible slots of the data structure, defining the parameters and their ranges, and giving default values (Fig. 9). Another library contains the declaration and definition of the slots. A modification of the syntax will be a modification of both of the mentioned libraries. The editor of our system is based on the C programming language under UNIX, additionally using a macro preprocessor to combine the definitions of the slots of the data structure to one large program dealing with one concept. The data structure shown in Fig. 8a has turned out be appropriate to represent different kinds of knowledge whether objects or motion or diagnoses. A short explanation of the slots will follow:

```
BEGINNE_KONZEPTDEFINITION(NAME= ?,
GRADE= ?,INFO= ?,0)

    KONZEPT_VON(NIL)

    GENERALISIERUNG(?)

    SPEZIALISIERUNGEN(?)

    AEHNLICHKEITEN(?)

    KONTEXT(?)

    CF_PROZEDUR(?)

    SEMANTISCHER_TEIL_VON(?)

    NOTWENDIGER_TEIL_VON(?)

    START_SEMANTISCHE_TEILE(?,MODALITAET())
    ENDE_SEMANTISCHE_TEILE

    START_SEMANTISCHE_ATTRIBUTE(?,MODALITAET())
    ENDE_SEMANTISCHE_ATTRIBUTE

    START_SEMANTISCHE_STRUKTUREN(?,MODALITAET())
    ENDE_SEMANTISCHE_STRUKTUREN

    START_NOTWENDIGE_TEILE(?,MODALITAET())
    ENDE_NOTWENDIGE_TEILE

    START_NOTWENDIGE_ATTRIBUTE(?,MODALITAET())
    ENDE_NOTWENDIGE_ATTRIBUTE

    START_NOTWENDIGE_STRUKTUREN(?,MODALITAET())
    ENDE_NOTWENDIGE_STRUKTUREN

BEENDE_KONZEPTDEFINITION(?)
```

Fig. 8a Syntactical structure of a node

```
        TEIL(FUNKTIONALE_ROLLE(?),
           DEFINITIONSBEREICH(KONZEPT,?),
           DIMENSION(1),
           WERTBERECHNUNG= UNDEFINIERT,
           RESTRIKTIONEN= NEIN,
           MODIFIZIERT= ?,
           MODIFIZIERTE_BERECHNUNG= NEIN,
           DEFAULTWERTE= NEIN)
```

```
ATTRIBUT(FUNKTIONALE_ROLLE(?),
    DEFINITIONSBEREICH(?),
    DIMENSION(?),
    WERTBERECHNUNG= ?,
    RESTRIKTIONEN= NEIN,
    MODIFIZIERT= ?,
    MODIFIZIERTE_BERECHNUNG= ?,
    DEFAULTWERTE= NEIN)

STRUKTUR(FUNKTIONALE_ROLLE(?),
    RELATION= ?,
    DEFAULTWERTE= NEIN,
    DEFINITIONSBEREICH(),
    MIT_DEN_KOMPONENTEN(?))
```

Fig. 8b Substructures of a node

names of the slots	parameter	defaults
INFO	string of text	-
GRADE	number	-
KONZEPT_VON	concept/instance	NIL
GENERALISIERUNG	concept/instance	-
.	.	.
.	.	.
.	.	.

Fig. 9 Structure of the syntax library

NAME: name of the data structure

GRADE: level of abstraction within the associative network

INFO: short description of the knowledge being represented
           by the actual node

KONZEPT_VON(NIL): link between modules MODEL and INSTANCES
           (when creating the knowledge base this slot will be
           unused)

GENERALISIERUNG: pointer to another concept being more
           general

SPEZIALISIERUNGEN: pointer to concepts being specializations

AEHNLICHKEITEN: possibility to refer to similar concepts (unused)

KONTEXT: pointer to a concept being the context of the actual one

CF_PROZEDUR: pointer to a function for assessing the instance of the actual concept

SEMANTISCHER_TEIL_VON: list of concepts which have the actual one as a semantic part

NOTWENDIGER_TEIL_VON: list of concepts which have the actual one as a necessary part

START_SEMANTISCHE_TEILE: number of semantic parts, and specification of optional parts

START_SEMANTISCHE_ATTRIBUTE: number of semantic attributes, and specification of optional attributes

START_SEMANTISCHE_STRUKTUREN: number of semantic structures, and specification of optional structures

START_NOTWENDIGE_TEILE: number of necessary parts, and specification of optional parts

START_NOTWENDIGE_ATTRIBUTE: number of necessary attributes, and specification of optional attributes

START_NOTWENDIGE_STRUKTUREN: number of necessary structures, and specification of optional structures

using the following substructures:

parts

> FUNKTIONALE_ROLLE: selector of the substructure (name)

> DEFINITIONSBEREICH: concept being part of the actual one

> MODIFIZIERT: hint whether the actual substructure should superimpose a substructure with the same name referenced in the generalization

attributes

> FUNKTIONALE_ROLLE: selector of the substructure (name)

DEFINITIONSBEREICH: specification of the space of definition

DIMENSION: dimension of the attribute

WERTBERECHNUNG: pointer to a function calculating values from actual input data

MODIFIZIERT: hint whether the actual substructure should superimpose a substructure with the same name referenced in the generalization

MODIFIZIERTE_BERECHNUNG: pointer to a more special function than referenced in the generalization

structures

FUNKTIONALE_ROLLE: selector of the substructure (name)

RELATION: pointer to a test function

MIT_DEN_KOMPONENTEN: list of the arguments of the test function

Substructures are referred to by names called `selectors`. Since there is the possibility of more than one substructure with the same name in different concepts, a special data base is designed listing all concepts which refer to substructures with identical names. This data base supports the facility of explanations of the human interface. A query language needs such a source of knowledge in favour of a rapid access. For instance, the attribute `certainty` is referred to in each of the concepts describing medical diagnoses assessing the admissibility of such a hypotheses in relation to actual input data. Then, queries like `Give me the certainty of all possible diagnoses` can be performed in a quick and userfriendly way.

The library of concepts contains the names of all concepts referred to in the knowledge base and gives labels for those who are not actually defined that is there is no node in the network. Fig. 10 shows a listing of that kind. The procedure for starting an analysis offers this listing to the user who chooses one concept to be verified. If this concept has some specialisations, these ones will also be instantiated that is the request for the verification of a more general concept results in instantiation of a set of goal concepts. The corresponding relations are shown by the editor function `SHOW`, which points out the context of a concept alphanumerically and/or graphically. The latter are graphics like Fig. 3.

A deletion of a concept results in a modification of the concept library by changing the length of that concept to 0 Byte. A replacement of a concept is the combination of the ADD- and DELETE-operator.

name of concept	comment	defined	length of concept	.
motion	description of motion (general concept)	true	1000 Byte	
cycle		false	0 Byte	
.	.	.	.	
.		.		
.		.		

Fig. 10 Library of concepts

Fig. 11 shows all data bases which are created during model generation. The

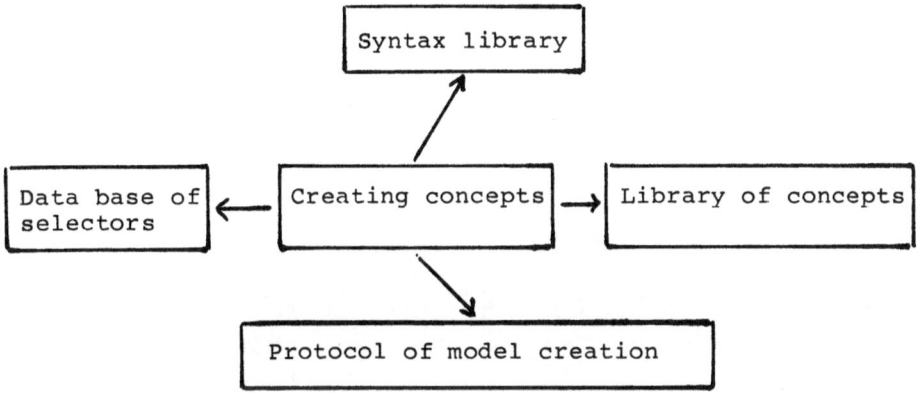

Fig. 11 Data bases accompanying model creation

functions of the editor use those data bases in order to fulfill their tasks mentioned above.

The explanation and justifying facility uses the knowledge base and its accompanying data bases to represent and explain results computed from actual input data. In medical routine at least a physician's letter is needed to describe the diagnosis gotten by an analysis of data of the patient. During an automatic analysis a protocol (search space) is generated which documents the history. So, it is possible to trace the path of decisions. The representation of results and intermediate results is supported by graphics. For instance, contours are superimposed to the original image sequence, the interpretation of volume curves uses medical terms (Fig. 12), or the

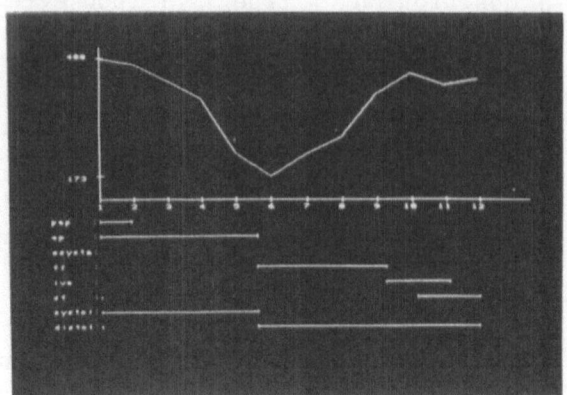

Fig. 12 Medical interpretation of a volume curve

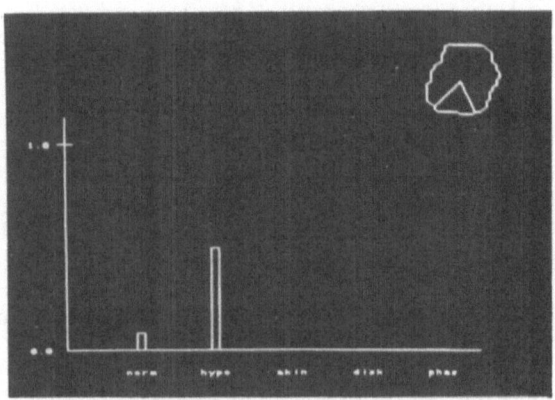

Fig. 13 Presentation of diagnosis concerning the
inferioapical segment

presentation of diagnosis is done by bar graphs (Fig. 13).
Further developments will improve the facilities of the human
interface and expand the knowledge base to offer the

possibility of solving more difficult problems like the comparison of different image sequences taken before and after heart surgeries, for example.

References

[BUC84] Buchanan, B. G.; Shortliffe, E.: Rule-Based Expert Systems: The MYCIN Experiments of the Heuristic Programming Project, Massachussetts, Addison-Wesley, 1984

[BUN82] Bunke, H. et al: Smoothing, Thresholding and Contour Extraction in Images from Gated Blood Pool Studies, Proc. 1st IEEE Comp. Soc. Int. Symposium on Medical Imaging and Image Interpretation, Berlin, 1982, pp. 146-151

[BUN84a] Bunke, H.; Grebner, K.; Sagerer, G.: Syntactic analysis of noisy input strings with an application to the analysis of heart-volume curves, Proc. 7th ICPR, Montreal, 1984, pp. 1145-1147

[BUN84b] Bunke, H.; Sagerer, G.: Use and Representation of Knowledge in Image Understanding Based on Semantic Networks, Proc. 7th ICPR, Montreal, 1984

[BUN84c] Bunke, H.: Segmentation of the Left Ventricle in Scintigraphic Image Sequences, Proc. of Int. Conf. on Digital Signal Processing, Florenz, 1984

[HOF85] Hofmann, I.; Niemann, H.; Sagerer, G.: Model Based Interpretation of Image Sequences from the Heart, Proc. Pattern Recognition in Practice, Amsterdam, to appear 1985

[MIL82] Miller, R. A.; Pople, H. E.; Myers, J. D.: INTERNIST-I, an experimental computer-based diagnostic consultant for general internal medicine, New England Journal of Medicine, August 19, 1982, pp. 468-476

[MIT84] Mittal, S.; Chandrasekaran, B.; Sticklen, J.: Patrec: A knowledge-directed database for a diagnostic expert system, COMPUTER, Sep. 1984

[NIE81] Niemann, H.: Pattern Analysis, Berlin, Springer-Verlag, 1981

[NIE85] Niemann, H.; Bunke, H.; Hofmann, I.; Sagerer, G.; Wolf, F.; Feistel, H.: A Knowledge Based System for Analysis of Gated Blood Pool Studies, IEEE Transactions on Pattern Analysis and Machine Intelligence, vol. PAMI-7, no. 3, May 1985

[PAT85] Patel-Schneider, P.; Brachman, R. J.; Levesque, H. J.:
ARGON: Knowledge Representation meets Information
Retrieval, Proceedings of the CAIA 1984, pp. 280-286

[SAG85] Sagerer, G.: Darstellung und Nutzung von
Expertenwissen fuer ein Bildanalysesystem, Dissertation,
Lehrstuhl fuer Informatik 5, Universitaet Erlangen-
Nuernberg, in preparation to appear 1985

[WEI81] Weiss, S. M.; Kulikowski, C. A.: Expert consultation
systems: The EXPERT and CASNET projects, Machine
Intelligence, Infotech State of the Art Report 9, no. 3,
1981

ULTRASONIC TISSUE CHARACTERIZATION USING A DIAGNOSTIC EXPERT SYSTEM

D.SCHLAPS, U.RÄTH, J.F.VOLK, I.ZUNA, A.LORENZ, K.J.LEHMANN, D.LORENZ, G.VAN KAICK, W.J.LORENZ

1.INTRODUCTION AND BACKGROUND

Conventional gray scale B-mode ultrasound is a commonly applied and useful method for a large number of diseases. The operator dependency, however, is limiting its clinical usefulness as well as the reproducability of an examination.

Due to this, varying diagnostic accuracies have been reported by several authors (1,5,8). A computer assisted approach to ultrasonic tissue characterization therefore should provide means for the extraction of quantitative data from an ultrasound examination in order to obtain reliable diagnostic information or other data indicating subtle changes meaningful for the planning or follow-up of therapies.

Two different approaches can be chosen to achieve this goal:

The physical measurement of ultrasonic tissue properties attempts to quantify

ultrasonic velocity

and attenuation properties

from reflected or transmitted ultrasound signals (3,4,18,20,21,22) . Due to various distortions occurring within the nonhomogeneous medium and because of reflections from many irregularly shaped interfaces, any physical characterization method will be faced with several problems:

When reflection signal data is used, sufficient signal segments must be available for radiofrequency data analysis (at least 3 cm). But this is not guaranteed in small organ applications as kidney and thyroid. Even in the liver application, problems occur since local inhomogeneities (e.g. vessels) do exist and have to be avoided. Additionally, only diffuse tissue alterations can be examined, thereby excluding the clinically interesting analysis of tumor tissue for therapy follow-up studies.

On the other hand, Kuc (20,21,22) has shown promising results in the differentiation of diffuse liver tissue patterns (i.e. fatty, normal and cirrhotic tissues) using frequency-dependent attenuation parameters.

Another approach for the in-vivo characterization of tissues using ultrasound data is based on image pattern analysis techniques (2,5,7,8,13,14,15,17). Here, the complex patterns in the greyscale ultrasound image are used to define tissue specific signatures, which can be used for tissue type identification. Because the two spatial dimensions are used in the analysis, the minimum data requirements are less restrictive than in the physical approach and the range of potential clinical applications is extended towards tumor recognition, classification and therapy follow-up.

The limitation of this method is the greylevel texture being dependent on the physical and electronic processing characteristics of the ultrasound system components. Although some of these problems can be reduced by deconvolution preprocessing with system transfer functions, standardized system settings as well as regular inspection of the system functions using ultrasound phantoms are necessary to obtain reliable tissue analysis results.

In a clinical study Räth et al. (5,8) have shown, that under these provisions, computer – assisted tissue characterization using image analysis even is superior to independent human observers in the diagnosis of hepatocellular disease.

In the following an integrated approach to ultrasound tissue characterization is presented based on the dual-mode analysis of radiofrequency and image data. The quantitative information obtained from the parameter extraction modules is stored in a diagnostic knowledge base and can be retrieved for diagnostic or therapeutic purpose. The system design features a statistical learning concept in order to make the system adaptive to changing clinical environments.

Thanks to microminiaturization, the system is running on a Hewlett Packard HP-1000/A600 microcomputer being interfaced to a Hewlett Packard HP 77020A electronic sector scanner employing a 3.5 MHz transducer (see Fig. 1). The examination of a patient typically takes 10 to 30 minutes and a diagnostic report is printed after the examination is finished.

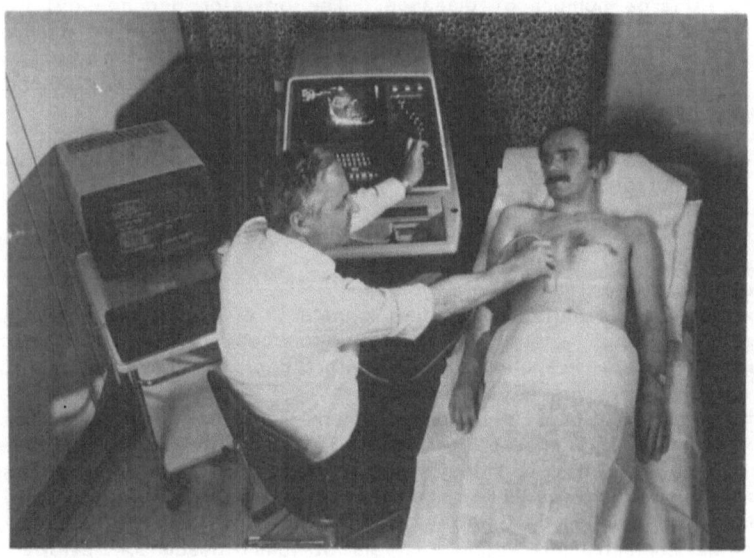

FIGURE 1. Ultrasound system and computer terminal arrangement

2. MATERIALS AND METHODS
2.1 The data acquisition step

During the patient's examination, the physician designates a region of interest in the image using the softkeys of the computer terminal (see Fig. 2). When the region-of-interest has been accepted, the video image sector is acquired in 120 consecutive signals of 396 points each, with an amplitude resolution of 6 bits. After this, the radiofrequency data is accessed from the output of the time gain compensation amplifier at a frequency of 16 MHz and an amplitude resolution of 8 bits within the selected region-of-interest.

From the video data, a 128*128 ultrasound image matrix is reconstructed. Every single line is transferred into the correct position within the image frame. Gaps between neighboring video lines are filled by interpolation (Interpolation Scan Conversion). Finally, the region-of-interest coordinates are mapped into the image frame defining the matrix area from where texture parameters will be extracted.

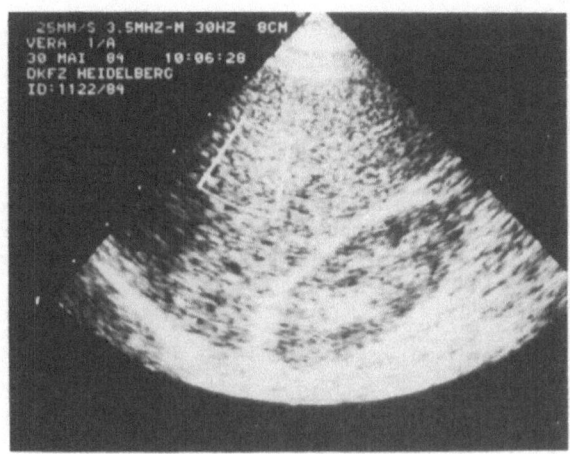

FIGURE 2. Ultrasound image with region-of-interest

2.2 The parameter extraction step

   2.2.1 Image texture parameters. Psychophysicists have classified image textures into the groups of first order and higher order textures (19). Here, first order texture is the type of spatial greylevel distributions which can be characterized in full extent by their greylevel histogram, displaying the occurrence frequencies of the greylevels in the image.

   The second order textures, however, are not sufficiently characterized by their greylevel histogram. In addition to the greylevel profile the spatial distribution (i.e. the spatial interdependencies between the image elements) must be specified for unambiguity. Therefore when texture features like contrast, local inhomogeneities and microstructures are of interest, the second order greylevel statistics should be analyzed (9,10,11,12).

   On the following pages, image texture analysis methods using first order as well as higher order greylevel statistics will be presented.

   2.2.1.1. Parameters from the first order greylevel distribution. These parameters are derived from the sampled greylevel histogram. They describe the shape of the first-order greylevel distribution without considering spatial interdependencies.

The mean greylevel

$$g_{ave} = (1/N) * \sum_{(i,j) \in R} g(i,j)$$

   using

   $g(i,j)$: Greylevel in pixel (i,j)
   R   : Region-of-Interest; selected
             by the operator

The variance of greylevels

$$v_g = (1/N) * \sum_{(i,j) \in R} (g(i,j) - g_{ave})^2$$

The skewness of the greylevel distribution

$$s = \frac{(1/N) * \sum_{(i,j) \quad R} (g(i,j) - g_{ave})^3}{\left(\sqrt{\sum_{(i,j) \in R} g(i,j)^2 - g_{ave}^2}\right)^3}$$

The skewness or the third central moment characterizes the deviation of the greylevel distribution from a symmetrical reference distribution. A positive s-value therefore characterizes a left-skew distribution, whereas a negative value indicates skewness to the right.

The curtosis of the histogram

$$c = \frac{(1/N) * \sum_{(i,j) \in R} (g(i,j) - g_{ave})^4}{\left(\sqrt{\sum_{(i,j) \in R} g(i,j)^2 - g_{ave}^2}\right)^4}$$

The curtosis value c characterizes the steepness of the greylevel distribution. A positive e-value indicates a distribution function which is steeper than the corresponding normal density function, a negative value characterizes a flat distribution function.

Percentiles of the greylevel histogram

Another approach to quantify the shape of the greylevel histogram is to use the percentiles representation method. The percentiles p_1 , ... ,p_{10} are the greylevel bounds, such that 10*i percent of all pixels have lower greylevels. The first percentile p_1 therefore corresponds to the greylevel which is a (minimum) upper bound for 10 percent of the pixels. The value p_5 corresponds to the median of the greylevel distribution. The p_{10} - value finally gives the smallest upper bound for all greylevels in the selected region-of-interest R (see Fig.3).

Formal definition:

Choose p_i such that

$$\sum_{j=0}^{p_i - 1} h_j < (i/10) * N =< \sum_{j=0}^{p_i} h_j$$

using

R = $\{(i,j)\}$ Selected Region-of-Interest
N = cardinality (R)
h_0 ,...,h_6 : Greylevel histogram in R
h_k = cardinality $\{ (i,j) \in R \mid g(i,j) = k \}$
k= 0,...,G : Greylevels
g(i,j) : Greylevel in pixel (i,j)
G+1 : Number of greylevels

New parameters can be calculated from this elementary parameter set to specify range (p_{80} - p_{20}) and variation coefficient v_g /g_{ave} .

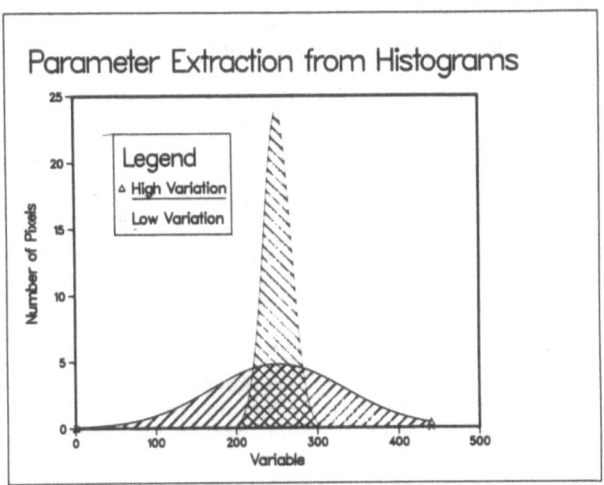

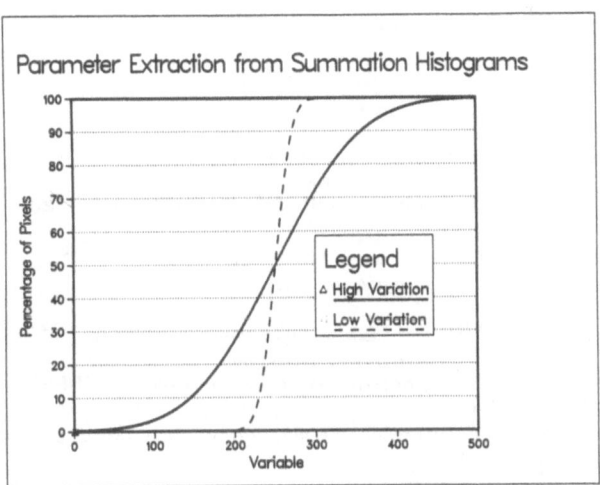

FIGURE 3. Parameter extraction from histograms:
  a) Histograms
  b) Integrated Histograms
   The percentage values preserve the shape of the distributions

2.2.1.2 <u>Parameters</u> <u>from</u> <u>the</u> <u>first-order</u> <u>gradient</u> <u>distribution</u>. The image gradient analysis which characterizes the local greylevel differences, offers a very efficient way to obtain limited second-order greylevel statistics. The absolute values and directions of the gradients (i.e. the directions of maximum greylevel change) can be obtained by the Roberts Operator.

In each pixel (M) a rectangular neighborhood is used to calculate the gradient:

$$\begin{array}{ccccc} A & B & C & D & E \\ F & G & H & I & J \\ K & L & M & N & O \\ P & Q & R & S & T \\ U & V & W & X & Y \end{array}$$

Using this labeling of pixels, the absolute value of the gradient is given by:

$$absv = \sqrt{(W-C)^2 + (O-K)^2}$$

Direction of the gradient:

$$dir = atan((O-K)/(W-C))$$

Sometimes it is necessary to represent gradient direction rather in discrete values than in degrees (e.g. edge images), therefore a strategy for the discretization of the gradient direction has to be defined:
Discretization of the gradient direction into 1,2, ... ,8:

$$w = NearestInteger\left[(4 * dir)/\pi\right] + 1$$

Several parameters can be obtained to characterize the distribution of the gradients:
Mean gradient absolute value:

$$absv_{ave}^+ = (1/N) * \sum_{(i,j)\in R} absv(i,j)$$

$$absv_{ave}^- = (1/N^-) * \sum_{(i,j)\in R, absv(i,j)>0} absv(i,j)$$

Variance of gradient values — with (+) and without (−) zero gradients

$$absv_{var}^+ = (1/N) * \sum_{(i,j)\in R} (absv(i,j) - absv_{ave}^+)^2$$

$$absv_{var}^- = (1/N^-) * \sum_{(i,j)\in R, absv(i,j)>0} (absv(i,j) - absv_{ave}^-)^2$$

Relative frequency of gradient elements in region R (RFE)

$$RFE = N^- / N$$

Most dominant edge direction (MDE); edges are derived from gradients and coded into 1, ..., 4$\left[- \diagup \mid \diagdown\right]$.
Relative frequency of the most dominant edge with respect to the number of gradient elements in the image (RFMDE).

Choose MDE and RFMDE such that

$$
\text{RFMDE} = \text{cardinality} \left\{ (i,j) \mid (i,j) \; \varepsilon \; R, \; \text{absv}(i,j) > 0, \right.
$$
$$
\left. (w(i,j) = \text{MDE or } w(i,j) = \text{MDE} + 4) \right\} =
$$

$$
= \max_{k=1,\ldots,4} \left\{ \text{cardinality} \left\{ (i,j) \mid (i,j) \; \varepsilon \; R, \; \text{absv}(i,j) > 0, \right. \right.
$$
$$
\left. \left. (w(i,j) = k \text{ or } w(i,j) = k+4) \right\} \right\}
$$

using

$$
N^- = \text{cardinality} \left\{ (i,j) \; \varepsilon \; R \mid \text{absv}(i,j) > 0 \right\}
$$

Number of pixels in region R with a nonzero gradient value

2.2.1.3 Parameters from the greylevel cooccurrence matrix.

The cooccurrence matrix Cd (greylevel spatial dependence histogram), first proposed by Haralick (10,11), is a two-dimensional histogram characterizing the occurrence of greylevel combinations in pairs of spatially related pixels. The matrix entry Cd(i,j) thereby specifies, how often two pixels which are separated by a given displacement vector d=(dx,dy) display greylevels i and j respectively. The displacement vector d is specified a priori, limiting the spatial relationships that can be analyzed. Fig. 4 displays a typical cooccurrence matrix in a 3D plot. The one dimensional distributions that result from projection on either of the axes are identical and represent the first-order statistic, the greylevel histogram.

Formal definition:

$$
Cd(i,j) = \text{cardinality} \left\{ ((k,l),(m,n)) \; \varepsilon \; R \times R \mid \right.
$$
$$
|k-m|=dx, \; |l-n|=dy,
$$
$$
\text{sign}((k-m)*(l-n)) = \text{sign}(dx*dy),
$$
$$
\left. g(k,l)=i, \; g(m,n)=j \right\}
$$

using

R : Region-of-interest

g(i,j) : Greylevel in pixel (i,j)

Before statistical parameters are obtained from the cooccurrence matrix, the matrix entries are normalized with respect to the total number of entries. This creates a matrix similar to a Markovian transition probability function for a (dx,dy)- transition :

$$
Cd \longrightarrow Pd : \left\{ p(i,j) \right\} \; ; \quad \sum p(i,j) = 1
$$

Several characteristic features can be extracted from Pd (9,10) :

Contrast

$$
CON = \sum_{i,j} (i-j)^2 * p(i,j)
$$

Angular second moment

$$
ASM = \sum_{i,j} p(i,j)^2
$$

Entropy

$$
ENT = - \sum_{i,j} p(i,j) * \log p(i,j)
$$

The Cooccurrence Matrix

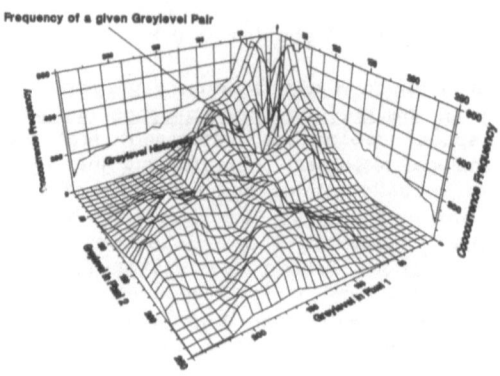

FIGURE 4. The greylevel cooccurrence matrix
Correlation

$$COR = \frac{(\sum i*j*p(i,j) - m_x *m_y)}{\sqrt{s_x^2 * s_y^2}}$$

using

$$m_x = \sum_i i \sum_j p(i,j)$$

$$m_y = \sum_j j \sum_i p(i,j)$$

$$s_x^2 = \sum_i i \sum_j p(i,j) - m_x^2$$

$$s_y^2 = \sum_j j \sum_i p(i,j) - m_y^2$$

CON is characterizing the contrast in the region-of-interest. Frequently occurring large greylevel differences increase the CON – value, whereas soft texture results in small CON – values. ASM and ENT characterize the distribution of cooccurrence matrix entries in a greylevel – independent way. ASM increases when the cooccurrence matrix values are clustering around a major greylevel transition. This corresponds to a situation where only a small number of different greylevel transitions exist. ENT measures the homogeneity or uniformity of the p(i,j) – values, and therefore it increases with increasing coarseness of the image texture. COR finally measures the linearity of the relationship of the greylevels in d – related pixels; this corresponds to an edge in Figure 4.

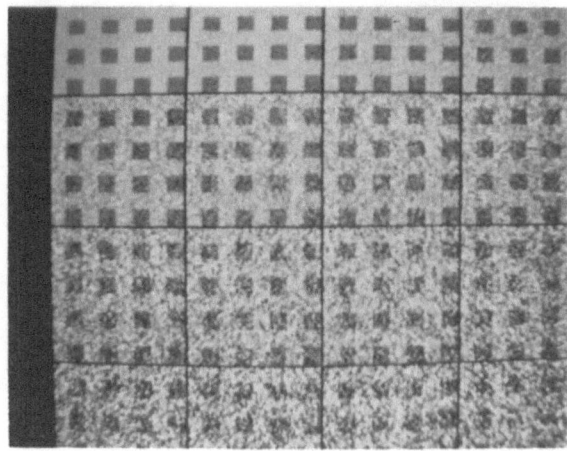

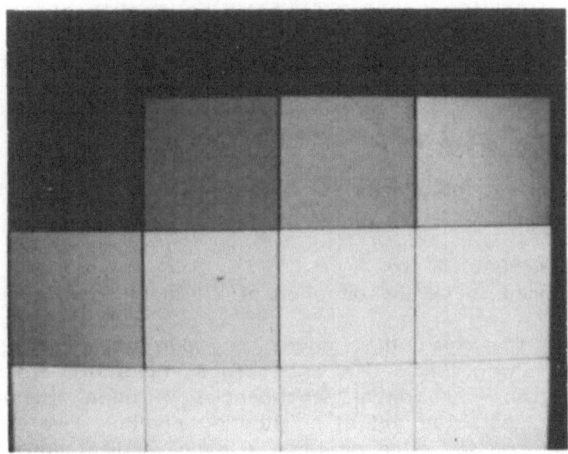

FIGURE 5. The response of the parameters Contrast and Entropy to additive noise
   a) The test images
   b) Response of Contrast (CON)

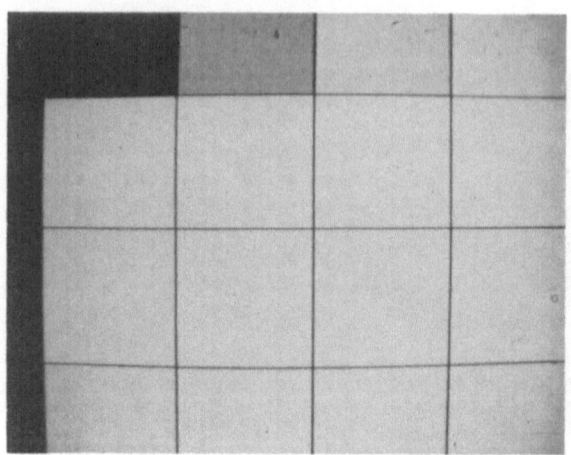

FIGURE 5. c) Response of Entropy (ENT)

Although CON and ENT seem to be very similar, they demonstrate very different sensitivities. This is demonstrated in a series of artificial images in Fig. 5. Beginning with a noisefree image (Fig.5a), the amount of noise is increased linearly in 16 steps. Figures 5b and 5c demonstrate the response of the CON and ENT parameters. It is obvious, that ENT is very much more sensitive to subtle deviations from regular patterns than the contrast parameter.

In our study, eight displacement vectors were chosen:

  a.) Close displacement between neighboring pixels
     (dx,dy ε $\{0,2\}$)
     East-West,North-South,Northwest-Southeast,Northeast-Southwest

  b.) Wide displacement between spatially separated pixels
     (dx,dy ε $\{0,4\}$)
     E-W, N-S, Nw-Se, Ne-Sw

East-West is assumed to be the direction of the incident ultrasound beam in the image.

2.2.1.4. Parameters from the edge cooccurrence matrix. The edge cooccurrence matrix along edges (Ka) and across edges (Kl) are two-dimensional histograms characterizing the spatial dependencies of edge directions obtained in gradient pixels with a selected set of neighboring pixels. Two sets of neighbors are chosen depending on the edge direction in each gradient pixel (11) .

Definition of neighborhood:
   The two hour-glass shaped patterns display the set of neighbors which are chosen for each one of 8 edge directions. The edge direction can be obtained from the gradient direction by a rotation of -90 degrees.
a.) Along edges

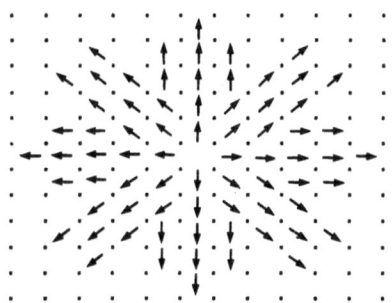

b.) Across edges

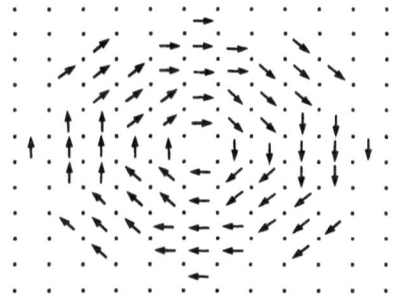

   In the calculation of the edge cooccurrence matrix, the corresponding set of neighbors is determined for each gradient pixel ((i,j) (absv(i,j) > 0)) edge laterally as well as edge axially and the cooccurrence matrix is updated. After completion of this procedure, the cooccurrence matrices are normalized and the parameters CON, ASM, ENT and COR are calculated.
   This set of parameters is characterizing the shape of contours near local inhomogeneities in the ultrasound image (Vessels, tumours, metastases, cysts etc.)
   2.2.1.5 Parameters from the greylevel cooccurrence matrix based on edge maxima. Using the earlier introduced method of neighborhood selection, greylevel cooccurrences can be determined in gradient pixels (11). Two greylevel cooccurrence matrices are obtained and characterized by CON, ASM, ENT and COR values. This set of parameters allows the quantification of enhancement characteristics of local inhomogeneities in the ultrasound image.
   2.2.1.6 Parameters from the greylevel runlength histograms. The two-dimensional greylevel runlength histogram counts the number of greylevel runs by their length and greylevel range. A run hereby corresponds to a set of vertically or horizontally neighboring pixels displaying similar greylevels.

The Greylevel Runlength Matrix

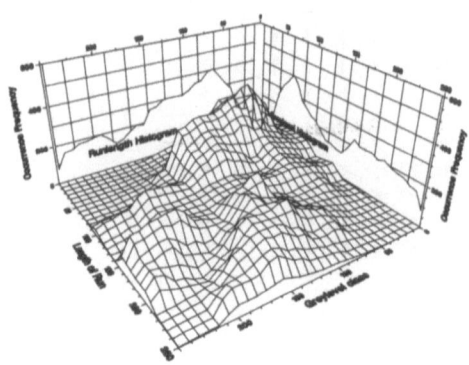

FIGURE 6. The greylevel runlength matrix

Although Figure 6 seems to suggest considerable similarities between the greylevel runlength histogram and the cooccurrence matrix, the concepts are quite different:

The greylevel runlength histogram is a nonsymmetric matrix. The projection on the runlength axis yields a runlength histogram, whereas the projection onto the greylevel axis again produces a greylevel histogram. Therefore, the greylevel runlength histogram in fact joins the two properties: spatial distribution and spectral intensity.

The count distribution of the histograms can be characterized by the following parameters:

Run percentages

$$RPERC = (1/N) * \sum_{l,g} GRHIST(l,g)$$

Long-run emphasis

$$LREM = (1/N) * \sum_{l,g} l^2 * GRHIST(l,g)$$

Greylevel distribution

$$GDIST = (1/N) * \sum_{g} \left[\sum_{l} GRHIST(l,g) \right]^2$$

Runlength distribution

$$RLDIST = (1/N) * \sum_{l} \left[\sum_{g} GRHIST(l,g) \right]^2$$

using

N : The number of pixels in region-of-interest R

GRHIST(l,g): The number of runs of length l and greylevel g in region R

RPERC characterizes the distribution of runs; this parameter increases with increasing inhomogeneity of the texture. In a homogeneous image, when only a small number of runs is present, the run percentages are small. The long-run emphasis LREM is largely dependent on the occurrence of long runs. The greylevel distribution GDIST characterizes the greylevel uniformity of the runs, whereas the length uniformity is expressed by the run length distribution parameter RLDIST. A texture pattern displaying uniformly coloured or uniformly spaced greylevel runs will be characterized by a high GDIST or a high RLDIST value respectively.

2.2.1.7 Parameters from the two-dimensional power spectrum. In this study, the two-dimensional power spectrum was obtained by the Fourier transformation of the 2D autocorrelation function (Wiener–Khinchin Theorem)(12).
Autocorrelation function

$$a'(u,v) = (1/N(u,v)) * \sum\sum_{((x,y),(x+u,y+v)) \, \epsilon \, RxR} g(x,y)*g(x+u,y+v)$$

using
$$N(u,v) = \text{cardinality} \left\{ ((x,y),(x+u,y+v)) \, \epsilon \, RxR \right\}$$

for u,v : $-16 =< u,v =< 15$
Fourier transforming $a'(u,v)$ yields the power spectral density $S'(r,f)$.

$$S'(r,f) = (1/32) \sum a'(u,v) * \exp(-j*2\pi(ru+fv)/32)$$

$$-16 =< u,v =< 15$$

for r,f: $-16 =< r,f =< 15$
After $S'(r,f)$ has been calculated, several parameters are extracted describing the three-dimensional shape of the power spectral density.

The power spectrum ring sums R_1 , ... ,R_4 characterize the distribution of energy with respect to frequency. The inner ring sum R_1 measures the low-frequency energy contents in the image signal, whereas the outer ring sum R_4 is expressing the high frequency contribution.

RING SUMS   SECTOR SUMS

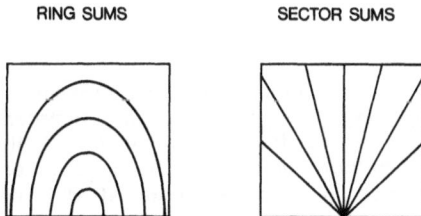

FIGURE 7: a) Power spectrum ring and sector sums
The power spectrum sector sums S_1 to S_8 characterize directional differences in the energy contribution. Anisotropic texture yields highly different sector sums, whereas in isotropic texture the sector sums are similar.

2.2.1.8 Parameters analyzing the speckle texture. As in radar images, speckle texture is typical for ultrasonic images. Although it is well known that speckles are largely device – dependent, the speckle texture still might contain some information about the tissue. To characterize the distribution of speckles in the image, a set of one-dimensional slices through the two-dimensional power spectrum is obtained. For each one-dimensional spectrum a level-crossing analysis is performed yielding the expected number of level crossings. In our approach we use the 60 percent greylevel threshold for speckle extraction.

Formal approach:

According to the theory of stochastic processes, the 2i-th moments of a spectral density $F(\lambda)$ of a real-valued stationary process $x(t)$ which is normally distributed with mean 0 are given by:

$$\lambda_{2i} = \int \lambda^{2i} \; dF(\lambda) \; ; \quad i=0,1,2,3, \ldots$$

A level crossing event at time t_x is characterized by:

$$\exists \exists_{t1<tx, t2>tx} \left[(x(t_1) - u) * (x(t_2) - u) < 0 \right]$$

A random variable D_u can be defined representing the number of u – crossings during the time interval $[0,T]$. The expectation value of $D_u (0,T)$ is given by:

$$E\left\{ D_u (0,T) \right\} = (T/\pi) * \sqrt{\lambda_2 / \lambda_0} * \exp(-u^2 / 2\lambda_0^2)$$

NUMBER OF 60%-LEVEL CROSSINGS
for given Spectral Density Slices
Orientation of Slices :

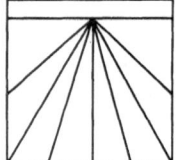

FIGURE 7: b) The spectral slicing applied for level crossing analysis

2.2.2 Radiofrequency parameter extraction. In comprehensive articles Kuc (20,21,22) has proposed a method for the estimation of the slope of acoustic attenuation. Basically the method relies on the calculation of the logarithmic difference of spectra obtained in data segments at different depths. Since the first studies, the tissue property of a low – pass filter for ultasonic energy is well known for causing a downshift of the far data segment spectrum towards lower frequencies. Looking at the logarithmic difference of the two spectra as a function of frequency, a linear relationship can be assumed. This is justified by the linear attenuation property of the tissue. Applying regression analysis to the logarithmic difference data therefore will yield the slope-of-attenuation coefficient.

Another approach to the measurement of attenuation is the spectral shift method. Here, the immediate frequencies are obtained in the near and the far data segment. An estimate of the acoustic attenuation can be obtained using the relationship (22) :

$$beta_{shift} = (4.34*(F_n - F_f))/(B^2 *D) \quad dB/MHz/cm$$

using

F_n , F_f : Frequencies in near and
far data segments

B : Bandwidth measure

D : Segment displacement in cm

The immediate frequencies can be estimated using the number of zero crossings in the raw data or in the autocorrelation function. The frequency is related to the number of zero level crossings by the formula:

$$F = N_z / (2 * M * T)$$

using

N_z : Number of zero crossings

M : Number of samples of the signal
(resp. maximum lag of autocorrelation function)

T : Time Interval

Another method for the estimation of the immediate frequency is to use the median value of the power spectrum (Center frequency method).

2.3 The decision making step

When the parameters are calculated, the list of the currently most discriminating parameter subset is selected from the knowledge base and a linear discriminant classification rule is applied. According to the discriminant scores and the prior probability settings, the most likely diagnosis is calculated (6,16).

As soon as the histology result becomes available, the patient parameter data eventually needs to be reordered within the knowledge base. This occurs if the patient was misclassified in the past, requiring the knowledge base to reorganize itself automatically in order to maintain data consistency (see Fig. 8).

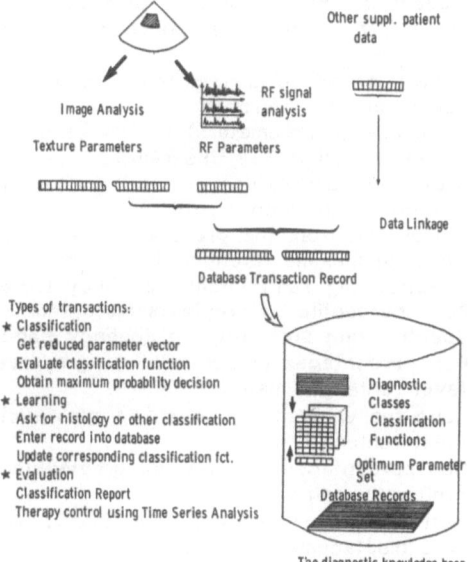

FIGURE 8. The knowledge base of the ultrasonic tissue characterization system

When the parameter set yielding maximum classification performance needs to be reevaluated, the following processing steps are activated:

1. Forty parameters yielding the highest T-test rankings over all groups are determined.

2. Twenty parameters are excluded from the original start set, if they are contributing to high entries in parameter crosscorrelation matrix. Parameters are excluded in a step-by-step manner.

3. The remaining twenty parameters are checked out in a series of discriminant analyses. In every single analysis one parameter will be dropped temporarily in order to obtain the corresponding classification accuracy (Hit rate). When every parameter of the current parameter set has been tried, the hit rates of all parameters that were dropped tentatively will be compared and a decision is made whether a parameter should be dropped permanently. When a parameter can be identified to minimize the classification accuracy, it will be eliminated and the correspondingly reduced parameter set will be carried into the next iteration. The parameter reduction process finishes when every potential parameter removal yields an accuracy lower than the current hit rate.

The extracted parameter list is presented to the physician who then decides whether or not the decision functions in the knowledge base should be updated.

3. RESULTS

For the evaluation of the texture analysis parameters 44 histologically well defined patients with a broad spectrum of liver disease and 13 healthy controls were examined. In the patient group, 27 persons were suffering from diffuse liver disease (i.e. cirrhosis and/or fibrosis), and 17 persons being tumor patients. No biopsy was performed on the group of normals, but strict selection criteria make liver disease in this diagnostic class very unlikely. Up to 3 parallel ultrasound images were acquired from each patient. Therefore, the sample numbers displayed in the following figures and tables always refer to the number of images actually used in the analysis. Statistical dependencies between the images of a patient are reduced by ultrasound slice-to-slice gap generally exceeding 1 cm.

The results of the liver tissue discrimination using image analysis are shown in Figure 9. Depending on the number of parameters used, the classification accuracies vary from 87% (9 parameters) to 60% (1 parameter).

The following parameter ranking was observed:

(Best:)   IM1 Grey level distribution in rows; 64 greylevels, from the greylevel runlength matrix

         IM2 Correlation from the greylevel cooccurrence matrix based on edge maxima (along edge)

         IM3 Spectral ring sum, upper frequency band

         IM4 70 - percentile of greylevel histogram

         IM5 Spectral ring sum, lower frequency band

         IM6 Run percentages in columns, 64 greylevels, from the grey-level runlength matrix

         IM7 Long run emphasis in rows, 64 greylevels, from the grey-level runlength matrix

         IM8 Run percentages in rows, 64 greylevels, from the greylevel runlength matrix

         IM9 Correlation from the greylevel cooccurrence matrix, short W-E displacement

         IM10 Spectral sector sum 36 - 45 degrees

         IM11 Spectral sector sum 45 - 64 degrees

         IM12 Spectral sector sum 90 -116 degrees

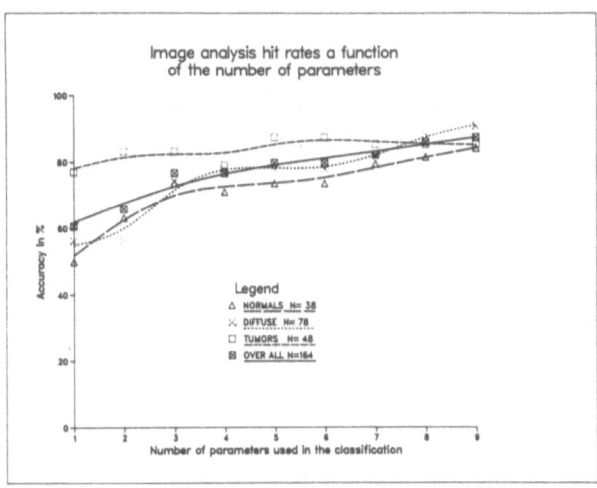

FIGURE 9. Image analysis hit rates as a function of the number of parameters

When the radiofrequency parameters are evaluated for tissue discrimination, the classification accuracies are consistently lower than for the image analysis approach. As mentioned above, the severe limitations of this approach do require minimum lengths of the radiofrequency segments being analyzed. In our study, the size of the region-of-interest was very often not sufficient for the physical parameter extraction method. Therefore, 3 patient subgroups corresponding to the minimum Near-to-Far segment displacements of 1.5 cm, 2 cm and 2.5 cm had to be defined. The population of the subgroups meeting the most rigorous requirement (2.5 cm) therefore was reduced to 9 normal images and 12 images from fibrotic or cirrhotic patients.

The classification results depending on the minimum displacement requirements are displayed in Figure 10. The classification accuracies that were obtained using 4,4 and 7 parameters leveled at 81%, 69.5% and 69% for the subgroups 1.5cm, 2cm and 2.5cm. The sample numbers N displayed in Figure 10 now refer to the number of near and far signal segment pairs that were obtained applying the minimum displacement requirements.

The most discriminating parameter subset was found to be:

(Best:)   RF1   Near segment immediate frequency, from the raw data zero crossing method

                RF2   Slope-of-attenuation from the log (power) spectral difference method

                RF3   Frequency shift from the raw data zero crossing method

                RF4   Near segment immediate frequency from the auto-correlation zero crossing method

                RF5   Far segment immediate frequency from the raw data zero crossing method

When the joint set of radiofrequency and image parameters is used in the discriminant analysis, then only 4 image texture parameters are needed to obtain a classification accuracy of 94% (see Table 1). When discriminant analysis is forced to use RF parameters only, a reduced classification rate of 86% is obtained (see Table 2).

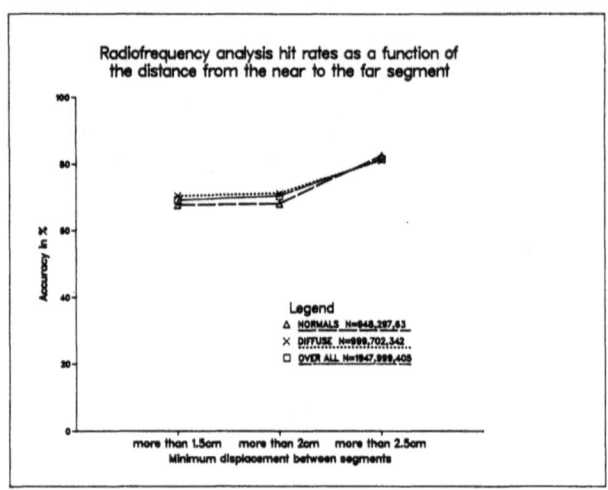

FIGURE 10. Radiofrequency data analysis hit rates as a function of the minimum displacement requirement

From group	Diffuse	Normals	Total
Diffuse	12 (100.0%)	0 (0.0%)	12 (100.0%)
Normals	1 (11.1%)	8 (88.9%)	9 (100.0%)
Total	13 (61.9%)	8 (38.1%)	21 (100.0%)

Overall accuracy: 95.2 %

TABLE 1. Classification rates using 4 image texture parameters

From group	Diffuse	Normals	Total
Diffuse	10 (83.3%)	2 (16.7%)	12 (100.0%)
Normals	1 (11.1%)	8 (88.9%)	9 (100.0%)
Total	11 (52.4%)	10 (47.6%)	21 (100.0%)

Overall accuracy: 85.7 %

TABLE 2. Classification rates using 2 radiofrequency parameters

It is interesting to notice a significant negative correlation between the key parameters of both approaches. Figure 11 shows a plot of the values of the parameters Spectral Sector Sum 26-45 degrees versus the radiofrequency parameter Immediate Frequency In Near Segment; the correlation is −.84.

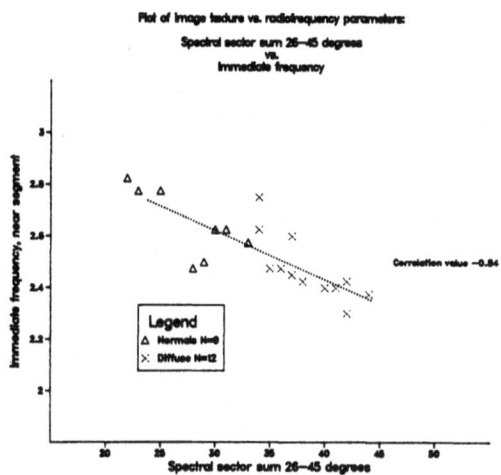

FIGURE 11. Plot of the image texture parameter Spectral Sum in the 26 to 45 degrees sector vs. the immediate frequency of the near radiofrequency segment.

4. DISCUSSION

The superiority of the image analysis approach that has been observed in this study may be due to several reasons:

The ultrasound system being used is an electronic sector scanner and therefore is difficult to characterize in terms of its physical properties. It is using a dynamic focussing method with ten focussing zones which may blurr the attenuation characteristics of the tissue measured from the reflected signals. This is the reason why we were not able to measure attenuation values that are in the range found by other authors. On the other hand, the values that we measured should be highly correlated with the true attenuation characteristics of the tissue. To verify this and to measure the system specific diffraction characteristics, a tissue-like phantom with well-defined attenuation properties is being developed.

The region sizes that we used were smaller than the regions used by other authors (20-22). On the other hand, we are convinced that region sizes exceeding 4cm are not feasible in a clinical routine use of the system; especially with tumor therapy follow-up in mind.

Finally, the time gain compensation characteristics of the system have been neglected. But it is generally accepted that potentially existing inherent nonlinearities should have only minor effects on the attenuation measurement.

The dual mode analysis of ultrasonic radiofrequency and image signal data has shown that there exists a definite relationship between the two approaches. It therefore should be possible to identify system − dependent as well as system −

independent information in the texture pattern of the tissue. This separation of the statistical knowledge base into system – dependent and system – independent domains represents a prerequisite for the transferability of ultrasound tissue characterization methods from one ultrasound machine to another. If transferability can be established, then the approach will become a diagnostic valuable tool as a noninvasive, sensitive and specific clinical test.

5. ACKNOWLEDGEMENTS

The authors are much endebted to Hewlett (Pete) Melton, Paul Magnin and Heinrich Beckermann from Hewlett Packard Medical Division Andover, Mass. and Böblingen, West Germany for the loan of the computer equipment and their contributions to the radiofrequency data acquistion system.

6. REFERENCES

1.Gosink BB, Lemon SK, Scheible W, et al.: Accuracy of Ultrasonography in Diagnosis of Hepatocellular Disease. AJR 133:19–23,1979.

2.Lerski AR, Barnett E, Morley P, et al.: Computer Analysis of Ultrasonic Signals in Diffuse Liver Disease. Ultrasound Med Biol 5:341–350,1979.

3.Sommer GF, Joynt LF, Carroll BA, et al.: Ultrasonic Characterization of Abdominal Tissues via Digital Analysis of Backscattered Waveforms. Radiology 141: 811–817,1981.

4.Jones JP, Leeman S: Ultrasonic Tissue Characterization and Quantitative Ultrasound Scatter Imaging: Methods and Approaches. Proc Int Workshop on Physics and Engineering in Medical Imaging. IEEE Cat.#1751-7,247-258,1982.

5.Räth U, Limberg B, Schlaps D, et al.: Ultrasonic Tissue Characterization in Chronic and Malignant Liver Disease: Subjective Evaluation versus Compu-terized A–Scan and B–Scan Analysis. Abstracts. Ultrasonic Imaging and Tissue Characterization Symposium. Ultrasonic Imaging 5:188, 1983.

6.Schlaps D, Zuna I, Lorenz A, et al.: Comparison of Mathematical Models Used in Diagnostic Computerized Echography. Proc World Congr Med Phys Biomed Eng Hamburg, 1982.

7.Schlaps D, Zuna I, Lorenz A, et al.: Tissue Characterization by Texture Analysis of Ultrasonic B–Mode Images. Abstracts. Ultrasonic Imaging and Tissue Characterization Symposium. Ultrasonic Imaging 5:189, 1983.

8.Räth U, Schlaps D, Limberg B, et al.: Diagnostic Accuracy of Computerized B–Scan Texture Analysis and Conventional Ultrasonography in Diffuse Paren-chymal and Malignant Liver Disease. J Clin Ultrasound 13: 87–99, February 1985.

9.Haralick RM: Statistical and Structural Approaches to Texture. Proc IEEE 67: 786–804, 1979.

10.Haralick RM, Shanmugam K, Dinstein I: Textural Features for Image Classifi-cation. IEEE Trans Syst Man Cybern, Vol SMC-3, No 3, May 1980.

11.Connors RW, Harlow CA: A Theoretical Comparison of Texture Algorithms. IEEE Trans Patt Anal Mach Intell, Vol PAMI-2, No 3,May 1980.

12.Kay SM, Marple SL: Spectrum Analysis – A Modern Perspective. Proc IEEE 69: No 11, Nov 1981.

13.Finette S, Bleier AR, Swindell W: Breast Tissue Classification Using Diagnostic Ultrasound and Pattern Recognition Techniques: I. Methods of Pattern Recognition. Ultrasonic Imaging 5: 55–70, 1983.

14.Finette S, Bleier AR, Swindell W, et al.: Breast Tissue Classification Using Diagnostic Ultrasound and Pattern Recognition Techniques: II. Experimental Results. Ultrasonic Imaging 5: 71–86, 1983.

15.Nicholas D, Nassiri DK, Bamber M, et al.: Classification of Diffuse Liver Disorders by Quantitative Evaluation of Conventional B-Mode Echograms. Proc 5th World Congress of Ultrasound in Medicine and Biology, Brighton 1982.

16.Lachenbruch PA: Discriminant Analysis. New York Hafner Press. Macmillan Publ Co 1975.

17.Lerski RA, Smith MJ, Morley P, et al.: Discriminant Analysis of Ultrasonic Texture Data in Diffuse Alcoholic Liver Disease. Ultrasonic Imaging 3: 164-172, 1982.

18.Lizzi FL, Rorke M, Feleppa EJ, et al.: Characterization of Liver Using Families of Parameters Derived from Spectrum Analysis. Abstracts. Ultrasonic Imaging and Tissue Characterization Symposium. Ultrasonic Imaging 5:188,1983.

19.Julesz B: Visual Pattern Discrimination. IRE Transactions on Information Theory, Vol IT-8, 84-92, 1982.

20.Kuc R, Taylor KJW: Variation of Acoustic Attenuation Coefficient Slope Estimates for In Vivo Liver. Ultrasound Med Biol 4: 401-412, 1982.

21.Kuc R: Clinical Application of an Ultrasound Attenuation Coefficient Estimation Technique for Liver Pathology Characterization. IEEE Trans Biomed Engin, Vol BME-27, No 6, June 1980.

22.Kuc R: Estimating Reflected Ultrasound Spectra from Quantized Signals. IEEE Trans Biomed Engin, Vol BME-32, No 2, February 1985.

AUTOMATIC SEGMENTATION OF CORONARY VESSELS FROM DIGITAL SUBTRACTED ANGIOGRAMS: A KNOWLEDGE-BASED APPROACH

S.A. STANSFIELD

CIS Dept., University of Pennsylvania, Philadelphia, Pa. 19104

ABSTRACT

This paper presents a rule-based expert system for identifying and isolating coronary vessels in digital angiograms. The system is written in OPS5 and LISP and uses low level processors written in C. The system embodies both stages of the vision hierarchy: The low level image processing stage works concurrently with edges (or lines) and regions to segment the input image. Its knowledge is that of segmentation, grouping, and shape analysis. The high level stage then uses its knowledge of cardiac anatomy and physiology to interpret the result and to eliminate those structures not desired in the output.

INTRODUCTION

Diagnosis of the narrowing of coronary vessels via angiographic studies is subject to large inter- and intra-observer variability. A computer-based system for the automatic quantification of arteriograms, however, would be able to create a reproducible measurement of stenosis. Critical to any such process is the segmentation of the coronary vessels from the digital images. Unfortunately, classical pattern classification and segmentation techniques do not perform well on angiographic images. Noise, overlapping structures, variations in background contrast, and variations in the structures themselves, all combine to make the use of such well established techniques inadequate. This paper describes ANGY, an expert system which combines the traditional methods of image processing with techniques from the field of Artificial Intelligence to solve the problem of identifying and isolating the coronary vessels in digital angiograms.

The ANGY system is divided into three separate and independent stages: the preprocessing stage and the two stages embodied in the expert itself. During the preprocessing stage, low level specialists written in C are applied sequentially to the input image. Both an edge and a region analysis are performed; the two representations are then combined, with the edge analysis serving to verify and refine the region segmentation. Finally, the regions are divided into *strips* based on their shape. These strips, along with the edge segments created by the edge anaysis, serve as input to the low level stage of the expert system.

It is the purpose of the expert to isolate the coronary vessels in the segmented image, while eliminating any noise structures which may have arisen from variations in background contrast, imperfect subtraction, or irrelevant anatomical detail. The system is rule-based and is written in OPS5, a high-speed production system interpreter. Some user-defined functions are also written in LISP and/or C. Control within the system is bottom-up or data-driven.

Briefly, a rule-based, or production, system consists of three major components: a data base or short-term-memory (STM); a knowledge-base or long-term-memory (LTM); and a rule interpreter which controls the problem solving process. Knowledge is represented within such a system by condition-action pairs of the form If <conditions> then <actions>. When control is bottom-up, the process works in the following way: The left-hand-sides (LHS) of all productions are evaluated to see which are satisfied given the current state of STM; a production with a satisfied LHS is selected; the actions specified in its right-hand-side are performed and the STM is updated. This cycle is repeated until no rule's LHS can be satisfied. This data-driven approach was chosen for the ANGY system because noise and the natural diversity of the cardiac anatomy make variations in the input image the major consideration.

The expert system itself is separated into two independent stages. In the low level stage, a domain independent knowledge of image segmentation, grouping, and geometric relations is applied to the segmented image created by the preprocessing stage. Rules are applied to join line segments, to merge regions, and to establish such relations as adjacent and parallel. The result is a refined segmentation and a set of relations between the objects in the segmented image.

The high level stage then applies a domain dependent knowledge of cardiac anatomy and physiology to interpret this segmented image. Rules are applied to label objects as vessel or as noise. The labels are then used to either retain or eliminate the labelled object and to guide the system in further processing. Anatomical knowledge is embodied within the system in the form of the spatial relations between objects and the expected characteristics of the objects themselves.

Once the high level stage has labelled the structures in the segmented image, a final binary image may be created containing only those structures which have been labelled as vessel. One application of ANGY is the use of this binary image by a system which automatically quantifies arteriograms based on measurements of video density [7].

THE LOW LEVEL SPECIALISTS

Inputs to the ANGY system are 2-D digital subtracted angiograms of the chest. The low level specialists, a collection of image processing routines written in C, are used to preprocess this input data and to create a representation to be used as input to the expert system. This entails the creation of a segmented image containing both edges and regions and the construction of a 2-D geometric model of the objects it contains.

Below, we describe in detail each of the low level specialists, including their component procedures and the techniques employed.

Edge Segmentation

The input image may be viewed as an array of numeric values in the range 0 to 255. These numbers represent the grey level intensity at each pixel in the digital angiogram. The first intermediate represenation we have chosen to create is the intrinsic image consisting of edge elements or edgels. The edge operator used is a simplified version of one developed by John Canny at MIT [4]. Figure 1b shows the results of running the Canny operator on figure 1a.

The output of the edgel detection process is a binary image with pixels containing edgels set to 255 and all other pixels set to 0. A segmentation procedure is now applied to this intrinsic image. Edge segments are created by applying a recursive subdivision algorithm to approximate series of adjacent and nearly linear edgels as straight line segments. These line segments are parameterized by the coordinates of their endpoints, their slopes, and their lengths.

Region Segmentation

Region analysis is a multi-phase process which begins with the creation of a binary image via thresholding. The inputs to the thresholder are the original image, the average and standard deviation for some background patch in the image, and a grid size. The thresholding proceeds as follows: Given a grid size N, the input image is divided into N X N windows. For each N X N window, the statistics (average and standard deviation of greyscale) within the window are calculated. Based upon these statistics, a decision is made as to whether there is an object within the window. If so, the greyscales are thresholded. Figure 2a shows the results of running the thresholder on figure 1a with a window size of 30 X 30. Note from figure 2a, that the thresholding process tends to create a lot of "salt-and-pepper" noise in the final binary image. The second step in the region analysis is to find the connected components, while eliminating these spurious noise points. This is the job of the region finder.

The region finder looks consecutively at each object point in the binary output of the thresholder. It assumes that each is a valid region point and attempts to find the connected region of which it is a part. Four point connectivity is used. The output of the region finder is a binary image, a file of region points, and a file of region descriptors. Figure 2b shows the results of the region finder run on figure 2a.

The next step is to grow the regions detected by the last two processes within the original image. In this way we may compensate for the gaps in larger objects left as a result of the thresholding process. For each region discovered by the region finder, the region grower attempts to grow the region by adding new points which it believes are also a part of the region. This time, however, a new point is accepted as part of the region if the greyscales of all four of its neighbors fall within a range determined by the average and standard deviation of the greyscale of the original region. The result of the region growing process is yet another binary image, to which the region finder is then reapplied.

Converging The Evidence

A quick look at figures 1a and 3a (which shows the final region and edge analyses combined) will show that the edge analysis gives us too much information, while the region analysis gives us too little. A sensible thing to do at this point, then, is to bring together the two representations, letting one serve to refine and verify the other. We call this step "converging the evidence." Accepting the regions created by the region analysis as indicative of "real" objects in the original image (we choose the region analysis over the edge analysis because it tends to be more "conservative" in its operation,) we now combine the two representations and attempt to use the edge analysis to guide us in the refinement of the region analysis. The process works as follows: The edges and regions are combined and input into a set of processes which attempt to detect which edges correspond to region boundaries and then, where necessary, to "fill out" and grow these regions to meet their boundaries. In cases where boundaries correspond to two or more atomic regions, a merging of the regions will take place. Figure 3b shows the results of the application of these processes.

We are now ready to determine the final regions and to create the 2-D represenation which will be used by both stages of the expert system.

The Strip Detector

The input to the strip detector is a binary image created by the edge/region analysis. Its purpose is to segment the regions into what we have chosen to call "strips." A strip is defined as a set of runs of similar width which are adjacent either above or below. A run is a set of region pixels which are adjacent either left or right. Strips are parameterized by elongation (length over wdith), length, width, average and standard deviation of greyscale, and by the trapezoid defined by the endpoints of the first and last run of the strip.

This representation was chosen because the primary objects of interest are coronary blood vessels -- in reality, long, thin strips! Because of the condition that the widths of runs within a strip not vary greatly, large regions whose shape varies greatly will be divided into many strips, while small and/or highly elongated regions will be comprised of only a few. Hence the strip representaion will split, based on shape, those objects which the region analysis, using a different set of criteria, viewed as one object. The output of the strip detector is a file of strips and a set of data records containing the above descriptors. These descriptors are the primary region representation used by the expert system. Figure 4a shows the trapezoidal representation of figure 1a.

THE EXPERT SYSTEM

The expert system portions of the ANGY system are rule-based and are written in OPS5, a high speed production system interpreter. The expert is divided into two separate and independent stages -- the low level image processing stage and the high level recognition or labelling stage. Within each stage, the rules are partitioned; a deterministic "meta-driver" participates in the transition from one subsystem to another.

Structure and Control in the ANGY System

The ANGY system is essentially a data driven, or bottom up, system. This approach was chosen for two reasons. First, while the images themselves are not complex (ie. the structure of the objects is simple and the number of objects is small), the images contain a great deal of noise (caused by variations in background contrast, subtraction artifacts, etc.) And second, the cardiac anatomy itself varies from subject to subject. (Variations in the visibility of the coronary structures arise from two sources. One is the natural diversity of the cardiac anatomy. The other is due to the fact that the contrast medium must circulate through the system. Those structures which do not contain contrast when the image is created will probably not be visible or will be only partially visible.)

Unfortunately, when images serve as the input to a data driven system, problems can arise. Unlike other forms of input, images tend to produce large amounts of data and hence large numbers of options for the system which must deal with it. Almost immediately -- even with a manageable number of rules -- the problem of influencing the interactions among productions becomes a difficult one to handle.

This problem also arises in production systems which have a large number of productions; and we have chosen a solution which is often used in these systems. Within each stage of the ANGY system, the productions are partitioned into subsystems. Some of the rules in each subsystem are dedicated to the task of arranging transfer to another subsystem. To be more specific, each of the productions within a given subsystem has, as an additional LHS condition, the requirement that the "goal" to be within that subsystem be active. None of the rules within that subsystem can fire unless this active goal is in working memory. The top level control has the task of generating these goals. Within each subsystem, control is purely data driven. When none of the rules in the active subsystem can be matched, control is returned to the top level which then causes the transition to the next subsystem.

The Low Level Stage

The low level stage of the expert contains the domain independent knowledge. It is similar (although on a much smaller scale) to that designed by Nazif and Levine [9]. In general, the knowledge embodied here is that of image segmentation, grouping, and geometric relations. It works concurrently with the edge and region representations developed by the preprocessors. The knowledge in this stage is divided into two classes: that which operates on lines and that which operates on regions.

Lines input into the system are parameterized by their slope, length, and the coordinates of their endpoints. The OPS5 memory element has the form

```
(literalize line
   key slope length
   x1 y1 x2 y2)
```

Regions are similarly defined.

Because the data structures and type of processing done by this stage are not easily implemented in OPS5, many of the actions in the RHSs of the rules are written in LISP and C. These routines are controlled via the OPS5 productions. Below, we discuss the knowledge and actions in this stage and provide some examples of its rules.

Line Relations. The system attempts to establish geometric relations between the lines in STM. These relations are then used by the system to make further processing decisions. The line relations currently implemented are linked-to (eg. two lines share a common endpoint or have endpoints within some neighborhood of each other), parallel-to, perpendicular, and intersects. The "knowledge" that a relation exists is in the form of a memory element. For example, the intersects relation looks like this

```
(literalize intersects
   line1 line2
   ix iy)
```

where line1 and line2 are the intersecting lines and (ix, iy) is the point of intersection.

A typical example of a production in this class is

```
(p link-e1e1
   (goal ^type run-lines ^status active)
   (line <k1> {} {} <ex1> <ey1> {} {} )
   (line {<k2> <> <k1>} {} {} <ex1> <ey1> {} {} )
  -(lghost <k1>)
  -(lghost <k2>)
  -(linked-to ^line1 <k2> ^line2 <k1> {} {})
  -->
   (make linked-to ^line1 <k1> ^line2 <k2> ^del-dist 0.0
                   ^config e1e1 ^type s))
```

This production is attempting to discover lines for which endpoint1 of line1 is the same as endpoint1 of line2. It may be translated as saying "If there are two distinct lines which are not already related by a linked-to relation, and if they have a common endpoint, and if this endpoint is endpoint1 for both of them, then establish a linked-to relation for these lines.*

Line Operations. The only operation performed on lines is to join two line segments into a longer segment. An example is the following production, which joins two lines if they are linked and if their slopes are sufficiently close

```
(p join-lines
  (goal ^type run-lines ^status active)
  (linked-to <k1> <k2> {} <config> {})
 -(lghost <k1>)
 -(lghost <k2>)
  (parallel-to <k1> <k2>)
  (line <k1> <s1> <l1> <x1-1> <y1-1> <x2-1> <y2-1>)
  (line <k2> <s2> <l2> <x1-2> <y1-2> <x2-2> <y2-2>)
 -->
  (make lghost <k1>)
  (make lghost <k2>)
  (call make-new-line <x2-1> <y2-1> <x2-2> <y2-2>))
```

Trapezoid Relations. Two relations between regions exist. These are adjacent and similar. Two regions are similar if their greyscales are within some delta of one another. They are adjacent in the usual sense of the word. There are two types of adjacency: above and right (below and left are redundant.) Like many of the line relations, the adjacent relation is really established by a set of LISP routines. The production which invokes these routines is

```
(p get-adjrel
  (goal ^type run-traps ^status active)
  (trap <key1> {} {} {} {}
        <ux1-1> <ux2-1> <uy2-1> <lx1-1> <lx2-1> <ly2-1>)
  (trap {<key2> <> <key1>} {} {} {} {}
        <ux1-2> <ux2-2> <uy2-2> <lx1-2> <lx2-2> <ly2-2>)
 -(tghost <key1>)
 -(tghost <key2>)
 -(adjrel {} <key1> <key2>)
 -->
  (call lget-adjrel <key1> <ux1-1> <ux2-1> <uy2-1> <lx1-1>
                    <lx2-1> <ly2-1> <key2> <ux1-2> <ux2-2>
                    <uy2-2> <lx1-2> <lx2-2> <ly2-2>))
```

where lget-adjrels is the user defined function which does the work.

Trapezoid Operations. The operation performed on trapezoids is the merge. Two trapezoids are merged into a new trapezoid if they are adjacent, their greyscales are sufficiently similar, and they are *positioned* correctly with respect to one another. One production which carries out this task looks like

```
(p try-merge-above
  (trap <key1> <e1> <l1> <w1> <a1> <ux1-1> <ux2-1>
```

```
          <uy2-2> <lx1-1> <lx2-1> <ly2-1> )
   (adjrel ^position above <key1> <key2>)
  -(tghost <key1>)
  -(tghost <key2>)
   (trap <key2> <e2> <l2> <w2> <a2> <ux1-2> <ux2-2>
          <uy2-2> <lx1-2> <lx2-2> <ly2-2> )
 -->
   (call try-merge-above <key1> <e1> <l1> <w1> <a1>
              <ux1-1> <ux2-1> <uy2-1>
              <lx1-1> <lx2-1> <ly2-1> <key2> <e2>
              <l2> <w2> <a2> <ux1-2> <ux2-2>
              <uy2-2> <lx1-2> <lx2-2> <ly2-2> )).
```

The High Level Stage

The high level stage contains the domain dependent knowledge. This includes knowledge of cardiac anatomy and physiology and of the image creation process. The high level stage takes as input the segmented image and the relations determined by the preprocessors and the low level stage. Its purpose is to label objects as either vessel or noise (our use of the term noise is meant to encompass such things as irrelevent anatomical structures and subtraction artifacts, as well as actual noise created by the image formation process.)

Stated simply, the coronary arteries may be viewed as cylindrical segments arranged in a tree-like structure which originates at the aorta. This simple anatomical knowledge is embodied within the system by the spatial relations among objects and the expected characterists of the objects themselves. Because of the great variability of the input, no attempt is made to identify individual vessels. Objects are labelled as either vessel or as noise. Surprisingly, the knowledge required at this stage for the system to perform successfully is quite simple. The region representation and the spatial relation adjacent have proved to be sufficient for the task.

The system works along the following lines: It finds the largest region in the input and assumes that this is the aorta. It then navigates the rest of its investigation by this landmark. Once it has found the aorta, it eliminates all structures which could not possibly be coronary vessels due to their position relative to the aorta. One production which carries out this task is

```
(p too-high
  (goal ^type init-id ^status active)
  (region ^cat aorta {} {} {} <uly> {} {} {} {} {} {})
  {(trap ^cat unknown {} {} {} {} {} {} {} { <= <uly>}
       {} {} {}) <t>}
 -->
  (modify <t> ^cat noise))
```

which finds structures which are higher than the highest point of the aorta.

It then turns its attention to those unknown regions which, due to their position, might be vessels. Again, the criteria which the system uses for identifying vessels are the same which you or I might use -- the shape of the unknown object and its position relative to objects already known to be vessel. The following are two examples

```
(p adj-vessel-1
  (goal ˆtype id-vessel ˆstatus active)
  {(trap ˆcat unknown <key2> {} {} {} {}
      {} {} {} {} {} {}) <t>}
  (adjrel ˆposition {} <key2> <key1>)
  (trap ˆcat vessel <key1> {} {} {} {}
      {} {} {} {} {} {})
  -->
  (modify <t> ˆcat vessel))

(p aorta-above-vessel-thin
  (goal ˆtype cleanup ˆstatus active)
  {(trap ˆcat aorta <key1> {} { < 25} {} {}
      {} {} {} {} {} {}) <t>}
  (adjrel ˆposition above <key1> <key2>)
  (trap ˆcat vessel <key2> {} {} {} {}
      {} {} {} {} {} {})
  -->
  (modify <t> ˆcat vessel)).
```

In the first production, an unlabelled region which is adjacent to a region labelled vessel receives the label vessel; in the second, the system is attempting to relabel regions of specific shape and position which may have been mistakenly labelled as aorta in the initial attempt at identification.

In much the same way, the system attempts to label noise structures. For example

```
(p adj-noise-1
  (goal ˆtype id-noise ˆstatus active)
  {(trap ˆcat unknown <key2> {} {} {} {}
      {} {} {} {} {} {}) <t>}
  (adjrel ˆposition {} <key2> <key1>)
  (trap ˆcat noise <key1> {} {} {} {}
      {} {} {} {} {} {})
  -->
  (modify <t> ˆcat noise))
```

labels as noise any unknown structure adjacent to a known noise structure. While the production

```
(p just-noise
  (goal ˆtype cleanup2 ˆstatus active)
```

```
{(trap ^cat unknown {} {} {} {} {}
     {} {} {} {} {} {}) <t>}
->
(modify <t> ^cat noise))
```

which will not be allowed to fire until after the system has determined all those
structures which it believes are vessel, has the task of labelling isolated and still
uncatagorized structures as noise.

RESULTS

The ANGY system is currently running on a VAX 11/750 under Berkeley
UNIX. It has been applied to a number of digital subtracted angiograms of the
chests of swine. Figures 1a, 4b, and 5 through 9 show the original angiogram and
the resulting segmentation for these images. As can be seen, the system is quite
successful in identifying the coronary vessels. The two recurring failures seem to be

1. The labelling of some noise structures (most notably, non-coronary
   vessels and motion artifacts) as vessel if they are of the right shape and
   are too close to a vessel or the aorta

2. The labelling of some portions of vessel as noise if they are not
   elongated and the segmentation process has resulted in their being
   isolated from any vessel.

The first problem might be alleviated if the boundary of the heart were
known -- this was something we had hoped to include in our system. However, at
the time of this work, no effective technique for obtaining a mask of the heart had
been implemented. As to the second, there is no doubt that the performance of the
system can be improved by "tuning." The addition of a few, well thought out
rules might possibly solve this problem. As with all systems, the quality of the
input image greatly effects the results of the output.

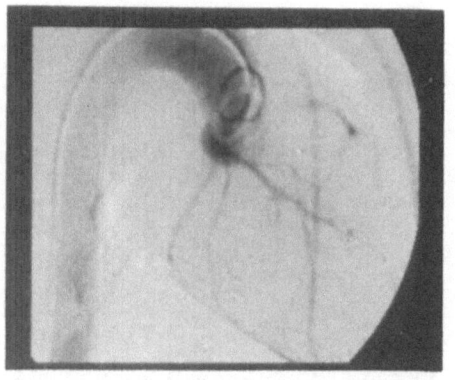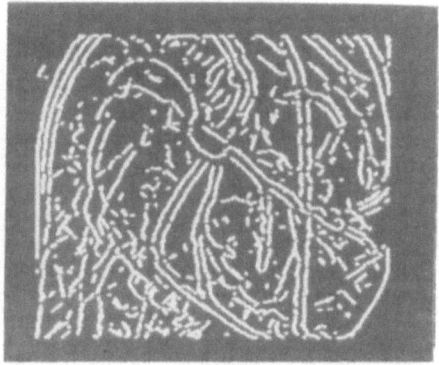

Figure 1: a. Angiogram b. Edge Segmentation

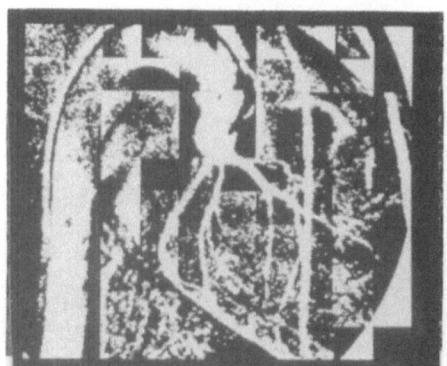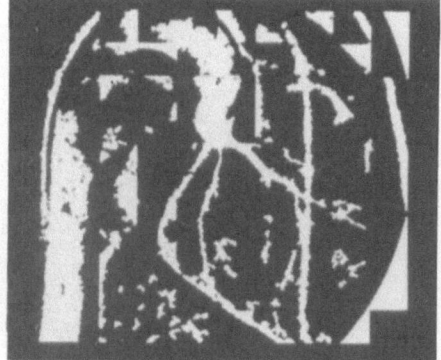

Figure 2: a. Thresholding b. Connected Components

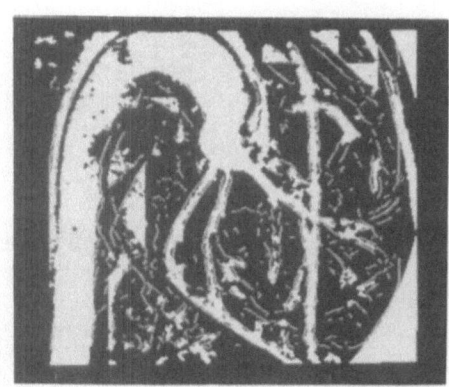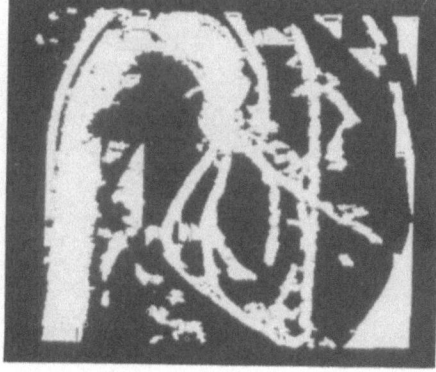

Figure 3: a. Regions/Edges b. After Converging

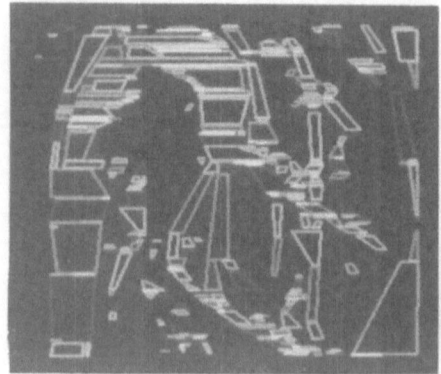 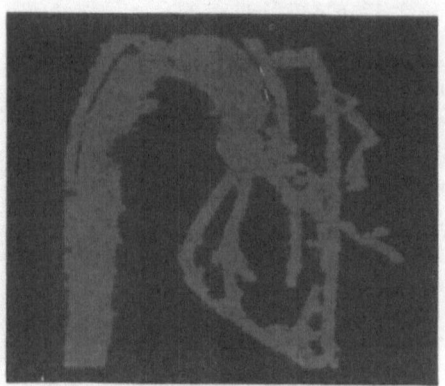

Figure 4: a. Trapezoid representation b. Final Segmentation

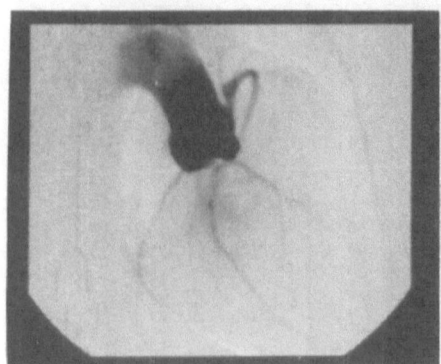 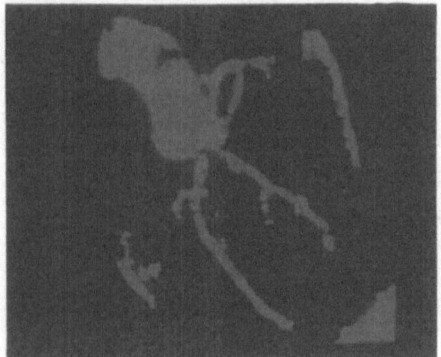

Figure 5: a. Angiogram b. Final Segmentation

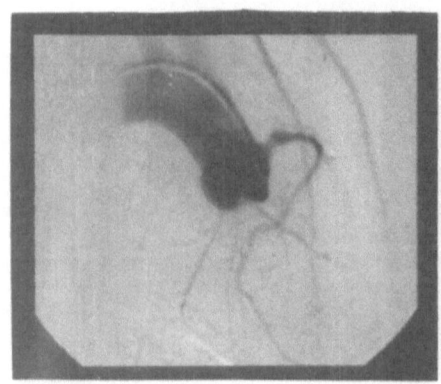 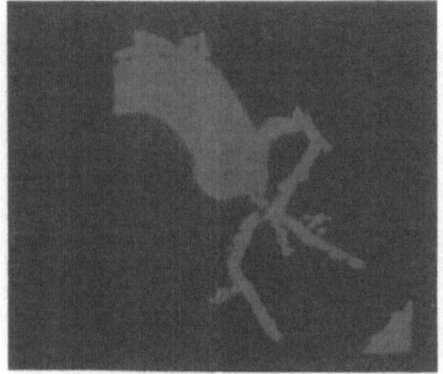

Figure 6: a. Angiogram b. Final Segmentation

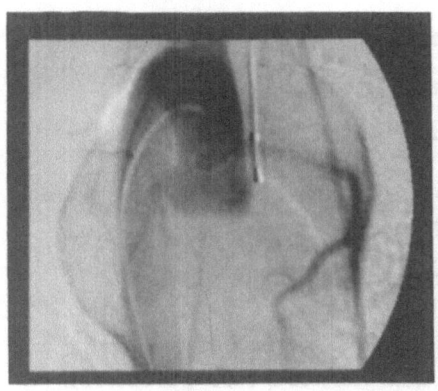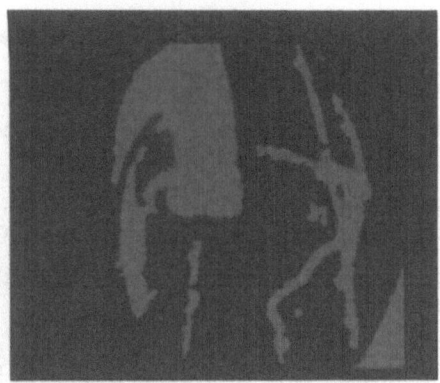

Figure 7: a. Angiogram b. Final Segmentation

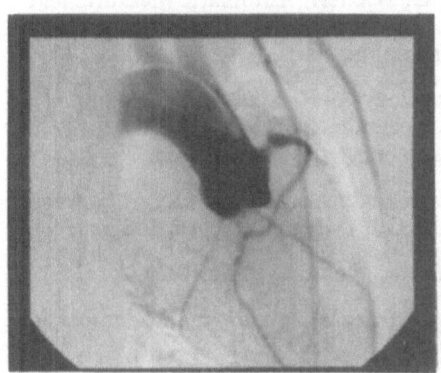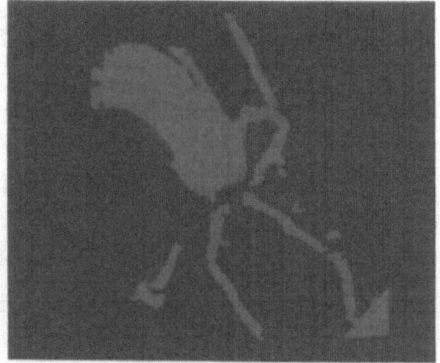

Figure 8: a. Angiogram b. Final Segmnetation

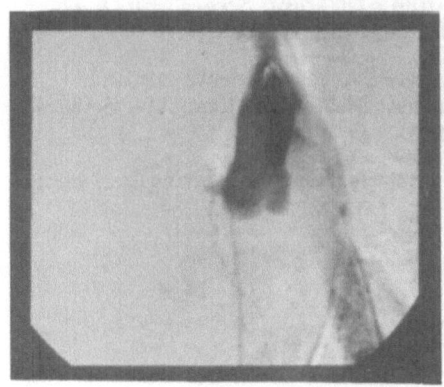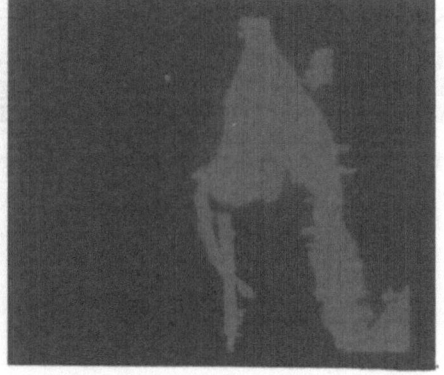

Figure 9: a. Angiogram b. Final Segmentation

References

1. D. Ballard and C. Brown. *Computer Vision*. Prentice-Hall, Inc, 1982.

2. M. Brady. Representing Shape. Proceedings of the International Robotics Conference, 1984, pp. 256-265.

3. B. Buchanan and R. Duda. Principles of Rule-Based Expert Systems. Department of Computer Science, Stanford University, August, 1982.

4. J. Canny. Finding Lines and Edges in Images. Artificial Intelligence Laboratory, MIT, June, 1983.

5. R. Davis and J. King. An Overview of Production Systems. In *Machine Intelligence 8*, E. Elcock and D. Michie, Ed., Ellis Horwood, 1977, pp. 300-332.

6. C. Forgy. *OPS5 User's Manual*. Department of Computer Science, Carnegie-Mellon University, 1981.

7. G. Herman, S. Rossnick, J. Udupa, and G. Waxler. Automatic Measurement of Coronary Vessels from Digital Angiograms. Presented to the Cardiovascular System Dynamics Society Conference, Philadelphia, Pa.

8. D. Kenepp. Cardiac Anatomy and Physiology As Related To Detection of Coronary Arteries with Digital Subtraction Techniques. Internal Memo, Department of Radiology, Hospital of the University of Pennsylvania.

9. A. Nazif and M. Levine. Low Level Image Segmentation: An Expert System. Computer Vision and Robotics Laboratoy, McGill University, April, 1983.

10. P. Pick and R. Howden. *Gray's Anatomy*. Running Press, 1974.

11. E. Potchen, P. Koehler, and D. Davis. *Principles of Diagnostic Radiology*. McGraw-Hill, 1971.

12. U. Shani. *Understanding Three-Dimensional Images: The Recognition of Abdominal Anatomy From Computed Axial Tomograms (CAT)*. Ph.D. Th., Computer Science Department, University of Rochester, 1980.

13. K. Sloan. *World Model Driven Recognition of Natural Scenes*. Ph.D. Th., Computer Science Department, University of Pennsylvania, 1978.

14. S. Stansfield. ANGY: A Rule-Based Expert System for Identifying and Isolating Coronary Vessels in Digital Angiograms. Master Th., Computer Science Department, University of Pennsyvania, 1984.

15. P. Wells. *Scientific Basis of Medical Imaging*. Churchill Livingston, 1982.

UTILIZATION OF NON-NEGATIVITY CONSTRAINTS IN RECONSTRUCTION OF EMISSION
TOMOGRAMS

E. TANAKA, N. NOHARA, T. TOMITANI and M. YAMAMOTO
National Institute of Radiological Sciences, Anagawa, Chiba-shi, Japan

1. INTRODUCTION

Emission computed tomography (ECT) has gained recognition in the past
decade as a valuable tool in nuclear medicine imaging. The ECT falls into
one of two categories: positron ECT and single-photon ECT(SPECT)[1]. The
ECT has the advantage of higher object contrast than planar imaging, but at
the same time has often suffered from a lack of sufficient count densities
to achieve statistically smooth images. The poor counting statistics is
due to limited isotope dosage to patients, limited counting time and limited count rate capability of the imaging devices. Fast dynamic studies
require reduction of total number of counts to be accumulated per image,
and high resolution imaging further reduces count density per resolution
cell. The magnitude of statistical noise of an image depends on various
factors such as the radionuclide distribution, the total number of counts,
the number of resolution cells in the object area, etc., but it also
depends on the reconstruction algorithm, because the statistical noise is
amplified in the stage of image reconstruction.

A common problem in the reconstruction of ECT images is the correction
for attenuation of photons in patients. For positron ECT, the attenuation
is independent of position along a projection line and the correction is
performed for projections using transmission scan data. Then, convolution-
backprojection algorithms are widely used for image reconstruction. In
SPECT, the correction is more difficult, because the attenuation of photons
depends on the depth in the body. For non-uniform attenuation objects, an
adequate correction is performed by means of iterative reconstruction
techniques. In most of the clinical applications, however, algorithms
based on the convolution principle with approximate attenuation correction
are used assuming a uniform attenuation in the body contour[2-4].

It has been pointed out that the incorporation of a priori information
on radionuclide distribution in the reconstruction process may be effective
to reduce the statistical noise artefacts[5]. The most useful a priori
information is the non-negativity constraints, that is any reconstructed
radionuclide image should not have negative densities. The convolution
method with poor counting statistics may produce many negative pixels so
that it is expected that a modification using the non-negativity constraints will be useful to improve signal-to-noise ratio in the low density
area of an image.

The non-negativity constraints are used in some iterative reconstruction algorithms. In EM (estimation maximization) algorithms based on
maximum likelihood concept, the constraints are automatically included[5-
8], but its performance on statistical noise has not been fully investigated. The method also has a drawback of computational slowness.

The major objectives of this paper are to find a practical reconstruction method involving the non-negativity constraints, and to evaluate its effectiveness in terms of improvement of image quality. The methods discussed are a modification from a convolution method, the EM algorithm and a hybrid method of convolution and EM-algorithm. Throughout this work, we assume that the detector system has an ideal spatial resolution and effects of scattering and attenuation of photons in patients are neglected.

2. MODIFICATION FROM CONVOLUTION-BACKPROJECTION IMAGES
2.1. Negative smoothing and image dividing technique

In an image reconstructed by a convolution method, statistical fluctuation of a pixel density has a negative correlation with those of the surrounding pixels[9]. If a pixel has a negative density it may be compensated with positive densities of the surrounding pixels. The compensation can be performed by convolving a two-dimensional filter to the negative pixel. The treatments for all negative pixels will result in local compensations between positive and negative fluctuations without excessive loss of spatial resolution. In the simulation study shown later, the filter function shown in Fig. 1 was used and the filtering was performed 8-times repeatedly. We call this procedure "negative smoothing".

1/12	1/6	1/12
1/6	0	1/6
1/12	1/6	1/12

FIGURE 1. Filter used for negative smoothing.

The simple negative smoothing is effective in the image area where the true density is zero or very low, but not in high density areas. If the image is divided into a number of sub-images and all the sub-images are summed after being treated by the negative smoothing individually, the non-negativity constraints may become more effective, because the number of negative pixels increases with decreasing the total number of events involved. This method is named "image dividing technique".

A series of sub-images may be obtained as time lapse images in a dynamic study mode. This is applicable when we obtain an average image in a certain period of time from a series of dynamic images. Another simple method is the division by angular views. For example, the total number of views is even and is sufficiently large, two sub-images can be reconstructed from even number views and odd number views, respectively.

When only a set of projection data is available and the number of views is not sufficiently large to perform the angular division mentioned above, the set of projections can be divided into two sub-sets by a binomial distribution law. The law states that a count number, n, is divided into n_1 and n_2 ($n_2 = n - n_1$) with a probability:

$$P(n_1, n) = \frac{n!}{n_1! \, n_2!} \left(\frac{1}{2}\right)^n. \tag{1}$$

In practice, a read-out table producing n_1 from a given value of n and a random number generated by a computer is prepared once and is stored in a memory. For a large n-value, eq.(1) is approximated by a Gaussian probability distribution function, and n_1 and n_2 are obtained by

$$n_1 = n/2 + q\sqrt{n/2}, \qquad n_2 = n - n_1, \qquad (2)$$

where q is a variable following a Gaussian probability distribution with a standard deviation of unity and zero mean. A read-out table producing q-value from a random generator is also stored.

By repeating the "binomial dividing method", an original set of projection data can be divided into $2,4,8\cdots$ sub-sets, from each of which an image is reconstructed.

2.2. Simulation experiments

Simulations were performed with two mathematical phantoms shown in Fig. 2. The phantoms are 20 cm in diameter. Sixty projections are generated from the phantom with a bin width of 0.42 cm, and images are reconstructed in a 60 x 60 matrix. The pixel size is 0.42 cm. Shepp-Logan filter is used as the convolution kernel with linear interpolation.

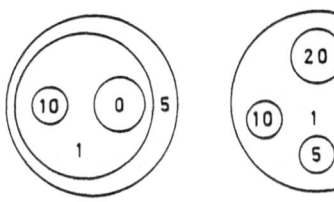

Phantom #1　　　Phantom #2

FIGURE 2. Mathematical phantoms used for simulation experiments. The diameters of the phantoms are 20 cm. Values in the figures are the relative activities.

Figures 3 and 4 show the results of the simulation. In both the figures, (a) is the image reconstructed by convolution method without noise, (b) is the convolution image with noise, (c) is the image obtained by cutting negative pixels from (b). Image (d) is obtained by the negative smoothing from image (b). Images (e) and (f) are obtained by image dividing technique from 8 sub-images using the binomial dividing method. Image (e) is the simple sum of the 8 sub-images treated by the negative smoothing each, and (f) is obtained by additional negative smoothing from (e).

It is seen that the simple negative smoothing is effective to reduce the noise at low density areas but positive streak-like artefacts still remain. On the other hand, the artefacts decrease by the image dividing technique. A major drawback of the image dividing method is, however, that it needs a longer computation time for convolution reconstruction in proportion to the number of sub-images.

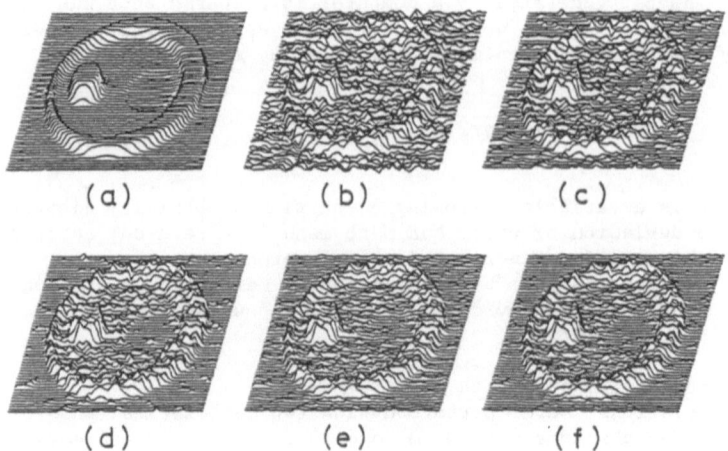

FIGURE 3. Images obtained by modifying convolution image of
Phantom #1.
(a) Convolution image without noise.
(b) Convolution image with statistical noise. The total
    number of events is 100,000.
(c) Image obtained by cutting negative pixels from (b).
(d) Image obtained by negative smoothing from (b).
(e) Image obtained by summing 8 sub-images treated by
    negative smoothing. The sub-images are obtained by
    binomial dividing technique.
(f) Image obtained by additional negative smoothing from (e).

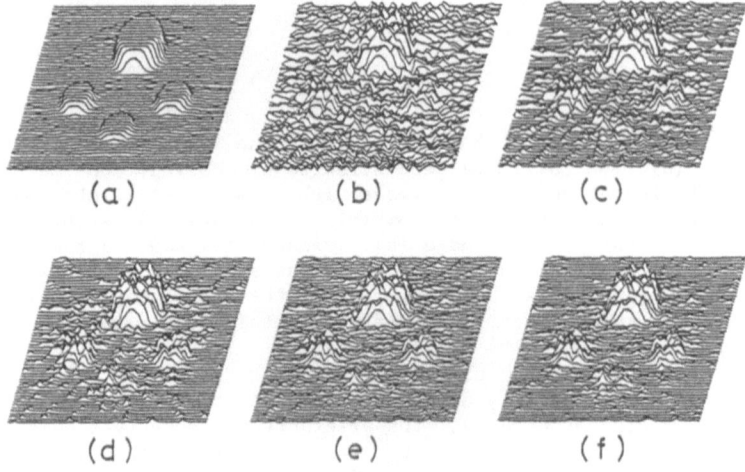

FIGURE 4. Images obtained by modifying convolution image of
Phantom #2. (a)-(f) are the same as those in Fig. 3 except
that the total number of events is 30,000.

3. EM ALGORITHM AND ITS MODIFICATION

3.1. EM algorithm (Mode A)

The EM algorithm proposed by Shepp and Vardi and others[6-8] is an iterative reconstruction technique for finding a maximum likelihood estimate. Letting s(b) be the image density in a pixel b (see Fig. 5), the iteration process is expressed by

$$s^{new}(b) = s^{old}(b) \; C(b), \qquad (3)$$

where C(b) is a correction factor to be multiplied to an old image. The correction factor C(b) is obtained by

$$C(b) = \sum_d \frac{n(d)}{m(d)} \, p(b,d), \qquad (4)$$

$$m(d) = \sum_{b'} s^{old}(b') \; p(b',d), \qquad (5)$$

where d is a "detector tube" or a "projection bin", n(d) is the number of detected events in bin d, and m(d) is the "forward projection" on bin d calculated by eq.(5) from an old image. The function p(b,d) is the probability that emission in a pixel b is detected in bin d.

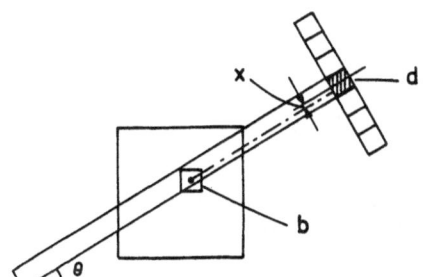

FIGURE 5. Illustration of pixel, b, and detector tube, d. x is the central distance between the pixel and the detector tube. θ is the view angle.

The choice of p(b,d) is important to discuss the performance of the EM algorithm. We assume that emission density is uniform in a square pixel, and that p(b,d) is proportional to the overlapping area between the pixel b and the detector tube d. The probability p(b,d) can be expressed as a function of the view angle θ and the central distance x between the pixel and the detector tube on the projection (see Fig. 5). Then we have

$$p(b,d) = p(\theta,x). \qquad (6)$$

We can calculate $p(\theta,x)$ for all view angles and various values of x, and store it as a two-dimensional table in a computer. The size of the table is not large because $p(\theta,x)$ has non-zero value only for a limited range of x.

In practice, for each view angle, forward projection of an image is obtained with a sufficiently fine pitch (1/15 of the bin width) assuming that the emission of a pixel is concentrated at the center of the pixel, and the obtained projection is convolved with $p(\theta,x)$.

A simpler $p(\theta,x)$ function, which is independent of view angle θ, was tested, but it produced small artefacts in images due to the interference between pixels and projection bins. Then, the following studies are performed with the more sophisticated $p(\theta,x)$ function described above.

General features of the EM algorithm are as follows. (a) Non-negativity constraints are automatically involved as long as the initial image is positive. (b) Speed of recovery of a source distribution is inversely proportional to the spatial frequency of the distribution, that is, a lower frequency component is reconstructed by a fewer iteration cycles than a higher frequency component. (c) The DC component is recovered by the first iteration, and the total number of events is preserved in the following iterations. (d) Spatial resolution generally increases with added iteration cycles, but it depends on many other factors such as the source distribution, the number of pixels in the reconstruction area, the average density of the point of interest, etc.

3.2. Speeding up of EM algorithm and simulation experiments

A drawback of the EM algorithm is slow speed of execution. Most of the computation time is spent in the calculation of forward projections and a matrix of correction factors $C(b)$ for all the pixels. A simple method of speeding up is "angle skipping". For example, if iterations are performed using only odd number views and even number views in turn, the computation time per iteration is roughly halved.

Another effective method is the amplification of $C(b)$ by replacing it with $C(b)^k$ in eq.(3) where $k > 1$. With this amplification, however, the total number of events is not preserved and the image tends to oscillate at a low spatial frequency for a large k-value. To prevent the oscillation of the D.C. component, eq.(3) is modified as follows:

$$s^{new}(b) = s^{old}(b) \ [C(b)]^k [N_T / \sum_{b'} s^{old}(b')]^{k-1}, \qquad (7)$$

where N_T is the total number of events of the observed projections. With this modification, the iteration was quite stable for a k-value less than about 3.5. The total number of events is preserved in the estimate at each iteration. The speed of convergence is almost proportional to the k-value. Thus, combining the angle skipping and the $C(b)$ amplification, the computation time is effectively reduced. Following studies were performed by odd-even angle skipping with the $C(b)$ amplification with k=3.

Computer simulations have been made to investigate the performance of the EM algorithms for mathematical phantoms. We assume that 60 projections are measured with an equal angular interval in an angular range π, and we assume 60 detector tubes equally spaced and closely packed in a projection. The "measured" data, $n(d)$, are generated by calculating emission density in each detector tube. Blurring due to spatial resolution of actual photon detectors or collimators is not taken into account. Attenuation and scattering of photons in the phantoms are again neglected. Images are reconstructed in a 60 x 60 matrix. The pixel size and the bin (detector tube) width are 0.42 cm.

First, we have studied the convergence rate. Figure 6 shows the rms error of images as a function of iteration cycle for Phantom #1 shown in Fig. 2 without noise. The iteration was started from a uniform image. The curve A is obtained with the original EM algorithm, and curve A-S is obtained by applying 1:6:1 smoothing in the measured projections before

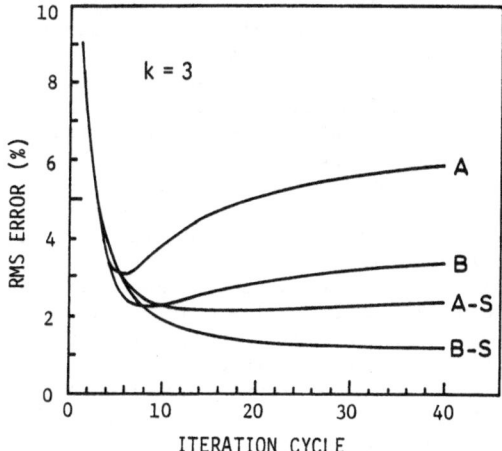

FIGURE 6. Root mean square error of noise free images obtained by EM
algorithms as a function of iteration cycle.   The iterations are
speeded up with k=3.   The phantom is Phantom #1 shown in Fig. 2.
Curve A   : Mode A (Original EM algorithm)
Curve A-S : Mode A with projections smoothed by 1:6:1 filter
Curve B   : Mode B (Modified EM algorithm)
Curve B-S : Mode B with projections smoothed by 7-point averaging
                  after 5-point expanding

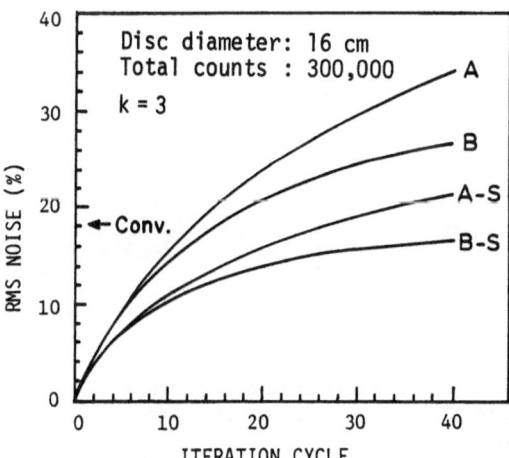

FIGURE 7. Root mean square noise of images obtained by EM algorithms
as a function of iteration cycle.   The phantom is a uniform disc of
16 cm in diameter.   Total number of events is 300,000.   The rms
noise is calculated in a circular area of 12 cm in diameter.
Curves A, A-S, B, and B-S are the same as those in Fig. 6.

iterations.   The rms error shown in the figure is the difference from the convolution image.   The value is the average of all pixels in the object region, and is normalized by the maximum value of the emission density.

Figure 7 shows the rms noise of a uniform disc phantom of 16 cm in diameter.   The rms value is an average value in the area of 12 cm in diameter.   The number of total events is 3×10^5.   The curve A is the original EM algorithm and A-S is obtained with the smoothed projections. The rms noise of the convolution image is 18.1 % (shown by an arrow in the figure).   Figure 8 shows the images after 40 iterations.

These results indicate that the original algorithm enhances the edge of the phantom excessively with the increase of iteration cycles unless suitable smoothing is applied to the projections.   With noisy projections, the root mean square noise of the reconstructed image increases beyond the noise level of the convolution image.   The main reason for this is con-sidered as follows.   An iteration cycle involves two steps of interpo-lations of data points represented by $p(b,d)$ in eq.(4) and $p(b',d)$ in eq.(5), respectively.   Nevertheless, the iterative correction works in such a way that the "smoothed" forward-projections agree with "un-smoothed" measured-projections, and accordingly the image converges to the one having excessive high-frequency component.

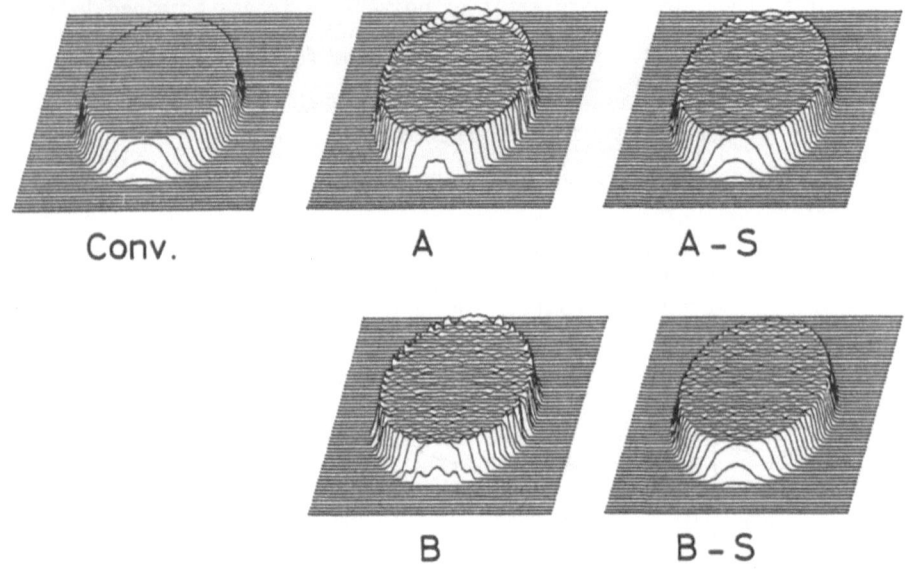

FIGURE 8. Images of a uniform disc phantom without statistical noise.   The phantom diameter is 16 cm and pixel size is 0.42 cm. Number of iterations is 40 (k=3).
Conv.: Convolution-backprojection method with Shepp-Logan filter
(linear interpolation)
A   : Mode A (Original EM algorithm)
A-S : Mode A with projections smoothed by 1:6:1 filter
B   : Mode B (Modified EM algorithm)
B-S : Mode B with projections smoothed by 7-point averaging
after 5-point expanding

3.3. Modified EM algorithm (Mode B)

To overcome the drawback of the original EM algorithm, a modified algorithm has been developed. As shown in Fig. 9, we consider an imaginary detector tube array, in which one of the detector tubes directly faces to the center of the pixel b. Letting d_i be an imaginary detector tube, eqs.(4) and (5) are replaced by

$$C(b) = \sum_{d_i} \frac{n(d_i)}{m(d_i)} \, p(b,d_i), \tag{8}$$

$$m(d_i) = \sum_{b'} s^{old}(b') \, p(b',d_i), \tag{9}$$

where $n(d_i)$ is the number of counts in bin d_i estimated from measured counts $n(d)$ by linear interpolation.

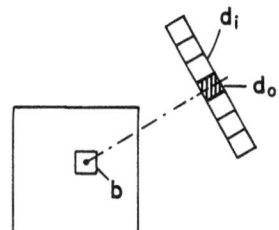

FIGURE 9. Illustration of imaginary detector tube array, d_i, for a pixel, b, in the modified EM algorithm. A detector tube, d_o, faces directly to the pixel.

For a projection at a view angle, $p(b,d_i)$ has the largest value for the directly facing bin, d_o, and the $p(b,d_i)$ for the other bins is negligibly small compared to $p(b,d_o)$ as long as the pixel size is equal to or smaller than the bin width. Then, we can assume that $p(b,d_o)$ is constant for all view angles and is equal to $1/N$ where N is the number of views. Under this condition, eq.(8) is further simplified and we have

$$C(b) = (1/N) \sum_{d_o} n(d_o)/m(d_o), \tag{10}$$

$$m(d_o) = \sum_{b'} s^{old}(b') \, p(b',d_o). \tag{11}$$

With this modification, the smoothing effect in an iteration cycle is small and the correction factor C(b) is obtained from the ratios of "smoothed" measured-projections to "un-smoothed" forward-projections. We call this algorithm "Mode B" and the original one "Mode A" in the following discussions. The computation time is nearly equal for both the modes.

The results of simulation experiments using Mode B are shown in Figs. 6 and 7 as curves B. Note that the rms noise in Mode B tends to saturate more rapidly to a smaller value than Mode A. Even with Mode B, however, the rms noise increases beyond the noise level of the convolution image as

388

the number of iterations increases.   Edge sharpening effect is still seen
in the reconstructed image (see Fig. 8). The reason for this is considered
as follows.   The pixels have a finite size, in which emission density is
assumed to be uniform, and hence neighboring two projection bins should
have a certain correlation in their values, while the statistical fluctuations occur independently.   This results in the excessive enhancement of
high frequency noise.

To reduce this effect, an additional smoothing of projection data is
required.   The observed projections are expanded in a finer pitch (1/5 of
the bin width) by linear interpolation, and 7-point running average is
applied to them.   The rms error and the rms noise are shown in Figs. 6 and
7 as curves B-S, and the 40-th iteration is in Fig. 8.   It is seen that
Mode B with the smoothed projections gives comparable noise and resolution
as the convolution method.

4. HYBRID METHOD OF CONVOLUTION AND EM ALGORITHM

The EM algorithm needs a large number of iterations to recover the
spatial resolution even with a suitable speed-up method if the iterations
are started from a uniform image.   The required number of iterations will
be greatly reduced by starting the iteration from a convolution image.
The initial image must be positive, then the convolution image is treated
by a non-linear operation to remove negative or zero density.   In this
"hybrid method", the spatial resolution is fully recovered by the convolution reconstruction and the density distortion caused by the non-linear
operation will be corrected by a small number of iterations.

The non-linear operation used here is expressed by

$$
\left.
\begin{aligned}
s_o &= s_i & (s_i \geq s_t) \\
&= s_t \exp[(s_i/s_t) - 1] & (s_i < s_t),
\end{aligned}
\right\} \tag{12}
$$

where s_i and s_o are the pixel values before and after the operation,
respectively, and s_t is a threshold value.   We call this operation "Diode
cut" from the similarity to the diode characteristics.   Note that the
distortion produced by the diode cut occurs mainly in low spatial frequencies for which the iterative correction is very fast.

Examples of images of Phantom #1 reconstructed by the hybrid method
are shown in Fig. 10.   In the figures, (a) is the phantom, (b) is the
convolution image, (c) is the initial image of iteration (processed by the
diode cut) and (d)-(f) are the images after 2, 4, 6, 8 iterations.   In the
EM algorithm, Mode B is used with smoothed projections described before (7-
point averaging for expanded projections).   The threshold value s_t in the
diode cut is a half the maximum density.   Figure 11 shows another example.
The lower-row images were obtained by applying 9-point weighted smoothing
to the upper-row. Note that 4 or 6 iterations yield reasonable images, and
that the signal-to-noise ratio in the low density area is greatly improved
compared to the convolution method.

5. NOISE REDUCTION BY MEANS OF NON-NEGATIVITY CONSTRAINTS

It is of interest to compare noise magnitude between images reconstructed with the EM algorithm and the convolution method with an identical
spatial resolution.   The reconstruction resolution of the EM algorithm can
not be uniquely defined, but in the present test, Mode B with 40 iterations
from smoothed projections seems to yield almost the same resolution as the
convolution method (see Fig. 8).   As shown in Fig. 7, no appreciable

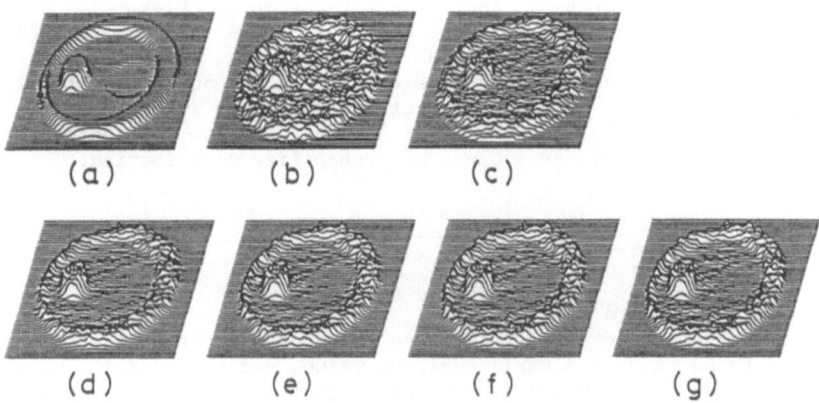

FIGURE 10. Images of Phantom #1 obtained with hybrid method.   The total number of events is 100,000.
(a)   Convolution image without noise
(b)   Convolution image with noise
(c)   Initial image of iteration obtained by diode cut from (b)
(d-g) Images after 2, 4, 6, 8 iterations, respectively

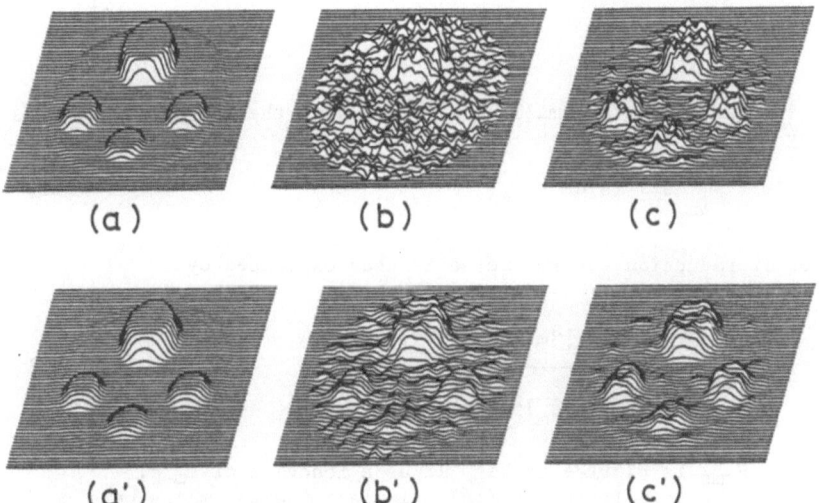

FIGURE 11. Images of Phantom #2 obtained with hybrid method.   The total number of events is 30,000.
(a)   Convolution image without noise
(b)   Convolution image with noise
(c)   Image after 6 iterations with noise
(a')-(c') are obtained by 9-point weighted smoothing from (a)-(c).

difference is observed in the rms noise between the two methods where the non-negativity constraints are not effective. The texture of noise is also similar in the two images. In low density areas in Figs. 10 and 11, however, the EM algorithm produces much less noise than the convolution method, which is apparently due to the non-negativity.

To estimate the effect of non-negativity on the noise, we shall consider a simple model. When the constraints are not involved as in the convolution images, the density, s, of a pixel tends to fluctuate around a mean value, s_m, according to a Gaussian probability distribution:

$$P(s) = \frac{1}{\sqrt{2\pi}\ \sigma} \exp\left[-\frac{1}{2}\left(\frac{s - s_m}{\sigma}\right)^2\right], \tag{13}$$

where σ is the standard deviation.

When non-negativity constraints are incorporated, the negative pixels are forced to be zero or a small positive value, and the positive values of pixels are compressed toward zero value in such a way that the mean value is kept constant. Assuming that the compression occurs linearly, the new distribution will be expressed by:

$$
\begin{aligned}
P'(s) &= \frac{1}{\sqrt{2\pi}\ \gamma\sigma} \exp\left[-\frac{1}{2}\left(\frac{s - \gamma s_m}{\gamma\sigma}\right)^2\right] & (s > \varepsilon) \\
&= \int_{-\infty}^{\varepsilon} P(s)\ ds & (s = \varepsilon) \\
&= 0, & (s < \varepsilon)
\end{aligned}
\tag{14}
$$

where ε is a sufficiently small density and γ is the factor of compression defined by

$$\int_{-\infty}^{+\infty} s\ P'(s)ds = s_m. \tag{15}$$

The factor of reduction for rms noise is then expressed by

$$F_{rms} = \left[\frac{\int_0^{+\infty} (s - s_m)^2 P'(s)\ ds}{\int_{-\infty}^{+\infty} (s - s_m)^2\ P(s)\ ds}\right]^{1/2} \tag{16}$$

The value of F_{rms} is plotted in Fig. 12 as a function of s_m/σ.

To check the validity of eq. (16), simulation experiments were performed with two mathematical phantoms. The one is a uniform disc phantom of 20 cm in diameter, and the other is a 20 cm diameter disc with an annular hot area of 2 cm width at the periphery. The rms noise is calculated in the central area of 12 cm in diameter. The two experimental points are plotted in Fig. 12, which indicates reasonable agreements with the theoretical model. The distributions of pixel values are shown in Fig. 13.

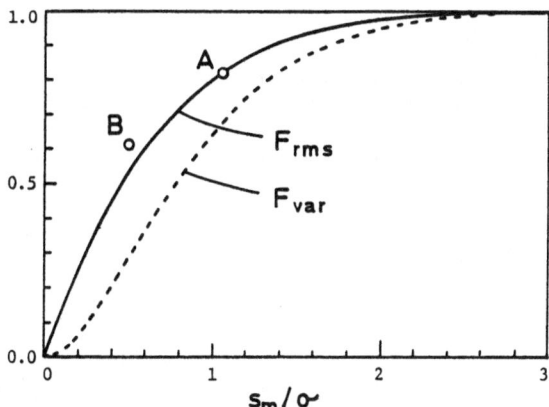

FIGURE 12. Factor of reduction for rms noise, F_{rms}, and for variance, F_{var}, by the use of non-negativity constraints. Points A and B represent the results of simulation experiments.

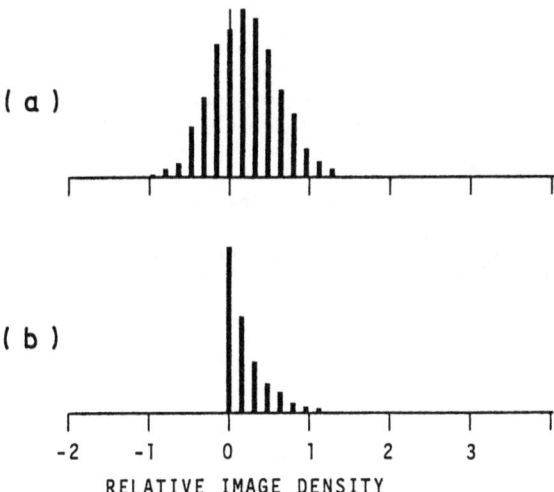

FIGURE 13. Distributions of pixel densities in the simulation experiment shown as point B in Fig. 12.
(a) Convolution image
(b) EM algorithm (Mode B with projection smoothing)

6. SUMMARY AND CONCLUSIONS

We have tested various methods of image reconstruction involving the use of non-negativity constraints. The negative smoothing of convolution images is the most simple and rapid method, but it is difficult to suppress positive streak artefacts. The image dividing method with the negative smoothing is effective to improve the above drawback. The method may be useful when an average image is obtained from a series of dynamic images.

The EM algorithm essentially satisfies the non-negativity constraints, but the convergence is very slow. To improve the computation speed, two methods have been developed; the one is angle skipping and the other is the amplification of correction factors. The original algorithm has an effect of edge sharpening, and it causes excessive increase in the noise magnitude in high density areas. To improve the convergence characteristics, a modified algorithm, Mode B, has been developed. With this mode, however, the rms noise still increases beyond the noise level of the convolution images as increasing iteration cycle. This fact implies that the maximum likelihood estimates achieved by the EM algorithms are not the most likely as practical emission images. A suitable smoothing must be applied to the measured projections to suppress the excessive noise amplification and to make the reconstruction resolution comparable to the convolution method.

In the present studies, the most promising method is the hybrid method which is composed of a convolutional reconstruction, a non-linear operation for removing negative pixels (diode cut) and several cycles of iterations of the modified EM algorithm. By using the speed up techniques in the iterations, the computation time is about 3-4 times longer than the simple convolution reconstruction.

The relative magnitude of rms noise has been evaluated between the convolution method and the EM algorithm with a similar reconstruction resolution. The rms noise in low density areas is apparently reduced with the EM algorithm by virtue of the non-negativity constraints, although no essential difference has been observed in high density areas.

It is concluded that the use of non-negativity constraints dramatically increases the signal-to-noise ratio in low density area of images and it improves the quality of high contrast images obtained with poor counting statistics. This is particularly important in the future developments of ECT technique because the count density per pixel decreases appreciably as one attempts to develop higher resolution imaging devices or to perform faster dynamic studies.

This work was supported in part by grants from the Ministry of Education and the Ministry of Health and Welfare, Japan.

REFERENCES

1. Budinger TF, Derenzo SE, Gullberg GT, Greenberg WL and Huesman RH : Emission computer assisted tomography with single-photon and positron annihilation photon emitters. J Comput Assist Tomogr 1:131-145, 1977
2. Sorenson JA : Quantitative measurement of radioactivity in vivo by whole-body counting. In : Instrumentation in Nuclear Medicine, Vol.2. Ed. by GJ Hine and JA Sorenson, New York, Academic Press, 1974, pp 311-348
3. Chang LT : A method for attenuation correction in radionuclide computed tomography. IEEE Trans Nucl Sci NS-25:638-643, 1978

4. Tanaka E, Toyama H and Murayama H : Convolutional image reconstruction for quantitative single photon emission computed tomography. Phys Med Biol 29:1489-1500, 1984

5. Snyder DL : Utilization of side information in emission tomography. IEEE Trans Nucl Sci NS-31:533-537, 1984

6. Rockmore AJ and Macovski A : A maximum likelihood approach to emission image reconstruction from projections. IEEE Trans Nucl Sci NS-23:1428-1432, 1976

7. Shepp LA and Vardi Y : Maximum likelihood reconstruction for emission tomography. IEEE Trans Med Imag MI-1:113-122, 1982

8. Lange K and Carson R : EM reconstruction algorithms for emission and transmission tomography. J Comput Assist Tomogr 8:306-316, 1984

9. Tanaka E and Murayama H : Properties of statistical noise in positron emission tomography. In : Proceedings of International Workshop on Physics and Engineering in Medical Imaging (Pacific Grove, 1982), IEEE Comput Soc 82CH1751-7, 1982, pp 158-164

IMAGE RECONSTRUCTION IN TIME-OF-FLIGHT POSITRON EMISSION TOMOGRAPHY

C. T. Chen and C.E. Metz
Department of Radiology and The Franklin McLean Memorial Research Institute
The University of Chicago, Chicago, IL   60637

1.   ABSTRACT

Five algorithms for image reconstruction in time-of-flight assisted positron emission tomography (TOFPET) have been studied. These algorithms include three approaches previously described in the literature and two new methods recently developed in our institute. Computer simulation studies have been performed to evaluate the relative merits of these various techniques. Performance indices such as computational efficiency, reconstructed image resolution, and signal-to-noise ratio (SNR) have been investigated. Results from the analysis suggest that the two new methods may offer some potential advantages over other algorithms.

2.   INTRODUCTION

Positron emission tomography (PET) has received considerable attention in the past decade for its use in physiological studies and for its potential role in medical diagnosis. In the past, most PET systems have employed only the coincidence detection of two annihilation photons to reconstruct tomographic images. There is an additional kind of potentially useful information for image reconstruction in PET, however: the difference between the times at which two annihilation photons arrive at opposing detectors, i.e., time-of-flight (TOF) measurements. The inclusion of this type of information in PET image reconstruction had been delayed until recently largely by the limitations of electronic and detector technologies. Recent advances in these two areas now permit more accurate measurements of differential TOF information in PET [1,2]. The feasibility of TOF assisted PET (TOFPET) systems incorporating these new technologies has been demonstrated recently [3,4].

Using TOF data, the location at which an annihilation event occurred along a line connecting the positions of the two coincident photon detections--and thus the interaction site where a nearby positron emission took place--can be estimated with an uncertainty governed by the resolving time of detectors if the positron range is negligibly small (Fig. 1). In contrast to conventional PET systems, which provide no spatial resolution in the transverse direction along the coincidence detection line, TOFPET systems can employ these TOF data in new image reconstruction strategies that potentially can improve image quality [5-9]. Although the transverse spatial resolution achieved by utilizing TOF measurements is still relatively poor to date, presently available TOFPET systems have demonstrated their capability of providing increased system sensitivity [10], improved correction schemes for photon attenuation [11] and scatter radiation [12], and better image quality [13,14] when compared to those obtained by some of the conventional PET systems.

Several algorithms for TOFPET image reconstruction have been suggested in the literature. These techniques can be broadly classified into two general categories: filtering methods and recursive methods. The filtering techniques include the most-likely position (MLP) method and the confidence weighting (CW) method. The MLP method is a simple and direct filtering scheme that suffers from poor noise properties [6,7]. The CW method employs a smoothing process which improves signal-to-noise ratio (SNR) at the expense of more computation time [6,7]. One possible recursive approach, the estimated posterior-density weighting (EPDW) method, employs the EM (expectation-maximization) algorithm to calculate a maximum likelihood estimate of the distribution of annihilation events [15]. The EPDW method can provide improved image quality but requires much more processing time than even the CW method.

Two new algorithms, one a filtering approach and the other a recursive method, are proposed and investigated in the present study. These new methods offer potential advantages over the other three algorithms in terms of computation time and/or image quality.

3. MATHEMATICAL MODEL OF TOFPET IMAGES

For an idealized TOFPET system, in which both TOF resolution and detector spatial resolution for all coincidence-detection pairs are invariant within an effective imaging region, the projection data $m(\xi,\eta;\theta)$ collected at angle θ is a two-dimensional (2-D) image expressed by (Fig. 2):

$$m(\xi,\eta;\theta) = \int\int_{-\infty}^{\infty} f(\xi',\eta';\theta)w(\xi-\xi',\eta-\eta') \cdot a(\xi',\theta)d\xi'd\eta' \tag{1}$$

where $f(x,y)$ is the in vivo spatial distribution of the administered positron emitter and $f(\xi,\eta;\theta) = f(\xi\cos\theta - \eta\sin\theta, \xi\sin\theta + \eta\cos\theta)$; η is distance in the direction of the coincidence detection line or TOF measurement; ξ is distance in the lateral direction in which detector spatial resolution is measured; and θ is the angle from the x-axis to the ξ-axis. The kernel $w(\xi,\eta)$ summarizes the effects of TOF uncertainty and detector uncertainty. The term $a(\xi,\theta)$ in eqn. (1) is the attenuation factor:

$$a(\xi,\theta) = \exp[-\int_{-\infty}^{\infty}\mu(\xi,\eta;\theta)d\eta] \tag{2}$$

where $\mu(\xi,\eta;\theta) = \mu(\xi\cos\theta-\eta\sin\theta,\xi\sin\theta+\eta\cos\theta)$ is the linear attenuation coefficient expressed in the rotated coordinate system. $a(\xi,\theta)$ can be either estimated from a transmission scan or calculated from an analytical approximation of the physical configuration of the object.

The detector resolution of a typical TOFPET system is about 4 to 8 mm full-width-at-half-maximum (FWHM), equivalent to about 8 to 15 mm full-width-at-tenth-maximum (FWTM). If within this small distance the variation of $a(\xi,\theta)$ is negligible, or $a(\xi,\theta)$ can be approximated by an average value, this term can be factored out of the integral as a constant:

$$m(\xi,\eta;\theta) = a(\xi,\theta)\int\int_{-\infty}^{\infty} f(\xi',\eta';\theta)w(\xi-\xi',\eta-\eta')d\xi'd\eta' . \tag{3}$$

Defining an attenuation-corrected projection image array, $p(\xi,\eta;\theta)$, by

$$p(\xi,\eta;\theta) = m(\xi,\eta;\theta)/a(\xi,\theta) \qquad (4)$$

one has

$$p(\xi,\eta;\theta) = \int\int_{-\infty}^{\infty} f(\xi,\eta;\theta)w(\xi-\xi',\eta-\eta')d\xi'd\eta' \qquad (5)$$

$$= [f**w](\xi,\eta;\theta)$$

where "**" denotes 2-D convolution. Equation (5) states that the attenuation-corrected image array $p(\xi,\eta;\theta)$ at projection angle θ is merely a noisy 2-D image blurred by a spatial resolution function w that represents relatively poor TOF resolution in the direction of the coincidence detection line and better detection resolution in the lateral direction.

Averaging $p(\xi,\eta;\theta)$ over angles from 0 to π, one obtains a rotationally averaged estimate of $f(x,y)$:

$$\hat{f}(x,y) = RA\{p(\xi,\eta;\theta)\}$$

$$= (1/\pi)\int_{0}^{\pi} p(\xi,\eta;\theta)d\theta$$

$$= (1/\pi)\int_{0}^{\pi} [f**w](\xi,\eta;\theta) \qquad (6)$$

$$= f(x,y)**\{(1/\pi)\int_{0}^{\pi} w(\xi,\eta;\theta)d\theta\}$$

where $\xi = x\cos\theta+y\sin\theta$, $\eta = -x\sin\theta+y\cos\theta$, and RA is the rotational average operator. Defining a point spread function (PSF) as:

$$psf(x,y) = (1/\pi)\int_{0}^{\pi} w(\xi,\eta;\theta)d\theta \qquad (7)$$

one can write

$$\hat{f}(x,y) = f(x,y)**psf(x,y) \qquad . \qquad (8)$$

Thus, the rotationally averaged estimate, $\hat{f}(x,y)$, obtained by averaging all pre-image arrays, $p(\xi,\eta;\theta)$, is the convolution of the original distribution (the true or real object), $f(x,y)$, and an effective, rotationally symmetric PSF of the data formation process, $psf(x,y)$.

If TOF uncertainty and detector uncertainty can be approximated by Gaussian functions with standard deviations σ_T and σ_D, respectively, then $w(\xi,\eta)$ can be written in the form:

$$w(\xi,\eta) = u_D(\xi)u_T(\eta) \qquad (9)$$

where

$$u_D(\xi) = (1/\sqrt{2\pi}\sigma_D)\exp(-\xi^2/2\sigma_D^2) \qquad (10)$$

$$u_T(\eta) = (1/\sqrt{2\pi}\sigma_T)\exp(-\eta^2/2\sigma_T^2) \qquad . \qquad (11)$$

In this case, eqn. (7) gives psf(x,y) as the rotational average of the resolution function $u_D \cdot u_T$ over 180°. The resulting PSF is:

$$psf(r) = (1/2\pi\sigma_D\sigma_T)\exp[-r^2(1/\sigma_D^2+1/\sigma_T^2)/4]$$
$$I_0[r^2(1/\sigma_D^2-1/\sigma_T^2)/4] \tag{12}$$

where $I_0(x)$ is the zero-order modified Bessel function of the first kind. Equation (8) can be rewritten as:

$$\hat{f}(r,\theta) = f(r,\theta)**psf(r) \quad . \tag{13}$$

In the Fourier (frequency) domain, eqn. (14) can be represented by:

$$\hat{F}(\nu,\theta) = F(\nu,\theta)OTF(\nu) \tag{14}$$

where $\hat{F}$ and F are the 2-D Fourier transforms (FT) of $\hat{f}$ and f, respectively. Here OTF(ν) is the FT of psf(r), or the optical transfer function (OTF) of the data formation process, and can be calculated by:

$$OTF(\nu) = 2\pi\int_0^\infty psf(r)J_0(2\pi\nu r)r \, dr \tag{15}$$

where $J_0(x)$ is the zero-order Bessel function of the first kind. For the case of Gaussian resolution, eqn. (15) yields:

$$OTF(\nu) = \exp[-\pi^2\nu^2(\sigma_T^2+\sigma_D^2)]$$
$$\cdot I_0[\pi^2\nu^2(\sigma_T^2-\sigma_D^2)] \quad . \tag{16}$$

In this way, the TOFPET image reconstruction task can be viewed as either a deconvolution problem in the spatial domain [i.e., solution of eqn. (13)], or an inverse filtering problem in the frequency domain [i.e., solution of eqn. (14)]. Thus, image reconstruction for TOFPET can be regarded as nothing more than a classical image processing task: to compensate for a known resolution function. Figure 3 illustrates examples of PSF for TOFPET and Fig. 4 demonstrates examples of the magnitude of OTF, i.e., the modulated transfer function (MTF), for TOFPET. Conventional PET imaging with a simple backprojection scheme, which is approximated by assuming a very large σ_T, is also shown in these figures.

4. FILTERING METHODS
4.1. The MLP method
The rotationally averaged estimate $\hat{f}(x,y)$ in eqn. (6) is now called the MLP pre-image array [6]. Defining a reconstructed resolution function with Gaussian shape and standard deviation σ_R as:

$$U_R(\nu) = \exp(-2\pi^2\sigma_R^2\nu^2) \tag{17}$$

and using eqn. (14), one can reconstruct the image by:

$$F_{R(MLP)}(\nu,\theta) = \hat{F}(\nu,\theta)[U_R(\nu)/OTF(\nu)] \tag{18}$$

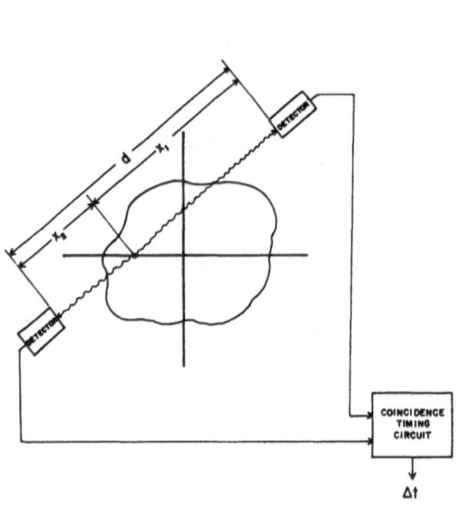

$$x_1 = \frac{1}{2}(c\Delta t + d)$$

where: c = speed of light

FIGURE 1. TOF measurements can provide transverse positional information along the coincidence detection line.

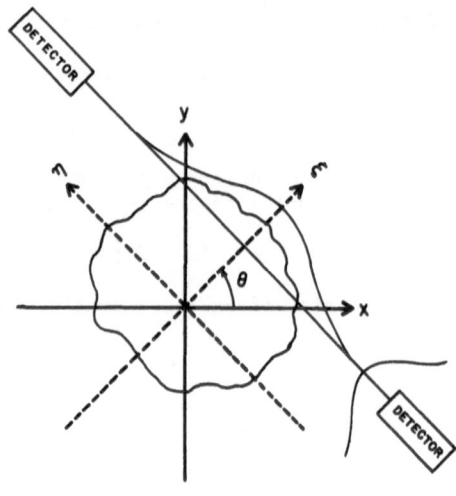

$\vec{\eta}$: TOF RESOLUTION

$\vec{\xi}$: DETECTOR RESOLUTION

FIGURE 2. TOFPET image data formation.

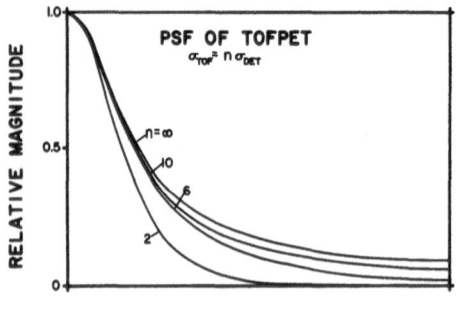

RELATIVE DISTANCE

FIGURE 3. Examples of PSF for TOFPET.

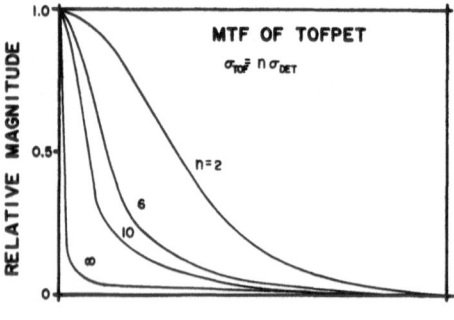

RELATIVE FREQUENCY

FIGURE 4. Examples of MTF for TOFPET.

The ratio in the bracket can be defined as the MLP filter:

$$H_{MLP}(\nu) = U_R(\nu)/OTF(\nu) \quad . \tag{19}$$

Hence, eqn. (18) can be rewritten as:

$$F_{R(MLP)}(\nu,\theta) = \hat{F}(\nu,\theta)H_{MLP}(\nu) \quad . \tag{20}$$

The reconstruction is done simply by filtering $\hat{F}(\nu,\theta)$ with the MLP filter $H_{MLP}(\nu)$. The MLP algorithm has the following steps:

1. $\hat{f}_{MLP} = RA\{p\}$

2. $\hat{F}_{MLP} = FT_2\{\hat{f}_{MLP}\}$

3. $F_{R(MLP)} = \hat{F}_{MLP} \cdot H_{MLP}$

4. $f_{R(MLP)} = FT_2^{-1}\{F_{R(MLP)}\}$

$$\tag{21}$$

The function $U_R(\nu)$ not only specifies the expected reconstructed resolution that one intends to achieve, but also serves to roll-off the high frequency noise components that are amplified by the monotonically increasing nature of $1/OTF(\nu)$ in eqn. (18). In principle, $U_R(\nu)$ represents the resolution that one can achieve in the reconstructed image. In practice, however, because of the discrete nature of the data matrix used in computation, the true spatial resolution function of final reconstructed image deviates from $U_R(\nu)$.

4.2. The CW method

If each event in the attenuation-corrected data is first smoothed by a weighting function before it is entered into the pre-image array, one has:

$$P_{CW}(\xi,\eta;\theta) = \int\!\!\int_{-\infty}^{\infty} f(\xi',\eta';\theta)t(\xi-\xi',\eta-\eta')d\xi'd\eta' \quad . \tag{22}$$

The kernel $w(\xi,\eta)$ in eqn. (1) now is replaced by a new kernel:

$$t(\xi,\eta) = w(\xi,\eta)**s(\xi,\eta) \tag{23}$$

where $s(\xi,\eta)$ is the weighting function for the smoothing process. It has been shown [7] that optimal image quality, in a signal-to-noise ratio (SNR) sense based on an amplitude model for a point source on a uniform background, is achieved if one chooses the weighting function $s(\xi,\eta)$ equal to $w(\xi,\eta)$. This choice of the weighting function $s(\xi,\eta)$ is a generalized form of "matched filtering." For this "confidence weighting" approach, the PSF is given by:

$$psf_{CW}(r) = (1/4\pi\sigma_D\sigma_T)\exp[-r^2(1/\sigma_D^2+1/\sigma_T^2)/8]$$
$$\cdot I_0[r^2(1/\sigma_D^2-1/\sigma_T^2)/8] \quad . \tag{24}$$

In the frequency domain, one has:

$$OTF_{CW}(\nu) = \exp[-2\pi^2\nu^2(\sigma_T^2+\sigma_D^2)]$$
$$\cdot \; I_0[2\pi^2\nu^2(\sigma_T^2-\sigma_D^2)] \quad . \tag{25}$$

Similar to the MLP method described by eqn. (20), the CW method for TOFPET image reconstruction can be described by:

$$F_{R(CW)}(\nu,\theta) = \hat{F}_{CW}(\nu,\theta)H_{CW}(\nu) \tag{26}$$

where

$$H_{CW}(\nu) = U_R(\nu)/OTF_{CW}(\nu) \tag{27}$$

is the CW filter and $\hat{F}_{CW}(\nu,\theta)$ is the FT of the new rotationally averaged image now called the CW pre-image array.

In summary, the CW algorithm for TOFPET image reconstruction first employs a smoothing process by convolving the attenuation-corrected image array at each projection angle with the uncertainty kernel $w(\xi,\eta)$ itself to form a weighted image array. Then the rotational average of these weighted image arrays, or the CW pre-image array, is filtered by the CW filter function $H_{CW}(\nu)$. The CW algorithm can be described as follows:

1. $p^\Delta = p**(u_D \cdot u_T)$

2. $\hat{f}_{CW} = RA\{p^\Delta\}$

3. $\hat{F}_{CW} = FT_2\{\hat{f}_{CW}\}$ (28)

4. $F_{R(CW)} = \hat{F}_{CW} \cdot H_{CW}$

5. $f_{R(CW)} = FT_2^{-1}\{F_{R(CW)}\}$.

Because of the smoothing process performed in the CW method, the reconstructed images are expected to be less noisy and the computation time longer, compared to the MLP method.

4.3. A new filtering approach: the "Metz filter" (MF) method

As stated earlier, the TOFPET image reconstruction problem can be viewed as either a deconvolution task [eqn. (13)] or an inverse filtering task [eqn. (14)]. Thus, the generalized iterative deconvolution technique-- and its equivalent filters--developed by Metz [16] for radionuclide image processing are readily applicable to the MLP pre-image array for TOFPET image reconstruction. This "Metz filter" (MF) method has been used in conventional radionuclide image processing [16-20], single-photon emission computed tomography (SPECT) [21], and digital radiology [22]. In the present study, it is applied to TOFPET image reconstruction [23,24]. Essentially, the proposed MF method is a modified version of the MLP method with different filter functions that provide potential advantages.

To understand this generalized deconvolution scheme, one can rewrite eqn. (14) as:

$$F(\nu,\theta) = \hat{F}(\nu,\theta)/OTF(\nu) \quad . \tag{29}$$

A series expansion of $1/OTF(\nu)$ can be written as:

$$1/OTF(\nu) = OTF^*(\nu)/|OTF(\nu)|^2$$

$$= OTF^*(\nu)/[1-(1-|OTF(\nu)|^2)] \tag{30}$$

$$= OTF^*(\nu) \sum_{k=0}^{\infty} [1-|OTF(\nu)|^2]^k$$

where the superscript "*" denotes the complex conjugate. This series converges if and only if $|OTF(\nu)| < \sqrt{2}$. Since $|OTF(\nu)| \leq 1$ in TOFPET (Fig. 4), this convergence criterion is satisfied. With an nth order approximation—namely, the nth order Metz filter—given by:

$$H_{MF}^{(n)}(\nu) = OTF^*(\nu) \sum_{k=0}^{n} [1-|OTF(\nu)|^2]^k$$

$$= OTF^*(\nu)\{[1-(1-|OTF(\nu)|^2)^{n+1}]/|OTF(\nu)|^2\} \tag{31}$$

$$= [1-(1-|OTF(\nu)|^2)^{n+1}]/OTF(\nu) \quad,$$

an nth order reconstruction scheme can be defined by:

$$F_{R(MF)}^{(n)}(\nu,\theta) = \hat{F}(\nu,\theta)H_{MF}^{(n)}(\nu) \quad. \tag{32}$$

The filtering process described above is equivalent to an iterative reconstruction scheme performed in the spatial domain as follows:

$$f^{(0)}(r,\theta) = psf(-r,\theta)**\hat{f}(r,\theta)$$

$$f^{(1)}(r,\theta) = 2psf(-r,\theta)**\hat{f}(r,\theta)$$

$$-psf(-r,\theta)**psf(-r,\theta)**psf(r,\theta)**\hat{f}(r,\theta) \tag{33}$$

$$\bullet$$
$$\bullet$$
$$\bullet$$

$$f^{(n)}(r,\theta) = psf(-r,\theta)**\hat{f}(r,\theta)+f^{(n-1)}(r,\theta)$$

$$-psf(-r,\theta)**psf(r,\theta)**f^{(n-1)}(r,\theta) \quad.$$

For TOFPET, $psf(r,\theta)$ is rotationally symmetrical; hence $psf(-r,\theta) = psf(r,\theta)$. One can note that, for a noise-free image, the initial estimate, $f^{(0)}(r,\theta)$, is actually the rotationally averaged CW pre-image array discussed earlier.

Rearranging the formula of the last iteration in eqn. (33), one has:

$$f^{(n)}(r,\theta) = f^{(n-1)}(r,\theta)+psf(-r,\theta)**$$
$$[\hat{f}(r,\theta)-psf(r,\theta)**f^{(n-1)}(r,\theta)] \quad. \tag{34}$$

This can be viewed as an iterative reconstruction algorithm with an additive correction scheme as follows:

1. $\hat{f} = RA\{p\}$

2. $n = 0; f^{(n)} = \hat{f}$

3. $\hat{f}^{\Delta} = f^{(n)}**psf$

4. $\Delta = \hat{f} - \hat{f}^{\Delta}$

5. $\Delta = \Delta**psf$

6. $f^{(n+1)} = f^{(n)}+\Delta$

7. $n = n+1$; GO TO 3. $\hspace{4cm}$ (35)

Fortunately, the time-consuming iterative process described above can be carried out by a single filtering step represented by eqn. (32) in frequency space. Therefore, in practice, the MF algorithm can be executed by:

1. $\hat{f}_{MLP} = RA\{p\}$

2. $\hat{F}_{MLP} = FT_2\{\hat{f}_{MLP}\}$

3. $F_{R(MF)}^{(n)} = \hat{F}_{MLP} \cdot H_{MF}^{(n)}$

4. $f_{R(MF)}^{(n)} = FT_2^{-1}\{F_{R(MF)}^{(n)}\}$. $\hspace{3cm}$ (36)

The MF approach promises the following advantages. (1) It provides excellent resolution enhancement at low frequencies where the spectral signal-to-noise ratio is large; hence large structures can be recorded with good quantitative accuracy. (2) It offers good noise suppression at high frequencies where the spectral signal-to-noise ratio is small; thus, high frequency noise is controlled automatically. No reconstructed resolution function, U_R [eqn. (17)], is needed for the purpose of noise suppression. (3) The amplitude and phase response of Metz filters change smoothly as functions of frequency; thus "ripple" or "ringing" effects (e.g., the Gibbs phenomenon) in the processed image are small. (4) Because the MF method employs the MLP pre-image array for image reconstruction, the time-consuming "confidence weighting" procedure is avoided. The MF approach is implemented by its equivalent filters in frequency space, thus requiring no more computation time than the MLP method.

5. RECURSIVE METHODS
5.1. The EPDW method

Maximum likelihood estimation has been under intensive study in recent years for its potential versatility in tomographic image reconstruction. It has received particular attention since the EM algorithm for maximum likelihood estimation was reported by Dempster, Laird, and Rubin [25]. Recently, this approach has been applied to image reconstruction in emission computed tomography (ECT) [26,27], transmission computed tomography (TCT) [27], PET [28,29], SPECT [30], and TOFPET [15,31], and to functional parameter estimation in tracer kinetic studies [32,33].

Maximum likelihood estimation calculates the values of unobserved parameters of some theoretical model that make the measured data most likely. Broadly speaking, a likelihood function can be defined by the joint probability function of measured data in terms of the unobserved parameters to be estimated in the task. Maximizing this likelihood function with respect to the unobserved parameters yields the source distribution estimate with which the data are most consistent. The virtue of the maximum likelihood approach is that, in principle, it can take into account in the reconstructed image every physical and statistical process in the sequence of events leading to data collection. Unlike most of other image reconstruction algorithms, in which factors such as attenuation, scatter radiation, radio-activity decay, detector sensitivity, geometry of the tomograph, detector resolution, TOF resolution, chance coincidence, etc. are either compensated for by a cascade of approximated correction schemes or sometimes assumed to be negligible, maximum likelihood reconstruction algorithms can include all the factors to be considered in a single probability function that is employed in the reconstruction process. Therefore, the maximum likelihood approach potentially can provide more accurate reconstructions.

However, using maximum likelihood estimation to perform image reconstruction usually involves iterative schemes requiring a substantial amount of computation. This is the major reason that this approach was not favored for image reconstruction in the past. Nevertheless, the current advancement of computer technology suggests that these presently time-consuming methods may be very promising in the future, when very fast computers will significantly diminish the disadvantage of long computations.

The calculations associated with the maximization step in a maximum likelihood approach may be very complicated. The EM algorithm generally employs a postulated, unobservable "complete data set" to facilitate the maximization process. This complete data set is sampled from a larger or richer space which can be related easily to the subspace from which the measured data set, now called the "incomplete data set," is sampled. A new likelihood function then can be defined by the joint probability function of the elements of this complete data set. The expectation value of this new likelihood function, given the measured data set and some initial or current estimates of the parameters to be determined in the task, is formulated in the expectation step (E-step) of the EM algorithm. The maximization step (M-step) that follows gives the formula used to calculate new estimates. The combination of the E-step and the subsequent M-step, which involves the likelihood function defined on the complete data set, is equivalent to the original task of maximizing the likelihood function defined on the measured or "incomplete" data set [25-27]. Therefore, the EM algorithm provides a practical way to approach iteratively the maximum of the likelihood function of the measured data.

For convenience in the following discussion, assume that the activity distribution function $f(x,y)$ in eqn. (5) is discrete and represented by an NxN matrix, with f_k representing the kth element ($0 < k \leq N^2$). Assume also that the attenuation-corrected image arrays $p(\xi,\eta;\theta)$ are also discrete and represented by an NxNxM matrix, with p_{ij} representing the measured data in the jth element ($0 < j \leq N^2$) at the ith angle ($0 < i \leq M$). The EPDW method employs the attenuation-corrected image arrays $\{p_{ij}\}$ as the measured or "incomplete" data set, and devises a "complete data set," s_{ijk}, which is the number of events emitting from f_k and detected in p_{ij}. It is obvious that:

$$p_{ij} = \sum_k s_{ijk} \quad . \tag{37}$$

Assuming that positron annihilation is an isotropic process, the expectation value of s_{ijk}, given f, can be written as:

$$E[s_{ijk}|f] = N_{ijk}$$
$$= w(\xi_j-\xi_k,\eta_j-\eta_k;\theta_i)f_k \tag{38}$$
$$= w_{ijk}f_k$$

where w is the kernel used in eqn. (1), and the expected count density within each pixel is assumed to be uniform. Governed by the Poisson nature of the process, the probability density function of s_{ijk} is:

$$Pr[s_{ijk}|f] = (N_{ijk})^{s_{ijk}} \exp(-N_{ijk})/s_{ijk}! \quad . \tag{39}$$

Because all s_{ijk} are independent from each other, the likelihood function, $q_L(s|f)$, of the complete data set can be expressed in terms of the joint probability density function by:

$$q_L(s|f) = \prod_i \prod_j \prod_k Pr[s_{ijk}|f] \quad . \tag{40}$$

Substituting eqn. (39) into eqn. (40), one can write the log likelihood function as:

$$\ln q_L(s|f) = \sum_{ijk} [-N_{ijk} + s_{ijk}(\ln(N_{ijk})) - \ln(s_{ijk}!)] \quad . \tag{41}$$

Using eqns. (37) and (41), one can also formulate the log likelihood function, $\ln g_L(p|f)$, of the measured or the "incomplete" data set as:

$$\ln g_L(p|f) = \sum_{ij} [-\sum_k N_{ijk} + p_{ij}(\ln(\sum_k N_{ijk})) - \ln(p_{ij}!)] \quad . \tag{42}$$

In the E-step of the EM algorithm, the conditional expectation of $\ln q_L(s|f)$ with respect to the measured data, p, and the current estimate, $f^{(n)}$, is formulated by:

$$Q_E(f|f^{(n)}) = E[\ln q_L(s|f)|p,f^{(n)}]$$

$$= \sum_{ijk} \{-N_{ijk} + E[s_{ijk}|p_{ij},f^{(n)}]\ln(N_{ijk})$$

$$- \ln[(E[s_{ijk}|p_{ij},f^{(n)}])!]\} \quad . \tag{43}$$

By noting that all s_{ijk} are independent variables and by using the definition of conditional expectation and eqn. (37), one can derive:

$$E[s_{ijk}|p_{ij},f^{(n)}] = E[s_{ijk}|\sum_k s_{ijk},f^{(n)}]$$

$$= \{(\sum_k s_{ijk})E[s_{ijk}|f^{(n)}]\}/\{\sum_m E[s_{ijm}|f^{(n)}]\}$$

$$= \{p_{ij}E[s_{ijk}|f^{(n)}]\}/\{\sum_m E[s_{ijm}|f^{(n)}]\} \quad . \tag{44}$$

Replacing f and f_k in eqn. (38) by the current estimate $f^{(n)}$ and its kth element $f_k^{(n)}$, one obtains:

$$E[s_{ijk}|f^{(n)}] = N_{ijk}^{(n)} = w_{ijk}f_k^{(n)} \quad . \tag{45}$$

From eqns. (37), (43), (44), and (45), it follows that:

$$Q_E(f|f^{(n)}) = \sum_{ijk}\{-w_{ijk}f_k + [w_{ijk}f_k^{(n)}P_{ij}/(\sum_m w_{ijm}f_m^{(n)})]\ln(w_{ijk}f_k)$$

$$-\ln[(w_{ijk}f_k^{(n)}P_{ij}/(\sum_m w_{ijm}f_m^{(n)}))!]\} \quad . \tag{46}$$

The M-step that follows is now straightforward. First, the partial derivatives are taken as follows:

$$(\partial/\partial f_k)Q_E(f|f^{(n)}) = \sum_{ij}[-w_{ijk}+w_{ijk}f_k^{(n)}P_{ij}/(f_k\sum_m w_{ijm}f_m^{(n)})] \quad . \tag{47}$$

Setting the right-hand side to zero yields the new, i.e., the (n+1), estimate:

$$f_k^{(n+1)} = (f_k^{(n)}/\sum_{ij}w_{ijk})[\sum_{ij}w_{ijk}(P_{ij}/\sum_m w_{ijm}f_m^{(n)})] \quad . \tag{48}$$

Equation (48) is the formula derived from the EM algorithm to calculate the next generation of estimates. It can be viewed as an iterative reconstruction algorithm with a multiplicative correction scheme as follows:

1. n = 0; assume an initial estimate $f^{(0)}$

2. i = 0; SUM = 0

3. a = $f^{(n)}$**w

4. b = p/a

5. d = b**w

6. SUM = SUM + d

7. If i = N(angles) GO TO 9

8. i = i + 1; GO TO 3

9. $f^{(n+1)}$ = $f^{(n)}$·SUM

10. n = n + 1; GO TO 2 (49)

where N(angles) is the number of projection angles.

As indicated by steps 2 through 8, the EPDW method is an angle-by-angle operation. Combined with its iterative nature, the computation time demanded by this approach is even greater than that required by the CW method. On the other hand, since this algorithm is based on the maximum likelihood estimation it can, in principle, provide more accurate reconstructions.

5.2. A new recursive approach: The "simple EM" (SEM) method

As indicated by eqns. (8) and (13), the rotationally averaged estimate $\hat{f}(x,y)$ is the convolution of the original distribution function, $f(x,y)$, and a rotationally symmetric PSF, $psf(r,\theta)$. A new reconstruction method, also based on the EM algorithm, can be designed if the rotational average operation [eqn. (6)] is executed as a preprocessing step before performing any EM step. In this new "simple EM" (SEM) method [31], the rotationally averaged estimate, $\hat{f}(x,y)$, is defined as the measured or "incomplete" data set. It can be also discretized into an NxN matrix with $\hat{f}_j$

representing the jth element $(0 < j \leq N^2)$. Notice that the dimension of the projection angle variable specified by the index i for the measured data p_{ij} in the EPDW method is now no longer needed. A complete data set, z_{jk}, is now defined as the number of events emitting from f_k and detected in $\hat{f}_j$. It can be related to the incomplete data set by:

$$\hat{f}_j = \sum_k z_{jk} \quad . \tag{50}$$

The expectation value of z_{jk}, given f, is:

$$\begin{aligned} E[z_{jk}|f] &= N_{jk} \\ &= psf(x_j-x_k, y_j-y_k)f_k \\ &= psf_{jk}f_k \quad , \end{aligned} \tag{51}$$

where psf is the rotationally symmetric PSF defined by eqn. (12) [or, more generally, by eqn. (7)], and the expected count density within each pixel is assumed to be uniform. The probability density function for z_{jk}, given f, is again a Poisson distribution as follows:

$$Pr[z_{jk}|f] = (N_{jk})^{z_{jk}} exp(-N_{jk})/z_{jk}! \quad . \tag{52}$$

Following the derivation for the case of the EPDW method in the previous section, one can obtain the log likelihood function of the complete data set as:

$$\ln q_L(z|f) = \sum_j\sum_k [-N_{jk}+z_{jk}(\ln(N_{jk}))-\ln(z_{jk}!)] \quad ; \tag{53}$$

the log likelihood function of the incomplete data set as:

$$\ln g_L(\hat{f}|f) = \sum_j [-\sum_k N_{jk}+\hat{f}_j(\ln(\sum_k N_{jk}))-\ln(\hat{f}_j!)] \quad ; \tag{54}$$

and the conditional expectation of $\ln q_L(z|f)$ with respect to $\hat{f}$ and the current estimate $f^{(n)}$ as:

$$\begin{aligned} Q_E(f|f^{(n)}) &= E[\ln q_L(z|f)|\hat{f}, f^{(n)}] \\ &= \sum_j\sum_k \{-N_{jk}+E[z_{jk}|\hat{f}_j, f^{(n)}]\ln(N_{jk}) \\ &\quad -\ln[(E[z_{jk}|\hat{f}_j, f^{(n)}])!]\} \\ &= \sum_j\sum_k \{-psf_{jk}f_k+[psf_{jk}f_k^{(n)}\hat{f}_j/(\sum_m psf_{jm}f_m^{(n)})]\ln(psf_{jk}f_k^{(n)}) \\ &\quad -\ln[(psf_{jk}f_k^{(n)}\hat{f}_j/(\sum_m psf_{jm}f_m^{(n)}))!]\} \quad . \end{aligned} \tag{55}$$

Equating the first derivative of $Q_E(f|f^{(n)})$ to zero results in the criterion for calculating the new estimate in this SEM method as:

$$f_k^{(n+1)} = (f_k^{(n)}/\sum_j psf_{jk})[\sum_j psf_{jk}(\hat{f}_j/\sum_m psf_{jm}f_m^{(n)})] \tag{56}$$

which gives a maximum of $Q_E(f|f^{(n)})$. In the continuous space, eqn. (56) can be written as:

$$f^{(n+1)} = f^{(n)} \cdot \{(\hat{f}/(f^{(n)} **\text{psf})) **\text{psf}^-\} \tag{57}$$

where $\text{psf}^- = \text{psf}(-r,\theta)$. For a rotationally symmetric PSF, $\text{psf}(-r,\theta) = \text{psf}(r,\theta)$; therefore, $\text{psf}^- = \text{psf}$.

Based on the above derivation, the SEM algorithm can be summarized as follows:

1. $\hat{f} = RA\{p\}$
2. $n = 0$; assume an initial estimate $f^{(0)}$
3. $a = f^{(n)} **\text{psf}$
4. $b = \hat{f}/a$
5. $d = b **\text{psf}$
6. $f^{(n+1)} = f^{(n)} \cdot d$
7. $n = n + 1$; GO TO 3. $\tag{58}$

Equation (57) is identical to the formula in the "iterative biased smearing" technique proposed previously for image processing in conventional scintigraphy by Metz and Pizer [17,18]. The same formula was later derived independently in a Bayesian-based iterative method for image restoration by Richardson [34,35]. The SEM method proposed here for TOFPET image reconstruction produces this same formula on the basis of the EM algorithm.

The most important advantage of the SEM method over the EPDW method is that the angle-by-angle calculations required in steps 2 through 8 of the latter method [eqn. (49)] are now reduced to a single operation specified by steps 3 through 6 in eqn. (58). For an image reconstruction study with M projection angles, the new SEM method requires only 1/M of the computation time demanded by the EPDW method. Like the EPDW method, this new reconstruction algorithm is also based on maximum likelihood estimation; therefore, it should provide more accurate reconstructions.

6. EVALUATION OF ALGORITHMS

Computer simulation studies have been performed to evaluate the relative merits of these five algorithms for image reconstruction in TOFPET. Computational efficiency, reconstructed image resolution, and SNR have been used as performance indices.

6.1. Computational efficiency

The number of floating point operations (addition and multiplication) required for each algorithm has been discussed and estimated in [24]. The actual computation times for reconstructing an image on a 256x256 matrix with 72 projection angles (and 10 iterations for the EPDW and SEM methods) in the simulation studies using a Perkin-Elmer 3254 computer were in the ratio MLP:CW:MF:EPDW:SEM = 1:80:1:1500:20.

6.2. Reconstructed image resolution

Two spatial resolution indices are used to specify the reconstructed image resolution: the commonly used FWHM and the equivalent width (EW) defined as:

$$EW \equiv \int_{-\infty}^{\infty} PSF(x)\,dx/PSF(0) \quad . \tag{59}$$

For a non-Gaussian PSF, EW can represent spatial resolution more adequately than can FWHM [31,36].

An ideal point source was generated using 72 projection angles on a 256x256 matrix with 0.25 cm pixels. The detector resolution was assumed to be Gaussian with a 1.2 cm FWHM; the TOF resolution, Gaussian with a 400 psec FWHM.

Figure 5a illustrates the resolution of the point source response function (PSRF) as a function of the standard deviation, σ_R, of the reconstructed resolution function, U_R [eqn. (17)], when the MLP or CW method is used with various weighting and filtering approaches. Two different weighting processes can be employed: a 1-D weighting that smoothes only along the direction of TOF resolution [indicated by W(T) in Fig. 5a]; or a 2-D weighting that smoothes along directions of both TOF and detector resolutions [W(T,D)]. There are four factors that can be incorporated into the filter function: TOF resolution [F(T)]; detector resolution [F(D)]; weighting along the direction of TOF resolution [F(W(T))]; and weighting along the detector resolution [F(W(D))]. A closer examination reveals that EW/FWHM = 1.06 for all curves plotted in Fig. 5a, suggesting that PSRFs in these cases are Gaussian in shape.

Figure 5b shows the resolution of the PSRF obtained with the MF method as a function of the order of Metz filter. It covers a range similar to that of Fig. 5a. The resolution of the PSRF achieved by the EPDW or SEM method is plotted in Fig. 5c as a function of the number of iterations. The advantage of using the SEM method can be better demonstrated in Fig. 5d, where the PSRF resolution is replotted as a function of relative computation time. One should note that the SEM method can provide excellent PSRF resolution in a calculation time less than that required for a single iteration in the EPDW method. The ratios of EW to FWHM for the MF, EPDW, and SEM methods deviate from 1.06, indicating that the PSRFs resulting from these algorithms are no longer truly Gaussian.

6.3. SNR

For the evaluation of noise, a circular source 30 cm in diameter was simulated with approximately 10^6 counts and the matrix configuration specified in the previous section. Two SNR models were used in the present study. The common "amplitude" model is defined by:

$$SNR^2 \equiv \left\{ \iint_{-\infty}^{\infty} SS^2(\nu_x,\nu_y)d\nu_x d\nu_y \right\} \bigg/ \left\{ \iint_{-\infty}^{\infty} WS(\nu_x,\nu_y)d\nu_x d\nu_y \right\} \tag{60}$$

where $SS(\nu_x,\nu_y)$ is the 2-D signal spectrum and $WS(\nu_x,\nu_y)$ is the 2-D noise Wiener spectrum. A "statistical decision theory" model, which has been demonstrated to provide better correlation between detectability and SNR than the amplitude model [37,38], is defined by:

$$SNR^2 \equiv \left\{ \iint_{-\infty}^{\infty} SS^2(\nu_x,\nu_y)d\nu_x d\nu_y \right\}^2 \bigg/ \left\{ \iint_{-\infty}^{\infty} SS^2(\nu_x,\nu_y)WS(\nu_x,\nu_y)d\nu_x d\nu_y \right\} \quad . \tag{61}$$

Relative SNRs for the five algorithms under investigation are illustrated in Fig. 6. The results have been normalized to the case of a 1.2 cm FWHM (i.e., 1.27 cm EW) PSRF achieved by the MLP method. Some improvement can be seen with the MF or SEM method under certain conditions. Different rankings of various algorithms using these two SNR models suggest that the selection of an appropriate SNR model is an important issue in the evaluation of image reconstruction algorithms and needs to be investigated further.

7. DISCUSSION

As mentioned earlier, image reconstruction can be thought of as a classical 2-D image processing task in which one attempts to restore an image with the knowledge of a well-defined PSF. This point of view is substantially different from that of conventional tomographic image reconstruction, in which one-dimensional (1-D) projection profiles from various angles are normally filtered and backprojected. The broader perspective opens new avenues for image reconstruction in TOFPET. In principle, all 2-D image processing schemes that have been developed in other areas are potentially applicable to TOFPET image reconstruction. The MF and SEM methods proposed in this paper are two examples of many such possibilities. The potential usefulness of other 2-D image processing methods in TOFPET image reconstruction should be explored in future research.

The CW method employs a generalized "matched filtering" process that operates angle-by-angle on the attenuation-corrected image arrays. If SNR values based on the amplitude model are used as the criterion for evaluation, then the CW method can be shown to be the optimal approach among all linear schemes [7]. However, as discussed in the previous section, evidence exists to suggest that other SNR models correlate better with visual signal detectability [37,38]. Thus, conclusions regarding the superiority of the CW method, which are based on the amplitude model, may not accurately predict visual detectability. Other linear algorithms, such as the MF method, and non-linear algorithms, such as the EPDW and SEM methods, may, in fact, provide better visual detectability. Furthermore, quantitative accuracy is often of greater concern in tomographic imaging. These issues require further investigation before the relative merits of different TOFPET image reconstruction algorithms can be clearly established.

Generalization of the MF and SEM methods to applications other than TOFPET image reconstruction must be undertaken with caution. For example, in the case of conventional PET (or x-ray CT) imaging with a simple backprojection scheme, the PSF is proportional to $1/r$ if perfect detector resolution is assumed. Neither the MF nor the SEM method is directly applicable in that situation due to the singularity of the corresponding OTF at $\nu = 0$.

8. SUMMARY

Two new algorithms for image reconstruction in TOFPET have been developed. Their performance has been examined and compared to three other algorithms. The MF method provides a good compromise between computational efficiency and reconstructed image quality. When a need for excellent spatial resolution can justify additional computation time, the SEM method may be preferable.

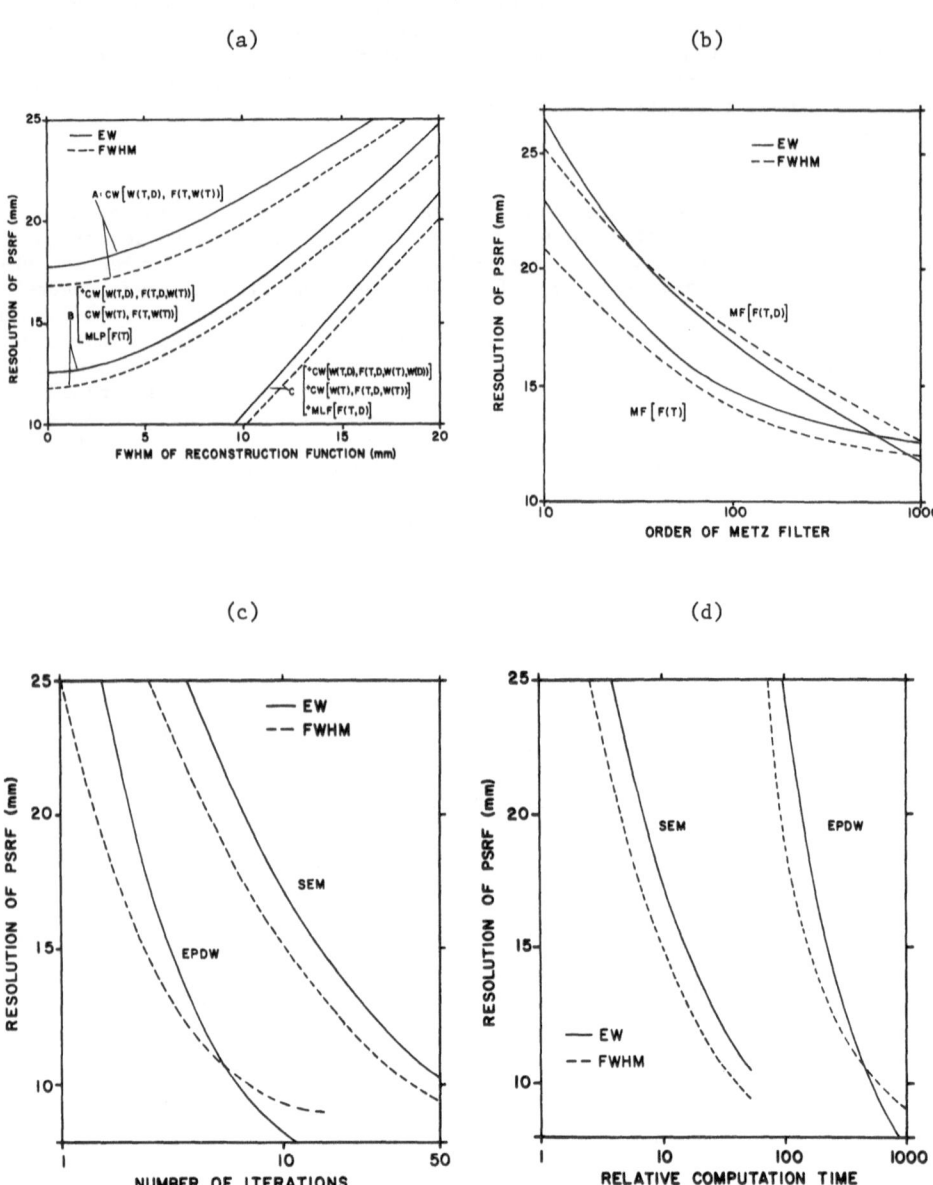

FIGURE 5. Reconstructed spatial resolution achieved by various image reconstruction algorithms for TOFPET.

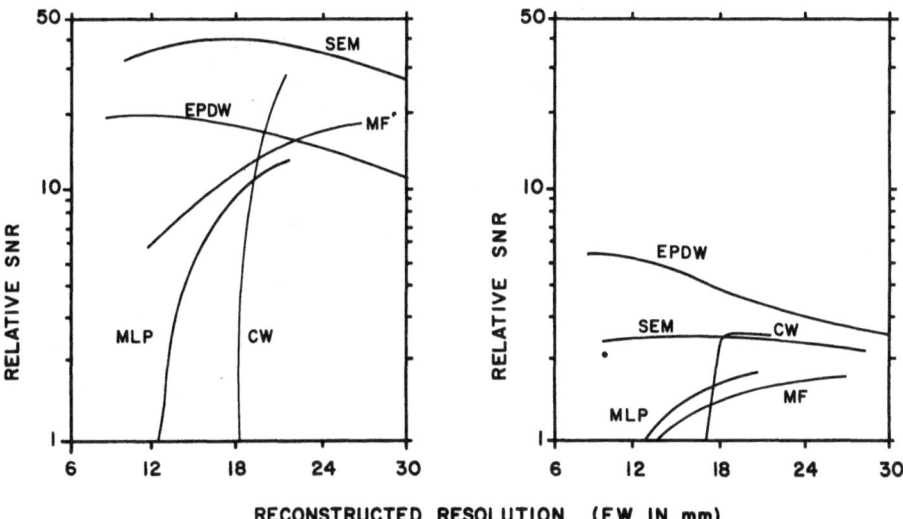

FIGURE 6. Relative SNR as a function of reconstructed spatial resolution (EW). The left is based on the amplitude model [eqn. (60)], the right on a statistical decision theory model [eqn. (61)].

REFERENCES

1. Campagnolo, R.E., Garderet, P. and Vacher, J.: Tomographic par emmetteurs positrons aves mesure de temps de vol. In: Proc. of the Communication au Colloque international sur le traitement du signal. Nice, May 1979.

2. Allemand, R., Gresset, C. and Vacher, J.: Potential advantages of a cesium fluoride scintillator for a time-of-flight positron camera. J. Nucl. Med. 21:153-155, 1980.

3. Mullani, N.A., Markham, J. and Ter-Pogossian, M.M.: Feasibility of time-of-flight reconstruction in positron emission tomography. J. Nucl. Med. 21:1095-1097, 1980.

4. Ter-Pogossian, M.M., Mullani, N.A., Ficke, D.C., Markham, J. and Snyder, D.L.: Photon time-of-flight-assisted positron emission tomography. J. Comput. Assist. Tomogr. 5:227-239, 1981.

5. Budinger, T.F.: Instrumentation trends in nuclear medicine. Semin. Nucl. Med. 7:285-297, 1977.

6. Snyder, D.L., Thomas, L.J. and Ter-Pogossian, M.M.: A mathematical model for positron emission tomography having time-of-flight measurement. IEEE Trans. Nucl. Sci. NS-28:3575-3583, 1981.

7. Tomitani, T.: Image reconstruction and noise evaluation in photon time-of-flight assisted positron emission tomography. IEEE Trans. Nucl. Sci. NS-28:4582-4589, 1981.

8. Snyder, D.L.: Some noise comparison of data collection arrays for emission tomography systems having time-of-flight measurements. IEEE Trans. Nucl. Sci. NS-29:1029-1033, 1982.

9. Wong, W.H., Mullani, N.A. and Gould, K.L.: Image improvement and design optimization in the time-of-flight PET. J. Nucl. Med. 24:52-60, 1983.

10. Mullani, N.A., Wong, W.H., Hartz, R., Philippe, E.A. and Yerian, K.: Sensitivity improvement of TOFPET by the utilization of the inter-slice coincidences. IEEE Trans. Nucl. Sci. NS-29:479-483, 1982.

11. Yamamoto, M., Ficke, D.C. and Ter-Pogossian, M.M.: Effect of the software coincidence timing window in time-of-flight assisted positron emission tomography. IEEE Trans. Nucl. Sci. NS-30:711-714, 1983.

12. Bendriem, B., Soussaline, F., Campagnolo, R., Verrey, B., Wainberg, P. and Syrota, A.: Contrast improvement by reduction of the scatter contribution in a PET system using TOF information. J. Nucl. Med. 26:P36, 1985. (Abstract)

13. Ter-Pogossian, M.M., Ficke, D.C., Yamamoto, M. and Hood, J.T.: Design characteristics and preliminary testing of SUPER PETT I, a positron emission tomograph utilizing photon time-of-flight information (TOFPET). In: Proc. of Workshop on Time-of-Flight Tomography, St. Louis, May 1982, IEEE Computer Society Press, Silver Spring, Maryland, 1982, pp. 37-41.

14. Mullani, N.A., Wong, W.H., Hartz, R.K., Yerian, K., Philippe, E.A., Gaeta, J.M. and Gould, K.L.: Preliminary result with TOFPET. IEEE Trans. Nucl. Sci. NS-30:739-743, 1983.

15. Snyder, D.L. and Politte, D.G.: Image reconstruction from list-mode data in an emission tomography system having time-of-flight measurements. IEEE Trans. Nucl. Sci. NS-30:1843-1849, 1983.

16. Metz, C.E.: A mathematical investigation of radioisotope scan image processing. Ph.D. Dissertation, University of Pennsylvania, Philadelphia, Pennsylvania, 1969. Ann Arbor, Michigan, University Microfilms (order no. 70-16, 186).

17. Metz, C.E. and Pizer, S.M.: Nonstationary and nonlinear scintigram processing. Presented at the Second International Conference on Data Handling and Image Processing in Scintigraphy, Hanover, Germany, October, 1971. (Unpublished manuscript)

18. Pizer, S.M., Correia, J.A., Chesler, D.A. and Metz, C.E.: Results of nonlinear and nonstationary processing. In: Proc. of the Third International Conference on Data Handling and Image Processing in Scintigraphy, Cambridge, Massachusetts, June 6-9, 1973, pp. 93-101.

19. Pizer, S.M. and Todd-Pokropek, A.E.: Improvement of scintigrams by computer processing. Semin. Nucl. Med. 8:125-146, 1978.

20. King, M.A., Doherty, P.W., Schwinger, R.B., Jacobs, D.A., Kidder, R.E. and Miller, T.R.: Fast count-dependent digital filtering of nuclear medicine images. J. Nucl. Med. 24:1039-1045, 1983.

21. King, M.A., Schwinger, R.B., Penney, B.C. and Doherty, P.W.: Two-dimensional filtering of SPECT images using the Metz and Wiener filters. J. Nucl. Med. 25:P14, 1984. (Abstract)

22. Chan, H.-P., Doi, K. and Metz, C.E.: Digital image processing: Effects of Metz filters and matched filters on detection of simple radiographic objects. Proc. SPIE 454:420-432, 1984.

23. Chen, C.-T. and Metz, C.E.: A new image reconstruction method for positron emission tomography with time-of-flight information (TOFPET). Med. Phys. 10:731, 1983. (Abstract)

24. Chen, C.-T. and Metz, C.E.: Evaluation and comparison of image reconstruction algorithms for positron emission tomography with time-of-
flight information (TOFPET). Presented at the 2nd International Symposium on Medical Images and Icons, July 1984. In: Proceedings of
ISMII 1984, pp. 388-393.
25. Dempster, A.P., Laird, N.M. and Rubin, D.B.: Maximum likelihood from
incomplete data via the EM algorithm. JRSS 39:1-38, 1977.
26. Shepp, L.A. and Vardi, Y.: Maximum likelihood reconstruction for emission tomography. IEEE Trans. Med. Imaging MI-1:113-122, 1982.
27. Lange, K. and Carson, R.: EM reconstruction algorithms for emission
and transmission tomography. J. Comput. Assist. Tomogr. 8:306-312,
1984.
28. Shepp, L.A., Vardi, Y., Ra, J.B., Hilal, S.K. and Cho, Z.H.: Maximum
likelihood PET with real data. IEEE Trans. Nucl. Sci. NS-31:910-913,
1984.
29. Vardi, Y., Shepp, L.A. and Kaufman, L.: A statistical model for positron emission tomography. J. Amer. Statist. Assoc. 80:8-37, 1985.
30. Miller, M.I., Snyder, D.L. and Miller, T.R.: Maximum likelihood reconstruction for single-photon emission computed-tomography. IEEE Trans.
Nucl. Sci. NS-32:769-778, 1985.
31. Chen, C.-T. and Metz, C.E.: A simplified EM reconstruction algorithm
for TOFPET. IEEE Trans. Nucl. Sci. NS-32:885-888, 1985.
32. Carson, R.E.: Two image-wide parameter estimation methods for positron
emission tomography: Theory and application to the measurement of
local cerebral blood flow in humans. Ph.D. Dissertation, University of
California at Los Angeles, 1983.
33. Snyder, D.L.: Parameter estimation for dynamic studies in emission-
tomography systems having list-mode data. IEEE Trans. Nucl. Sci.
NS-31:925-931, 1984.
34. Richardson, W.H.: Bayesian-based iterative method of image restoration. J. Opt. Soc. Am. 62:55-59, 1972.
35. Raeside, D.E.: Bayesian statistics: a guided tour. Med. Phys. 3:1-
11, 1976.
36. Knoop, B., Jordan, K., Judas, R. and Schober, D.: Spatial resolution
in imaging systems: equivalent width, a realistic measure to replace
FWHM. J. Nucl. Med. 25:P22, 1984. (Abstract)
37. Wagner, R.F.: Decision theory and the detail signal-to-noise ratio of
Otto Shade. Photog. Sci. and Engr. 22:41-46, 1978.
38. Loo, L.-N., Doi, K. and Metz, C.E.: A comparison of physical image
quality indices and observer performance in the radiographic detection
of nylon beads. Phys. Med. Biol. 29:837-856, 1984.

THREE DIMENSIONAL RECONSTRUCTION OF VASCULAR BEDS

Dennis L. Parker, David L. Pope, Keith S. White, Lawrence R. Tarbox, and Hiram W. Marshall

Department of Medical Biophysics and Computing, LDS Hospital/University of Utah, Salt Lake City, Utah 84143

This chapter discusses the mathematics and computer processing required to generate three dimensional representations of vascular beds from multiple digital angiographic projections. In order to compensate for the deficiencies of conventional reconstruction techniques, a method is presented which directly reconstructs a vascular tree structure. This method appears to take good advantage of vessel characteristics such as connectivity and uniform internal density. Direct reconstruction takes full advantage of the information contained in multiple images, using a dynamic programming technique to determine the vessel centerline, edges, and densitometric profiles in each of the views. With the knowledge of the artery locations from each projection, reconstruction of the arterial tree centerline is overdetermined and averaging or least squares techniques can be used. The vessel lumen geometry may be estimated using the edge information and attenuation profile. The lumen geometry can then be refined by densitometric reprojection of the vascular tree and comparison with original profiles. Examples of direct reconstruction and perspective display of a pig heart coronary artery cast are given.

1. INTRODUCTION

The three dimensional reconstruction of a vascular bed from multiple projections may be of significant clinical benefit. Perspective views of the vessel tree could assist interventional radiologists and cardiologists with catheter placement during angioplasty procedures. Such views may also be of assistance to the surgery team during conventional cardiac bipass surgery. Orientation information is essential for accurate densitometric cross-sectional area measurements as well as for time of flight flow analysis (1,2,3). Three dimensional reconstructions of the coronary arteries at various points in time during the cardiac cycle has been shown to be useful in studying the absolute motion of the myocardium (4).

The potential for reconstruction of vascular beds from multiple projections has been studied by various groups. The geometrical mathematics for reconstructing the centerline of vessels from two non-coplanar views has been presented by Kim, et al. (5). This included mathematical transformations from the object coordinate system to the two projected planes, as well as the property of matching points in the two views. This technique was also used by MacKay et al. (6), in the three dimensional position determinations used for motion analysis.

The reconstruction of an arterial cross-section is a more complicated problem. In general, arbitrary points within a cross-section cannot be matched between views. In this case, reconstruction requires the utilization of edge location and densitometric information from the vessel profiles. The general mathematics for object reconstruction from multiple views of totally arbitrary orientation has been presented (7,8,9). An iterative approach which allows small numbers of views of arbitrary orientation has also been developed (10,11,12). In general, densitometric reconstruction requires more than two views, with the number of views being directly related to the desired spatial resolution of the vessel cross-section. Attempts have been made to reconstruct the three-dimensional left ventricle using densitometric information obtained from bi-plane' views (13,14,15). Reiber et al. developed similar algorithms for reconstructing the cross-section of an artery segment from two views (16). Ambiguities inherent in these reconstructions may be reduced by including out of plane information corresponding to the structure of interest.

This chapter reviews two alternative basis function structures which can be used to represent vascular beds. The merits of a tree structure (possibly similar to the structure used by Mol et al. 17) are presented and compared with the standard rectangular matrix. We explore an algorithm which recognizes vessel information, matches the information for corresponding vessels in multiple images and reconstructs the three dimensional vessel structure. Given this information, it is possible to rotate, translate and scale individual images to achieve optimal alignment. The geometrical mathematics required to orient images, match corresponding points and perform the reconstruction are also presented. The problems associated with reconstructing the vessel cross-section are discussed. Examples of such reconstructions are given.

2. LIMITATIONS OF CONVENTIONAL RECONSTRUCTION TECHNIQUES

Reconstruction of the vascular beds could in principle be accomplished using convolution, backprojection techniques. Conventional image reconstruction from projection, as performed in standard CT scanners, uses as explicit knowledge the orientation of each projection and the measured x-ray attenuation along each path. Errors in orientation (angle, translation, etc.) result in significant artifacts such as streaking and blurring. Inconsistencies in density measurements (polychromatic beam hardening, scatter, etc.) also lead to streaks between regions of generally different atomic number (bone, iodine, etc.). Finally, conventional reconstruction requires a large number of views, and limiting this number results in non-compensated streaks radiating away from dense objects.

Due to the wide availability C-arm angiography systems it is important to find a reconstruction technique which is compatible with their limitations. Such systems cannot acquire more than two simultaneous views but are capable of obtaining views from totally arbitrary (non-coplanar) angles. The acquisition of further views will require additional time and thus may not be practical for reconstruction of the moving coronary arteries.

The reconstruction of vascular beds by conventional algorithms will be subject to all of the above sources of artifacts. If imaging is performed with C-arm x-ray systems geometric distortions can be significant. Ambiguities introduced by the geometric instabilities of C-arm based systems can be reduced by matching corresponding vessel points and performing the required transformations to achieve optimal alignment. However, it is unlikely that the artifacts due to geometric inconsistencies will be completely eliminated. Additionally, x-ray scatter, beam hardening, veiling glare, etc. can all make the densitometric measurements inconsistent. For all of these reasons, conventional reconstruction of vessel images would be extremely artifactual. Finally, we note that the ratio of vessel volume to reconstruction volume is typically very low. Thus, even were the convolution/backprojection reconstruction process to be non-artifactual, much time would be wasted in reconstructing non-vessel information.

3. TREE STRUCTURE VS. VOXELS

In the absence of motion artifacts and if only the vasculature of interest is opacified, several aspects of arterial bed imaging are unique. These unique aspects tend to simplify and reduce the large number of calculations required to reconstruct the vascular bed. First, the vessels of interest are often widely separated, resulting in a reconstruction matrix which is somewhat sparse. The iodine density is relatively constant within the vessels and is ideally zero elsewhere. Points along the centerline (e.g. densitometric center of mass) of the vessels can be logically connected in a structure resembling a tree. Because of this sparseness and connectivity, it appears advantageous to perform pre-processing operations which remove all extraneous information from each projected image. The fundamental vessel information which remains can be combined to form an appropriate three-dimensional vascular tree structure.

The unique structure that has been applied in this work is illustrated in Table I. The tree itself consists of branches which begin and terminate at node points. Each branch is connected to a parent branch and may or may not connect to children. The initial node is treated as a special case. As indicated in the table, the fundamental unit of each branch is the element structure which consists of the x,y,z coordinates of the element, the orientation angles, θ and φ, and the various radii around the element within the plane defined by the orientation angles.

The reconstruction process consists of specifying the three dimensional tree structure. It is not necessary to perform backprojection over the entire three dimensional volume representing the reconstructed object. It is only required to matched corresponding segments, generating a three dimensional tree structure, and then perform the reconstruction operations in the immediate vicinity of the tree structures. Although this process leads readily to an iterative reconstruction technique, other possibilities such as the algorithm developed by Reiber, exist and are being investigated.

General three dimensional imaging requires that the effects of motion and geometric distortions be negligible. Because of the time between projections in conventional systems and because of cardiac motion, this condition is not generally met in such systems and image distortions will be

TABLE I
Vascular Tree Structure

TREE

    Number of Branches
    BRANCH
        NODE
            Parent node
            Next Brother
            Number of Children
            First Child
        Number of elements
        ELEMENT
            Center Position (x,y,z)
            Plane Orientation (θ, φ)
            Average Radius
            Cross-sectional Area
            Cross-sectional Radii

ELEMENTS OF 3D TREE STRUCTURE

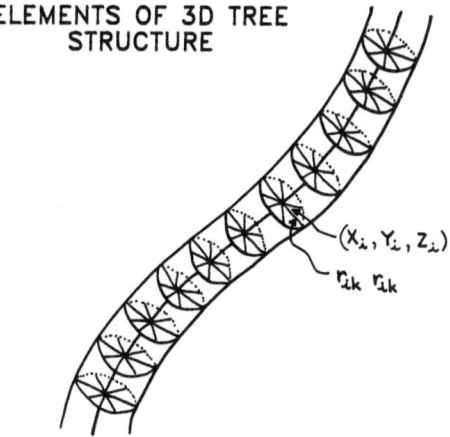

FIGURE 1. Example tree elements.

significant. Reconstruction mathematics can be applied only after some initial pre-processing of each projection image to correct for the distortions. Corrections may be accomplished by matching identical points in each view of the artery tree and then developing 3D rotation, translation and warping transformations to align the projected image of each segment relative to the segments in other views.

4. PROJECTION IMAGES

To demonstrate the concepts of three dimensional reconstruction, 3 x-ray projection images of a pig heart coronary artery phantom were obtained. The phantom and 3 images are shown in Fig. 2. These images were obtained with axial angle increments of 30 degrees (thus a total of 60 degrees between first and last image). The images will be used for graphic illustration of the concepts presented below.

5. MATHEMATICS OF RECONSTRUCTION

This section presents the mathematics and geometric transformations essential to reconstructing the vessel centerlines in a vascular bed. The further complexities involved in determining the complete vessel cross-section are discussed.

5.1 Centerline Determination

The tree structure lends itself to the specification of the arterial segments in each view. In the present implementation, approximate node points on the first view are entered using a graphics tablet. If necessary some indication of the vessel path between nodes is also provided. In this manner, a target consisting of the node points and segments between node

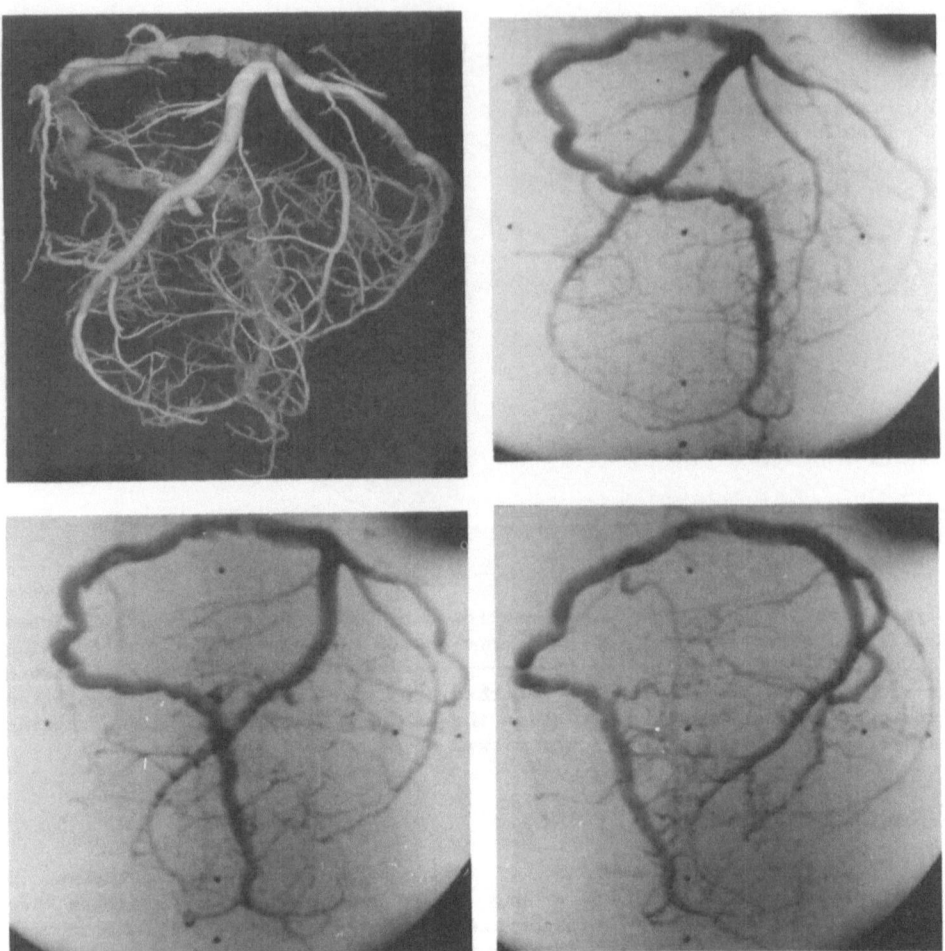

FIGURE 2. a) Pig coronary artery phantom. b-d) X-ray images with $\theta = 90°$ and $\varphi = 0, -30°$, and $-60°$ respectively

points is generated (see Fig. 3a). Using this target, the edges and center of the vessel are found by application of a dynamic search process which has been described previously (18,19,20). The likelihood of a point being part of the vessel edge or center is established using a one dimensional matched filter applied orthogonal to the target. The matched filter outputs are searched with a dynamic program to establish the optimal paths for the two edges and centerline. Resulting centerlines from Fig. 3a are shown in Fig. 3b.

5.2 Centerline Reconstruction

We limit ourselves at the onset to projections of objects obtained along lines diverging from a single point (the x-ray source). A point in three-dimensional space is assigned the coordinates (x,y,z) relative to a

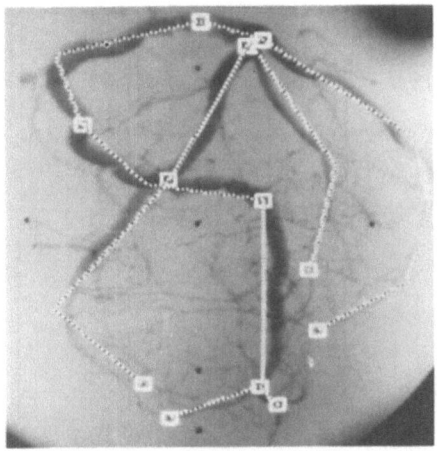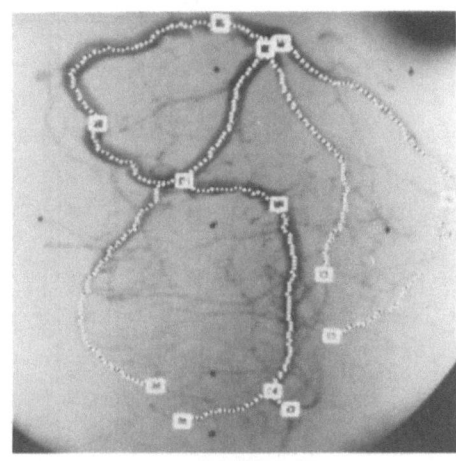

FIGURE 3. a) Hand entered target. b) Result of dynamic search.

conventional Cartesian three-dimensional coordinate system. For convenience it is assumed that the z-axis is vertical. The x-ray source location is specified by the polar angle θ, the axial angle, φ, and the distance, D_s, of the source from the center of rotation (i.e. the origin) as indicated in Fig. 4a. Note, that although a true 'iso-center' makes a natural origin for the coordinate system, it is not generally true that a point from the x-ray source through the center of rotation, will always pass through the same point on the projected image. In fact, effects of the earth's magnetic field are sufficient to cause image distortion on conventional image-intensification, television camera acquisition systems. It is essential that the projection of the origin of the coordinate system be determined in each projected image, as well as the distance, D_s, of the x-ray source and D_I, of the image receptor from the specified origin.

Within each image, the location of a point is specified by the two orthogonal coordinates, (u,v). If the projected location of the origin of the three dimensional coordinate system is known, then the point (u,v) can be specified relative to that system. It is finally necessary to specify the angle of rotation, α, within the plane of the image. Because of magnification due to x-ray divergence the distance between points in the (u,v) coordinate system depends on the relative locations of the points in the original 3D coordinate system. It is convenient to define an intermediate coordinate system, (x',y',z') where x' and y' are parallel to the u and v axes, respectively, and z' is perpendicular to the image plane along the direction toward the x-ray source. In this coordinate system the location of the x-ray source is:

$$\underline{x}'_s = (x'_s, y'_s, z'_s) = (0, 0, D_s). \qquad (1)$$

The location of a point in 3D space can be expressed in terms of either the primed or unprimed coordinate systems and the coordinates are related by the rotation matrix, R:

$$\underline{x}' = R \underline{x}. \qquad (2)$$

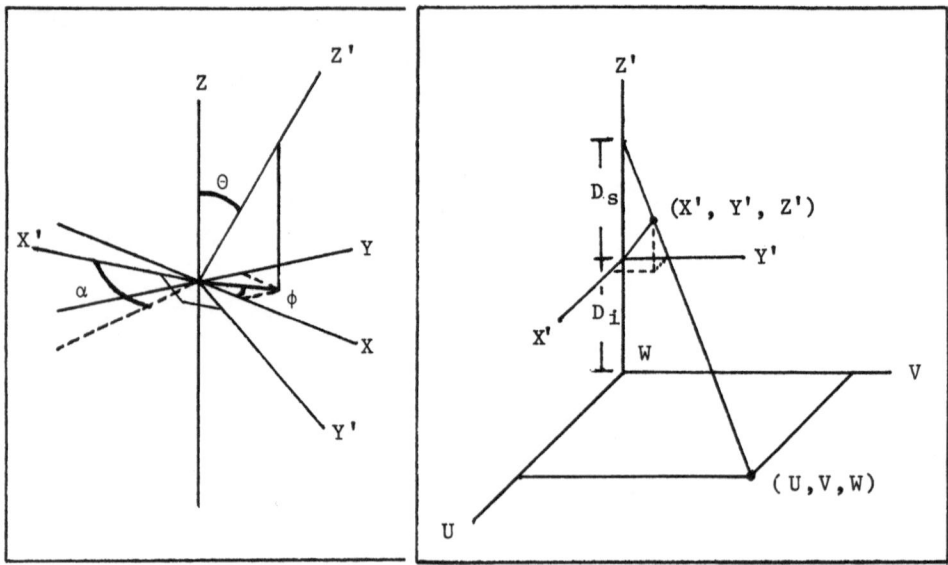

FIGURE 4. a and b) Conversion geometry from 3D to projection image.

The matrix, R, is given by the composition of the rotations:

$$R = \begin{bmatrix} \cos\alpha & -\sin\alpha & 0 \\ \sin\alpha & \cos\alpha & 0 \\ 0 & 0 & 1 \end{bmatrix} \begin{bmatrix} 1 & 0 & 0 \\ 0 & \cos\theta & \sin\theta \\ 0 & -\sin\theta & \cos\theta \end{bmatrix} \begin{bmatrix} -\sin\varphi & \cos\varphi & 0 \\ -\cos\varphi & -\sin\varphi & 0 \\ 0 & 0 & 1 \end{bmatrix} \quad (3)$$

The conversion of the point (x',y',z') to the coordinates (u,v,w) is then simply a matter of scaling. With the source at $(x',y',z') = (0,0,D_s)$ and the image plane at $(x',y',z') = (0,0,-D_I)$, the coordinates (u,v) are simply the coordinates (x',y') multiplied by the ratio of the relative z' distances of the source to the image and the source to the point:

$$(u,v) = \frac{D_s+D_I}{D_s-z'}(x',y'). \quad (4)$$

This relation between (x',y',z') and (u,v,w) is illustrated in Fig. 4b. In general an offset, (u_o,v_o), will be required to translate from the measurement coordinates of each plane to the coordinates (u,v). For the present, we assume that this offset is known and that the translation is performed before comparative analysis.

Equation (4) is that of a line passing through the point (x',y',z'), where (u,v) are linearly related to the distance D_{sI} ($D_{sI} = D_s + D_I$). As pointed out by Kim et al.(5) and Potel et al.(4), a line segment between the x-ray source and a point (u,v) in one image plane will map to a line segment in the image plane for any other view. Thus it is possible to designate a specific point in a single view (which corresponds to a uniquely determined point in the 3D space such as an intersection of recognizable vessels) and to then generate and display the line segment corresponding to this structure in another view. In the absence of geometric distortions, motion, etc. the image of the point in the second view will be found at some position along this line segment. The designation of this position in the second view then completely determines the location of the point in the three dimensional space.

We first let $^1\underline{u} = (^1u, ^1v, ^1w)$ represent the (x',y',z') coordinates of the image point in the first view. Note that ^1w is simply the distance, ^1D_I. The coordinates of this point with respect to the (x,y,z) coordinate system are given by:

$$^1\underline{x} = {}^1R^{-1} \ {}^1\underline{u}. \tag{5}$$

Likewise, the source position is given as:

$$^1\underline{x}_s = {}^1R^{-1} \ {}^1\underline{u}_s. \tag{6}$$

The coordinates of these points in the second projected coordinate system are then obtained as:

$$^{12}\underline{x}' = {}^2R \ {}^1\underline{x} \tag{7}$$

$$^{12}\underline{x}'_s = {}^2R \ {}^1\underline{x}_s. \tag{8}$$

Finally, the $\underline{x}'$ coordinates of these two points in the second image coordinate system are scaled to the image coordinates $(^2u, ^2v)$ and $(^2u_s, ^2v_s)$ using the transformation of Eq. (4). The line between these two points is then explicitly determined. The set of 'node' points illustrated in Fig. 3a are transformed into the line segments shown in Fig. 5a. In the absence of geometric errors or distortions, the location of a node point in the second view is found along the corresponding line segment. Thus, as shown in Fig. 5b, the nodes on the second view have been moved to the appropriate position. Where necessary the path between the nodes has also been altered to more closely follow the true artery path in the second view. This set of paths is then used with the dynamic search algorithm to find the location of the centerlines in the second view as shown in Fig. 5c. The edge determinations are shown in Fig. 5d.

If the projected location of a point within an object in three dimensional space is accurately identified in two non-coplanar projections of the object, the exact three dimensional location of the point is overdetermined. This is true because the locations of the points in the projected images define lines from the respective source points through the object. In the absence of geometric inaccuracies, these lines intersect at

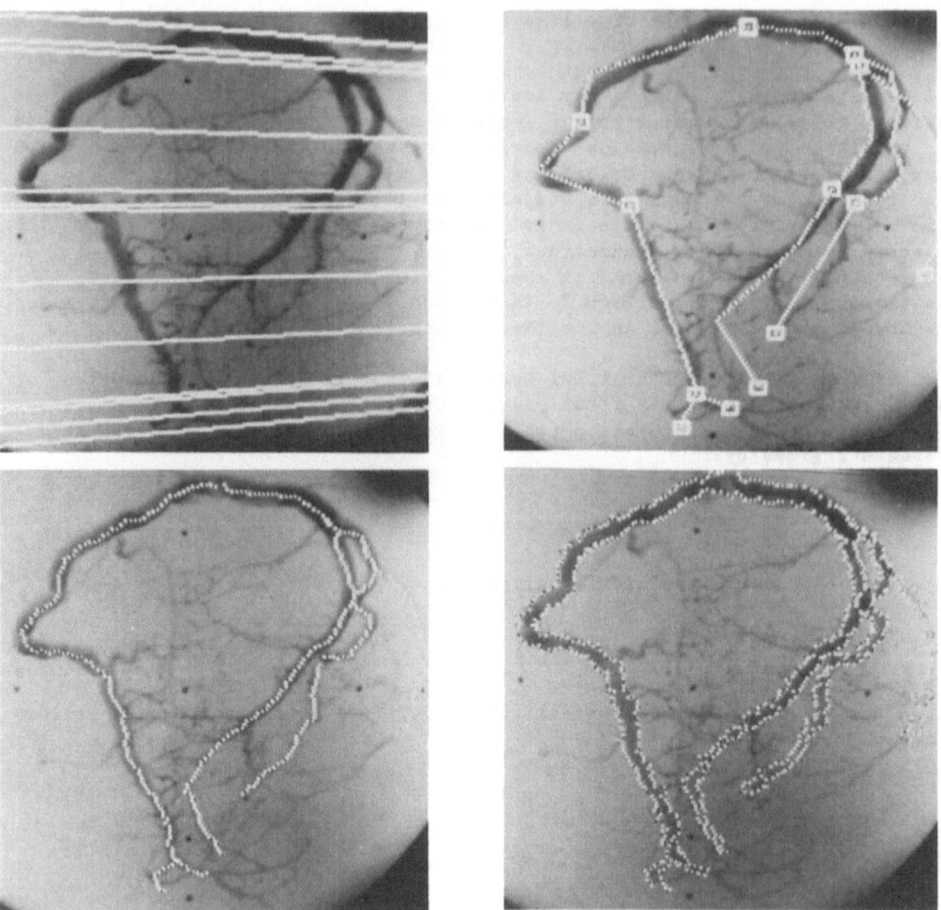

FIGURE 5. a)Lines on 2nd view corresponding to nodes of Fig. 3a. b) Manually positioned node points and target centerlines. c) Vessel centerline determined with dynamic search. d) Edges determined with dynamic search.

the original three dimensional location of the point. Because each line contributes two equations (resulting in 4 total equations) the 3 unknown coordinates of the point location are overdetermined. These lines may not intersect due to inaccuracies or geometric distortions and an exact solution to the three-dimensional location of the point may not exist. The matching of points therefore implies that the orientation of one view may have to be shifted relative to another.

5.3 Multiple Projections and Optimality

Two views overdetermine point locations and it is necessary to adopt some optimality criteria in order to resolve these locations. The optimality criteria are applied in two related processes: the images are geometrically aligned relative to each other and then the optimal 3D coordinates of matching points are determined. For both processes, it is convenient to formulate the optimality conditions so that more than two views can be utilized. Using the relations (5) and (6), we define the line for the jth point in the kth plane as:

$$ {}^k\underline{x}_j = {}^k\underline{r}_j s + {}^k\underline{a}_j \tag{9} $$

where:

$$ {}^k\underline{r}_j = {}^k\underline{x}_j - {}^k\underline{x}_s = {}^kR^{-1}({}^k\underline{u}_j - {}^k\underline{u}_s) \tag{10} $$

and:

$$ {}^k\underline{a}_j = {}^k\underline{x}_s - {}^k\underline{x}_o = {}^kR^{-1}({}^k\underline{u}_s - {}^k\underline{u}_o). \tag{11} $$

The vector $\underline{u}_o$ accounts for any required shift in coordinates between those used and the true origin of $\underline{x}'$. If the points $\underline{u}_s$ and $\underline{u}$ are measured relative to the 'true' origin of the $\underline{x}'$ coordinate system, $\underline{u}_o$ is zero. Registration is accomplished by shifting one plane relative to the others. This may be logically accomplished in a serial fashion by registering each view in turn to the others.   The goal is to minimize is the sum of the squared distances between each line for each corresponding point. We define ${}^{ik}d_j^2$ as the squared distance between the lines for the jth point in the ith and kth planes respectively:

$$ {}^{ik}d_j^2(s,t) = ({}^k\underline{r}_j s + {}^k\underline{a}_j - {}^i\underline{r}_j t - {}^i\underline{a}_j)^2. \tag{12} $$

Differentiation with respect to s and t separately, gives for the points of minimum separation:

$$ s = \left[({}^k\underline{a}_j - {}^i\underline{a}_j)\cdot({}^{ik}r_j\,{}^i\underline{r}_j - {}^i r_j^2\,{}^k\underline{r}_j) \right] \Big/ ({}^k r_j^2\,{}^i r_j^2 - {}^{ik}r_j^2) \tag{13} $$

and

$$ t = \left[({}^k\underline{a}_j - {}^i\underline{a}_j)\cdot({}^k r_j^2\,{}^i\underline{r}_j - {}^{ik}r_j\,{}^k\underline{r}_j) \right] \Big/ ({}^k r_j^2\,{}^i r_j^2 - {}^{ik}r_j^2) \tag{14} $$

where:

$$ {}^{ik}r_j = {}^i\underline{r}_j \cdot {}^k\underline{r}_j. \tag{15} $$

Substitution of Eqs. (13) and (14) into (12) yields the minimum separation:

$$^{ik}d_j^2 = \left[{}^i\underline{r}_j \cdot ({}^k\underline{a}_j - {}^i\underline{a}_j){}^k\underline{r}_j - {}^k\underline{r}_j \cdot ({}^k\underline{a}_j - {}^i\underline{a}_j){}^i\underline{r}_j \right]^2 \Big/ ({}^{ik}r_j^2 - {}^ir_j^2\,{}^kr_j^2)$$

$$- |{}^k\underline{a}_j - {}^i\underline{a}_j|^2. \tag{16}$$

For the kth plane we want to minimize the quantity:

$$^kD^2 = \sum_{i \neq k}^{N} \sum_{j=1}^{M} {}^{ik}d_j^2. \tag{17}$$

Note that from Eqs. (10) and (11), the dependence of $^kD^2$ on θ, φ, and α does not facilitate linear least-squares techniques. Iterative or non-linear techniques are apparently required. On the other hand, $^k\underline{u}_o$ can be determined using linear techniques. The resulting expression is

$$^k\underline{u}_o = {}^k\underline{u}_s - M^{-1}\underline{v}. \tag{18}$$

The matrix elements, M_{qp}, are given by:

$$M_{qp} = \sum_{i \neq k}^{N} \sum_{j=1}^{M} \left[{}^kr_j^2\,{}^i\xi_{jq}\,{}^i\xi_{jp} - {}^{ik}r_j\,{}^i\xi_{jq}\,{}^k\xi_{jp} - {}^{ik}r_j\,{}^k\xi_{jq}\,{}^i\xi_{jp} \right.$$

$$\left. + {}^ir_j^2\,{}^k\xi_{jq}\,{}^k\xi_{jp} + ({}^kR^{-1}\,{}^kR^{-1})_{qp} \right] \tag{19}$$

where

$$^i\xi_{jq} = ({}^i\underline{r}_j \cdot {}^kR^{-1})_q. \tag{20}$$

The qth element of the vector, $\underline{v}$, is given by:

$$\underline{v} = \sum_{i \neq k}^{N} \sum_{j=1}^{M} \left[({}^kr_j^2\,{}^i\underline{r}_j \cdot {}^i\underline{a}_j - {}^{ik}r_j\,{}^k\underline{r}_j \cdot {}^i\underline{a}_j){}^i\xi_{jq} \right.$$

$$\left. + ({}^ir_j^2\,{}^k\underline{r}_j \cdot {}^i\underline{a}_j - {}^{ik}r_j\,{}^i\underline{r}_j \cdot {}^i\underline{a}_j){}^k\xi_{jq} \right] \tag{21}$$

After the planes have all been registered, it remains to find the 'best' 3D point, $\underline{x}_j$, which corresponds to the matching points, $^i\underline{u}_j$ for all planes, i. This is accomplished by finding the point that minimizes the quantity:

$$D_j^2 = \sum_{k=1}^{N} (\underline{x}_j - {}^k\underline{r}_j s - {}^k\underline{a}_j)^2. \tag{22}$$

Again, s is first found to be dependent on $\underline{x}_j$, $^k\underline{r}_j$, and $^k\underline{a}_j$:

$$s = {}^k\underline{r}_j \cdot ({}^k\underline{a}_j - \underline{x}_j) / {}^k r_j^2 \tag{23}$$

giving:

$$D_j^2 = \sum_{k=1}^{N} \left[{}^k r_j^2 |\underline{x}_j - {}^k\underline{a}_j|^2 - |{}^k\underline{r}_j \cdot (\underline{x}_j - {}^k\underline{a}_j)|^2 \right] . \tag{24}$$

Linear least-squares techniques can be used with Eq. (24) to find $\underline{x}_j$.

The above discussion applies specifically to points which are uniquely determined and matched in all views. If all vessel points were uniquely matched between views, the 3D reconstruction problem would now be solved. In practice, however, only the node or branch points are uniquely matched, leaving a sequence of unmatched points between nodes in each view. In general, because of the arbitrary orientations, the centerline of any branch will have a different number of points in each view. Each branch must have the same number of points in each view for the above reconstruction to work. If the longest centerline for a given vessel segment is used to generate the set of points in the 3D coordinate system, some interpolation process must be used to generate an equal number of matching points in each of the shorter branches. A modified nearest neighbor interpolation has been found to work adequately. This modification consists of a connectivity constraint which requires that the indices of subsequent matches can differ by at most one from the indices of previous matches. Matching the elements between two views is accomplished by minimizing the total squared distance between matched lines consistent with the connectivity requirement.

In practice the matching is accomplished by generating the matrix $^{ik}d_{lm}^2$, defined as the squared distance between the lines of points l and m of planes i and k respectively. Dynamic programming is then used to find the optimal matching of indices, l and m, consistent with the connectivity constraint mentioned above.

At the completion of this matching process, each corresponding branch in all views has the same number of points, with points of the same index assumed to match (i.e. correspond to the same 3D point). The three dimensional reconstruction of the vascular tree is then accomplished as outlined above. The reconstructed centerlines corresponding to the images of Fig. 5 are shown in Fig. 6.

5.4 Vessel Cross-section (Area vs. Shape)

The reconstruction of the vessel cross-section consists of determining the lumen radii as a function of angle around each element of the centerline. Information about the vessel lumen is contained in the edge locations in each image as well as the densitometric profile. With the assumption that the iodine density within the vessel is uniform, a general idea of the vessel shape can be obtained from the x-ray attenuation profile. In the case of views which are nearly orthogonal to each other, the edge information from one view can be used to calibrate the densitometric

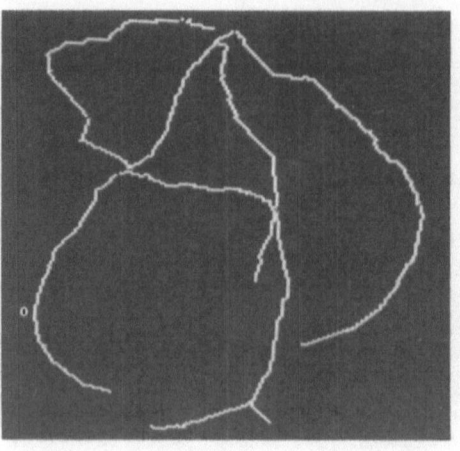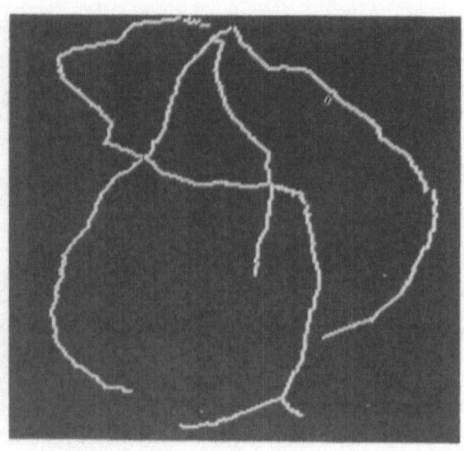

FIGURE 6. a and b) Stereo pair projection of reconstructed pig coronary centerline

information of the other. This allows absolute vessel thickness along the x-ray path to be determined from the densitometric profile. Should the x-ray paths in two or more views be nearly orthogonal to the vessel centerline, an iterative technique can be used to relax the vessel structure to one that matches the measurement data. To resolve the many possible structures a dynamic program similar to the algorithm of Reiber can be applied to constrain the shape changes between planes (16).

In the case of segments where views orthogonal to the segments are not available, the interconnecting relationships of the various radii with different orientations are more complex. Our present implementation only determines the average radius around the vessel centerline, based on edge detection information. This yields an estimate of the vessel cross-sectional area.

6. DISPLAY ALGORITHMS

There are many ways to display the information contained in the tree structure. Those we have used can be classified as centerline, densitometric and shaded surface.

The centerline technique simply uses Eqs. (2) and (3) to project each centerline position onto a two dimensional image matrix. This was illustrated in Fig. 6.

The densitometric projection simulates the x-ray attenuation process by computing the length of each x-ray path internal to the vessels. Currently this is accomplished by transforming each surface point of the vessel tree to the desired (u,v) coordinate system and thus obtaining the matrix element affected by the surface element. The length of the x-ray path through a vessel is obtained as the distance between the (x,y,z) coordinates of the first and last surface element along an x-ray path through a vessel segment. The total density for a picture element is the sum of all such x-ray paths for the pixel. A densitometric projection of a reconstruction of the pig coronary artery phantom is given in Fig. 7. In this case, only width information from edges was available to the algorithm and some artifactual increase in width is observed in the reconstruction of smaller vessels. This is indicative of the potential for improvements based on iterative techniques which compare such reprojections with the original images.

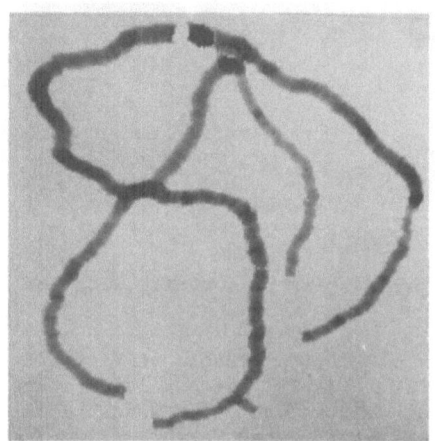 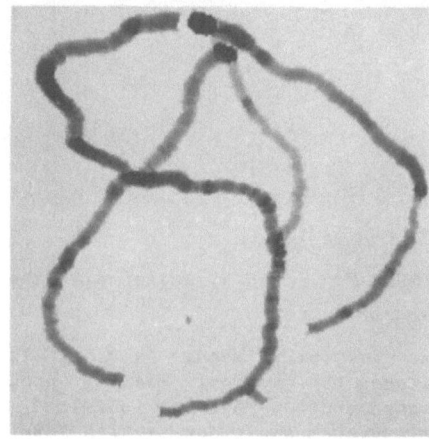

FIGURE 7. a and b) Stereo pair densitometric projections of the pig coronary arteries.

A visually pleasing shaded surface display can be obtained using the projected surfaces mentioned above. By computing the illumination of the surface element nearest the x-ray source as a function of orientation and proximity, depth and orientation cuing can be rendered. For the display of Fig. 8, a brightness function of the form:

$$I = A\cos\theta_p + B(R-s)/2R + C \qquad (25)$$

was used. The angle θ_p is the inclination of the surface computed relative to the x-ray path, 2R is the thickness of the display region, and s is the position of the point relative to the center of the display region (i.e. $-R \leq s \leq R$). The factors A, B and C represent the relative contribution of the three processes: illumination, fogging and background respectively. The values of A, B, and C, were approximately 0.6, 0.3, and 0.1.

7. ARTIFACTS

Artifacts are a major concern in any reconstructive imaging process. By imposing connectivity constraints and allowing operator control of node matching, a believable reconstruction is expected. If iterative techniques

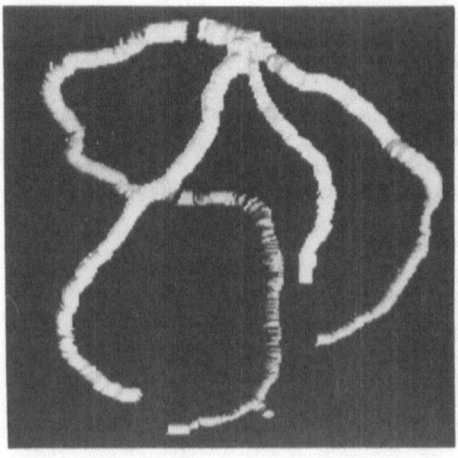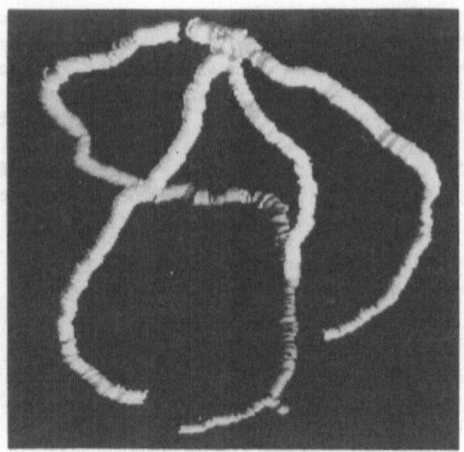

FIGURE 8. a and b) Stereo pair shaded surface display of coronary arteries.

are correctly used, (i.e. if the forward projection process sufficiently matches the physical imaging process) it is likely that a consistent reconstruction can be obtained. However, discrepancies in vessel size, orientation and cross-section are to be expected when errors in edge detection or centerline matching occur. Because of the limited number of views, it is not likely that exact vessel lumen cross-sectional geometry will be obtained. Those artifacts which do occur will not be as visibly obvious as streaks and rings. This indicates that strict quality control of the imaging and reconstruction processes will be essential to establish the credibility of these images.

8. SUMMARY

A method of three dimensional reconstruction of vascular beds has been presented based on the computation of a tree structure. Basic operator directed pattern recognition techniques are used to segment vessel images. Optimality constraints are used to align images, match points between views

and select the corresponding three dimensional point coordinates. Edge information, and ultimately densitometric profile information are then used to reconstruction the vessel cross-sectional geometry. The prelimary results have been very encouraging. The resulting reconstructions are expected to provide more accurate measures of vessel dimensions, flow as well as myocardial motion. It is also expected that perspective views will be of use during clinical procedures.

9. ACKNOWLEDGMENTS

The authors acknowledge the helpful support of Rudy Van Bree, Brendon Anderl, and Raj Desai. This work has been supported by grants from the Montana and Utah Heart Associations. Additional support was provided by Siemens Medical Systems.

REFERENCES

1. Parker DL, Pope DL, Petersen JC, Clayton PD, and Gustafson DE: Quantation in Cardiac Video-densitometry. Computers in Cardiology, 1984.

2. Bateman WA, Kruger RA: Blood flow measurement using digital angiography and parametric imaging. Med. Phys. 11(2):153-7, 1984.

3. Jaques P, DiBianca F, Pizer S, Koholt F, Lifshitz L, and Delany D: Quantitative Digital Fluorography. Inv. Radiol. 20:45-52, 1985.

4. Potel MJ, MacKay SA, Rubin JM, Aisen AM, Sayre RE: Three-Dimensional Left Ventricular Wall Motion in Man, Coordinate Systems for Representing Wall Movement Direction. Inv. Radiology, 19(6):499-509, 1984

5. Kim HC, Min BG, Lee TS, Lee SJ, Lee CW, Park JH and Han MC: Three-Dimensional Digital Subtraction Angiography. IEEE Trans on Med. Imaging Vol MI-1(2):152-158, 1982.

6. MacKay SA, Potel MJ and Rubin JM: Graphics Methods for Tracking Three-Dimensional Heart Wall Motion. Comp. Biom. Res. 15:455-473, 1982.

7. Pelc NJ and Chesler DA: Utilization of Cross-plane rays for three-dimensional reconstruction by filtered back-projection. JCAT 3(3):385-395, 1979.

8. Ra JB, Lim CB, Cho ZH, Hilal SK, and Correll J: A true three-dimensional reconstruction algorithm for the sperical positron emission tomograph. Phys. Med. Biol. 27(1):37-50 1982.

9. Deans SR: The Radon Transform for Higher Dimensions. Phys. Med. Biol. 23(6):1173-1175, 1978.

10. Bates JHT, McKinnon AE and Bates RHT: Subtractive image restoration. I: Basic theory. Optik 61(4):349-364, 1982.

11. Bates JHT, McKinnon AE and Bates RHT: Subtractive image restoration. II: Comparison with multiplicative deconvolution. Optik 62(1):1-14, 1982.

12. Bates JHT, McKinnon AE and Bates RHT: Subtractive image restoration. III: Some practical applications. Optik 62(4):333-346, 1982.

13. Onnasch DGW and Heintzen PH: A New Approach for the Reconstruction of the Right or Left Ventricular Form from Biplane Angiocardiographic Recordings. Computers in Cardiology, 1976, pp 67-73.

14. Chang SK and CHow CK: The Reconstruction of Three-Dimensional Objects from Two Orthogonal Projections and its Application to Cardiac Cineangiography. IEEE Transactions on Computers, c-22(1):18-28, 1973.

15. Slump CH and Gerbrands JJ: A Network Flow Approach to Reconstruction of the Left Ventricle from Two Projections. Computer Graphics and Image Processing. 18:18-36, 1982.

16. Reiber JHC et al.: Three-dimensional reconstruction of coronary

arterial segments from two projections. Digital Imaging and Cardiovascular Radiology, Edited by PH Heintzen and R. Brennecke, International Symposium, Kiel, 1982.

17. Mol CR, Colchester ACF, Hawkes DJ, O'Laoire SA, Hart G: 3-D reconstruction from biplane X-ray recordings: application to arterio-venous malformations (abstract). In Computer-Aided Biomedical Imaging and Graphics. Eds Jordan, MM and Perkins, WJ, London: Biol Engin Soc, 1984.

18. Pope DL, Parker DL, Gustafson DE, and Clayton PD: Dynamic search algorithms in left ventricular border recognition and analysis of coronary arteries. Computers in Cardiology, September, 1984.

19. Parker DL, Pryor TA: Analysis of B-scan speckle reduction by resolution limited filtering. Ultrasonic Imaging 4:108-125, 1982.

20. Pope DL, Parker DL, Clayton PD and Gustafson DE: Left Ventricular Border Recognition Using a Dynamic Search Algorithm. Radiology 155:513-518, 1985.

A SYSTEMATIC APPROACH TO THE DESIGN OF DIAGNOSTIC SYSTEMS FOR NUCLEAR MEDICINE

K. J. Myers[1,2] H. H. Barrett[1,2], M. C. Borgstrom[2], E. B. Cargill[1,2],
A. V. Clough[2], R. D. Fiete[1,2], T. D. Milster[1,2], D. D. Patton[2],
R. G. Paxman[3], G. W. Seeley[1,2], W. E. Smith[1,2], M. O. Stempski[2]

1 Optical Sciences Center, University of Arizona, Tucson, Az. 85721
2 Div. of Nuclear Medicine, Arizona Health Sciences Center, Tucson, Az. 85724
3 Environmental Research Institute of Michigan, P.O. Box 8618, Ann Arbor, Mi. 48107

1. INTRODUCTION

Diagnostic radiology has traditionally been based on the evaluation of images by human observers, but neither an image nor a human is absolutely essential to the problem. The best diagnostic system is not necessarily one that produces pleasing images or has a good MTF or good signal-to-noise ratio (SNR). Rather, the only meaningful measure of system performance is the correctness of the final diagnosis. The central question in system design is: How can one collect the best data set with which to make a diagnosis? To even attempt to answer this question, we must first decide what organs and what diseases are to be studied by a system or, in other words, what the precise task of the system is. In addition, a careful definition of "best" must be given. Finally, some strategy must be defined for realizing the best data-collection system. It is our purpose to show that such a systematic approach to total system design is possible in principle (although very difficult in practice), and to summarize current efforts at the University of Arizona towards realization of this goal.

2. OBJECT CLASS AND TASK

The general framework of our research program is illustrated in the flow chart of Figure 1. We have chosen to concentrate our initial efforts on the diagnosis of liver diseases and are currently developing a comprehensive mathematical model of normal and pathological livers to define the "object class" specified in the top box of this figure. By generating a digital model of the object, as opposed to an object set composed of clinical or phantom images, we have complete control over (and

thus knowledge of) the statistics of each object class before corruption by
an imaging system. For simplicity, the initial task will be to divide the
objects into two classes, normal and abnormal. Eventually a more detailed
differential diagnosis will be attempted.

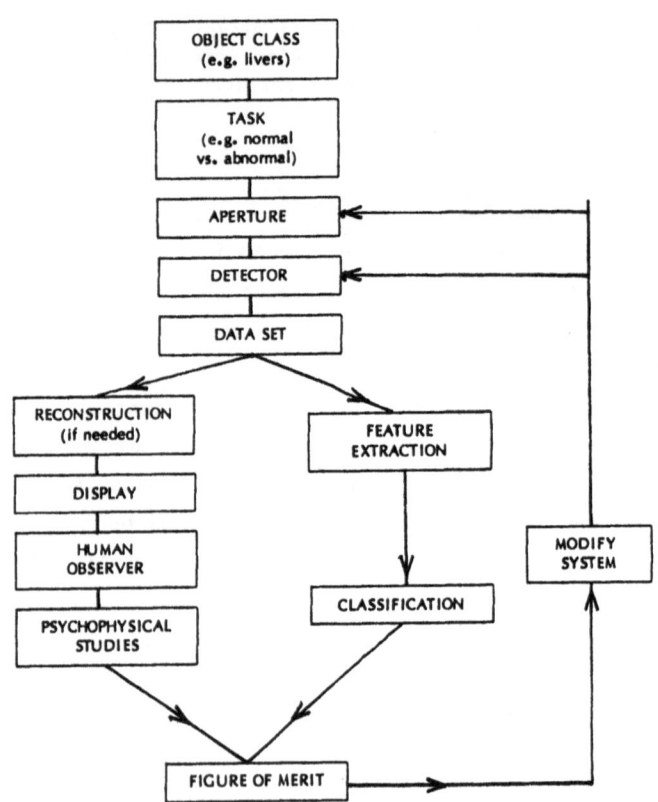

FIGURE 1. Flow chart showing steps involved in optimization of
diagnostic systems.

The liver model we are constructing will occupy a 64x64x64 voxel array. An outline of the liver is first obtained from actual anatomical data, resulting in the wire mesh of Figure 2. We then derive a continuous contour for the model by fitting a set of spherical harmonics to the sampled data. Liver pathology will be incorporated through probabilistic modeling of the physical processes involved in liver disease growth. The radiation emitted from each location within the liver will then be determined by simulation of the radiopharmaceutical uptake at each position.

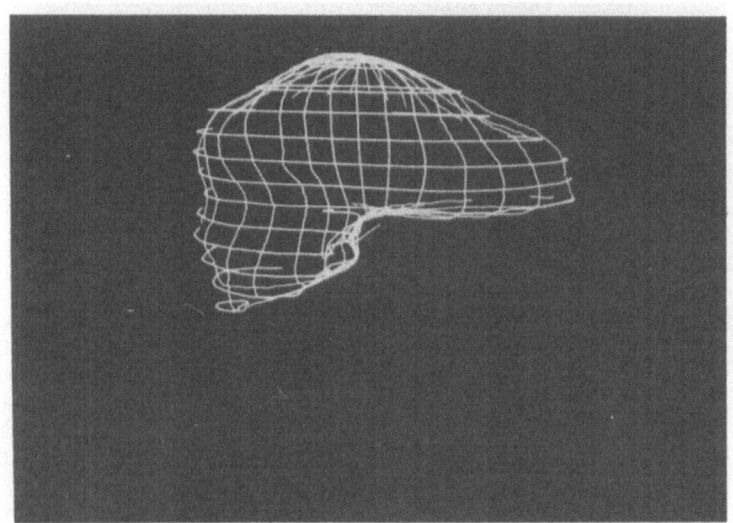

FIGURE 2. Contour of three-dimensional liver model.

Once our model is complete it will be verified by comparison with real anatomical data. The veracity of the model will also be confirmed through simulations of various imaging systems operating on our model. The resulting images must conform to those obtained for real livers and real imaging systems in the clinic. As an example, Figure 3 shows two simulated nuclear medical images of the liver model with tumors added to the object data. The image on the left is from a high-resolution system, while the image on the right is from a low-resolution system. The simulation performed to derive these images included scatter, attenuation, noise and blur.

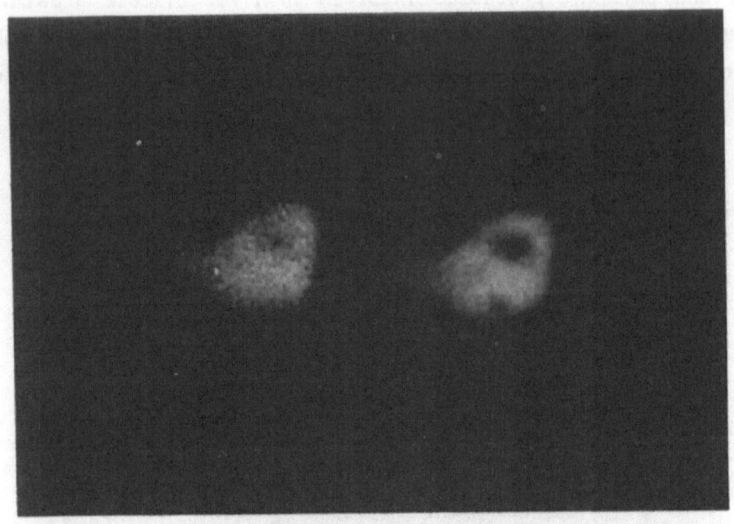

FIGURE 3. Two simulated nuclear medical images of the liver model with tumors.
a) Image obtained through a high-resolution, high-sensitivity system.
b) Image obtained through a low-resolution, low-sensitivity system.

3. APERTURE AND DETECTOR

The next boxes in our flowchart represent the operations of the aperture and detector on the object data. The aperture and detector could be a conventional collimator and Anger camera, but we are taking a broader view. The aperture is a general coded aperture, which could include a pinhole or collimator as special cases. Most of our work concentrates on multiple-view coded-aperture geometries to eliminate problems associated with limited-angle tomography. Using a multiple-view arrangement we can interrogate the entire object volume simultaneously, making this system suitable for dynamic studies. When using coded apertures the resulting data set often contains overlapping views. Multiplexed data is not necessarily a disadvantage for coded-aperture systems, however. We have found that when photon noise is included in the data, reconstructions obtained from multiplexed data are better than those obtained from unmultiplexed data, due to the higher photon count made available [1].

In order for the detector to be compatible with the coded-aperture geometries we are investigating, we must not limit the detector in our system to a single plane as with an Anger camera. Rather, we consider a wide variety of non-planar detector configurations composed of modular scintillation cameras currently under development in our laboratory [2]. The coded apertures and modular cameras are important elements in this work because they provide the flexibility to physically implement the optimum systems. The modifiable system parameters in the optimization routine are the locations of the modular cameras and the variables related to the coded-aperture design.

4. RECONSTRUCTION

The output from the detector is a data set that is not necessarily a recognizable image of the object. If the data are to be used by a human observer, as in the left branch of the flow chart, an image must be reconstructed and suitably displayed. We are currently investigating a Monte Carlo approach for obtaining tomographic reconstructions from coded data sets and a priori information. This approach defines a cost function related to how well the projection of the reconstruction agrees with the actual data and to how well the reconstruction agrees with the a priori knowledge. The algorithm can incorporate the process known as simulated annealing, a technique that searches for the global minimum of the cost

436

function. We have chosen to focus on this reconstruction technique because it can readily incorporate experimentally determined aspects of the imaging problem such as the detector characteristics, scattering, attenuation, radiometric effects, and the exact form of the aperture. Some results obtained using this reconstruction technique have been reported elsewhere [1,3,4].

5. HUMAN-BASED CLASSIFICATION

On the left-hand side of the flowchart the human observer is considered an integral part of the imaging system. We quantify the performance of the human observer in cascade with the physical imaging system using psychophysical methods such as ROC-based detectability studies. Psychophysical studies allow us to measure the ability of the human observer to perform a well-specified detection or discrimination task. The figure of merit we derive from the psychophysical experiments must be a simple scalar measure of system performance, such as d' or area under the ROC curve, which can then be used as the basis for our system optimization.

Unfortunately, to measure human performance accurately requires numerous images and observers, so that the procedure can be quite time-consuming. An alternative method is to use a model to predict the performance of the human observer and thus eliminate the need for lengthy psychophysical studies. With such a model a simple calculation derives the system figure of merit for a given set of system design parameters.

The model of the human we are investigating is the ideal observer, a concept found in the literature on statistical decision theory. The ideal observer is an optimum Bayesian observer designed to minimize the probability of making an incorrect decision. It has been shown that the human observer acts like an ideal observer, except for the human observer's inability to prewhiten correlated noise. The efficiency of the human observer relative to a non-prewhitening ideal observer is approximately constant over a wide range of noise correlation functions [5]. One possible figure of merit is therefore the signal-to-noise ratio at the output of a non-prewhitening ideal observer. The first stage of the system design could be performed using this figure of merit, presuming that a system optimized with respect to ideal-observer SNR would be at least approximately optimized for humans.

Both psychophysical techniques and the ideal-observer model suffer from still another limitation. That is, the signal is generally assumed to be deterministic. The theory becomes quite complicated when parameters of the decision problem, such as signal shape or location, vary in some non-deterministic way. Hence, the signal and the noise are often given very stylized forms to make the calculations tractable. Additionally, ROC techniques are not well suited to situations where there are more than two possible hypotheses. The ROC curve and metrics derived from it are basically binary.

6. MACHINE-BASED CLASSIFICATION

Because of the limitations of the signal-detection-theory techniques discussed in the previous section, we are giving special attention to system assessment based on automatic pattern recognition, denoted by the right branch of the flowchart. In this case, a set of features is derived from the initial data set (not from the reconstructed image), and an optimal discriminant function is determined for dividing the objects into K classes. (We are no longer restricted to the simple binary classification problem.) A figure of merit is then derived from the performance of this classifier.

Many different ad hoc figures of merit have been suggested in the literature on pattern recognition [6], most of them based on interclass and intraclass scatter matrices. We have chosen a figure of merit known as the Hotelling trace criterion [7] for further evaluation. We define the scatter matrices and the Hotelling trace criterion below.

We specify the object data set by the Mx1 column vector f. For example, the vector f might correspond to the lexicographic ordering of the pixel values of our mathematical liver model. The mean object vector of the kth object class is then $\bar{f}_k$. The grand mean is the average of all objects for all K classes, weighted by their probability of occurrence, P_k, and is written

$$\bar{f}_0 = \sum_{k=1}^{K} P_k \bar{f}_k \; .$$

(1)

The interclass scatter matrix S_1 measures the amount by which the means of the K classes are scattered about the grand mean:

$$S_1 = \sum_{k=1}^{K} P_k(\bar{f}_k - \bar{f}_0)(\bar{f}_k - \bar{f}_0)^T \quad , \tag{2}$$

where the superscript T denotes the transpose operation. The intraclass scatter matrix S_2 is the mean covariance matrix averaged over the K classes:

$$S_2 = \sum_{k=1}^{K} P_k C_k \quad , \tag{3}$$

where C_k is the covariance matrix of the kth class:

$$C_k = \langle (f - \bar{f}_k)(f - \bar{f}_k)^T \rangle \quad . \tag{4}$$

We can define the Hotelling trace criterion J in terms of the scatter matrices as follows:

$$J = Tr[S_2^{-1} S_1] \quad , \tag{5}$$

where Tr denotes the trace of the matrix.

The Hotelling trace criterion has the nice property that it is a scalar figure of merit that increases as the means of the classes become further apart and decreases as the scatter of each class about its own mean increases. It can be shown that J is related by a simple expression to d' in the appropriate limit (binary hypothesis, deterministic signal, Gaussian noise). However, there is sometimes a problem with using the Hotelling trace criterion as a measure of object-class separability. The intraclass scatter matrix S_2 is often singular, causing the value of J to go to infinity. The reason for the singularity is that the scatter matrix is often a sample covariance matrix determined by averaging over a small training set of objects, rather than an ensemble covariance matrix. When the number of objects in the training set is less than the dimension of the scatter matrix, S_2, the matrix is not full rank. Even when the number of objects in the training set is greater than the dimension of the scatter matrix, S_2 is not guaranteed to be full rank because the objects may be linearly dependent.

The Hotelling trace criterion provides us with a formalism for selecting linear features of the pixel data to reduce the dimensionality of the data space, without decreasing the intrinsic separability of the classes. The feature extractor is a non-unitary linear operator that simultaneously diagonalizes S_1 and S_2. The number of features needed to represent the data without compromising the object-class separability is just the number of linearly independent eigenvectors of the matrix $S_2^{-1}S_1$, which can be shown to be less than or equal to K-1 [8]. Thus, for a two-class problem only one feature is needed, even though the original data set contains N^3 pixels, where N is equal to 64 for the objects we are considering.

The expression of Eq. 5 tells us the intrinsic separability of the object classes. We can measure the loss in class separability due to the corruption of the object data by a diagnostic system in the following way. The data vector received at the output of the diagnostic system is denoted by the Lx1 column vector g, where

$$g = Hf + n \quad . \tag{6}$$

The LxM matrix H describes the action of the diagnostic system on the object data. In using this linear operator notation we are assuming that the system is linear, and the image-forming operator H in general represents space-variant blur. Usually L is much less than M, implying that there is some loss of information due to a data reduction associated with the imaging process. The Lx1 column vector n represents additive, zero-mean noise in the system and has associated with it the covariance matrix C_n. It is straightforward to show that the scatter matrices S_{1g} and S_{2g} associated with the data vector g are related to the scatter matrices for f by

$$S_{1g} = HS_{1f}H^T \tag{7}$$

and

$$S_{2g} = HS_{2f}H^T + C_n \quad . \tag{8}$$

The Hotelling trace criterion for g becomes

$$J_g = Tr[S_{2g}^{-1}S_{1g}] \quad . \tag{9}$$

The expression for J_g of Equation 9 defines a figure of merit for class separability at the output of a diagnostic system. The ideal system is one that delivers the object pixel values without blur or noise, hence without compromising the object-class separability specified by J_f. As the performance of an actual system nears the performance of an ideal system, J_g approaches J_f. The goal of system optimization is to maximize J_g.

6. SYSTEM MODIFICATION

Once a scalar figure of merit is found from either the human-based or machine-based approach, the system design can be modified to maximize it. Any system design parameter, such as the aperture code or the arrangement of the modular cameras, can be adjusted to get the largest figure of merit. Two general approaches to system optimization can be identified: analytic techniques and ad hoc methods.

If an analytic expression can be found that describes the system characteristics in terms of the figure of merit, in principle we could solve this expression to determine the optimum system parameters. For example, we might consider attempting to use an analytic approach to optimize a system in terms of J_g of Eq. 9, where the scatter matrices are computed from the liver model and the system matrix H is written in terms of the coded-aperture and detector design parameters. In practice this idea breaks down when we insist that the matrix H represent a realizable system. Usually we solve this problem by adjusting the system parameters according to some iterative algorithm that seeks the maximum value of the figure of merit, within the constraint of providing a physically meaningful solution. We have demonstrated the use of an iterative algorithm to optimize system design parameters using a mean-square-error figure of merit [9,10].

Alternatively, when the number of design parameters is constrained to a small enough set, we can replace the iterative algorithm with an exhaustive search through all possible system designs. We have found the best coded-aperture design from a limited configuration space using this method and the Hotelling trace criterion as the figure of merit [11]. As shown in Figure 4, the system geometry consisted of three identical code planes separated by 120 degrees, each containing eight possible pinholes. Behind each code plane was a detector in a known location and containing eighteen elements. With eight possible pinholes there are 2^8 or 256 possible code functions to be evaluated. Figure 5 is a plot of J_g as a function of the pinhole code, where the code is expressed as a number equivalent to the binary representation of the open and closed pinholes (open pinholes are ones, closed pinholes are zeros). The best and worst codes found by the search routine are also given in Figure 5.

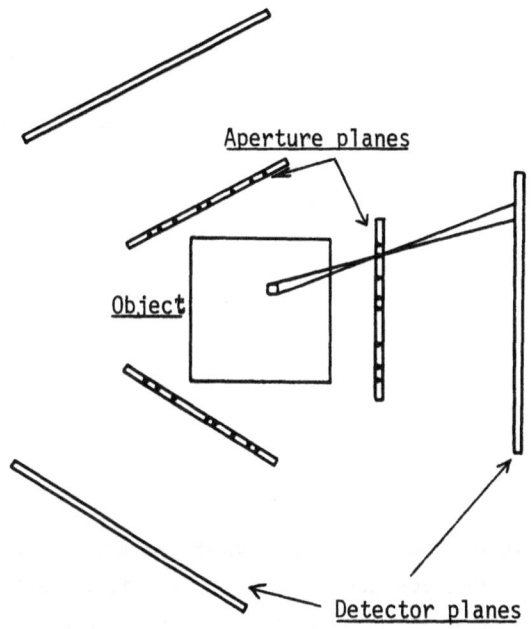

FIGURE 4. System geometry for optimization problem using Hotelling trace criterion as a figure of merit. An exhastive search procedure was used to determine the best possible pinhole configuration in the aperture plane.

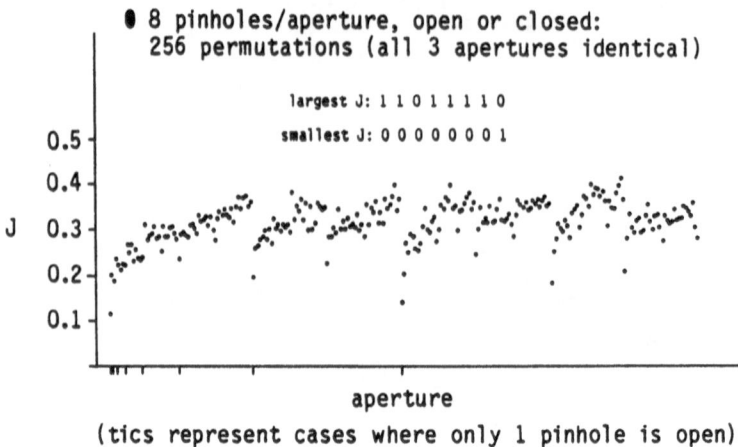

FIGURE 5. Results of exhaustive search for optimum pinhole code.

Finally, if it is found that some particular feature is very important in the task, then <u>ad hoc</u> methods can be devised to emphasize this feature. As an example, suppose that a narrow band of spatial-frequencies were determined to be very important in diagnosing liver disease, perhaps because of the information these frequencies might contain about the texture of the liver. We might imagine a diagnostic system consisting of a single coded aperture designed to optimally measure the signal intensity within this range of frequencies. The single number we measure at the output of this special coded aperture is our feature. Since we are measuring just a single number, rather than the, say, 4096 numbers we measure when we image the liver, we can obtain this number quite accurately with a substantially lower exposure time than is normally necessary for imaging. Thus we are much less sensitive to Poisson noise in the photon flux. We could imagine a nuclear medicine system in the future with a set of interchangable aperture plates, one for imaging and additional plates for measuring other features found to be of interest.

We are currently using a psychophysical method known as multidimensional scaling to determine what features in clinical images of livers are important when physicians make similarity judgments regarding their diagnostic evaluation. We would expect these same features to be utilized when a clinician classifies an image into the class of normals or abnormals. Once the important features have been determined, it may be possible to adjust the system design in an ad hoc way to emphasize these features in the final image.

7. CONCLUSION

We have presented an overall approach to the design of optimum diagnostic systems in nuclear medicine. We have defined a relevant clinical task and determined the important design parameters of the system hardware subject to optimization. These design parameters specify the code function of one or more coded apertures and the location of the apertures and detectors. Using either human observers or machine classifiers, a figure of merit for a medical system can be defined. A number of strategies exist for improving this figure of merit, leading to an optimum system configuration for the task at hand.

Probably the most important controversy in this approach is whether a system optimized for machine classification (maximum Hotelling trace criterion J) is optimized for human observers. We are currently investigating this question by running a psychophysical study that measures human classification performance as a function of J.

ACKNOWLEDGMENTS

This work was supported by the National Cancer Institute through Grant No. P01 CA 23417. In addition, one of the authors (KJM) was supported by a Kodak Graduate Fellowship and two (TDM and WES) were supported by IBM fellowships.

REFERENCES

1. Smith, W. E., R. G. Paxman, H. H. Barrett, "Image reconstruction from coded data: I. Reconstruction algorithms and experimental results," J. Opt. Soc. Am. A **4**, 399 (1985).

2. Milster, T. D., L. A. Selberg, H. H. Barrett, R. L. Easton, G. R. Rossi, J. Arendt, R. G. Simpson, "A modular scintillation camera for use in nuclear medicine," IEEE Trans. Nucl. Sci. **NS-31**, 578 (1984).

3. Smith, W. E., H. H. Barrett, R. G. Paxman, "Reconstruction of objects from coded images by simulated annealing," Opt. Lett. 8, 199 (1983).

4. Paxman, R. G., W. E. Smith, H. H. Barrett, "Two algorithms for use with an orthogonal-view coded-aperture system," J. Nucl. Med. **25**, 700 (1984).

5. Myers, K. J., "Visual Perception in Correlated Noise," Ph.D. dissertation, Univ. of Az. (1985).

6. Fukunaga, K., Introduction to Statistical Pattern Recognition, Academic Press, New York (1972).

7. Hotelling, H., "The generalization of Student's ratio," Ann. Math. Stat. **2**, 360 (1931).

8. Barrett, H. H., W. E. Smith, K. J. Myers, T. D. Milster, R. D. Fiete, "Quantifying the performance of imaging systems," Proceedings of the SPIE, **535**, 1985.

9. Paxman, R. G., "Coordinated Design of Restoration Algorithm and Coded Aperture," Ph.D. Dissertation, Univ. of Az. (1984).

10. Smith, W. E., R. G. Paxman, H. H. Barrett, "Application of simulated annealing to coded-aperture design and tomographic reconstruction," IEEE Trans. on Nucl. Sci. **NS-32**, 758 (1985).

11. Smith, W. E., H. H. Barrett, R. D. Fiete, K. J. Myers, T. J. Roney, "A scheme for the optimization of imaging systems based on object-class separability," Proceedings of Image Science '85, Helsinki, Finland, 11-14 June 1985.

SPECT IMAGING REQUIRED FOR RADIOIMMUNOTHERAPY DOSIMETRY
INVESTIGATIONS: IMPORTANCE OF COLLIMATION IN DEVELOPMENT OF
MATHEMATICAL MODELS TO CORRECT FOR RECOVERY COEFFICIENT (RC)
DEPENDENCE ON OBJECT SIZE, PHOTON ENERGY AND BACKGROUND

LAURENCE P. CLARKE, Ph.D.

1. INTRODUCTION

One of the objectives of radionuclide tomography is to relate
the measured radionuclide concentration (counts/cm2) to the
actual activity concentration (uCi/cm3), within sources of
varying size in the transverse tomographic plane. This
relationship has been found to be dependent on source size for
Positron Emission Tomography (PET) systems, the relative image
contrast or Recovery Coefficient (RC) decreasing with object
size as it approaches the system's spatial resolution (FWHM)
(1). Larger integration areas or Regions of Interest (ROI),
chosen to fully enclose the image of each source in the
transverse plane are required, in order to maintain the
linearity of the Detector Response (LDR) (i.e. total
counts/uCi) (2). The dependence on the measured concentration
or RC has been demonstrated, both experimentally (1,2) and
theoretically (2), to be primarily related to the limited
spatial resolution of the PET systems employed.

Quantitative SPECT imaging in radioimmunotherapy using the
gamma camera, however, requires additional corrections relating
to the RC dependence on object size because of the wide photon
energy range involved (table 1) (3-5). These corrections
include the influence of: (a) geometrical spatial resolution of
each collimator type, (b) scattering effects at each photon
energy (6-8), (c) photon penetration effects across the full
sensitive area of the collimated detectors and (d) level of
background activity surrounding each source (9,10). In
addition the influence of photon penetration and scatter on the
LDR should be investigated, particularly for the presence of
multiple sources and surrounding background activity in the
transverse tomographic plane (10-12).

The feasibility of developing a mathematical model to correct
for the RC and LDR dependence on object size over a wide range
of photon energy (140-364 keV) was, therefore, investigated.
An experimental approach was taken because of current practical
limitations of using computer simulating techniques to correct
for detector resolution characteristics, where both photon
penetration and scatter effects in the collimator and detector
are significant (12,13). Furthermore, simulation methods do
not account for the practical problems of SPECT imaging with
heavy collimators such as associated center of rotation (COR)
artifacts (6). The importance of collimation in RC and LDR
measurements was, therefore, demonstrated by comparing data at
low and medium photon energy (Tc99M (140 keV), I-131 (364

keV)), to partially differentiate between photon penetration
and scattering effects. Data for conventional and specially
designed long bore thick septa collimators were obtained using
a Multiple Source Size (MSS) Phantom similar to the phantom
used in evaluating PET systems (1).

Table 1: Representative examples of radionuclides proposed for
radioimmunotherapy, reflecting the wide range of photon energy
and non-monoenergic gamma emissions involved. I-131 is
currently being used in clinical trials.

Nuclide (Parent)	Particulate Energies	Gamma Energies (%)
I-131 (T1/2=8d) (Beta-)	0.25 MeV 0.33 MeV 0.61 MeV	364 keV (82) 637 keV (7) others
Br-77 (T1/2=57h) (EC)	10.1 keV 1.15 keV 11.7 keV	239 keV (23) 520 keV (22)
Bi-212 (T1/2=60m) (Beta-/Alpha)	2.25 MeV 6.09 MeV 6.05 MeV	727 keV (6) others
Cu-67 (T 1/2=62h) (Beta-)	577 keV 484 keV 395 keV	91 keV (7) 93 keV (17) 184 keV (47) others

2. MATERIALS AND METHODS
  A SPECT system (Picker International Dyna Camera 5) with a
3/8 inch NaI(Tl) crystal and 511 keV detector shielding was
employed. This system was interfaced to a Computer Design
Applications (CDA) mini computer system (Micro Delta) with a 30
Mbyte disc and array processor. The SPECT gantry was designed
to support heavy collimators of up to 250 lbs weight.
Collimators employed included a High Sensitivity Low Energy
Collimator (HSLEC) or ultrafine collimator, a High Sensitivity
Medium Energy Collimator (HSMEC) designed for conventional
diagnostic investigations with I-131, and a Low Sensitivity
Medium Energy Collimator (LSMEC) designed to minimize septal
penetration using I-131 (9,10). Sensitivity considerations are
not as critical in radioimmunotherapy with I-131 because of the
larger radiation doses involved (4). Collimator dimensions are
shown in Table 2. Their corresponding measured transverse
plane spatial resolution (FWHM, FWTM) and NEMA sensitivity are
tabulated in table 3 (10).

The MSS phantom dimensions are shown in table 4. Its design was similiar to that employed by Hoffmann et al (1) for a PET System, except that the source dimensions were increased to allow for the more limited spatial resolution (FWHM) of the SPECT system. Each source in the MSS phantom contained a uniform and equal activity concentration of either Tc99M or I-131, the remainder of the phantom being filled with water. In addition, the phantom was later uniformly filled with water containing Tc99M or I-131 activity at a concentration of 0.2 times that within the sources (i.e. Source/Background (S/B) activity concentration ratio = 1:0, or 5:1). The MSS phantom was imaged with each collimator using similar acquisition and reconstruction parameters as outlined in Table 5.

Table 2: Collimator dimensions (mm) and theoretical leakage through their septa. Diameter of holes are approximate due to varying hole geometry with each collimator type.

Collimator	HSLEC	HSMEC	LSMEC
Dia. Hole	1.3	3.8	3.4
Length	25.4	50.8	68.3
Septa	0.18	1.35	1.39
Theoretical	1.0	8.0	3.0
Leakage	(140 keV)	(364 keV)	(364 keV)

Table 3: Measured spatial resolution (FWHM, FWTM) in the transverse plane for each collimator and radionuclide. The spatial resolution was found to remain within the experimental error of measurement ($\pm$ 10%), across the tomographic plane (linear sampling = 128).

Collimator	Transverse Plane (mm)		NEMA
	FWHM	FWTM	Sensitivity
(Tc99M)			
HSLEC	15.9	27.3	181
HSMEC	22.5	36.8	-
LSMEC	16.9	31.4	-
(I-131)			
HSMEC	25.6	45.0	202
LSMEC	17.0	31.8	75

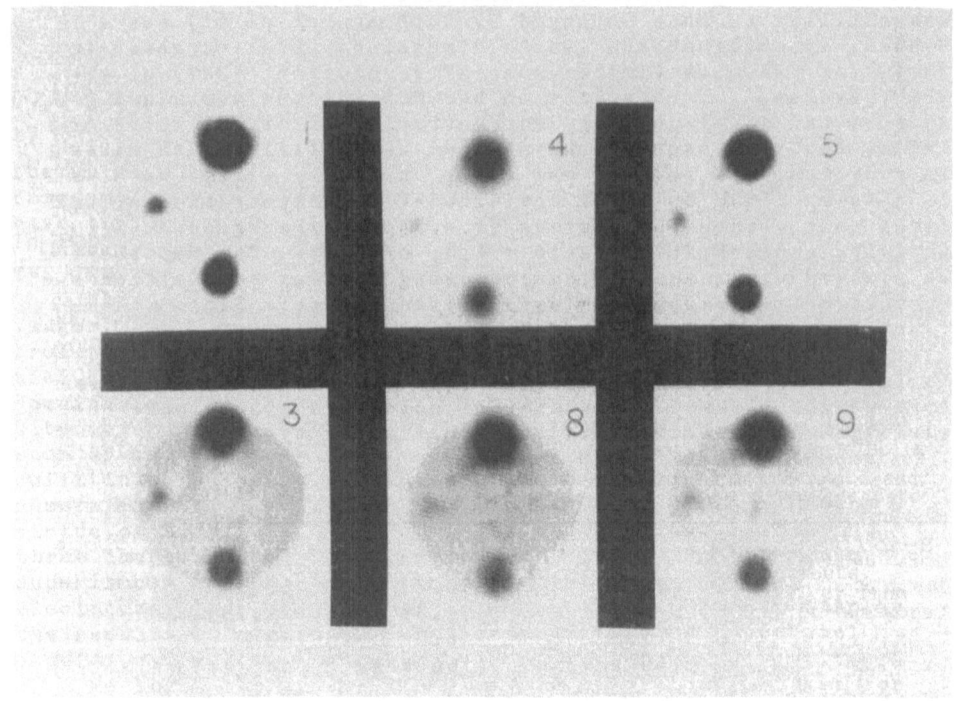

FIGURE 1. Representative transverse images of the MSS phantom, demonstrating loss of image contrast or RC with object size. LHS: HSLEC/Tc99M. Middle: HSMEC/I-131. RHS: LSMEC/I-131. Images are shown for signal/background (S/B)=1:0, 5:1 respectively.

3. RESULTS

Representative transverse images of the MSS phantom are shown in Fig. 1 for the three collimators evaluated and with S/B activity concentration of 1:0 and 5:1 respectively. The loss of image contrast or RC with object size was visually well demonstrated for the smaller sources imaged. In the quantitative analysis, the RC data was measured for each source by computing the maximum counts/pixel. The relative variation of RC was computed by setting the value for source number 1 (4 x FWHM) to 1.0, as proposed by Hoffman et al (1); in this case for the isolated source without background activity. Similiarly the LDR was measured using circular ROI's fully enclosing the image of each source. Relative variation in LDR was then computed as above.

Table 4: Dimensions of four cylindrical sources of varying
diameter, contained within the water filled MSS phantom (ID =
20 cm). Each source was positioned with its centroid at 5 cm
radial distance from the central axis. The sources were 8 cm
long to allow a thick traverse slice (4 cm) to be selected,
reducing systematic errors in measuring RC and LDR data.

Source	1	2	3	4
Diameter (cm)	5.7	3.75	1.8	1.0
Diameter (FWHM)	4X	2X	1X	0.5X

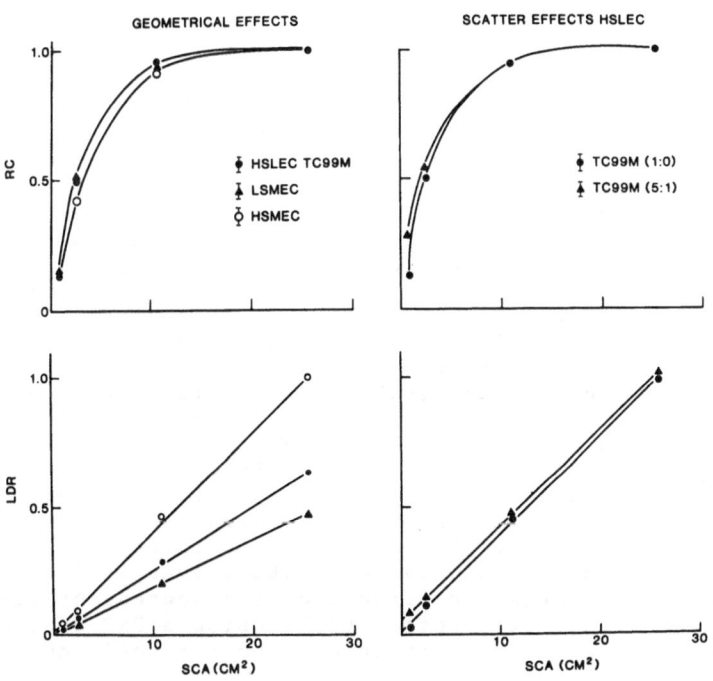

FIGURE 2. Measured RC and LDR dependence on Source Cross
sectional Area (SCA): Influence of geometrical resolution and
photon scattering. LHS: HSLEC, HSMEC, and LSMEC using Tc99M
with S/B =1.0. RHS: HSLEC using Tc99M wih S/B=1:0, 5:1.
Representative systemic errors in measurement are indicated.

Table 5: SPECT acquisition and processing parameters used to evaluate each collimator. Parameters were fixed to allow comparison of measured data. The filter parameters in parenthesis were later used to measure influence of filter type.

Energy Window	13%
Flood Correction	30 x 10(6)
Linear Sampling	64 x 64
Angular Sampling	30/360
Total Counts/View	100K
Radius of Rotation (cm)	16
Butterworth Filter	
(order)	4 (7)
(cut off FN)	16 (16)
Attenuation Correction	(cm -1)
(Chang first order)	
Tc99M (140 keV):	0.13
I-131 (364 keV):	0.101

3.1   INFLUENCE OF (GEOMETRICAL) SPATIAL RESOLUTION

The experimentally measured RC and LDR dependence on object size without background is plotted in Fig. 2 for each collimator using Tc99M activity. The plotted RC data primarily reflect the influence of the different geometrical spatial resolution of each collimator since septal penetration effects are not significant and photon scattering conditions to a first approximation are similar. Hence, the RC curves for both the HSLEC and LSMEC were almost identical because of their similar resolution characteristics (table 3) at this photon energy. The HSMEC, however, showed a reduced RC dependence on object size as expected. The effect of using a different reconstruction filter (table 5) had only a minor effect on the shape of the RC curves. The filter type slightly modifies the measured spatial resolution in the tomographic plane (6). The LDR was maintained with the relative sensitivity of each collimator varying in accordance to its geometrical efficiency. The above results obtained using isolated sources of Tc99M were in agreement with that reported (1,2) using a PET system with varying degrees of lead collimation used for positron annihilation detection.

3.2   INFLUENCE OF PHOTON SCATTERING

Fig. 2 also shows the RC and LDR data obtained for the HSLEC or ultrafine collimator, for both the isolated sources and with the presence of background activity (S/B=1:0, 5:1). Since the same collimator was used, the RC data primarily reflect the increase in count contribution due to photon scattering from the background activity region. The LDR data also reflect a small count contribution due to background activity included with the ROI, particularly for the smaller sources imaged. The influence of the above effects was, however, not very significant except for the smallest source, particularily when compared to the data acquired at higher photon energy using conventional collimation.

3.3 INFLUENCE OF PHOTON PENETRATION

Fig. 3 shows a comparison of the results obtained for the HSMEC and LSMEC respectively, when imaging the higher photon energies of I-131. The results obtained for Tc99M are also plotted to compare the shape of the geometrical response curves. The RC dependence on object size was significantly photon energy dependent for the HSMEC, the RC values being greatly reduced for the smaller sources. A plateau was not reached in the RC curve for this collimator for the largest source (4 X FWHM) imaged. This observation was attributed to the continued influence of the photon penetration effects through the collimator septa with larger sources as demonstrated previously for planer imaging methods (11). Furthermore, the presence of background activity (S/B=5:1) introduced a large overestimation of the RC values; the uncertainty introduced frequently being greater than 50%. Similarity, the level of background activity introduced an overestimation of the LDR values, although a linear response was still maintained.

In contrast to the above, the RC data for the LSMEC was not significantly photon energy dependent and object size dependence remained similar to the ultrafine collimator at lower photon energy. The level of background activity in turn did not greatly modify the RC or LDR values, except for the smallest source. The data observed for this collimator, therefore, suggest that its RC dependence on object size could be equally well characterized by a mathematical model as for the ultrafine collimator. It has the added advantage of not being photon energy dependent for the energy range described.

4. DISCUSSION

The objectives of this work was to demonstrate the feasibility of generating a mathematical model to correct for the RC and LDR dependence of the SPECT system on object size. It's clear that unique corrections are required independent of photon energy and level of background activity surrounding the sources. These conditions cannot be met unless long bore collimators with uniform spatial resolution and with a low penetration fraction are employed, such as the LSMEC (table 2 and 3). Sacrifice in collimator geometrical efficiency is necessary . If conventional type collimators are employed at higher photon energies, the measurement uncertainties are large and inter-related, even for the rather idealized phantom used, where symmetrical sources and uniform background were present in a phantom of fixed dimensions. The same limitations apply to planer imaging techniques (11).

452

The generation of a comprehensive mathematical model to allow the broader objectives of absolute measurements in-vivo, as required for dosimetry estimations (4,14), requires attention to an additional range of factors not addressed. These factors include the uncertainty in applying attenuation corrections, measurement of patient thickness profile, non-uniform background and optimization of reconstruction filters (6,7). However, prior to addressing these primarily software related factors, it's clear that appropiate choice of collimator and SPECT hardware design is important, because of the relatively large uncertainties related to object size dependence. Emphasis on the detector response to small sources is required in dosimetry estimations, since the dose delivered to (small) tumors must be determined with a precision comparable to external beam therapy (ideally within $\pm$ 10%) (4,14).

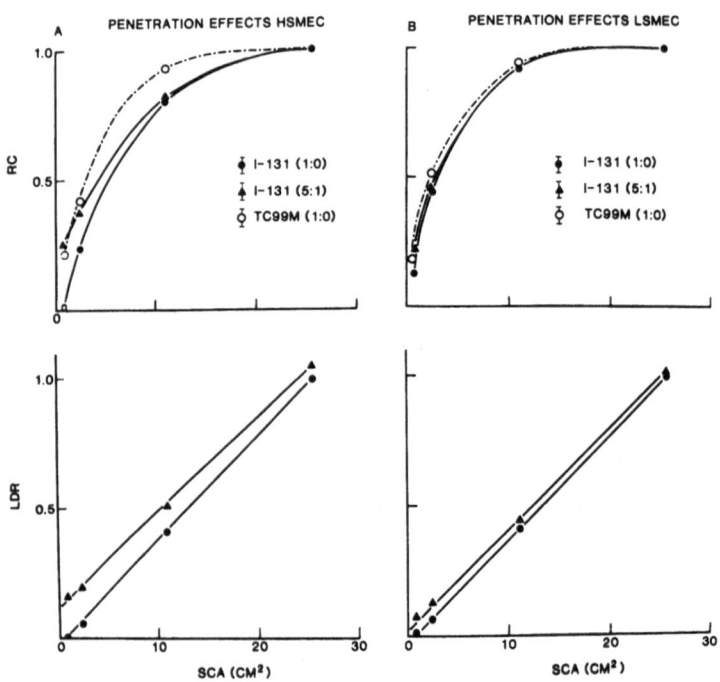

FIGURE 3. Measured RC and LDR dependence on Source Cross Sectional Area (SCA): Influence of photon penetration. LHS: HSMEC using I-131 and Tc99M. RHS: LSMEC using I-131 and Tc99M. Representative systematic errors in measurement are indicated.

Computer simulation techniques have recently been reported that calculate the dose delivered to the target site, based on the particulate and gamma radiations emitted by selective therapy nuclides (14). In this work, one of the greatest sources of uncertainties in dose calculations was the assumed biodistribution, which highlights the importance of accurate quantitative SPECT imaging techniques.

The experimental approach, using a recognized limited range of phantom measurements, therefore, provided a useful guide in identifying the appropriate choice of long bore collimator and an acceptable tolerance of theoretical leakage levels for quantitative measurements (9-11). Although the data might initially be considered to be somewhat predictable based on common principles of collimator design, it is not readily possible to accurately predict the measured leakage through collimator septa or its integrated effects (penetration fraction) at high photon energy, throughout the object volume, using either analytical or computer simulation methods (8,12,13). Simulation techniques cannot be used as an optimization procedure in collimator design (12) and furthermore, they cannot readily predict the subsequent quantitative RC or LDR charcteristics as experimentally measured here, since the measurement uncertainties are not accounted for (9,10).

Important practical considerations unique to SPECT imaging at high photon energies include the COR variation with collimator weight and possible related registration shifts in linear sampling due to translation motion of heavier collimated detectors. In our preliminary investigations for a wide photon energy range (140-511 keV) none of the artifacts were found to be significant (9,10). The above results were attributed to the design of the SPECT gantry and heavily shielded detector.

In this work, the RC and LDR dependence on object size was considered for the two dimensional (2D) case in the traverse tomographic plane, in order to minimize the systematic errors in the proposed measurement parameters. It's clear that partial volume effects, related to the differences in object size and slice thickness were not addressed. Measurements are currently in progress for the 3D case using edge detection methods. Differences in the RC and LDR curves are expected to be greater as predicted elsewhere for PET (2). This data will further support the importance of collimator choice before the development of mathematical models for antibody biodistribution measurements in-vivo.

REFERENCES

1. Hoffman EJ, Cheng H, and Phelps ME. Quantitation in Positron Emission Tomography: 1. Effect of Object Size. J Comp Assist Tomography 3:299-308, 1979.
2. Kessler RM, Ellis JR, Eden M. Analysis of Emission Tomographic Scan Data: Limitations Imposed by Resolution and Background. J Comp Assist Tomography 8(3):514-522, 1984.

3. Larson S, Brown JP, Weight PW, et al. Imaging of Melanoma
    with I-131 Labeled Monochonal Antibodies. J Nucl Med 24:
    123-129, 1983.
4. Leichter PK, Klein JL, Garrison JB, et al. Dosimetry of
    I-131 Antiferritin in Hematoma: A Model for
    Radioimmunogoblin in Dosimetry. Int J Radiat Oncol Biol
    Phys 7:323-333, 1981.
5. Berche C, Mach JP, Lumbroso JD, et al. Tomoscintigraphy
    for Detecting Gastrointestinal and Medullary Thyroid
    Cancer: First Clinical Results Using Radiolabeled
    Monoclonal Antibodies Against Carcinoembryonic Antigen.
    Br Med J 285:1447-1451, 1982.
6. Jaszczak RJ, Coleman RE, and Whitehead FR. Physical
    Factors Affecting Quantitative Measurements Using Camera
    Based Single Photon Emission Computed Tomography (SPECT).
    IEEE Trans Nucl Sci NS-28, 69-78, 1981.
7. Moore SC, Brunelle JA, Kirch CM. Quantitative
    Multidetector Emission Computed Tomography Using
    Interactive Attenuation Compensation. J Nucl Med 23:
    706-714, 1982.
8. Floyd CE, Jaszczak RJ, Greer KL, et al. Deconvolution of
    Compton Scatter in SPECT. J Nucl Med 26:403-408, 1985.
9. Clarke LP, Cheng CB, Leong LK, et al. SPECT Imaging of
    I-131 (364 keV): Importance of Collimation. Nucl Med Comm
    6:41-47, 1985.
10. Clarke LP, Gentile M, Saw CB, et al. SPECT Collimation for
    Medium-High Photon Energy: Influence of Spatial Resolution
    and Image Contrast with Traverse Tomographic Plane. Nato
    Advanced Study Institute. Proc. Meeting: Physics and
    Engineering of Medical Imaging; Maratea, Italy; October,
    1984.
11. Clarke LP, Malone JF, Casey M. Quantitative Measurement of
    Activity of Small Sources Containing Medium Energy
    Radionuclides. Br J Radiol 55:125-133, 1982.
12. Jahns MF. The Influence of Penetrating Radiation on
    Collimator Performance. Phys Med Biol 26:113-124, 1981.
13. Clarke LP, Duffy GJ, Malone JF. An Improved Uptake Probe
    Collimator for a Large Crystal Rectilinear Scanner.
    Phys Med Biol 23:118-126, 1978.
14. Wessels BW and Rogus RD. Radionuclide Selection and Model
    Absorbed Dose Calculations for Radiolabeled Tumor
    Associated Antibodies. Med Phys 11(5):638-645, 1984.

Methodology for Predicting the Performance of Different PET Camera Designs.

M.Defrise, F.Deconinck, S.Kuijk+, A.Bossuyt, V.Lacroix, M.Waligorski*

Vrije Universiteit Brussel, +Aspirant van het N.F.W.O., *Institute of Nuclear Physics, Krakow

1.Introduction

The evaluation of the performance of a given positron camera design is an extremely complex problem; since so many physical (photon scattering, detector parallax...), and algorithmic (deconvolution filter, image post-processing) factors interfere to produce the final image to be used for medical diagnosis. The assessment of the quality of a given final image is also far from trivial, this problem being influenced by physical, physiological and psychological factors.

An objective comparison of the performances of different camera designs requires an accurate evaluation of the camera characteristics, such as sensitivities for unscattered, scattered, and accidental coincidences. The distribution of these coincidences must also be determined. Monte-Carlo simulation techniques seem best suited for solving such a problem and have indeed been used by several authors (cf. § 2.1). These works, however, were only devoted to one type of positron camera : either based on scintillation crystal rings (1), or on multi-wire proportional chambers (MWPC, 2). We have written a Monte-Carlo program to simulate these two types of positron cameras, and, therefore, to compare them on an objective basis. The simulation, which is described in detail in Chapter 2, includes the transport of the annihilation photons in a user-specified phantom (§ 2.2) and the detection of these photons in the MWPC (§ 2.3) or crystal ring (§ 2.4) detectors. Using this method, we can integrate the influence of the Compton and photoelectric interactions of photons in the phantom and shielding, of the geometrical efficiency, and of the energy dependence of the detectors' intrinsic efficiency correctly. We have not yet taken into account the influence of the positron range and $\gamma\gamma$ acolinearity, which degrades the resolution of the imaging system seriously (§ 2.2.4), but does not affect the camera sensitivity.

The Monte-Carlo simulation yields, for any positron camera design, a certain number of quantitative characteristics. In order to compare different possible designs, we determine the criteria that should be used to decide which design is to be prefered for a given imaging purpose. Chapter 3 is devoted to that problem. In the context of previous works (3,4,5), a quality factor (5) is presented, and its limitations discussed. Possible improvements, which should allow one to account for the complexity of the imaging system better, are proposed. The methods defined in Chapters 2 and 3 are then used in Chapter 4 to compare two particular, but typical positron cameras : one based on multi-wire proportional chambers, the other on a single crystal ring.

2. The Monte-Carlo method for the simulation of positron cameras

2.1. The need for a Monte-Carlo simulation of positron cameras

This chapter is devoted to the study of the output signal of a positron camera, namely, to the evaluation of the count rates for true, scattered and random coincidences with a given phantom and camera design. Even this limited problem is difficult to tackle by means of purely analytical methods: the exact integration of the detector's solid angle, of the energy dependence of the detector's efficiency, of the attenuation due to Compton and photoelectric effects - just to mention a few problems - is impossible, except perhaps in the case of a centred point source in air.

It is nevertheless tempting to draw very qualitative design considerations from the use of simple analytical expressions, like e.g. (6) :

true rate	~	$\Omega \; \varepsilon^2$
scattered rate	~	$\Omega^2 \; \varepsilon^2$
random rate	~	$\Omega^2 \; \varepsilon^2$
single rate	~	$\Omega \; \varepsilon$

where Ω is the fractional solid angle sustented by the detectors and ε the detector efficiency.

The results of several Monte-Carlo simulations - including this one - have shown that these expressions may lead to erroneous conclusions regarding for instance the compared efficiency of ring and plane detector positron cameras. It is of course possible to improve the reliability of analytical computations markedly (see e.g. 7). The obtained expressions for the various counting rates then become extremely unwieldy and lose the appealing and intuitive character of the crude formulae given above, still without approaching the reliability of a Monte-Carlo calculation.

The versatility of the Monte-Carlo method allows much more than the mere evaluation of count rates: the achievable resolution (8), the homogeneity of scattered and random events, and many other factors can be studied accurately. Realistic data for testing reconstruction algorithms can be generated too.

Although this falls beyond the scope of this paper it is interesting to notice that the Monte-Carlo method can also be used to perform image reconstruction in medical imaging, as was shown by H.H. Barrett et al. for coded-aperture tomography (9,10).

Finally, a Monte-Carlo simulation can yield information about variables which cannot be obtained experimentaly with a real camera: the photon's exact energy, the number of scatterings, the true origin of a given photon pair... For those reasons the Monte-Carlo simulation is the method of choice to evaluate count rate characteristics.

The need for a Monte-Carlo simulation of positron cameras has been recognized by several authors. Particularly interesting are the works of Lupton and Keller (1) and Perez-Mendez, Del Guerra, Nelson and Tam (2) which are briefly described below. References 12,13,14,15,16 refer to related works.

Lupton and Keller study single-slice crystal ring cameras. They restrict themselves to tracking the photons in the several parts of the experimental set-up: the phantom, the shields, the crystals and inter-crystal septa. This means that the influences of positron range and $\gamma\gamma$ acollinearity are not taken into account, although they could be, by using previous experimental data or other Monte-Carlo simulations (see 2.3.5). They have studied the influence over the count rates of several design factors like the fan-angle, the septa width, or the patient port-radius in detail (17).

Perez-Mendez, Del Guerra, Nelson and Tam study positron cameras based on large multi-wire proportional chambers. Their simulation is based on the code EGS (Electron Gamma Shower), which simulates the electromagnetic interactions of photons and leptons up to 100 GeV. This allows them to simulate the transport of positrons before their annihilation, of the photons, and also of the photoelectrons in the detectors converter. Particularly interesting in their study is the analysis of the different factors which limit the resolution .

An important problem remains unanswered by these previous Monte- Carlo studies: the comparison of the performances of the positron cameras using crystal rings and those using Multi-Wire Proportional Chambers. Most statements to be found in the literature about this problem are based on crude analytical expressions, and are therefore questionable. The main purpose of this chapter is to provide some sound quantitative data for such a comparison.

2.2. Description of the Monte-Carlo program for the simulation of positron cameras

2.2.1. Overview

The Monte-Carlo method simulates a large number - typically 10^6 - of individual positron "histories". Each "history" is a succession of a certain number of "events" like for instance :

- positron emission at a given point
- annihilation with an electron, giving 2 photons with given momenta
- Compton and photoelectric interactions of the photons in the specified phantom
- detection or loss of the photons

(The number and types of "events" vary of course from "history" to "history"). The choice between the different possible outcomes of any particular "event" (e.g. the coordinates of the positron emission point, or the scattering angle in some Compton interaction) is made at random, according to the known probability distribution function for that "event" (e.g. the user-specified radionuclide distribution, or the Klein-Nishina's differential cross section).

The generation of a large number of individual "histories" then reproduces these known distribution functions correctly, and allows one to determine how they combine to produce the characteristics of the global system (phantom + positron camera): for instance, by recording the number of Compton scatterings undergone by the photons for each "history", one can determine the scattered fraction of the coincidence rate. It is clear that a large number of different characteristics of positron cameras can be evaluated, using one unique simulation program. (Analytical methods, where possible, would in general require a separate calculation for each characteristic!).

2.2.2. Description of the simulated system

The system simulated by the Monte-Carlo program consists of three parts, which must be specified by the user :

1. The radionuclide distribution
It also specifies the type of radionuclide used, if some kind of positron tracking were to take place (see below).

2. The phantom is a set of regions with homogeneous properties. Each region is described by its electronic density and by 2 coefficients which determine a fit of the photoelectric cross section.

3. The detector characteristics, which will be described in sections 2.3 and 2.4. The routines consist of a purely geometrical part on one hand (will a photon with a given position and

momentum hit the detector ?) and of a dynamical part on the other hand (if a photon with a given energy hits the detector, will it be detected ?)

We will describe the modules in more detail, mentioning various methods which can be used to design them.

2.2.3. Generation of a positron

We generate the position of an emitted positron, according to a given radionuclide distribution. If the Monte-Carlo simulation is to take into account the motion of the positron before annihilation, we have to generate the following variables :
- The positron momentum's direction cosines, which are isotropically distributed
- The positron's energy, which should be generated using the known energy spectrum for the radionuclide. This latter parameter was not included in our simulations

2.2.4. Tracking the positron

We track the created positron until it annihilates with an electron to yield 2 photons, whose initial position, momenta and energies are then evaluated.

The interactions of the annihilation photons in the phantom and detectors have a primordial influence on the global characteristics of the positron camera, like for instance the true and accidental coincidences rates. The positron's interactions before annihilation, on the other hand, have a more restricted influence; they only affect the resolution, i.e. the form of the point response function of the camera. Two factors combine to produce this contribution to the blurring of the point response function :

1. The distance travelled by the positron before its slows down and annihilates with an electron

2. The acolinearity between the two annihilation photons. As shown by Del Guerra et al., this acolinearity is essentially due to the Fermi motion of the atomic electron, the fraction of the positrons which annihilates in flight being negligible.

It should be stressed that the simulation of the interactions with matter of a charged particle like the positron is much more complicated than the equivalent problem for a neutral particle like the photon: the mean free path for a 511 keV photon in water is of the order of 10 cm, which means that a relatively small number of discrete interactions have to be simulated. The positron momentum, on the other hand, is continuously modified by the long-range Coulomb forces and by brehmsstrahlung. The simulation of these interactions is far from simple, and was not included in our Monte-Carlo simulation.

The influence of the positron's motion has to be incorporated in the form of an experimentally determined distribution of the distance between the positron emission and annihilation points. Such distributions, which depend on the radionuclide being studied and on the absorbing medium, can be found e.g. in Derenzo (18). They also include the influence of the photon-photon acolinearity. Notice that the simulation of the influence of the electron's Fermi motion - which yields the major contribution to the photon- photon acolinearity - must always be based on experimental data : an "ab initio" simulation is impossible here. Although implemented, we have not yet used this part in our simulation.

2.2.5. Tracking the photons in the phantom

We track a photon in the phantom, until one of three events occurs :
- the photon reaches the boundary of the phantom
- it is absorbed by a photoelectric interaction
- its energy falls below a user-specified threshold by Compton scatter

During the tracking, two types of interactions are simulated :

- the Compton scattering, the cross section of which is given by a look-up table. This cross-section is further multiplied by the electronic density for the current region of the phantom to get the absorption coefficient in cm^{-1}.
- The photoelectric interaction with an atom. Like Lupton and Keller, we fit the total absorption coefficient (in cm^{-1}) for this reaction by

$$\Sigma \, photo \; = \; A \; x \; Energy^{-B}$$

where A and B depend on the region.
The coherent scattering on atoms has been neglected. Its importance is small, except for low energies and high Z elements.

2.3. The simulation of a detector based on multiwire proportional chambers

2.3.1. The detectors set-up

Typical positron cameras based on multiwire proportional chambers (2,8,19,20) consist of 2 to 6 large rectangular plane MWPC (typically 30 X 30 cm), all parallel to the Z-axis of the camera. Each detector plane contains a high Z converter (typically 6 mm lead), from which the inpinging photons extract Compton- or photoelectrons. The converter should have a very high surface to volume ratio to allow the electrons - which have a very short range in high-Z elements - to escape the converter volume. Such a high surface to volume ratio can be obtained by drilling a large number of small holes (± 1 mm diameter) in a lead plate (20). Another solution consists in forming a compact "honeycomb" by fusing together a large number of lead glass capillaries (8)
If an electron escapes the converter and gets into a hole or a capillary, it is submitted to a high voltage gradient which drifts it to the wire chamber itself, where it is detected. By piling up several layers of converter + wire chambers, it is possible to improve the detection efficiency without increasing the parallax error, as would be the case with a single but thicker converter .

2.3.2. The simulation

A more detailed description of these detectors and of the associated optimization problem is beyond the scope of this paper; let us only review the points which should be included in a Monte-Carlo simulation :

1. Geometrical efficiency.

2. Photon conversion.
Since the dimension of the holes or capillaries is small with respect to the resolution of the global system or even with respect to the parallax error, it seems reasonable for the present purpose to approximate the converter by means of a homogeneous lead plate with an appropriate lower density. It is then possible to track the photon in this simplified converter, using the same technique as that used in the photon routine (2.2.5). With this method we can determine :
- The photon conversion probability (for a given energy)
- The parallax error, caused by the distance between the point where the photon inpinges, and the point where the photo-electron is created.

3. Tracking the electron in the converter.
The overall detection efficiency also depends on the probability that a photoelectron with a given energy escapes to a hole. This probability can only be determined by simulating the electron interactions in the converter, this time taking the complete converter geometry into

460

account. This was done by Del Guerra et al. We restrict ourselves to a rough analytical simulation of this point which nevertheless yield satisfactory results.

4. Electron detection in the wire chamber

When an electron leaves the converter's volume and reaches a hole, it may be considered as detected with a probability 1. One must still take into account the intrinsic resolution of the wire chamber, which further degrades the global resolution of the system.

We have simulated the global detection process using a known efficiency, function of the photon's energy : $\varepsilon(E)$. When a photon with energy E hits the detectors plane, one generates a random number r uniformly distributed on (0,1). If $r < \varepsilon(E)$ the photon is considered detected. The efficiency should ideally depend on the photon's impact angle. However, since this angle is usually close to the normal, we have so far neglected this dependence. The efficiency curve used could be based either on a previous Monte-Carlo study, or on some experimental data . This simulation method was used in most of our simulations, and has the following advantages:
- it may be very accurate if a sufficiently accurate efficiency curve is used
- it is flexible, and economic regarding execution time
- by replacing the condition $r < \varepsilon(E)$ by $r < F.\varepsilon(E)$, where F is such that $F.\varepsilon_{max} = 1$, it is possible to improve the efficiency of the Monte-Carlo simulation significantly (the evaluated count rates must be corrected afterwards).

2.4. Crystal ring detectors

2.4.1. Description of the simulated detector

Lupton and Keller (1, 17) have studied a single slice crystal ring positron camera using the Monte-Carlo method. They have not used their simulation to compare such positron cameras with those based on multiwire proportional chambers. We adapted our Monte-Carlo program to allow the simulation of crystal ring cameras. (Only the routines relevant to the detection process have to be modified).
We have simulated the following cylindrical symmetrical geometry :

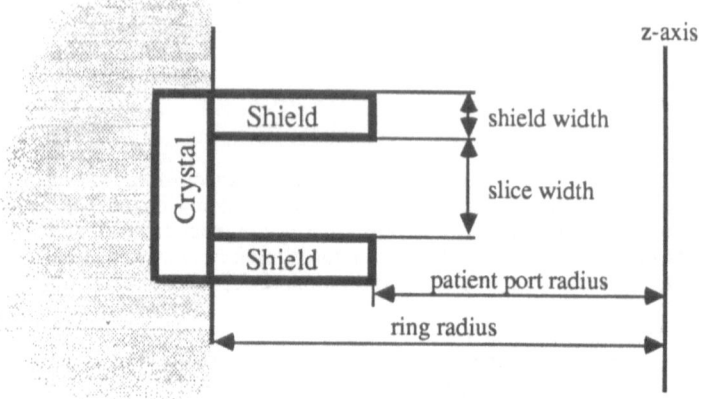

The shaded area is perfectly absorbing: a photon hitting this area is considered lost. In the shield, on the other hand, Compton and photoelectric interactions are simulated according to the method of section 2.2.5. Our simulation does not take into account inter-crystal septa and shadow-shields. This should not significantly affect global count rates (as is shown by comparing our results with those of Lupton and Keller) but only the resolution, which is not the main object of the present study.

The geometrical efficiency of a ring camera is very low: the fractional solid angle seen from the centre of the ring is of the order of a few percent. The efficiency of the Monte-Carlo simulation is therefore also very low if the annihilation photon pair is emitted isotropically, as it is in the real situation. In a typical situation, one would record only 2400 true unscattered coincidences for 10^6 generated positrons!

In order to improve the efficiency of the simulation, and therefore the statistical accuracy of the evaluated count rates, we have used importance sampling to generate the direction of the photon pairs preferably towards the ring (22).

This method improves the accuracy for some variables (in particular, the true coincidence rate) but degrades it for other variables (like the scattered rate); it must therefore be used with caution.

2.4.2. The crystal intrinsic efficiency

In order to simulate the detection efficiency, we use the same method as in section 2.3.2. We then need to know the efficiency - energy relationship for the particular crystal being considered. Some data can be found in the literature (e.g. 23). We have made a separate Monte-Carlo study of a cylindrical BGO crystal, having a depth of 3 cm and a radius of 1.35, such that the cylinder area equals the area of the crystal (1,9 cm x 3 cm) used by Lupton and Keller (the computed efficiency varies fairly slowly with the crystal radius).

Photons are "shot" against the crystal, at a random location on its surface and with a direction cosine uniformly distributed between cos 30° and cos 0° = 1. The photons are tracked in the crystal until they are absorbed or escape.

If the deposited energy is larger than a certain threshold, the photon is considered to be detected. (for BGO we use an electronic density of $1.678 \ 10^{24}$ cm^{-3} and, like Lupton and Keller, we fit the photoelectric absorption coefficient by $4.01 \ 10^6$ cm^{-1} x (energy in keV)$^{-2.6}$).

2.5. Evaluating count rates using the Monte-Carlo study

We have seen how the characteristics of a given positron camera design can be evaluated using the Monte-Carlo method. The program proceeds by simulating a large number of individual and independent positron "histories" . This means that the time factor is not included in the simulation; the output of the Monte-Carlo program does not consist of count rates but of probabilities that an emitted positron yields an event of a given type. For instance, we can determine:

q : the probability that a positron triggers no detector
s : the probability that a positron yields a single event
c : the probability that a positron yields an unscattered coincidence
c_s: the probability that a positron yields a scattered coincidence

Many other probabilities, and also distribution functions, can be evaluated. How can these probabilities be translated into count rates ?

The solution does not merely consist in multiplying the probabilities by the activity of the source; it is necessary to take into account the various dead times of the system, which eventually cause the saturation of the count rates when the activity grows.

Two types of dead times will be considered :

-the non-paralyzable dead-time due to the acquisition electronics

Suppose that coincidences are detected at a total rate λ, according to a Poisson distribution. Suppose also that the electronics are unable to acquire more than one coincidence per time interval t_D. A coincidence will be registered if it is separated from the last registered coincidence by a time interval larger than t_D. Otherwise it is lost.

The effective rate registered is then known to be (24):

$$\lambda_0 = \frac{\lambda}{1 + \lambda t_D} = \frac{1}{\int_0^\infty \lambda\, e^{-\lambda t'}\ (t' + t_D)\ dt'}$$

-the paralyzable dead-time, specific to the coincidence measurement in positron tomography.

Despite a much smaller characteristic time ($\pm$ 10 ns instead of 1 μs) this paralyzable dead-time will be shown to be quite important, in particular for cameras based on MWPC.

Suppose that a photon (call it γ_1) is detected at time t=0. The coincidence circuitry will be triggered if a second photon (γ_2) is (or was) detected during the time interval $(-\tau,+\tau)$, where τ is the time window, characteristic of the type of detector used. Suppose that a third photon (γ_3) is detected during this time interval . Even if the electronics were fast enough to record the coordinates of the three photons, this event would clearly be useless since it would in general be impossible to decide which pair of photons (if any) is originating from the same positron (in some particular cases, one could use the geometry of this multiple photons event to select the "good" pair with high probability).

Such events, therefore, must not be registered. This results, at high doses, in the saturation of the positron camera. The non-paralysable dead-time previously discussed causes the observed rate to tend to the limit value $1/t_D$, when the activity becomes large.The present saturation phenomenon, on the other hand, will eventually cause the useful coincidence rate to decrease to zero; this corresponds to the concept of paralyzable dead-time. The observed coincidence rate is now given by

$$\lambda = c\, A\, e^{-2\tau A (1-q)}$$

where c is the probability that a positron gives a coincidence, (1-q) is the probability that a positron triggers any detector and A is the total activity in the source. The exponential factor corresponds to the probability that no event (coincidence, single or multi-photon) is detected during the time interval 2τ.

Notice that this model for the saturation of a positron camera does not take into account the dead-time associated to the detector itself, but only the fact that multi-photon events are useless. A more accurate model for saturation would depend on the detectors' characteristics and on the precise description of the data acquisition procedure (see e.g. 25,26).

The random coincidence rate is calculated as usual by

$$R = (sA)^2\, 2\tau$$

where A is the activity of the source, τ the time window of the coincidence circuit. To study how these random coincidences are distributed, we simulate them in the Monte Carlo program as pairs of successive single events. This allows us e.g. to determine which fraction of the random is left over after eliminating the coincidence lines that do not cross the phantom: this often results in an important reduction of the effective random coincidence rate.

3. Evaluating the performances of positron cameras

Using the Monte-Carlo simulation described in the previous section, we can evaluate the count rates and other characteristics for different camera designs. The next question is, how can we compare their performances, how can we decide which design is to be prefered for a given imaging problem ? Two rather opposite approaches could be advocated:

Since the final product of the positron camera is the image, take a particular phantom, simulate data and perform the reconstruction. The two images should then be compared. As noted by Shosa and Kaufman (4),this first method mostly yields subjective information (although it could be argued that the final image is to be used subjectively anyway). Furthermore, it gives no information about the origin of the differences between the "qualities" of the two images.

The second approach consists in defining one - or a few - quantifiable quality factors which should somehow reflect the performances of a given camera design. It is clear that the definition of a useful quality factor is complex, and that no single number can ever account for the multidimensional quantity we call the "quality" of an image. Nevertheless, the use of such quality factors may prove extremely useful and complementary to the comparison of reconstructed images. In the next section we introduce the notion of effective count rate, which will be used in the following chapter. This quality factor (5, 27) takes into account the degradation of the signal-to-noise ratio due to the scattered and random coincidences. Its definition follows from the use of the formula of Rose naturally (3), which relates the detectable object contrast to the number of resolution elements and to the total coincidence count recorded. Limitations of the Rose's formula and of the "effective count rate" will be discussed and possible improvements (some of which are due to Shosa and Kaufman) outlined.

We shall consider that we want to optimize the ability of the camera to allow the detection of unhomogeneities (lesions for instance...) in the radioisotope distribution. The performance of a camera is then measured by the size of the smallest lesion that can be detected on an image obtained after a given imaging time, this lesion having a given contrast to the background. Notice that we would use a different way of evaluating the camera's performance if we were to quantify the activity in a given region of interest accurately.

Let $o(x)$ be the unknown radioisotope distribution (the "object") and $i(x)$ the corresponding image yielded by an imaging system which consists of the camera and the reconstruction algorithm. Suppose we want to detect the presence, or absence, of a contrast between two regions x_1 and x_2 of the object distribution. A criterium must be chosen to decide, using the reconstructed image, whether such a contrast exists. A natural criterium is (28) :

We decide that there is a contrast if and only if :

$$|i(x_2)-i(x_1)| > k_\varepsilon\, \sigma(\, i(x_2)-i(x_1)\,) \qquad (1)$$

where $\sigma^2(\, i(x_2)-i(x_1)\,)$ is the variance of the quantity $i(x_2)-i(x_1)$. In practice, $i(x_2)$ and $i(x_1)$ represent the image integrated over a volume corresponding to the lesion studied, but with a diameter at least equal to the FWHM of the point spread function of the imaging system. Two types of error might occur when using this criterium to detect the presence of a contrast :

1) The error of the first type ("false positive"), is related to the specificity of the test. The probability ε for such an error is related to the factor k_ε by (in the normal approximation) :

$$\varepsilon \;=\; 2 \int_{k_\varepsilon}^{\infty} \frac{e^{-1/2\ x^2}}{\sqrt{2\pi}}\ dx \quad .$$

As noted by Lim et al., the mean number of false alarms is equal to ε times the number of voxels studied. The choice of ε should therefore depend on the number of voxels.

2) The error of the second type ("false negative") is related to the sensitivity of the test, and occurs when the unequality (1) does not hold, although a certain contrast

$$C \;=\; (o(x_2) - o(x_1)) \,/\, o(x_1)$$

exists. The probability 1-p of such an error depends on C. By plotting 1-p versus ε for different values of k_ε (C being fixed), one would obtain the ROC curve of an observer who would blindly apply the criterium (1).

What is the requirement on the mean image contrast $<i(x_2)>-<i(x_1)>$ if we want to detect the presence of this contrast with a probability p, the risk of false alarm being ε ? The answer is, if $i(x_2)$ and $i(x_1)$ are distributed normally (and for C>0 and p>0.5):

$$<i(x_2)>-<i(x_1)> \;>\; (k_\varepsilon + k_{2(1-p)})\ \sigma\ (\ i(x_2)-i(x_1)\ ) \quad (2)$$

where $k_{2(1-p)}$ is defined as k_ε hereabove.

Let's apply this to an ideal imaging system in which $i(x)$ is equal to the number of detected photons in the pixel or voxel x, the mean number of photons $<i(x)>$ being proportional to the unknown object distribution at x, $o(x)$. If we suppose that different voxels are uncorrelated, the unequality reduces to the formula of Rose (4):

$$|C| \quad <i(x_1)>^{1/2} \quad > \quad k\ (2+C)^{1/2}$$

where the contrast C is defined by $(o(x_2)-o(x_1))/o(x_1)$ and $k = k_\varepsilon + k_{2(1-p)}$. This formula can be used to evaluate the maximum number of resolution elements in an image if the total number of detected photons, k and C are fixed.

Unfortunately, the situation is more complicated since the object contrast C is degraded in the image by the blurring effect of the imaging system. Furthermore, in tomography, the statistical fluctuations are not as easy to analyse, since the ramp type filters used in tomographic reconstruction algorithms amplify the high frequency components of noise (see e.g. Lim). We shall analyse these two problems.

1) the systematic error is the difference between the object distribution $o(x)$ and the mean image $<i(x)>$, i.e. the image obtained with an infinite number of counts. This error is among others due to photon scatter and attenuation, to the positron range and $\gamma\gamma$ acolinearity, to the limited spatial resolution of the detectors... Some of these factors could in principle be corrected for by the reconstruction algorithm, but this would require very high statistics since such corrections are usually equivalent to deconvolutions and are therefore unstable in the presence of noisy data.

Let's investigate how the formula of Rose should be modified if the image contains a background of scattered photons, which, in first approximation, may be considered as uniformly distributed:

$$i(x) = i_{unscattered}(x) + i_{scattered}$$

When the contrast is small, more precisely, when $C\, i_{scattered} << (2+C)\, i_{total}$, the effect of this uniform background can be accounted for by replacing $<i(x_1)>$ in the formula of Rose with an "effective" number of photons (5,27):

$$<i_{effective}(x_1)> = \frac{<i_{unscattered}(x_1)>^2}{<i_{unscattered}(x_1)> + <i_{scattered}(x_1)>}$$

The same approach can be applied for random coincidences in positron tomography, insofar as these random coincidences are uniformly distributed. In the next section, we shall use the effective count rate

$$Q = \frac{(\text{True count rate})^2}{\text{True + Random + Scattered count rate}}$$

as a quality factor to compare the performances of two types of positron cameras, as was done by other authors previously (17,27).

The systematic error $o(x)-<i(x)>$ can be studied more generally if the imaging system (camera + reconstruction algorithm) can be described by a space invariant point spread function $\rho(x)$:

$$<i(x)> = (\rho * o)(x)$$

Particular models may be used (e.g. a Gaussian PSF and a spherical or sinusoidal lesion) to evaluate the contrast degradation due to this effect (4,5).

2) The statistical fluctuations are due to Poisson noise, which is amplified by the deconvolution procedure applied to the backprojected data. If the reconstruction algorithm is linear, we can write :

$$i(x) = \Sigma_{j=1 \text{ to } M}\; n_j\; h_j(x)$$

where n_j is the number of photons (or coincidences) detected in the acquisition channel j; $h_j(x)$ depends on the reconstruction algorithm and contains among othersthe factors used to correct for scatter and attenuation.

If the n_j are distributed as independent Poisson variables, we can calculate for (2) :

$$\sigma^2(\,i(x_2)-i(x_1)\,) = \Sigma_{j=1 \text{ to } M}\; <n_j>\, (h_j(x_2)-h_j(x_1))^2$$

When the correlation between $i(x_1)$ and $i(x_2)$ can be neglected (which is true in many cases, though one should be careful when neighbouring pixels are compared), we get :

$$\sigma^2(\,i(x_2)-i(x_1)\,) = \sigma^2(i(x_2)) + \sigma^2(\,i(x_1))$$

If the sampling of the data is sufficiently fine, i.e. if the number of channels M is large enough, the discrete summation can be approximated by an integral. It is possible to evaluate the statistical fluctuations for instance at the centre of the image of a uniform disk or sphere.

In the case of 2-dimensional tomography, and using a ramp filter cut at the frequency A, one obtains for a disk of radius R :

$$\sigma^2(i(\text{centre of disk})) \approx 8 \pi^2 (R.A)^3 / 3 N_T$$

where N_T is the total number of photons (or coincidences) detected. This result was first obtained, in an equivalent form, by Budinger (29, see also 28). The frequency cut-off A being related to the size d of the resolution elements by $A \approx 1/2d$, this is equivalent to :

$$\sigma^2(i(\text{centre of disk})) \approx \sqrt{\pi} \; N_{resol}^{3/2} / 3 N_T$$

where N_{resol} is the number of resolution elements in the image of the disk. Whereas the numerical constant depends on the kind of filter used, and on the place on the disk where the variance is evaluated, the dependence $N_{resol}^{3/2} / N_T$ is a property of 2-dimensional tomography, which can be derived using different approaches (30,31) and reflects the ill-posedness of the inversion of the Radon transform.

In the case of 3-dimensional X-ray transform, which is relevant for positron cameras using plane detectors, we obtain for a sphere of radius R :

$$\sigma^2(i(\text{centre of sphere})) \approx 16 \; \pi^2 (R.A)^4 J(\Omega) / 3 N_T$$

where the constant $J(\Omega)$ depends on the solid angle sustended by the detectors. (We suppose that this solid angle is constant for every point of the object, which implies that we restrict ourselves to the "universal cone". For a discussion of this problem, see 32) In the ideal case of a full 4π detector one has $J(\Omega) = 1$. In terms of the number of resolution elements in the image of the sphere, we find :

$$\sigma^2(i(\text{centre of sphere})) \approx 2^{-8/3} \; 3^{1/3} \; \pi^{2/3} \; N_{resol}^{4/3} / N_T$$

Again, a more detailed analysis, including e.g. the influence of the attenuation correction, will modify the numerical factor, but not the main dependence on N_{resol} and N_T.

A few remarks :

1) The above analysis presupposes that the image of a uniform radioisotope distribution would be uniform itself. Practically this is not true since the imaging system introduces structured artifacts in the image. As proposed by Shosa and Kaufman (4), this can be accounted for by adding a term representing the "variance" due to structured noise to the right hand side of (1). This term, however, can only be evaluated experimentally, by imaging a flood field phantom.

2) Like Lim et al. (1982), we have treated the systematic and statistical contributions to the reconstruction error separately. This separation, however, is somewhat artificial since the reconstruction algorithm (e.g. the cut-off frequency A) should in practice depend on the signal-to-noise ratio, in such a way as to minimize the sum of the systematic error (decreasing function of A) and of the statistical error (increasing function of A).

A different approach consists in considering only this global error. This can be done in the framework of regularization theory (e.g. 33), by computing upper bounds for the global error

$$\int |o(x)-i(x)|^2 \, dx.$$

4. Comparison of a ring and a MWPC camera

4.1. Description of the compared camera design

This chapter is devoted to the comparison of the performances of two positron cameras: the first is a single-slice BGO crystal ring camera, the second is built from two pairs of oppositely faced multiwire proportional chambers. The comparison is based, on one hand on the Monte-Carlo technique described in chapter 2, and on the other hand on the effective count rate defined in chapter 3. We restrict ourselves to the comparison of global count rates and do not discuss the -essential - problem of resolution: indeed we think that there is a general agreement about the fact that the instrumental resolution of MWPC cameras is significantly better - particularly in the axial direction- than that of ring cameras.
The crucial problem is to determine whether the statistics - i.e. the count rate - will be high enough to allow this potentially high resolution to be used.

Both cameras are represented in the next figure :

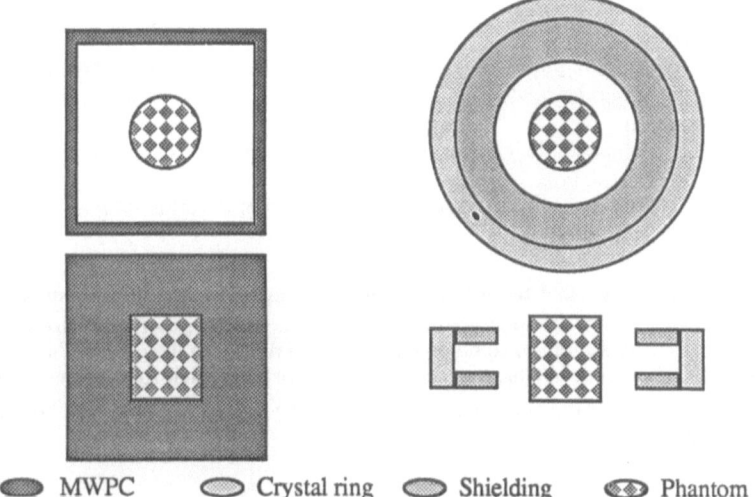

● MWPC　　◌ Crystal ring　◯ Shielding　◉ Phantom

The MWPC camera consists of two perpendicular pairs of opposite multi-wire proportional chambers. The sensitive area of each detector is 43 cm x 43 cm; two opposite detectors are parallel and separated by 45 cm. The efficiency is fitted by :

$$\varepsilon(E) = 0.16 - 0.49 \ e^{-0.0074 \ . \ E(keV)}$$

i.e. $\varepsilon(511 \ keV) = 0.15$ with a cut-off at 140 keV (this value is worse than the best one quoted by Jeavons ($\pm$ 20%) and Perez-Mendez (22.5%)). The non-paralyzable dead-time is 1 μs; the coincidence window is $2\tau = 40$ ns.

The ring camera consists of a single cylindrical ring of radius 26 cm and height 2.8 cm; no septa are simulated (i.e. the whole crystal ring surface is sensitive). The shielding is also cylindrical, and leaves a patient port radius of 16 cm. The lead shield's width is 2.1 cm on each side. the intrinsic crystal efficiency is fitted by :

$$\varepsilon(E) = 1 - 0.23 \cdot \log (E/140)$$

with a cut-off at 300 keV so that $\varepsilon(511) = 0.70$. The non-paralyzable dead-time is 1 μs, the coincidence window is $2\tau = 10$ ns.

4.2. Description of the method

The phantom is a water cylinder with radius 10.75 cm and a variable height (the standard value will be 12 cm). The source within the cylinder is uniform, but with a radius of 10 cm. The cylinder is centred with respect to the camera and has its axis along the camera z axis.
We generate 10^6 positrons for the ring camera, 5.10^5 for the MWPC camera (since the geometrical efficiency of the MWPC is larger) and the annihilation photons are tracked up to the detector. The following quantities are evaluated.

-C_0 : unscattered coincidence sensitivity
-C_s : scattered coincidence sensitivity
-S : single sensitivity
-f_R^{total}: fraction of the single pairs (used to simulated randoms) which must be registered
-f_R : fraction of the single pairs whose coincidence line crosses the phantom, i.e. the fraction used for reconstruction
-f_s : fraction of the scattered coincidences whose coincidence line crosses the phantom, i.e. the fraction used for reconstruction.
-q : the probability that a positron triggers no detector (i.e. it yields neither a single, nor a coincidence)

Sensitivities in cps/μCurie cm^{-3} are obtained by multiplying the output of the simulation (event per generated e$^+$) by: 37000 x source volume in cm^3. The quoted scattered sensitivity accounts for photon pairs detected in opposite modules (for the MWPC); in the case of the ring camera we suppose that coincidence channels are established only when their line crosses the phantom (this means that $f_s = 1$ for the ring). Denoting by "a" the source activity in μCurie cm^{-3}, we evaluate the paralyzable dead-time attenuation factor :

$$\exp (-(1-q) \, 2 \, \tau \, a \, V)$$

where V is the source volume. The true, scattered and random coincidence rates reduce to:

$$C_0 \, a \, e^{-(1-q)2 \, \tau \, a \, V} = \lambda_0$$

$$C_s \, a \, e^{-(1-q)2 \, \tau \, a \, V} = \lambda_s^{total}$$

$$(S \, a)^2 \cdot 2 \cdot \tau \cdot f_R^{total} \cdot e^{-(1-q)2 \, \tau \, a \, V} = \lambda_R^{total}$$

The total rate is :

$$\lambda^{total} = \lambda_0 + \lambda_s^{total} + \lambda_R^{total}$$

Due to the non-paralyzable dead-time t_D, the real registered rate will be further reduced by a factor

$$1/(1 + \lambda^{\text{total}} \cdot t_D)$$

Furthermore, the scattered rate is reduced by a factor f_s, the random rate by a factor f_R/f_R^{total} by the software cuts (i.e. the requirement that the coincidence lines must cross the phantom). Taking all factors into account, the count rates finally become :

$$\lambda_0 = C_0 \, a \, e^{-(1-q) \, 2 \, \tau \, a \, V} / (1 + \lambda^{\text{total}} \cdot t_D)$$

$$\lambda_S = C_s \, a \, f_s \, e^{-(1-q) \, 2 \, \tau \, a \, V} / (1 + \lambda^{\text{total}} \cdot t_D)$$

$$\lambda_R = (S \cdot a)^2 \, 2 \, \tau \, f_R \, e^{-(1-q) \, 2 \, \tau \, a \, V} / (1 + \lambda^{\text{total}} \cdot t_D)$$

From these figures we calculate the effective count rate, given in Chapter 3.

4.3. Results

4.3.1. The standard phantom

For a phantom 12 cm high, the Monte-Carlo simulation yieldsthe following results :

	MWPC	RING	
C_0	309	79	kcps/μCi cm^{-3}
C_s	218 #	33	kcps/μCi cm^{-3}
S	18200	4500	kcps/μCi cm^{-3}
f_R	0.14	0.27	
f_R^{total}	0.25	0.27	
f_s	0.68	1.0	
q	0.86	0.97	

The ratio of the unscattered coincidences sensitivity, $309/79 = 3.9$ is to be compared to the ratio which would be obtained using a rough analytical expression: ratio of solid angle x (ratio of efficiencies)^2 x (ratio of Fields Of Views). The solid angles seen from the centre are respectively $0.63 \times 4\pi$ and $0.054 \times 4\pi$ for the MWPC camera and the ring camera. The effective cylinder height in the FOV is 12 cm for the MWPC, it is 2.8 cm for the ring. One then obtains a ratio of 2.3 instead of 3.9. The difference is due to the fact that the solid angle seen fom the boundaries of the 2.8 cm slice, in the ring camera, is not 0.054 but zero!
Notice also that the scattered fraction $C_s \times f_s / C_0$ has about the same value in both cases : 0.48 for the MWPC camera; 0.42 for the ring.
As for f_R^{total}, it has the value $0.25 = 1$ module/4 modules for the MWPC camera, and $0.27 = 4$ x arctan (phantom radius/ring radius)/4π for the ring.
Now we are ready to evaluate the effective count rate Q as defined in the previous section . The result is shown in the figure, as a function of the activity a.

If the intrinsic efficiency of the MWPC were constant with the energy (i.e. 15%), the scattered and single sensitivity would be respectively 272 and 21000 kcps/μCi cm-3.

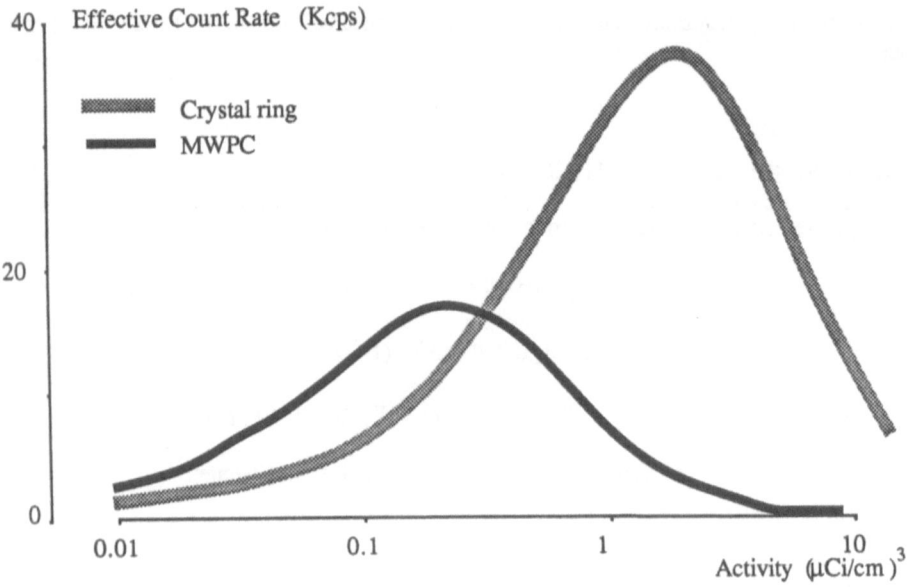

A few remarks :

1) For low activities (in this case, smaller than 0.3 $\mu Ci/cm^3$, which corresponds to a total dose of 1.1 μCi), the MWPC camera has a higher yield: the degradation due to accidental coincidences is still moderate at such activity levels and the dominating factor is the true unscattered coincidence sensitivity, which is higher for the MWPC camera.

2) The saturation of the effective count rate at higher activities is due to three factors :

- the increased rate of accidentals

- the non-paralyzable dead-time of 1 μsec

- essentially : the paralyzable dead-time 2τ, which eventually causes the count rates to vanish . As expected, the saturation occurs much earlier in the case of a MWPC camera. The maximum effective count rate is :

	Q_{max}	dose	total registered rate
MWPC	16.7 kcps	± 1 mCi	224 kcps
ring	36.8 kcps	± 7.4 mCi	282 kcps

The total registered rate are somewhat high. If we restrict ourselves to a total registered rate of about 50 kHz we obtain :

	Q	dose	total rate registered
MWPC	10.8 kcps	± 0.29 mCi	52.8 kcps
ring	16.9 kcps	± 1.45 mCi	47.9 kcps

3. We have seen that the use of the effective count rate is somewhat questionable in that it assumes a uniform distribution of random and scattered coincidences. It is therefore important

to know, for a given Q, the signal-to-noise ratio, i.e. the ratio of true coincidences to the total coincidences used in the reconstruction. This ratio has the value 0.52 for the MWPC, 0.59 for the ring camera, in the case of a total rate of 50 kHz (see the last table hereabove).

4. The effective count rate gives the total rate for equivalent random- and scattered-less coincidences, in other words it is the "information" rate. In the case of the ring camera, it is important to keep in mind the fact that this information is relative to the central slice of 2.8 cm only. In the case of the MWPC camera, the effective rate relative to this slice is about one fourth (2.8/12) of the quoted value.

5. Although the count rates degradation due to dead times is not very important for realistic total count rates (say < 100 kHz), it is nevertheless quite sizeable and must be incorporated in a correct simulation :

	$e^{-(1-q) 2 \tau a V}$	$(1 + \lambda_{total} \cdot t_D)^{-1}$	product
MWPC (52.8 kHz)	0.94	0.94	0.88
RING (47.9 kHz)	0.98	0.95	0.93

4.3.2. Influence of the phantom's volume

To what extent do the previous results depend on the size of the radionuclide source ? Let us consider for the phantom and source a cylinder of height 24 cm instead of 12 cm.
In the case of the ring camera, this does not significantly modify the sensitivities quoted above, since the added volume lies outside the ring's field of view, even for (unscattered) single events. Only the scattered and single sensitivities are expected to slightly increase; the change, however, was smaller than the accuracy of the Monte-Carlo simulation.
On the other hand, one would expect the MWPC camera to profit of the increased source's volume. As shown by the table below, however, the increased true coincidence sensitivity is more than compensated by the increase of the single sensitivity. The effective count rate is shown in the following figure :

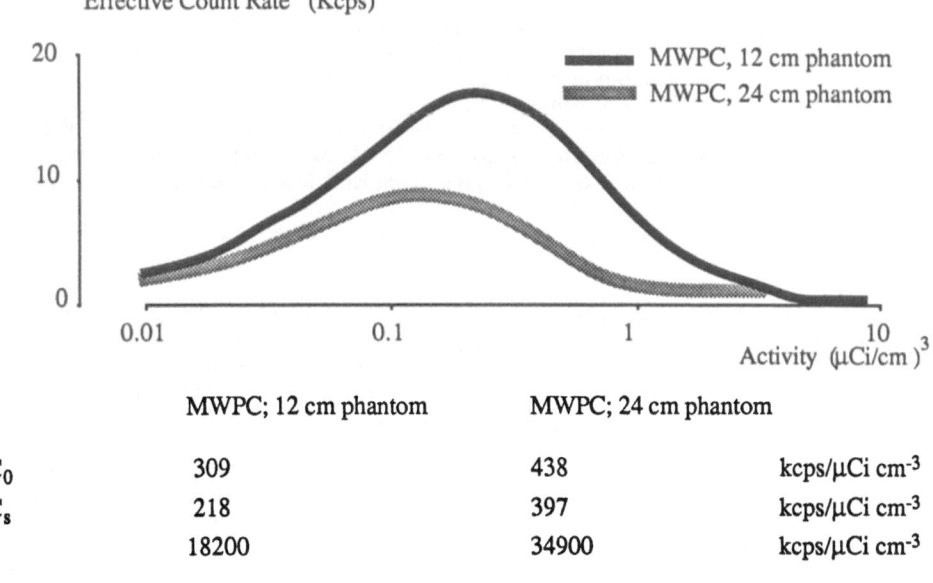

	MWPC; 12 cm phantom	MWPC; 24 cm phantom	
C_0	309	438	kcps/µCi cm^{-3}
C_s	218	397	kcps/µCi cm^{-3}
S	18200	34900	kcps/µCi cm^{-3}

f_R	0.14	0.19
$f_R{}^{total}$	0.25	0.25
f_s	0.68	0.81
q	0.86	0.87

The maximum effective rate is Q_{max} = 8.4 kcps for a total dose of 0.9 mCi; and a total rate of 176 kcps. For a total rate of 54 kcps we get Q = 6.9 kcps. The performance of the MWPC camera is thus clearly degraded when the source's volume is increased too much.

Reducing the height of the source to 2.8 cm, on the other hand, slightly improves the performance of the MWPC camera, at least if we assume that the source is known to be confined to this central slice; in this case, indeed, a larger fraction of the random and scattered coincidences may be rejected by software cuts.

As for the ring camera, although the true coincidence sensitivity does not change with respect to the 12 cm high source, the scattered and single sensitivities are significantly reduced, and the effective count rate is much larger than that with the 12 cm high source :

Source 2.8 cm ; Phantom 12 cm

	MWPC	RING	
C_0	59	79	kcps/μCi cm^{-3}
C_s	53	19	kcps/μCi cm^{-3}
S	4180	1650	kcps/μCi cm^{-3}
f_R	0.074	0.27	
$f_R{}^{total}$	0.25	0.27	
f_s	0.45	1	
q	0.87	0.95	

The maximum effective count rates are respectively 18 kcps (for a dose of 1.14 mCi and a total rate of 261 kcps) and 135 kcps (for a dose of 5.8 mCi and a total rate of 464 kcps). In the more realistic case of a total rate of about 50 kcps, one gets for the MWPC: Q = 10 kcps, for the ring: Q = 30 kcps.

Notice that the phantom and source set-up considered here is ideal for the ring camera, the source being confined to the central slice, namely to the field of view of that camera. It should also be stressed that the phantom used here still has a height of 12 cm, which attenuates the coincidences in the case of MWPC camera strongly.

If the attenuating medium (i.e. the phantom) is also reduced to a height of 2.8 cm, the true sensitivity for the MWPC leaps from 59 kcps up to 154 kcps! The effective count rate at 50 kHz is then 25 kcps. This case, of course, is quite unrealistic, but is given as an illustration of the importance of attenuation!

4.4. Conclusions

It is always dangerous to draw general conclusions from a study involving two particular positron camera designs. The choice of any parameter in the comparison (phantom size, detector set up, efficiency curves used...) can be questioned. For instance, supporters of the ring cameras could rightly criticize the choice of a single-slice ring. Advocates of MWPC cameras, on the other hand, would probably consider an efficiency of 15% for 511 keV photons as too conservative.

It is also clear, from the previous study, (cf. fig. in section 4.3.1.), that the conclusions of a comparison can be completely modified, simply by choosing a different value for the source activity. Despite these remarks, we think that a few qualitative and general conclusions can be drawn from our study.

1. The maximum effective count rate generally appears to be better for the ring camera, than for the MWPC camera. This difference should be even more pronounced if a multi-slice ring were to be considered.
However, the difference between the performance of these two types of cameras is much smaller than what would be expected from many statements in the literature, and also from previously published comparisons (e.g. 27). The efficiency of the MWPC camera thus appears sufficient to allow the high spatial resolution to be used effectively .

2. In terms of count rate the MWPC camera may prove more efficient than the ring camera if one is forced, for some technical or medical reason, to work at low activity levels.

3. The use of the MWPC camera is optimal for the imaging of medium size sources: if a thin slice only must be imaged, one should clearly advocates the use of a ring camera. On the other hand, the imaging of large source's volumes with a MWPC is made quite difficult by the saturation problem (cf. the worse performance with the 24 cm source than with the 12 cm source).

5. References

1-Lupton L.R. and Keller N.A. : A general purpose Monte-Carlo simulation for the design of single-slice PET ring cameras. Chalk River Nuclear Laboratories, Report AECL-7680 (1982)

2-Perez-Mendez V. et al. : The imaging performance of a MWPC positron camera. Proc. 1st International Symposium ISMIII 99-106 (1982)

3-Rose A. : Vision,Human and Electronic. Plenum Press 1974

4-Shosa D. and Kaufman L. : Methods for evaluation of diagnostic imaging instrumentation. Phys. Med. Biol. 26, 101-12 (1981)

5-Beck R.N. et al. : The theoretical advantages of eliminating scatter in imaging systems. In: Semiconductor Detectors in the future of Nuclear Medicine. P.B.Hoffer et al.editors, Society of Nuclear Medicine Inc. 1971

6-Phelps M.E. et al. : Design consideration in Positron Emission Tomography. IEEE Trans. Nucl. Sc. 26, 2746-51 (1979)

7-Tanaka E. et al. : Analytical study of the performance of a multilayer PCT scanner. Jour. Comp. Ass. Tomo. 6, 350-64 (1982)

8-Perez-Mendez V. et al. : Further improvements in the design of a positron camera with dense drift space MWPC's. Nucl. Instr. Meth. 217, 89-91 (1983)

9-Smith W.E., Barrett H.H., Paxman R.G.: Reconstruction of objects from coded images by simulated annealing. Optics Letters 8, p. 199 (1983)

10-Floyd C. et al. : Inverse Monte Carlo : a unified reconstruction algorithm for SPECT. IEEE Trans. Nucl. Sc. 32, 779-85 (1985)

11-Del Guerra A. et al. : Design consideration for a high spatial resolution PET with MWPC. IEEE Trans. Nucl. Sc. 30, 646 (1983)

12-Logan J. and Bernstein H.J. : A Monte-Carlo simulation of Compton Scattering in PET. Journ. Comp. Ass. Tomo. 7, 316-20 (1983)

13-Townsend D.W. and Jeavons A.P. : private communication 1984

14-Chan and Doi : The validity of Monte-Carlo simulation in studies of scattered radiation in diagnostic radiology. Phys. Med. Biol. 28, 109-29 (1983)

15-Guang Y.X. and Rogers J.G. : A Monte-Carlo calculation of detector design for PET. Nucl.Instr. Meth. A234, 382-87 (1985)

16-Bradshaw J. et al. : Application of Monte-Carlo methods to the design of SPECT detector systems. IEEE Trans. Nucl. Sc. 32, 753-7 (1985)

17-Lupton L.R. and Keller N.A. : Performance study of a single slice PET using Monte-Carlo techniques. IEEE Trans. Med. Imag. 2, 154-68 (1983)

18-Derenzo S.E. : Precision measurement of annihilation point spread function for medically important positron emitters. Proc. 5th Int. Conf. on positron annihilation, Lake Yamanaka, Japan April 1979 p. 819-823

19-Perez-Mendez V. et al. : The HISPET design. Submitted to Computerized Radiology (1984)

20-Jeavons A. et al. : The High Density Avalanche Chamber for PET. IEEE Trans. Nucl. Sc. 30, p. 640 (1983)

21-Webb S. et al. : Tumour localization in oncology using positron emitter radiopharmaceuticals and a MWPC positron camera. Nucl. Instr. Meth. 221, 233-41 (1984)

22-Hammersley J.M. and Handscomb D.C. : Monte-Carlo methods. Methuen, London 1964

23-Flugge S. : Handbook der Physik, vol. XLV Nuclear Instrumentation II. Springer-Verlag 1958

24-Sorenson J.A. and Phelps M.E. : Physics in Nuclear Medicine. Grune and Stratton,Inc, New York 1980

25-Holmes T.J. : Predicting count loss in modern PET systems . IEEE Trans. Nucl. Sc. 30, 723-28 (1983)

26-King S.E. and Lim C.B. : Pulse-pile up,dead time, derandomization and count rate in scintillation gamma cameras. IEEE Trans. Nucl. Sc. 32, 807-10

27-Derenzo S. : Methods for optimizing side shielding in positron-emission tomographs and for comparing detector materials. J. Nucl. Med. 21, 971-7 (1980)

28-Lim C.H. et al. : Image noise, resolution and lesion detectability in SPECT. IEEE Trans. Nucl. Sc. 29, 500-5 (1982)

29-Budinger T.F., Derenzo S.E., Gullberg G.T., Greenberg W.L., Huesman R.H. : J. Comp. Assist. Tomogr. 1, 131 (1977)

30-Natterer F. : Numer. Math., 30, p 81-91 (1978)

31-Defrise M. and De Mol C. : Resolution limits for full- and limited-angle tomography. Proc. 8th IPMI conference, Brussels 1983, F. Deconinck ed., Martinus Nijhoff 1984, 94-105.

32-Colsher J.G. : Fully three-dimensional positron emission tomography. Phys. Med. Biol. 25, 103-115 (1980)

33-Bertero M. et al. : in Inverse scattering problems in optics (H.P.Baltes ed.), Topics in Current Physics, vol 20, Springer Verlag 1980, 161-214

A TECHNIQUE FOR SCATTERED EVENT COMPENSATION IN A PET SYSTEM USING TOF INFORMATION

B. BENDRIEM, F. SOUSSALINE, R. CAMPAGNOLO*, B. VERREY, P. WAJNBERG, A. SYROTA. Service Hospitalier Frédéric Joliot, Orsay, France. *LETI, Grenoble, France.

1. INTRODUCTION

Positron Emission Tomography (PET) is a unique tool for the study of metabolism and biochemical mechanisms in human being. However clinical applications require that PET systems combine high resolution and low statistical fluctuations in order to provide an accurate quantitation of the radionuclide distribution in selected organs of the human body. Recently the Time of Flight (TOF) information has been shown to improve image quality (1,2,3,4) and is now used in different PET systems. Nevertheless the objectives of PET will only be reached when all physical aspects of positron emission and annihilation radiation detection are correctly taken into account.

Radiation scattering is one of these effects. Although it is a well-described physical phenomenon, its influence on tomographic images is complex (5) and depends on many parameters (mostly tomograph geometry, shielding, energy discriminator level, scattering medium and radioactivity distribution). Few correcting methods can be found in other literature (6,7,8). In this chapter, we propose a deconvolution technique for scattered radiation compensation in a PET system using TOF information. The study was carried out on such a system called "TTV01", built by the French group from the Laboratoire d'Electronique et de Technologie de l'Informatique (LETI, CEA Grenoble) and installed at the Service Hospitalier Frédéric Joliot (SHFJ, CEA Orsay) where it is used for clinical studies and physical measurements. Its temporal resolution is 500 ps (FWMH) and its transverse resolution is 12 mm (FWMH) for the medium resolution mode which was used in this study (9).

2. THE USE OF TOF IN PET

The time of flight information is the measure of the pathlength difference of the two annihilation photons reaching two coincident detectors. It allows the localization of the positron emission site on the line connecting the two detectors. Indeed, if the intrinsic resolution of the detector is neglected, the distribution of events generated by a point source is described by a 1-D gaussian centered on the source position with a standard deviation depending on the temporal resolution of the detection system. The combination of TOF information with conventional techniques of tomographic image reconstruction has been studied by the LETI (10) and other groups. Let's recall briefly the different steps of the image reconstruction.

The histogram of TOF measurements along a given path is called a "histopath". The set of all those corresponding to parallel paths is called a "histoprojection". A histoprojection is thus a 2-D matrix denoted $h(u,v)$ where u is the sampled position defined by the TOF measurement (TOF sampling interval 12 mm) and v is the sampled position on the perpendicular direction (linear sampling interval 4 mm). Figure 1 illustrates the localization in a histoprojection of a true coincidence and of a coincidence involving single radiation scattering.

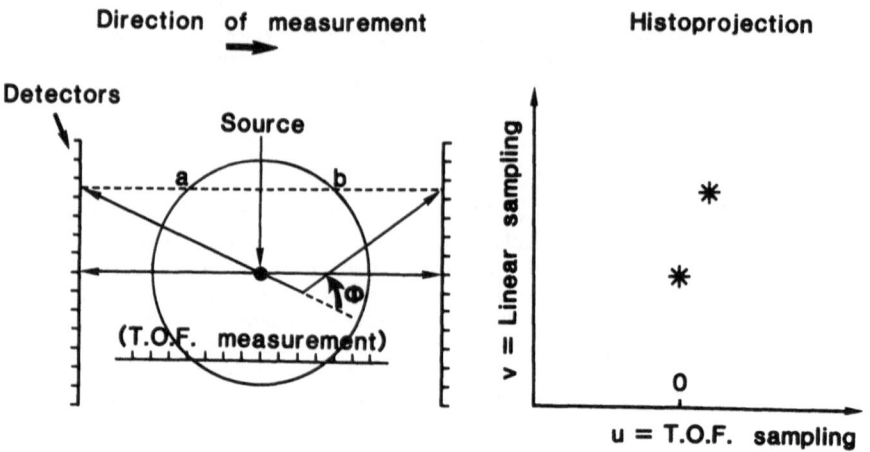

Fig. 1 : Localization in a histoprojection of a true
coincidence and of one involving single scattering.

The list mode data acquisition is used in TTVO1 and allows a great flexibility for a posteriori data processing. Once set up, the histoprojections are corrected for detector variations in sensitivity, for radiation auto-attenuation and for random coincidence registration. All correcting coefficients are obtained from measurements and stored in different tables. The corrected histoprojections are then convolved with an uncertainty function, then fitted to the final grid by 2-D interpolation and summed up to provide a "pre-image". This procedure, called confidence weighing, is equivalent to a non uniform backprojection of events in a limited area of the field of view, whose dimensions depend on the TOF measurement resolution. The optimal uncertainty function (which provides the best S/N ratio for the images) is equal to the TOF distribution function defined by :

$$ f(u,v) = \frac{1}{\sigma \sqrt{2\pi}} \exp\left(-\frac{u^2}{2\sigma^2}\right) \times \delta(v) $$

where σ is the standard deviation of the TOF measurement dispersion.
The TOF response of the system is then $f**f$ and the point spread function of the back-projected preimage is :

$$ p(r) = \frac{1}{\pi} \int_0^\pi f**f \ (r\cos\theta , r\sin\theta) \ d\theta = \frac{1}{\sigma' \sqrt{2\pi}} \ \frac{1}{r} \times \exp\left(-\frac{r^2}{2\sigma'^2}\right) $$

where r is the radial distance from the point source and σ' is equal to $\sigma\sqrt{2}$.

The modulation transfer function is :

$$P(\omega) = 2\text{-}F\ \{p\}\ (\omega) = \frac{I_0(\pi^2\sigma'^2\omega^2)}{\exp(\pi^2\sigma'^2\omega^2)}$$

where 2-F is the 2-D Fourier transform operator and I_0 is the zero-order modified Bessel function.
The 2-D filter used to restitute the final image is :

$$H\ (\omega) = \frac{1}{P(\omega)}$$

3. THE TECHNIQUE FOR SCATTERED RADIATION COMPENSATION

We defined a new response of the system including a component due to scattered radiations.

$$t\ (u,v) = (1\text{-}k).\ f^{**}f\ (u,v)\ + k.s\ (u,v)$$

where s is the scattered radiation component signal and k is the scattered to total event ratio. S was formulated from experimental measurements of a NA-22 linear source (2 mm in diameter) in a scattering medium (water-filled cylinder of 20 or 30 cm in diameter). Figure 2 shows the averaged histoprojection in all measurement direction of the events generated by the source centered in the homogeneous scattering medium. It turned out that the dispersion introduced in TOF measurements by Compton scattering is negligible compared with that of the detection system. If we assume that the contribution from scattered radiation is mainly due to measured coincidences in which only one of the two photons is scattered and only once (5), it implies that the probability for a photon to interact and to reach an adequate detector is higher near its emission site. This statement was verified by a numerical simulation similar to that described in ref 5. S was then chosen to be :

$$s\ (u,v) = \frac{1}{\sigma'\sqrt{2\pi}}\ \exp\ (-\ \frac{u^2}{2\sigma'^2})\ x\ \frac{\alpha}{2}\ \exp\ (-\ \alpha|v|)$$

α and k depend on the tomograph geometry, the nature of the scattering medium and on the position of the source in this medium. Mean values can be evaluated for measurements on a phantom simulating brain or cardiac situation.

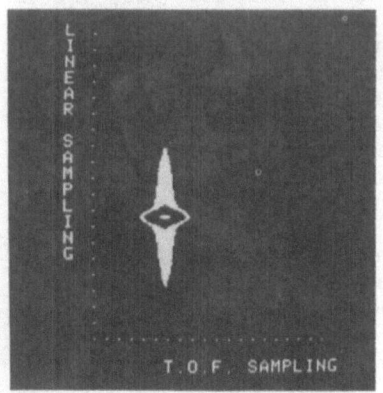

Fig. 2 : 2-D histogram of events generated by a point source in a scattering medium.

The new MTF function is derived :

$$P'(\omega) = (1-k) \; P \; (\omega) + \frac{k}{\pi} \int_o^\pi 2\text{-F} \; \{s\} \; (\omega \; \cos\theta \; , \; \omega \; \sin\theta \;) \; d\theta$$

and is represented in fig. 3 for $k = 0.2$ and $\alpha = 0.3 \; cm^{-1}$.

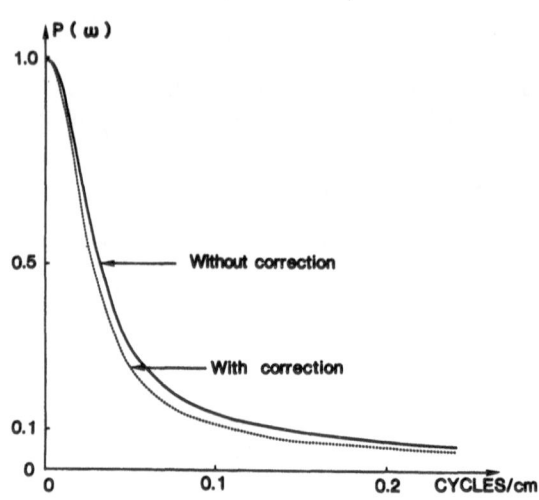

Fig. 3 : Modulation transfer functions.

4. RESULTS AND DISCUSSION

The method was tested on three GA-68 filled cylindrical phantoms (20 25 and 30 cm in diameter). The first one contained one concentric lucite insert (3 cm in diameter) and five smaller others placed 6 cm away from center. The second one contained three cold cylinders (4,5 and 7 cm in diameter) placed 6 cm off center and the third one a lucite cylinder (6 cm in diameter) placed in its center. The contrast was defined as the ratio of the measured activity in small Region of Interest (ROI) inside the cold spots (less than 40% of the insert diameter) over the measured background activity. It improved by more than 10% in corrected images (table 1) for cold spots with a diameter larger than twice the spatial resolution. Under this value the partial volume effect is predominant. The method was also tested on the recovery coefficients (measured activity over true activity) obtained with three cylinders (2,4 and 6 cm in diameter) located in an elliptical water-filled phantom (17 cm-long axis and 12 cm-short axis). The improvement in accuracy is shown in table 2. In all experiments adapted values of the different parameters were chosen. It was verified that the improvement obtained is not dependent on the activity concentration used. No significant deterioration of the S/N ratio was observed. The apparent activity outside the phantom can be almost totally removed. However we measured a 3% increase in the concentration at the periphery of a uniformly active cylinder of 20 cm diameter resulting from the choice of constant values for k and α (indeed the values decrease when the source is located at the edge of the phantom).

The method does not completely eliminate the distorsion due to scattered radiations but reduces it significantly. Its main advantage is that it does not require any additional computing time and can be integrated in the standard reconstruction procedure (18 sec for an image reconstructed from 500,000 events). The value of k and α must be previously evaluated, the filter can then be derived and stored in a table. The method is then flexible and parameters adapted to the tomograph and to the type of clinical study can be used. The use of an analytical or numerical function which approaches more the scattered radiation distribution is presently being studied.

TABLE 1 - CONTRAST IMPROVEMENT

Cold spot size (mm)		COMPENSATION	
		Without	With
in a Ø 20 cm cylinder	30	22%	8%
in a Ø 25 cm cylinder	40	22%	8%
	50	17%	4%
	70	12%	1%
in a Ø 30 cm cylinder	60	25%	10%

TABLE 2 - "HOT SPOT" MEASUREMENT

Hot spot size (mm)	Recovery coefficient	
	without compensation	with compensation
60	0.84	0.94
40	0.79	0.91
20	0.43	0.50

REFERENCES

1. Snyder DL, Thomas LJ and Ter-Pogossian MM : A mathematical model for positron-emission tomography systems having time-of-flight measurements. IEEE Trans. Nucl. Sci. NS-28 : 3575-3583, 1981.
2. Tomitani T : Image reconstruction and noise evaluation in photon time-of-flight assisted positron emission tomography. IEEE Trans. Nucl. Sci. NS-28 : 4582-4589, 1981.
3. Gariod R, Allemand R, Cormoreche E, Laval M and Moszynski M : The "LETI" positron tomograph architecture and time of flight improvements. In Proc. Workshop on time-of-flight tomography : 25-30, St Louis MO, May 1982.
4. Wong WH, Mullani NA, Philippe EA, Hartz R and Gould KL : Image improvement and design optimization of the time-of-flight PET. J. Nucl. Med. 24 : 52-60,1983.
5. Tanaka E, Nohara N, Tomitani T and Endo M : Analytical study of the performance of a multilayer positron computed tomography scanner. J. Comput. Assist. Tomogr. 6 : 350-364, 1982.
6. King PH : Noise identification and removal in positron imaging systems. IEEE Trans. Nucl. Sci. NS-28 : 148-150, 1981.
7. Bergstrom M, Eriksson L, Bohm C, Blomqvist G and Litton J : Correction for scattered radiation in a ring detector positron camera by integral transformation of the projections. J. Comp. Assist. Tomog. 7 : 42-50, 1983.
8. Endo M and Tinuma TA : Software correction of scatter coincidence in positron CT. Eur. J. Nucl. Med. 9 : 391-396, 1984.
9. Soussaline F, Comar D, Allemand R, Campagnolo R, Laval M and Vacher J : New developments in positron emission tomography instrumentation using the time-of-flight information. In the metabolism of the human brain studied with positron emission tomography edited by T. Greitz et al. Raven press, New York, 1985.
10. Garderet P and Campagnolo R : Image reconstruction using time-of-flight information in the LETI positron tomograph. In Proc. Workshop on time-of-flight tomography : 97-100, St Louis MO, May 1982.

ANALYSIS AND DISPLAY OF MEDICAL IMAGES OBTAINED WITH THE HIDAC POSITRON CAMERA

D. TOWNSEND , P. FREY , A. JEAVONS [*] , A. DONATH
A. CHRISTIN , M. WENSVEEN , H. J. TOCHON-DANGUY

Division of Nuclear Medicine , University Hospital , Geneva
* E.P. Division , CERN , Geneva , Switzerland

1. INTRODUCTION

The role of positron emission tomography (PET) in medical research, particularly in neurology [1] and cardiology [2], is now well-established, whereas its application in routine clinical diagnosis is less obvious. In recent years, major technological achievements include the availability of both low-priced, compact medical cyclotrons and ring-type positron cameras with greatly improved performance. Significant progress in radiopharmaceutical labelling and tracer-kinetic modelling has greatly extended the range of potential applications and the contribution of PET to basic clinical sciences such as neurophysiology.

The main developments in positron camera design have been the improvements in spatial resolution and sensitivity [3,4], and the imaging of multiple sections simultaneously. Better image quality and shorter imaging times have contributed to the advance of PET from a simple imaging modality to a unique tool for the *in vivo* study of human physiology both in health and disease. Multi-ring positron cameras based on bismuth germanate or barium fluoride crystals have played a dominant role in this progress.

Alternative technology, such as the high density proportional chamber (HDPC), although offering full three-dimensional imaging at high spatial resolution, currently has only moderate sensitivity for detection of 511 keV photons. As a consequence, the data acquisition times tend to be rather long, with low signal to noise in the image due to the presence of a significant fraction of accidental and scattered coincidences. Despite these drawbacks, however, some HDPC designs, and in particular the high density avalanche chamber (HIDAC) detector, are successful in certain clinical applications. Indeed, in cases such as the imaging of small, internal organs and complex structures with low radioisotope uptake, a HIDAC camera may be more suitable, and certainly less expensive, than a multi-ring crystal-based system. Thus, organs such as the thyroid and kidneys, brain structures such as the basal ganglia, and small tumours are particularly favourable imaging situations for the HIDAC camera. To take maximum advantage of the high spatial resolution, however, an uptake of at least 5 to 10 kBq/cm^3 is required, remaining static within the camera field of view for about ten minutes. Such conditions are not usually met by organs involving significant movement such as the heart and the lungs and by metabolic processes involving rapid radioisotope turnover. To image with short-lived isotopes such as O^{15} (2 min half-life) and Rb^{82} (75 sec half-life), it will be necessary to maintain a steady state situation by a continuous supply of radioisotope.

High resolution, three-dimensional positron imaging with a HIDAC camera offers unique possibilities for the analysis and display of organ function. Corrected for scatter and accidental coincidences and combined with physiologic data, the images yield absolute radioisotope uptake, the dimensions and volumes of interesting structures, and a precise localisation with respect to external landmarks. Powerful shaded graphics techniques may be used for display to give a global view of the functional structure with potential applications in both diagnosis and therapy.

In August, 1984, a prototype HIDAC camera was installed in the University Hospital of Geneva to undergo clinical evaluation. The performance of the camera will be summarised and the problems of data analysis and display discussed. The absence of an on-site medical cyclotron limits clinical applications to those using long-lived or generator-produced positron-emitters; some examples will be presented.

2. THE HIDAC CAMERA

The camera installed in the division of nuclear medicine consists of two HIDAC detectors, each of useful area 31cm x 31cm, mounted on a gantry that rotates under computer control in a step-and-shoot mode; detector separation is 54 cm. The principles of the design and construction of the HIDAC detector have been described elsewhere [5,6]. The current detectors are shown in Fig. 1, mounted on the gantry with the patient bed and head support positioned for a typical scan. The performance parameters are summarised in Fig. 2a, and the computer configuration shown schematically in Fig. 2b. ; details may be found elsewhere [7]. Data is collected in list

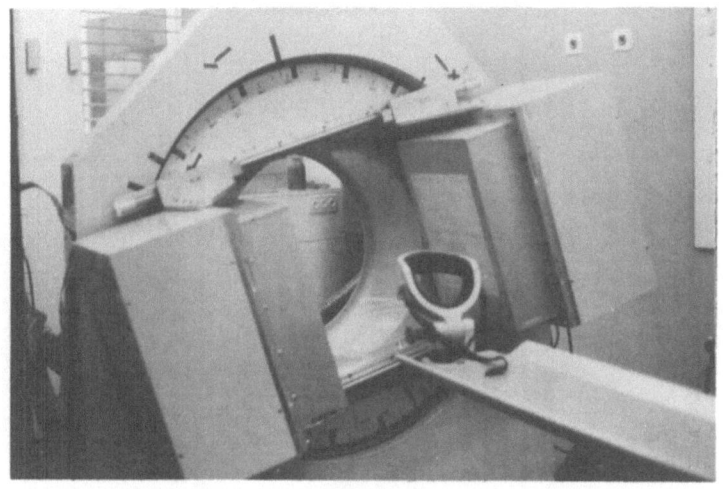

FIGURE 1. The HIDAC Camera

Number of detectors	2
Convertors per detector	4
Useful area	31 cm * 31 cm
Gas mixture	Ne-CO$_2$ (atmospheric)
Patient aperture	54 cm
Spatial resolution	2.5 mm (intrinsic)
	<4 mm (reconstructed)
Time resolution	20 nsecs
Singles Efficiency	12% per detector
Coincidence (Camera)	1.5%
Number of sections	16 or 64
Section thickness	>2 mm
Sensitivity (20 cm phantom)	2.8 * 10^4 cps/μCi/cc
Accidentals	~20% at 2 kHz
Scatter (thyroid)	~25%

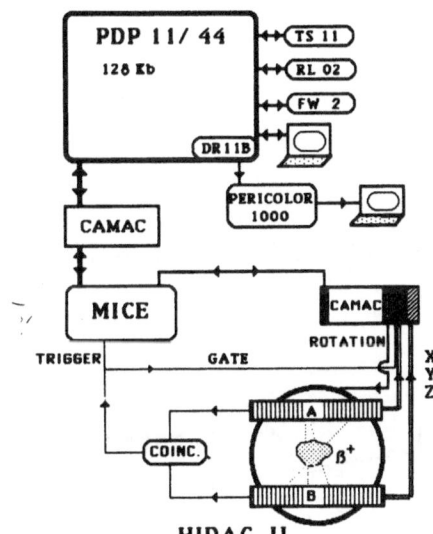

FIGURE 2. (a) HIDAC Specification (b) Computer Configuration

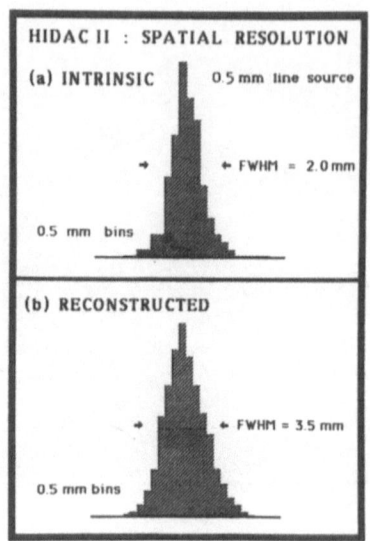

FIGURE 3. Spatial Resolution (a) Intrinsic (b) Reconstructed

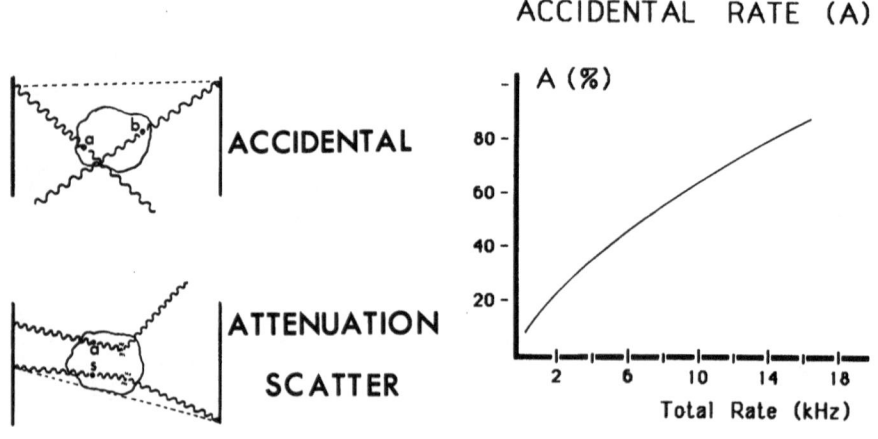

FIGURE 4. Background Events   FIGURE 5. Accidental Rate

mode and transferred to the PDP11/44 for storage on disc; maximum on-line storage capacity is sufficient for 3.5 million events. A significant advantage of the HIDAC camera is the reliable operation that has been a feature of both the current 31 cm x 31 cm detectors and the previous 20 cm x 20 cm prototype [6]. The latter required only minimal maintenance during the two years it underwent clinical evaluation in Geneva University Hospital.

2.1. Spatial resolution

The *intrinsic* spatial resolution, estimated from a profile through a 0.5 mm diameter line source of Ga^{68} in air is shown in Fig. 3a to have a full width at half maximum (FWHM) of 2 mm and a full width at tenth maximum (FWTM) of 5 mm. A profile through a *reconstructed* line spread function, shown in Fig. 3b, has a FWHM of 3.5 mm, a value which depends not only on the intrinsic camera resolution but also on the smoothing window used in the reconstruction to offset the effect of statistical fluctuations. In Fig. 3b a Hanning window was applied with a cut-off at the Nyquist frequency. The FWHM of 3.5 mm at the centre of the field of view increases slightly towards the edge.

2.2. Sensitivity

The sensitivity of the camera was measured for a standard 20 cm diameter phantom, 20 cm long. For an activity of 3.7 kBq/cm^3 of Ga^{68}, the coincidence rate was 2850 cps, at a chamber separation of 46 cm. This type of phantom, although an accepted standard for measuring the performance of a ring camera, is not necessarily the most appropriate choice for a volume imaging device.

2.3. Accidental Coincidences

The main contributions to the background in PET images (Fig. 4) are accidental and scattered coincidences. The accidental rate can be estimated from:

$$A = S^2 . 2t$$

where S is the singles rate on one detector and t is the coincidence resolving time. HIDAC detectors have a resolving time of about 20 nsecs, compared with a ring camera resolving time of less than 5 nsec. The measured accidental rate for the HIDAC camera is shown in Fig. 5, as a function of the total coincidence rate. In contrast to crystal-based cameras, the data acquisition rate for clinical imaging with a HIDAC camera is limited by accidental coincidences rather than by the singles rate. The significance of high accidental rates will be discussed in section 3.3.

2.4. Scattered Radiation

To fully exploit the volume imaging capability of the HIDAC detector, the use of shielding within the field of view should be avoided and thus the detectors are exposed to all scattered radiation falling within their acceptance angle. As a consequence of the conversion process, the incident photon energy cannot be measured and pulse-height rejection of scattered radiation is therefore not possible. However, the intrinsic efficiency of the HIDAC detector decreases with decreasing photon energy. Measurements [6] indicate a sensitivity reduction relative to 511 keV of 50% at 350 keV and of 85% at 200 keV. Nevertheless, a detected scatter fraction of 30% to 40% is unavoidable in typical clinical imaging situations involving the head and neck, increasing to more than 50% for the abdomen.

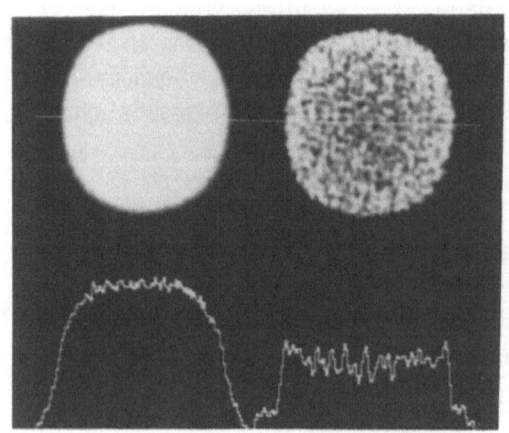

(a)   (b)

FIGURE 6. Uniform Cylinder
(a) unmodified back-projection   (b) filtered back-projection

2.5. Uniformity

Field of view uniformity was measured with a 20 cm diameter phantom filled with Ga^{68} and the image is shown in Fig. 6 for (a) the unfiltered back-projection and (b) the result after Fourier space filtering. A total of 500,000 counts were acquired corresponding to statistical fluctuations of about 13%. Although the filtering process increases the noise, Fig. 6b. indicates good uniformity throughout the field of view.

3.   IMAGE RECONSTRUCTION

Image reconstruction is based on three-dimensional back-projection and frequency-space filtering [8,9].   After reconstruction, a background level, estimated as explained below, is subtracted from the normalised, three-dimensional image to compensate for scatter and accidental coincidences.

3.1. Back-projection

During a full rotation of the camera, data is acquired at a number of discrete angular positions. At each position, a constraint [10] is applied to the data to ensure shift-invariance of the system point response function (p.r.f.) (Fig. 7). At least 50% of the data is discarded as a consequence of this constraint, the exact amount depending on the source distribution and the field of view required. Shift-invariance of the p.r.f. is necessary for the convolution formulation of the integral equation relating the back-projection to the source distribution. However, it is a condition that applies to the total back-projection (i.e. the sum of all angles), but need not be satisfied at each angular position separately.   The constraint in the xz-plane (Fig. 7) may be removed and back-projection weights used to compensate for the resulting variations in channel sensitivities.   The weight for a particular coincidence channel depends upon the perpendicular distance of the channel from the centre of rotation and is inversely proportional to the fraction of the total imaging time that that channel is *seen* by the detectors during rotation. The back-projection weights for detectors of side 20 cm as a function of the distance (r) from the centre of rotation are shown in Fig. 8 (solid curve, $\mu=0$) for an 18 cm diameter field of view.

The correction for attenuation may also be made by weighting the back-projection. For distributions of circular or elliptic cross-section, such as the head or neck, these weights act in opposition to the sensitivity equalizing weights discussed above, being greater for channels closer to the centre of rotation where the attenuation is more significant. For the simple example of a cylinder of diameter 15 cm, back-projection weights that correct both for attenuation and sensitivity have a dynamic range of only two (Fig. 8, dotted curve, $\mu=0.1$). This small dynamic range avoids the potential noise amplification inherent in such weighted back-projection

488

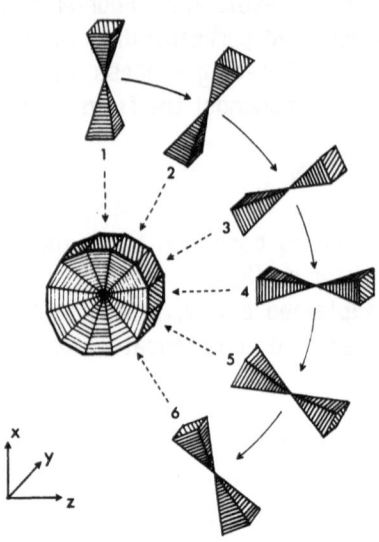

FIGURE 7. System Point Response Function

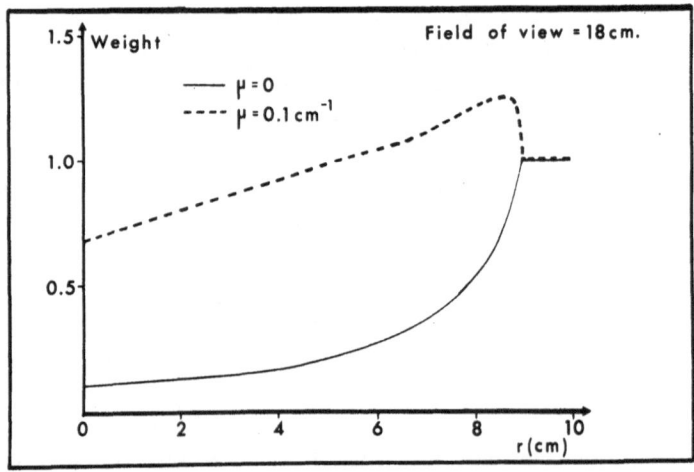

FIGURE 8. Back-Projection Weights with Attenuation Correction

approaches.

3.2. Frequency Filtering

For reasons of computational efficiency, the deconvolution of the system p.r.f. is implemented as a filtering operation in frequency space. The Fourier transform of the ideal p.r.f. may be reduced to [8]:

$$H(R,\beta,\emptyset) = D(\beta,\emptyset) / |R| \qquad (1)$$

where $R,\beta,\emptyset$ are polar coordinates in frequency space, and the angular function $D(\beta,\emptyset)$ is a one-dimensional integral over finite limits. The kernel of the integral includes a specification of the geometrical configuration of the camera i.e. it takes into account the support and functional behaviour of the ideal p.r.f.. The filter $H(R,\beta,\emptyset)$ has the form of a modified ramp function in three dimensions, the modification arising from the angular limitations of the camera ($<4\pi$ acceptance). As with other ramp filters, $H(R,\beta,\emptyset)$ cannot generally be used directly without amplifying excessively the noise in the high Fourier frequencies. Instead, it must be modified to:

$$H(R,\beta,\emptyset) = D(R,\beta) / |R| \cdot W(R,\beta,\emptyset) \qquad (2)$$

where $W(R,\beta,\emptyset)$ is a *window* function that supresses the noise dominated high frequencies. Usually, a simple Hanning window is adequate, with a cut-off at or below the Nyquist frequency. The lower the cut-off, the smoother and less noisy is the appearance of the reconstructed image. However, improvements in visual quality are often at the expense of quantitative accuracy. Excessive smoothing degrades the inherent spatial resolution, distorts local count density estimates and makes precise determination of regional boundaries more difficult.

These effects can be seen with the Hoffman brain phantom [11] imaged and reconstructed under different conditions. The phantom simulates the uptake of fluoro-deoxyglucose in a two-dimensional brain section at a level through the thalamus, putamen and the heads of the caudates. The four-to-one uptake ratio between grey and white matter is simulated in the phantom by a variable thickness of activity; only the lateral ventricles and the centrally-located third ventricle contain zero activity. The phantom was filled with 30 MBq of Ga^{68} and a total of four million counts acquired in about 30 minutes. The results are shown in Fig. 9 ; for comparison, a longitudinal back-projection with the phantom orientated parallel to the detectors is also shown (Fig. 9a), containing 1.5 million events. Transverse section reconstructions are shown in Fig. 9b to Fig. 9f; Figs. 9b, 9c and 9d contain four million counts, smoothed to spatial resolutions of 2.5 mm, 3 mm and 4 mm respectively, as defined by the maximum frequency cut-off. The actual resolution in the image will, of course, be worse than these values. Figs. 9e and 9f are each smoothed to an effective resolution of 4 mm, and contain 2 million and 1 million counts respectively. In all the images, however, about half the total counts are scattered and accidental

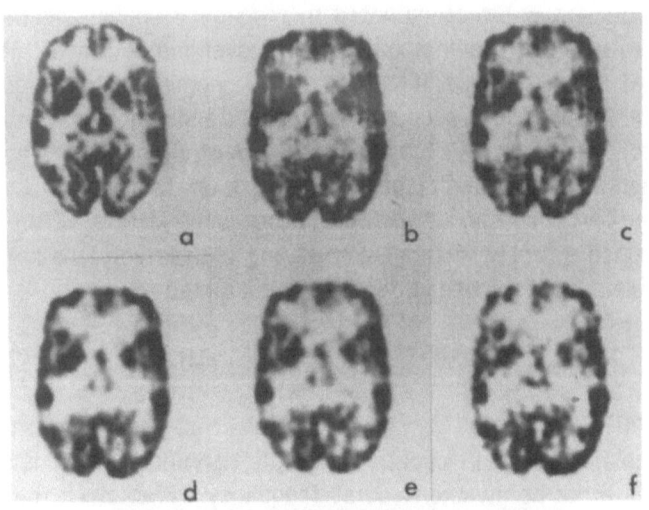

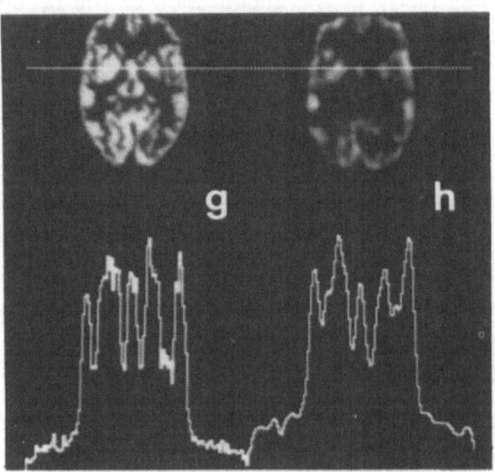

FIGURE 9. The Hoffman Brain Phantom

coincidences. The main cortical features and grey matter structures are clearly visible, although the poor contrast of the thalamus and caudates may be due to a suboptimal attenuation correction. For 4 million total counts (about 2 million true coincidences), statistical noise obscures detail for effective spatial resolutions of 2.5 mm and 3 mm. This is not unexpected as the measured resolution after reconstruction (Fig. 3b) is about 4 mm. Comparison of Fig. 9d and Fig. 9e shows that little improvement in visual quality is achieved by doubling the number of events, from two to four million, with 4 mm smoothing. However, at one million total counts (about 500k true), as shown in Fig. 9f, statistical noise begins to affect the cortex and even the larger grey matter structures such as the putamen. Using the reconstruction of Fig. 9e and defining regions of interest that contain grey matter, white matter and background, a grey to white uptake ratio of 3.8 is obtained, in good agreement with that expected. Profiles through Fig. 9a and Fig. 9d are shown in Fig. 9g and Fig. 9h, respectively. Some contrast reduction due to the reconstruction filtering can be seen, although significant grey-matter structures such as the putamen are easily identified.

3.3. Background Subtraction

The main contributions to the image background come from accidental and scattered coincidences. Ring-based cameras reduce accidentals by operating with a very short time resolution, and reduce scatter by the use of carefully designed lead shielding to eliminate photons that scatter out of the plane. These options are not available to the HIDAC camera, and thus a significant fraction of the total counts are background events, except for small objects imaged at low rates. Some background subtraction is therefore necessary even for the qualitative interpretation of the image.

Accidentals are, in general, distributed randomly throughout the full imaging volume, and even a comparatively high rate (30% to 40% of the total) divided among 256,000 voxels makes only a small contribution to each. A non-uniform distribution of accidentals may be taken into account by collecting both delayed and prompt coincidences and then subtracting the accidental map from the total image. A good discussion of the effect of accidentals in ring cameras may be found in [12].

A high rate of scattered coincidences is more serious because their distribution is not, in general, random but depends upon the radioisotope distribution, the distribution of the non-active scattering medium and the response of the camera to scattered photons. Measurement of the profile of a line source in a scattering medium shows characteristic long tails with little increase in the FWHM. Such an effect could be modelled and included in the p.r.f. to be deconvolved from the back-projection, although it would probably introduce a non-stationary component. Alternatively, methods which iterate on the projections have been proposed for section-imaging systems [13]. For the HIDAC camera, advantage is taken of the fact that it is a multi-section device and that some sections outside the signal volume, i.e. sections that contain only background, are imaged. The mean value determined from combining several of these background sections is taken as the mean background level for the whole image. This same value is then subtracted from all sections; in practice a slightly higher level is sometimes used to allow for statistical fluctuations.

The background subtraction procedure was applied to an image obtained with a phantom consisting of a 20 cm diameter cylinder containing three cold spots of diameter 1 cm, 3 cm and 5 cm; the phantom was filled with Ga^{68} and one million events acquired and reconstructed. The result is shown in Fig. 10, for a) a background plane and b) a plane through the cylinder. A profile through the centre of the 3 cm cold spot shows that the dip reaches the level of the background as determined from sections outside the cylinder. Thus, after background subtraction the 5 cm and 3 cm cold spots

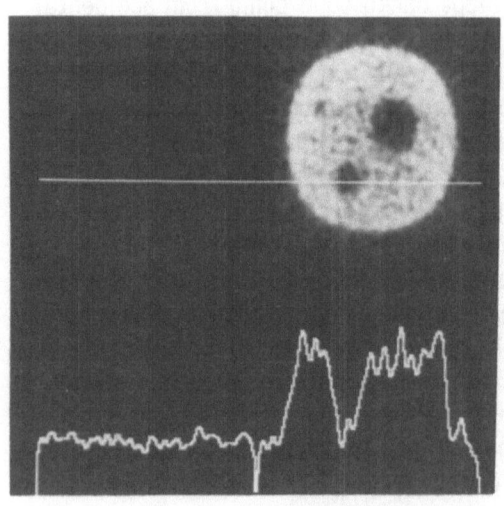

(b)

FIGURE 10. Uniform Cylinder with cold spots.
(a) background plane (b) plane through cylinder

both show zero activity. The 1 cm cold spot, barely visible in the upper left part of the cylinder, appears to contain about 30% of the activity in the cylinder. This effect is due partly to positron penetration of the plastic and partly to the smoothing effect at boundaries of the reconstruction filter.

4. CLINICAL APPLICATIONS

A complete evaluation of the clinical potential of the HIDAC positron camera requires cyclotron-produced radionuclides such as C^{11} (20 min half life) and F^{18} (110 min half-life), and the synthesis of metabolically interesting compounds such as labelled glucose, amino acids and neurotransmitters. In the absence of an on-site cyclotron, however, applications are limited to those involving longer-lived and generator produced nuclides. These include:

I^{124}: a positron-emitting substitute for I^{131} or I^{123} with a half-life of 4.2 days and a 25% positron emission. It is produced by 40 MeV alpha particle bombardment of a natural antimony target and the long half-life facilitates the transportation from a remote cyclotron. Thyroid imaging has been the main application.

Co^{55}: a positron-emitter with a half-life of 17.5 hours. Transport from a remote cyclotron is feasible with careful organisation. It is used to label bleomycin and the resulting radiopharmaceutical behaves as a tumour-seeking agent.

Ga^{68}: a positron-emitter with a 68 min. half-life that is obtained by elution with HCl of an in-house Ge^{68}-Ga^{68} generator. It may be used to label a variety of substances for imaging different internal organs. Examples include: EDTA as a vascular tracer, colloids for liver studies, microspheres for lung perfusion and diphosphonates for bone studies.

4.1. Thyroid Imaging

Thyroid imaging is performed between six and twenty-four hours after oral administration of 1 to 10 MBq of I^{124}, depending on the study and the clinical situation of the patient. The iodine uptake in the thyroid varies from about 10 kBq/cm^3 for hypothyroid patients, up to as much as 100 kBq/cm^3 in cases of Graves' disease. The PET scan lasts about 15 minutes, during which between 50,000 and 300,000 events are collected.

Data rates vary from 100 to 1000 cps. Although imaging at the higher rate for, say, 15 minutes yields 900,000 counts, up to 70% of them are eliminated by constraints and background subtraction. Firstly, the accidental rate at 1000 cps is around 15% (Fig. 5); secondly, during the image reconstruction approximately half the events are eliminated by the shift-invariance constraint in the yz-plane (Fig. 7, section 3.1); and finally, the scatter fraction, estimated from the background level (section 3.3), for thyroid imaging is about 25%. Thus, of the 900,000 events acquired, some 270,000 remain as signal. An enlarged thyroid of 50 cm^3 would therefore have 5400 counts/cm^3, or 43 counts in a voxel of size 2mm x 2mm x 2mm, corresponding to a theoretical statistical error of ≳15%. A thyroid of similar size imaged for 20 minutes at 100 cps will have only 800 counts/cm^3. In such cases, for the purpose of interpretation, the transverse section thickness is increased to 8 mm to give a statistical accuracy of around 20%. Most thyroid imaging lies between these two extremes, and a section thickness of 4 mm represents a reasonable compromise.

After background correction, the absolute regional radio-iodine uptake in the thyroid can be obtained by normalising the image to an independent measurement of total uptake using, for example, a single-crystal counter and well-counter measurements of blood activity levels. The normalised images are presented for interpretation as transverse sections viewed slightly from above and facing the patient (Fig. 13). Tomographic images contain considerably more information than conventional pinhole projections, particularly with respect to *local* function. Cold nodules of less than 1 cm are identified tomographically, whereas on a pinhole projection they are often obscured by overlapping activity. Absolute normalisation allows the important distinction to be made between a cold (non-active) region and a region of reduced uptake, at least when the activity level exceeds the statistical fluctuations.

4.1.1. Volume Estimation   An important advantage of a three-dimensional image is the possibility to estimate the dimensions of features of interest. In the case of the thyroid, a measurement of functional volume is useful for radio-iodine treatment planning, since the appropriate dose of I^{131} depends upon this volume. In principle, the volume may be estimated directly from the background-subtracted image by counting all voxels that contain non-zero values. In practice, however, the exact border of the thyroid tissue in the image is uncertain due to the partial volume effect and reconstruction smoothing, and, as confirmed by experiments with phantoms, the correct volume is obtained with a threshold somewhat higher than the mean background level discussed in section 3.3.

Determination of the appropriate threshold is not always straightforward, especially with noisy or heavily-smoothed images. Webb et al. [14] suggested that from observations with phantoms of known volume, the appropriate threshold corresponds to a slope-change or kink in

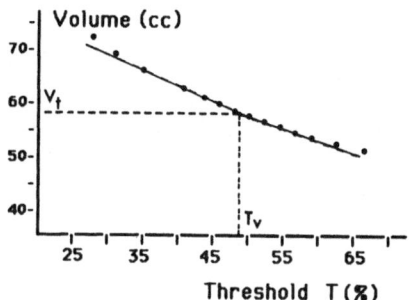

FIGURE 11. Volume Estimate vs Threshold for
a small phantom

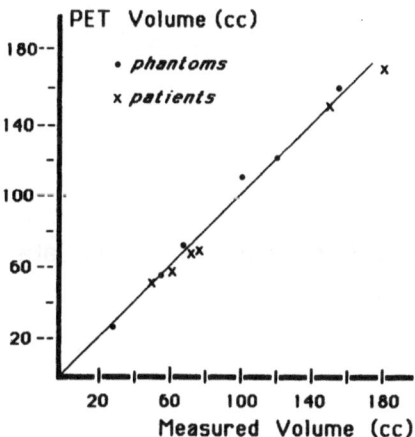

FIGURE 12. A Comparison of PET Volume Estimates with *in vitro*
measurements for phantoms and patients.

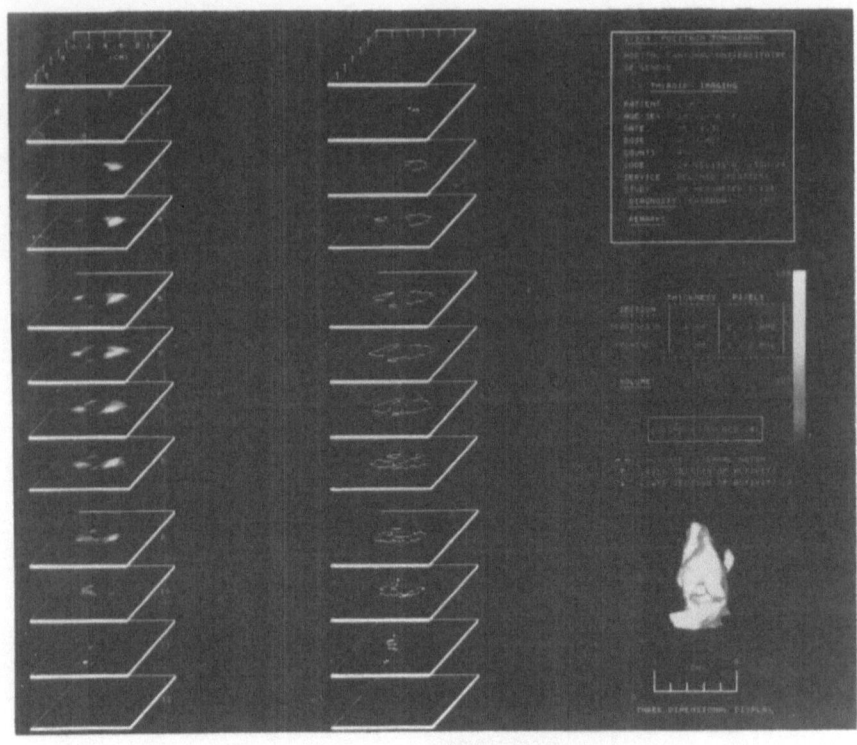

FIGURE 13. PET Thyroid Imaging: A Patient Data Summary

the plot of volume against threshold. Such a plot is shown in Fig. 11 for a phantom of 58 cm^3; a slope-change at a threshold of 48% is just discernable. Large variations in the magnitude of this effect, however, have been observed with both phantoms and thyroids of differing sizes. Thus, in some cases a distinct kink is seen, whilst in others an almost entirely smooth curve occurs; no obvious correlation with phantom size or the mean rate of change of volume with threshold has been found. Where a slope-change can be clearly identified, the resulting threshold corresponds roughly to the average value between the (zero) background and the maximum signal level.

The problem of verifying this technique in practice is that the true functional volume of the thyroid is unknown. However, in cases where a partial thyroidectomy is performed, the physical volume of the excised gland can be measured and compared with the volume estimated from the PET image. Obvious sources of discrepancy in this comparison are: (1) some part of the thyroid will remain within the patient, (2) PET estimates the functional thyroid volume, whereas the measurement is that of the physical volume and (3) parts of the thyroid, particularly fluid-containing nodules, may be damaged during the operation. The most important effect appears to be (2), so that the PET functional volume tends to be an *underestimate*. This effect can clearly be seen in Fig. 12 where the PET estimate is plotted against the measured volume for a number of phantoms and for six patients who underwent partial thyroidectomy. For volumes in the range 30 cm^3 to 180 cm^3, agreement with phantoms is good, whereas for patients the PET result is usually an underestimate. The PET thresholds for the volumes in Fig. 12 were obtained, where possible, from the slope-change in the V/T plot; an approximate error in the volume (ΔV) can be estimated from:

$$\Delta V \approx \langle dV/dT \rangle \Delta T$$

where $\langle dV/dT \rangle$ is the mean value at the point where the slope changes, and ΔT is the uncertainty in locating this point. For phantoms, ΔV increases from 4% at 32 cm^3 up to 10% at 156 cm^3; for patients, the error is slightly larger because of a greater uncertainty in locating the slope-change point. For therapy planning, a knowledge of the functional volume is more relevent than the physical volume, since it includes only those parts of the thyroid which actually capture and metabolise iodine.

4.1.2. Three-Dimensional Display. Figure 13 shows an example of a thyroid patient data summary that is presented to the referring clinician along with the clinical report. It includes the normalised, transverse

498

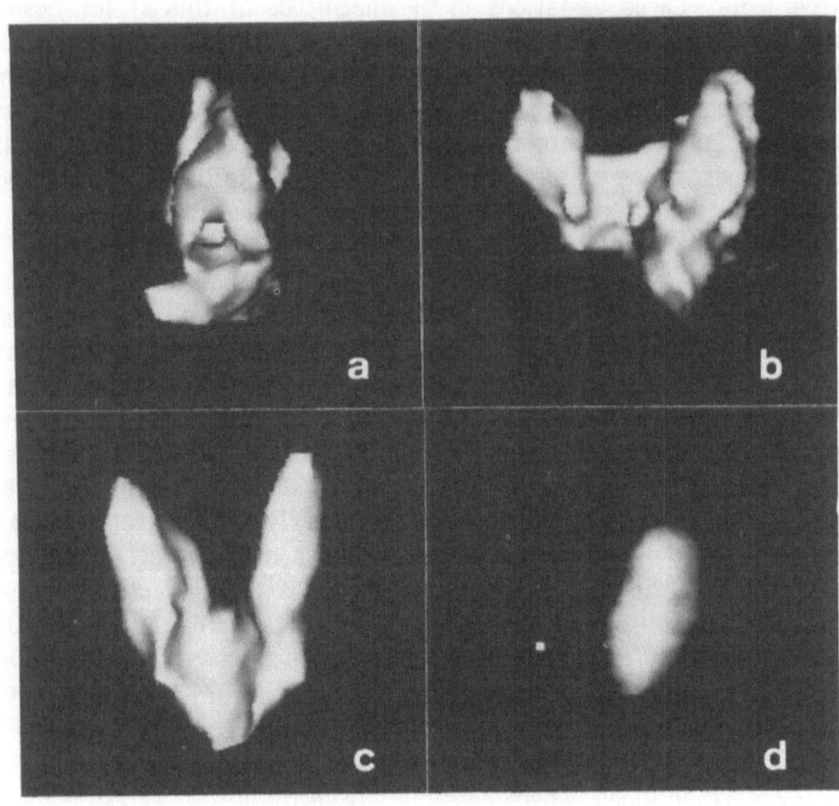

FIGURE 14. Three-Dimensional Thyroid Display

section images, the corresponding contours used for the volume estimation, the volume estimate and patient data, and either an enlargement of one section, or a shaded-graphics display of the complete thyroid. Points are marked on the transverse sections to locate specific anatomical landmarks such as the sternal notch. They are obtained by imaging small Na^{22} point sources that are fixed to the surface of the patient after thyroid imaging is complete and before the patient is allowed to move.

Typical examples of three-dimensional thyroid display are shown in Figure 14. They are obtained using image reconstructions with 2 mm x 2 mm x 2 mm, cubic voxels as input, after segmentation, to the shaded-graphics program MOVIE.BYU [15]. By rotating in space, cold regions may be easily located (Fig. 14a) and the presence of unsuspected features such as pyramidal lobes, or retro-tracheal extension identified. For diagnostic purposes, they may help to identify and localise both hot and cold nodules and as a guide in fine-needle biopsies, while for surgical purposes they provide a global view of the thyroid prior to the operation. Figure 14a shows a diagnosed Graves' disease, and Fig. 14b a goitre. Fig. 14c and Fig. 14d are images from the same patient, also with Graves' disease, taken, respectively, before and after partial thyroidectomy; the upper pole of the right lobe remained in the patient, and the follow-up scan was obtained with an activity of 1 MBq, eighteen months after the operation. The point in Fig. 14d marks the Adam's apple. These images are taken from an on-going follow-up study to provide feedback on the surgical procedure. Some case reports on imaging the human thyroid with I^{124} have been published elsewhere [16].

4.2. Tumour Imaging

The main difficulties with the imaging of tumours are firstly, that sufficient radiopharmaceutical must reach the tumour tissue to provide adequate signal and secondly the interpretation of the resulting tumour image. For a system of limited sensitivity such as the HIDAC camera, it is important to have sufficient background clearance before imaging to optimise the tumour to background ratio.

Co^{57}-labelled bleomycin has been demonstrated to be a tumour marker of good sensitivity and reasonable specificity for lung cancer [17]. Co^{55} is a positron-emitter with a convient 17.5 hour half-life, that allows imaging to be performed 20 hours after an intravenous injection of 40 MBq of labelled bleomycin. For tumours of the brain, hypopharynx and larynx, data rates in the HIDAC camera are variable, but sufficient to provide 50,000 to 80,000 counts in about 20 minutes imaging. Even with such low statistics, the high spatial resolution and low background ensures good signal to noise in the final image.

The problem of image interpretation is illustrated in Fig. 15a, which shows four, 4 mm thick frontal sections through the head of a patient with a metastatic brain tumour (arrowed). Although the tumour is clearly visible, the precise localisation is difficult because of the absence of recognizable topographic-anatomical structures; the skull contour is arbitrary and has been added for illustration purposes. As the objective of the cobalt study is not only to recognise malignancy but also to localise and stage the tumour, it is essential to mark well-defined features of surface anatomy. As for the thyroid, this is achieved by imaging a number of point sources fixed at known positions. The black square in Fig. 15a, bottom right, marks a point on the lower part of the right ear of the patient.

Similar difficulties of interpretation arise with tumours of the hypopharynx and larynx regions. Additional non-specific uptake in the surrounding soft tissue reduces signal to noise and tumour identification is

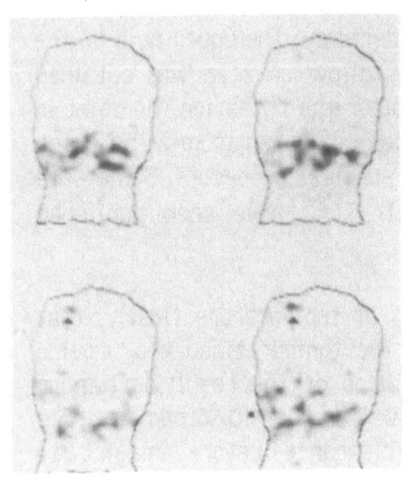
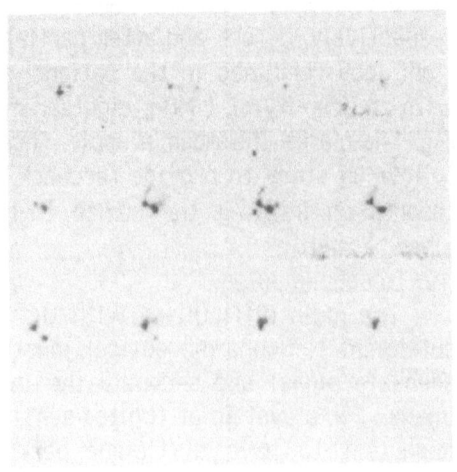

(a)   (b)

FIGURE 15. Co^{55} – bleomycin.
(a) Metastatic brain tumour
(b) Malignant tumour of the hypopharynx

less obvious than in the brain. An illustrative example appears in Fig. 15b showing sixteen, 4 mm thick frontal sections through a large tumour of the hypopharynx. Heterogeneous activity uptake is seen in the periphery of the tumour which has an inactive (probably necrotic) centre. Features such as the Adam's apple (cross in section 1), the right mastoid process and the tumour (black squares in section 7) were marked with external point sources.

4.3. Vascular Imaging.

Gallium-labelled pharmaceuticals are attractive because the positron emitter Ga^{68} can be obtained directly from an in-house generator, and has a half-life of only 68 minutes. Ga^{68}-EDTA, for example, is a vascular tracer and a well-known indicator of blood-brain barrier integrity [18]. Fig. 16 shows a sequence of 4 mm thick transverse (a) and frontal (b) sections through the head of a normal volunteer injected with 200 MBq of Ga^{68}-EDTA.

When imaging at a rate of 4000 cps, 2.4 million events are registered in about ten minutes, half of which are subsequently eliminated by the

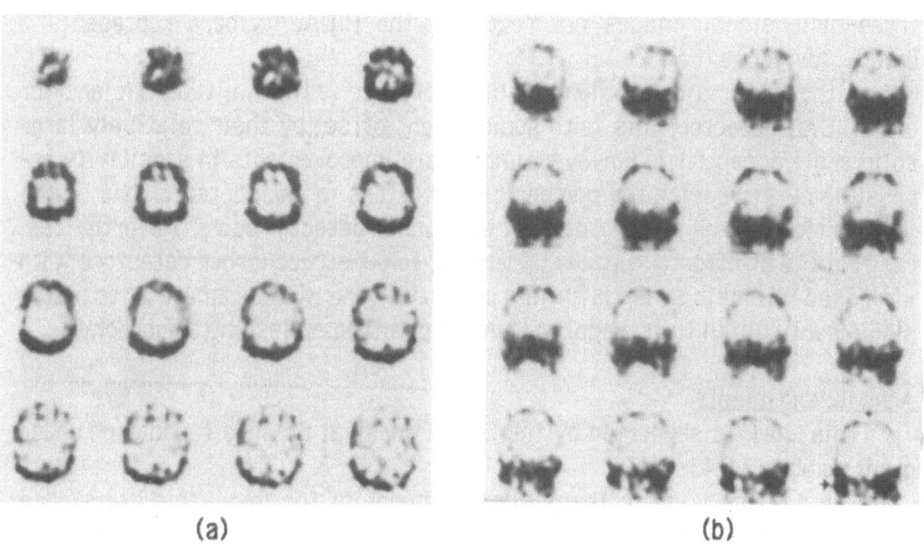

(a)   (b)

FIGURE 16. Ga^{68}-EDTA in a normal volunteer.
(a) 4 mm transverse sections
(b) 4 mm frontal sections

stationarity constraint (section 3.1). The accidental rate is about 30% (Fig.

5), and scatter, estimated from the background level, accounts for a further 35%. The images in Fig. 16 therefore contain only about 420,000 unscattered coincidences. As expected, a ring of vascular activity is seen surrounding the brain; the black arrows on section 16, Fig. 16b mark the vertex and the right ear.

5. CONCLUSION

This paper has summarised the status and performance of the HIDAC positron camera for clinical applications, and highlighted some of the associated problems of image analysis and display. Although full evaluation will require the availability of short-lived radioisotopes, the prototype has already demonstrated, during two years of reliable operation, considerable potential in certain, well-chosen clinical applications. Situations such as the imaging of small, internal organs and complex structures with low radioisotope uptake are particularly suitable for the HIDAC camera; examples presented include thyroid imaging and the localisation of tumours. Also, for the imaging of animals when *in vivo* high-resolution, fully three-dimensional images are required, the HIDAC camera represents a unique, low-cost tool.

Although a major problem of this prototype is the limited efficiency of each HIDAC detector, this is to some extent offset by their relatively large solid angle acceptance. However, immediate improvements in sensitivity are possible by increasing the number of converters in each detector and by the installation, on the same gantry, of additional detector pairs. Nevertheless, the success of efforts, already underway, to construct larger detectors with increased intrinsic sensitivity is a priority if the HIDAC camera is to play a significant role in future applications of positron emission tomography.

Acknowledgements

This work is supported by the Swiss National Science foundation under grant number 3.848-0.83.

The authors wish to thank Renato Magnanini for invaluable assistance in the construction of the detectors, A.Smith and H.Sharma from the Biomedical Physics Department, Manchester University for the supply of I^{124} and Co^{55}, and Andrew Long from the Royal Marsden Hospital, Sutton for the three-dimensional display of the thyroids. The authors are grateful to Rolf Clack of Dalhousie University, Canada for his critical reading of the manuscript.

REFERENCES.

1. Heiss W-D and Phelps ME. (ed): Positron Emission Tomography of the Brain. Springer-Verlag, 1983.
2. Ratib O, Phelps ME, Huang S-C, Henze E, Selim CE, Schelbert H: Positron Tomography with Deoxyglucose for estimating local myocardial glucose metabolism. J. of Nucl. Med. 23(7) 577, 1982.
3. Hoffman EJ, Ricci A, van der Stee L,Phelps ME: ECAT III – Basic design considerations. IEEE Trans. Nucl. Sci. NS-30,1,729, 1983.
4. Mullani NA, Wong WH, Hartz R, Philippe EA, Yerian K: Sensitivity improvement of TOFPET by the utilization of inter-slice coincidences. IEEE Trans. Nucl. Sci. NS-29, 479, 1982.
5. Jeavons AP, Schorr B, Kull K, Townsend D, Frey P, Donath A: A large area stationary positron camera using wire chambers. Proc. Conf. on Medical Radionuclide Imaging. Heidelberg, (IAEA Vienna) , 49, 1981.
6. Jeavons AP, Hood K, Herlin G, Parkman C, Townsend D, Magnanini R, Frey P, Donath A: The High density avalanche chamber for positron emission tomography. IEEE Trans. Nucl. Sci. NS-30, 640, 1983.
7. Townsend D, Clack R, Frey P, Donath A, Jeavons AP, Kulick J: Data Acquisition and image reconstruction for a high resolution positron camera. IEEE Frontiers of Computing in Medicine. 59, 1982.
8. Schorr B, Townsend D, Clack R: A general method of three-dimensional filter computation. Phys. Med. Biol. 28(9) 1009, 1983.
9. Townsend D, Clack R, Magnanini R, Frey P, Donath A, Schorr B, Jeavons AP, Froidevaux A: Image reconstruction for a rotating positron tomograph. IEEE Trans. Nucl. Sci. NS-30, 594, 1983.
10. Clack R, Townsend D, Jeavons AP: Increased sensitivity and field of view for a rotating positron camera. Phys. Med. Biol. 29(11) 1421, 1984.
11. Hoffman Brain Phantom: Data Spectrum Corporation, Chapel Hill, North Carolina.
12. Hoffman EJ, Huang S-C, Phelps ME, Kuhl DE: Quantitation in positron ECT:4. Effect of accidental coincidences. J. Comp. Assist. Tomogr. 5(3) 391, 1981.
13. Endo M, Iinuma T: Software correction of scatter coincidences in positron CT. Eur. J. Nucl. Med. 9, 391, 1984.
14. Webb S, Ott RJ, Flower MA, Leach M, Marsden P, McCready V:Verification of a technique for the measurement of functioning thyroid volume using positron emission tomography. Proc. of the VII ICMP, Espoo, Finland, 1985.
15. MOVIE.BYU: Shaded-graphics display program, Brigham-Young University

Provo, Utah, USA.

16. Frey P, Townsend D, Donath A, Jeavons AP: *In vivo* imaging of the human thyroid with a positron camera using I^{124}. Eur. J. Nucl. Med., 10, 472, 1985.

17. Nieweg O, Beekhuis H, Piers DA, Sluiter HJ, van der Wal AM, Woldring MG: Scintigraphy with Co^{57}-bleomycin in detection of lung cancer: A review of 268 well-documented cases. Cancer 53, 1675, 1984.

18. Hawkins R, Phelps ME, Huang S-C, Wapenski J, Grimm P, Parker R, Juillard G, Greenberg P: A kinetic evaluation of blood-brain barrier permeability in human brain tumours with ^{68}Ga-EDTA and positron computed tomography. J. Cerebral Blood Flow and Metabolism. 4, 507, 1984.

A COLORFUL ALTERNATIVE TO DIGITAL SUBTRACTION

W O'CONNELL, D ORTENDAHL, D FAULKNER, B ENGELSTAD,
M OKERLUND, E BOTVINICK, M DAE, J GARRETT

METHODS

It is often useful to compare two different, but related clinical images, I1 and I2. We may wish to compare dual isotope images of an organ, the end-diastolic and end-systolic frames of a gated blood-pool study, or T1 and T2 images from a magnetic resonance study. A particular pixel, p, specifies a value in each image, and so defines a vector (p1,p2). We can collapse the information to one dimension by forming the difference image D = I1 - I2, or the ratio image R = I1 / I2.

For the past two years we have been investigating a comparison technique which retains the two-dimensional nature of the image data. The vector (p1,p2) can be represented in polar coordinates as a magnitude (M) and an angle (A) where:

$$M = sqrt(p1^2 + p2^2)$$
$$A = arctangent(p2 / p1)$$

M is a measure of composite intensity and A measures the relative contributions of p1 and p2 to the composite. See Figure 1.

Figure 2 (top-left) shows a row and a column grey scale ramp. Their polar transform appears below, the magnitude image screen left and the angle image to its right. Figure 2 (top-right) shows a pair of clinical images. In the catheterization laboratory, macroaggregated albumin (MAA) particles labeled with In-111 and Tc-99m were injected into the right and left main coronary arteries respectively. Both arteries supply the septum which should comprise a region of overlap between the images. The polar transform of these images is shown below. The overlap region can be seen in the polar angle image.

The multidimensional nature of color suggests a way to show the polar transform as a single image. We can map M to intensity (I) and angle to hue (H) using an IHS model of color space. Saturation (S) is kept maximal. The IHS model is described in some detail below.

Figure 3 shows a color composite of the polar transformed ramp images. We call this composite a polar comparison image. In principle, it should be possible to reconstruct the original image pair from the polar comparison image. But real displays can show a limited

number of colors, n(C), simultaneously. On our display n(C)
= 248. Since each hue includes a full range of intensities
we have:

$$n(H) \times n(I) \leq n(C)$$

where

    n(H) = number of hues displayed.
    n(I) = number of intensity levels displayed.
    n(C) = number of color combinations available.

    The investigator chooses n(H). This choice sets n(i) =
int(n(C) / n(H)). Figure 3 results from setting n(H) = 5 and
n(i) = 49. The intensity gradient from lower-left to upper-
right is fairly smooth. The 0 to 90 degree range of A is
partitioned into five 18 degree isohue wedges. Figure 4
shows the comparison images built by setting n(H) = 11. The
22 isointensity arcs are now plainly visable.
    The implementing computer program reads images I1 and
I2 and produces two outputs:

1. A composite image in which each pixel encodes both M
   and A. For example when n(H) = 11, pixel values 0-21
   encode the 22 intensity levels of the first hue; values
   22-43 encode the levels of the second hue, etcetera.

2. Color translation tables which convert the IHS values
   to the RGB values which most displays require.

RGB COLOR SPACE
    Human color perception is a complex and long studied
area through which we will pick a narrow path. We begin by
describing the RGB cube. The retina responds to wavelengths
in the 400 to 700 nanometer range. Color perception depends
upon the response of three different retinal photopigments.
It is a remarkable fact that most colors can be realized as
weigted sums of just three wavelengths, (R,G,B) = (410,530,
650 nm.). Color monitors generate their range of colors in
this way. The human visual system is most sensitive to the
wavelengths which produce a yellow-green sensation, less
sensitive to those which produce red, still less to those
producing blue.
    Manufacturers balance monitors so that specifying equal
parts of R, G and B will a produce a combination perceived
as grey or white. So it is possible to describe any color
realizable by the display as a point in the cube generated
by three orthogonal axes, R (0 to 1), G (0 to 1), and B (0
to 1).

THE IHS COLOR SPACE
    Although the RGB axis wavelengths correspond roughly to
photoreceptor sensitivity peaks, this basis is not a natural
one for understanding color perception. People find it difficult to factor a perceived color into its RGB components.
Many animals lack color vision but can judge relative
intensitity reliably. People retain the ability to
see color images in 'black and white', that is, to extract

intensity information from them. In fact, the only black and white images we encounter are artificial - photographs or computer displays. In figure 5 the grey line from (0,0,0) to (1,1,1) is the locus of points with equal parts R,G and B, and so defines the grey scale or intensity (I) axis.

$$I = R + G + B$$

Now consider the set of planes normal to the I axis. These planes comprise points of equal intensity. Figure 6 shows the largest color wheel which can be fit into the color cube. This wheel contains the most vivid (saturated) colors obtainable in the cube, and lies in the transverse cut through the I axis at $(R,G,B) = (.5,.5,.5)$. This plane is the locus of points with $I = 1.5$.

Let p be a point in the plane. We can represent the p in polar coordinates (fig.7) with:

Saturation (S) = distance of p from the intensity axis.

Hue (H)   = angular distance around the wheel from an arbitrary starting angle.

Again the limit of 248 simultaneous colors forces us to quantize S into discrete bands and H into isohue wedges. The color wheel of figure 6 consists of the maximally saturated points of figure 7. The RGB cube can be viewed as a stack of similar color planes which form a double cone, one growing darker as it shrinks to the (0,0,0) vertex and one growing brighter as it shrinks to the (1,1,1) vertex.

Figure 8 shows some longitudinal cuts along the length of the lower cone. To build each slice we fix a particular hue (and its 180 degree complement) while varying S along the X axis and I along the Y axis. Finally, figure 9 represents points on the surface of the lower cone. These are the maximally saturated cone points. Hue varies around the periphery while intensity increases with distance from the center. We use only color combinations on the surface of the lower cone to build the comparison images. We transform (p1,p2) to (M,A). M is then mapped to I and A is mapped to H, while S is kept maximal.

IHS TO RGB TRANSFORMS
The polar representation of (p1,p2) specifies particular IHS values. But we must construct look-up tables which transform these to the RGB values required by most displays. We will deal only with points within the lower cone where $0 <= I <= 3/2$. The central idea is to control the RGB color guns with lagged cosine functions. The transforms appear below.

$$R = 1/3\ I\ (1 + S\ \cos(H))$$
$$G = 1/3\ I\ (1 + S\ \cos(H-120))$$
$$B = 1/3\ I\ (1 + S\ \cos(H-240))$$

where

$$0 <= R,G,B <= 1$$
$$0 <= I <= 3/2$$
$$-PI <= H < +PI$$

Figure 10 shows the RGB color tables used to display the uniform intensity color wheel. One can show, using trigometric identities, that the transformed coordinates do have the specified intensity, saturation, and hue.

THE TWO GUN APPROACH

There is another approach to making polar comparison images. Suppose we let the intensities of I1 directly control the intensities of, say, the Red gun while I2 intensities control the Blue gun. On a display with 248 color combinations we can let each gun take one of fifteen intensity levels. The top half of Figure 11 shows color comparisons of the ramps and of the MAA images which have been built in this fashion. Below are the corresponding polar comaparisons. This rectangular coordinate approach has the virtue of simplicity and can be extended to comparison of three images. This approach has been used in astronomy to superimpose images made using different bands of the electromagnetic spectrum, and in Nuclear Medicine to display the results of principle component analysis of blood pool studies.

We think the polar method offers several advantages for the comparison of two images. These follow from the fact that intensity and hue are perceptually separable variables which can be manipulated independently.

1. The rectangular approach limits us to two primary colors. The polar method lets us use all three. We can map any selected range of polar angles to any segment of the color wheel.

2. We can distribute hues over any interesting range of polar angles. If I1 and I2 contain negative values we can choose the range 0 to 360 rather than 0 to 90 degrees. To look for small differences we can display successively narrower bands of angles about 45 degrees.

3. We want color to reflect the relative contributions of I1 and I2. The polar method guarantees that particular ratio I1/I2 always yields the same hue regardless of intensity level. This is true for the rectangular method only in the special case that I1 equals I2.

4. Polar magnitude, M, is a simple function of I1 and I2 intensities. The polar method guarantees that a particular M will be displayed at constant intensity and saturation, regardless of hue. So a polar comparison image will show smooth intensity and hue contours.

5. Since I and H can be manipulated independently, we can let a third image, I3, set intensity. For instance, a map of hues representing T1 versus T2 times can be superimposed on an MRI composite intensity image.

6. For a particular image class we can trade off n(H) against n(I). For example, we have seen the ramp and MAA comparisons built with 5 and 11 hues.

DUAL ISOTOPE STUDIES

Let us look at some clinical and research protocols to which we have applied the polar comparison technique.

MAA STUDIES

We used this MAA study as an example in the previous section. Figure 13 maps coronary circulation imaged from three projections. The yellow regions of overlap mark the septum. N(H) = 5 and n(I) = 49. Notice that a difference image would eliminate exactly that interesting region of overlap.

We are now using MAA to investigate the effect of pre-existing collateral circulation on the clinical outcome of angioplasty intervention. Figure 14 shows the perfusion pattern of the left main coronary of a patient who underwent angioplasty to open an occluded right coronary. The image top-left shows the distribution of Tc-99m labeled MAA which was injected while the right coronary was occluded. The feint arc to the left marks collateral circulation to the right ventricle (RV).

After opening the right coronary, In-111 MAA particles were injected into the left coronary. This distribution pattern is shown top right. The polar comparison image (bottom-right) shows mostly Tc labeled MAA in the right ventricular region. The implication is that collateral circulation to the RV existed, and shut down after the right coronary was opened.

Bottom-left we see a histogram equalized version of TC labled MAA distribution. We use this image to set intensity in the polar comparison, since collateral distribution is feint relative to LV main distribution. Hues are defined by the original Tc and In images.

PARATHYROID STUDIES

Both Tc-99m pertechnitate and Tl-201 accumulate in the lobes of the thyroid gland. But Tl-201 also localizes in abnormal parathyroid glands while Tc-99m does not. In a series of 74 surgically confirmed cases, computer processing (which consisted of low-pass filtering, background correction, and polar comparison) increased sensitivity of adenoma detection by 6% and hyperplastic gland detection by 33% over diagnoses made from analog images alone.

Figure 15 shows a large parathyroid adenoma below the right-lower pole of the thyroid gland. We are currently studying the relative effectiveness of Tl - Tc difference images versus polar comparison images in the evaluation of parathyroid studies.

MONOCLONAL ANTIBODY STUDIES

Six nude mice grafted with human melenomas were injected with an In-111 labeled antibody reactive to the tumor and also with a nonreactive antibody of the same immunoglobulin subclass labeled with Ga-67. Images obtained in 20% windows about the 247 Kev photopeak of In and about the 93 Kev peak of Ga both showed uptake in the kidney, spleen, bone marrow and in the tumor. But preferential uptake in the 247 Kev image identified tumor sites in the comparison images.

These images display only polar angles in the range 10 - 60 degrees, since we are not looking for preferential localization of the nonreactive antibody. Pixels with angles outside this range are shown in grey. An angle of 10 degrees means that 85% of the counts detected in that pixel come from the 247 Kev (In) image.

MYOCARDIAL MAPS OF TL-201 AND I-123 MIBG

In another animal experiment dogs were injected with Tl-201 and metaiodobenzylguanidine (MIBG), and imaged in 20% windows about the 159 Kev photopeak of I-123 and the 80 Kev photopeak of Tl-201. MIBG maps myocardial adrenergic uptake against the perfusion map provided by Tl-201. Figure 17 shows anatomic slices from the normal hearts of two dogs. Notice the relative abundance of MIBG uptake (yellow) in the RV. This result accords with published reports of catecholamine distribution in the canine heart.

LABELED WHITE BLOOD CELLS

We will describe one last dual isotope example. UCSF has a large renal transplant service. The patient shown in Figure 18 developed an infection after his transplant operation. In-111 labeled white blood cells localized in a region between the transplanted kidney and bladder which were labeled by I-131 hippuran uptake. Upon re-operation, a large abcess was found in this region.

GATED BLOOD POOL STUDIES

The cardiac gated blood pool study is the Nuclear Medicine technique to which functional images have been applied most extensively . Goris, Maddox, and Holman pioneered the use of stroke volume, paradox, and ejection fraction (EF) images, and showed the EF image to be a sensitive indicator of segmental wall motion abnormalities.

Figure 18 shows the best septal end-diastolic (ED) and end-systolic (ES) frames of an normal study (top-left) and of a study showing pronounced apical dyskinesis (top-right). Below are the corresponding stroke volume, paradox, and EF images. Note the typically bright ejection shell of the normal EF image. As the wall contracts, pixels on the ED rim will show a 100% EF even though the involved blood volume is small.

Suppose that we plot the background corrected ES value

of a pixel against its ED value. Pixels with an EF of 100%
will lie on the ED axis since their ES value is zero. Pixels
with an EF of zero have equal counts at ED and ES and lie on
the line with slope of unity. So pixels with positive EF
have associated polar angles less than 45 degrees. Polar
angles greater than 45 degrees mark pixels with negative EF.
Distance from a pixel to the origin corresponds to the blood
volume involved. For instance the pixels with coordinates
(100,50) and (50,25) both have an EF of 50%. But the stroke
volume at the first pixel is twice that at the second.

Figure 20 shows polar comparison images built from the
ED and ES frames of the two studies shown above. Hue codes
for regional EF and intensity codes for the involved blood
volume. $N(H) = 12$ and $n(I) = 20$. The 12 hues are distributed
over the range 0 to 60 degrees since we are principally
interested in regions with positive EF. Red through yellow
through green hues mark regions of progressively higher EF.
Magenta marks regions with EF less than 16%, and blue regions show paradoxical EF. We let the ED image (rather than
$M = \text{sqrt}(ED^2 + ES^2)$) define intensity. This choice seems
the natural one, and choosing M will somewhat reduce the
intensity of high EF pixels.

The color EF map offers several advantages over one
dimensional functional images.

1. We can display regions with positive and negative EF in
   a single image.

2. Akinetic regions are also shown so that the anatomic
   contours of the cardiac chambers and the great vessels
   are apparent.

3. The color EF map shows the involved blood volume along
   with regional EF, so that it is possible to estimate
   global EF from the information in the EF map image.

These images are part of our standard gated blood pool
protocol. They have proved particularly useful in the evaluation of exercise studies. Figure 21 (top) documents the
increase in function of a patient with a normal response to
exercise. Below we see the EF map images of a patient with
an abnormal response.

FIRST FOURIER HARMONIC IMAGE

Figure 22 (top) shows first harmonic phase and amplitude images for the patient with apical dyskinesis. The
corresponding cosine and sine images are shown below. The
cosine-sine pair and the phase-amplitude pair are the rectangular and polar represntations of the same information.

This fact suggests building a first harmonic image
which displays amplitude as intensity and phase as hue. We
have chosen $n(H) = 20$ and $n(i) = 12$. These images are also
part of our clinical protocol and complement the EF map with
stroke volume and timing information. Extracardiac pixels
have low amplitude and so are suppressed in the display.

This is a mixed blessing, since cardiac regions with low amplitude are also suppressed. Bacharach and Green have shown that sufficient counting statistics can establish the phase of low amplitude regions reliably. To display phase in such regions we can let another image, say ED, define intensity, as shown in Figure 24. It would be interesting to let the error function directly establish pixel intensity.

The choice of twenty hues gives a temporal resolution of eighteen degrees, which is rather course. We can double the resolution by restricting our attention to ventricular pixels (-90 to +90 degrees). We can also use the course resolution to advantage. The map of hues segments the ventricle into natural regions of pixels with similar volume curves. We can sum the pixels in each region to obtain a single volume curve for each isohue region. These curves will have sufficient statistics to support multiharmonic curve fits. Figure 26 shows three harmonic curves fit to the volume curves of selected isohue segments within an operator defined region of interest. Some filling and emptying parameters derived from the fit curves are shown top-right.

THALLIUM-201 WASHOUT IMAGES

Figure 27 (top) shows the isotime LAO 45 exercise (EX) and redistribution (RE) images of a patient with a normal response to exercise. The images have been low-pass filtered and background corrected using a variant of the interpolative technique developed by Goris and others. The RE image has been rotated and translated to match the EX image using a registration technique described below. Figure 27 (bottom) shows a study with apparently less global washout.

Figure 28 shows the polar comparison images built from these EX and RE images. This time intensity codes for regional myocardial uptake of TL-201, and hue codes for percent washout (or washin) with time. $N(H) = 7$ and $n(I) = 35$, and we consider the range of polar angles 0 - 60 degrees. We are currently validating this technique against radial profile and catheterization labaratory results.

Figure 29 shows four normal washout images. Figure 30 shows four abnormal images. The image top-left shows a study with uniformly low washout. Top-right and bottom-left we see studies with segmental defects which re-perfuse. The image bottom-right shows a region of deficit at the base of the heart which persists in the RE image. Although washout is normal in the region, its relatively low intensity flags the region in the washout image.

REGISTRATION

Any pixel by pixel image comparison technique requires that the comparison images be properly matched with each other. This is a simple requirement to meet when dual isotope images are obtained simultaneously, but difficult when the images are acquired at different times. Our parathyroid, MAA, and TL-201 myocardial perfusion studies consist of two images acquired at different times. Like Watson and Beller we use a cross-correlation technique to register the images.

But we match operator defined outlines rather than the
images themselves, and we allow in-plane rotation to
influence the match.

There is a kind of paradox involved in using cross-
correlation for this purpose. We depend upon image similarities to match the images so that we can look for image
differences. For this reason we match outlines which are
drawn to bypass defects in the TL-201 EX image. Our technique aligns the geometric centroids of the two outlines, then
cross-correlates 90 radii drawn from the centroid to the
boundaries of each outline. We allow up to 44 degrees of
rotation in either direction. The best match defines a
linear transform, and the second image is resampled to match
it with the first. The outlines shown in figure 31 are from
an MAA study.

CARDIAC CINE CT

The IMATRON cine CT at UCSF can image 256x256 transverse slices at four levels every 50 milliseconds. A typical
study consists of 20 sets of four slices acquired in the one
second following injection of contrast material. Figure 32
(top) shows the ventricular ED and ES frames of a cine
reconstructed at one level. Below are the positive and
negative ED - ES difference images. The negative difference
shows atrial contrast material which at ventricular ES has
moved below the ED borders of the atria. Figure 33 shows
three polar images made from the ED and ES slices in progressively narrower bands about 45 degrees. In the 0-90
degree image only movement at the base and in the free LV
wall is apparent. This is the case since intensity changes
are small relative to image base intensities. As the focus
narrows about 45 degrees we can see changes marking movement
of all the walls and ejection of contrast material. Regions
with polar angles outside the selected range are shown as
grey shades.

DISCUSSION

The classical techniques of image comparison are to
difference or ratio the images. Each of these techniques
collapses two dimensional data to a single dimension. Polar
comparison adds a third technique, one which retains much of
the information in the original images while making their
interrelation clear. When should a particular technique be
used? Subtraction should be used when we wish to remove all
structure common to both images, as in digital angiography.
Ratios are also sometimes effective, as in the comparison of
multiband LANDSAT data. But the ratio image has two
drawbacks:

1. The ratio image makes no distinction between high and
   low error data unless ad hoc thresholding techniques
   are used. High error regions will be suppressed in
   polar comparison images since they have low magnitude.
   The arctangent error function is $U^2 = \sin(A)\cos(A)$
   $(\sin(A) + \cos(A)) / M$.

2. Ratios are asymmetric about unity. Ratios less than unity are in the range 0 - 1. Ratios greater than unity are in the range 1 to infinity. The inverse tangent function is symmetric about 45 degrees. The polar comparison image built from (I2,I1) is identical to the image made from (I1,I2) with color table inverted.

Because they describe two independent parameters simultaneously, polar comparison images require displays which can present a large number of simultaneous colors. But polar comparison images have several nice properties:

1. The polar image retains much of the original image data including anatomical landmarks. Misregistered images will show an excess of I1 hues 180 degrees opposite an excess of I2 hues. Misscaled images will show a tilt toward the hues of one image in the normalization region.

2. Since intensity and hue are perceptually separable, we can distribute the n(H) hues over interesting ranges of polar angles. We can also let a third image set intensity. For instance, we can paint a T1 versus T2 map of hues on an MRI composite intensity image.

3. It is our experience that people learn to interpret these images quickly, perhaps because they are based upon an underlying perceptual mechanism.

4. Finally, the polar representation often comprises clinically interesting pairs - regional blood pool volume and ejection fraction, first harmonic phase and amplitude, TL-201 myocardial uptake and percent washout.

REFERENCES
1. Ballard DH, Brown CM: Computer Vision. 1982 Prentice Hall Inc., Englewood Cliffs, N.J.
2. Buchanan MD, Pendergrass R: Digital image processing: Can intensity, hue and saturation replace red, green and blue? Electro-optical Systems Design, March 1980
3. Murch GM: Physiological Principles for the Effective Use of Color. IEEE C G & A, Nov. 1984
4. Baldwin, Lee: Color Considerations. BYTE, Sept. 1984
5. Cavailloles F, Bazin J, Di Paola R: Factor analysis in gated cardiac studies. J Nucl Med, 25: 1067-1079, 1984
6. Okerlund MD, Sheldon K, Corpuz S: A new method with high sensitivity and specificity for localization of abnormal parathyroid glands. ANNALS of SURGERY, Vol 200, No.3, Sept 1984
7. Angelakos ET: Regional distribution of catecholamines in the dog heart. CIRC RESEARCH, Vol XVI, Jan. 1965
8. Maddox DE, Holman BL, Wynne J, et al: Ejection fraction image: A non-invasive index of regional left ventricular wall motion. Amer J Cardiol 41:1230-1238,

1978
9. King MA, Doherty PW: Color coded ejection fraction
   images for following regional function throughout the
   cardiac cycle. In Functional Mapping of Organ Systems,
   New York. The Society of Nuclear Medicine 119-128, 1981
10. Adam WE, Tarkowska A, Bitter F, et al: Equilibrium
   gated radionuclide ventriculography. *Cardiovasc Radiol*
   2:161-173, 1979
11. Bacharach SL, Green MV, Dino V: A method for objective
   evaluation functional images. *J Nucl Med* 23:285-290,
   1982
12. Machac J, Horowitz SF, Broder D, et al: Accuracy and
   precision of multiharmonic Fourier analysis of gated
   blood-pool images. *J Nucl Med* 25:1294-1299, 1984
13. Goris ML: Nontarget activities: Can we correct for
   them? *J Nucl Med* 20:1312-1314, 1979
14. Watson DD, Campell NP, Read EK, et al: Spatial and
   temporal quantitation of plane thallium myocardial
   images. *J Nucl Med* 22:577-584, 1981

FIGURES AND IMAGES

All hue information is lost when polar comparison
images are photographed in black and white. Whenever
possible we have highlighted the intensity of one isohue
region in these images. A detailed explanation of each
figure and image can be found in the text where it is
referenced.

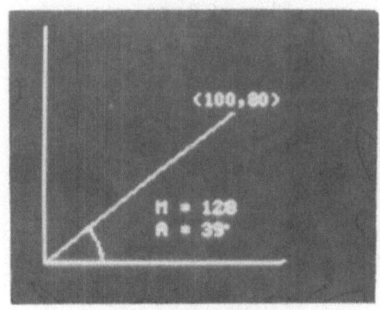

FIGURE 1
Rectangular and
polar coordinates.

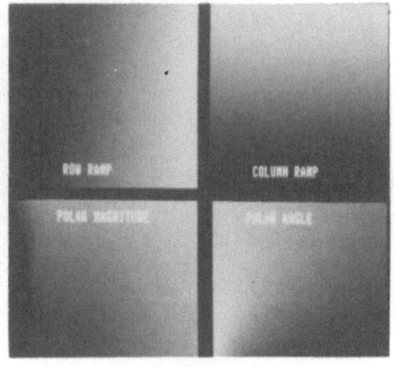

FIGURE 2A
Top - Grey scale ramps
Bottom - Polar transform

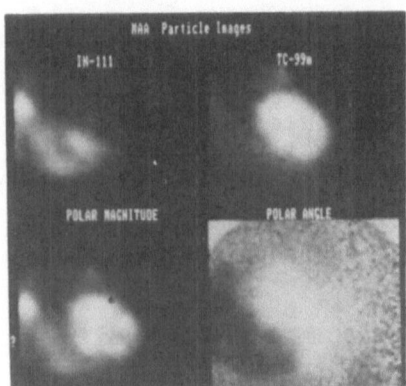

FIGURE 2B
Top - MAA particle images
Bottom - Polar transform

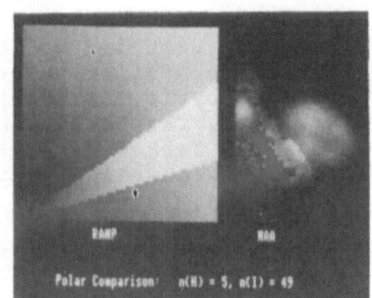

FIGURE 3
Polar comparison images
n(H) = 5, n(I) = 49

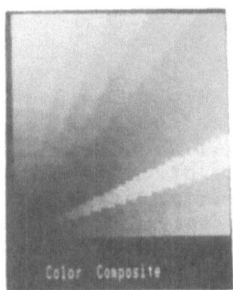

FIGURE 4
Polar comparison images
n(H) = 11, n(I) = 22

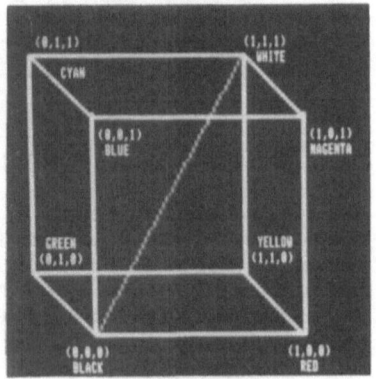

FIGURE 5
The RGB cube

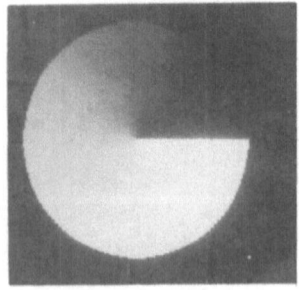

FIGURE 6
Color wheel
n(H) = 248

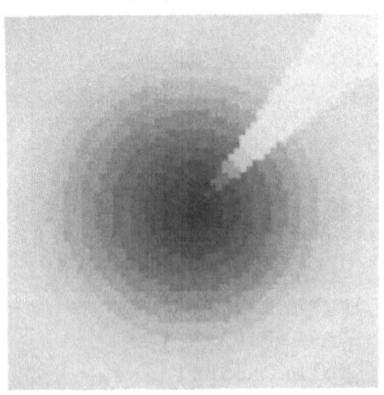

FIGURE 7
Color plane.
I=3/2, n(H)=20, n(S)=12

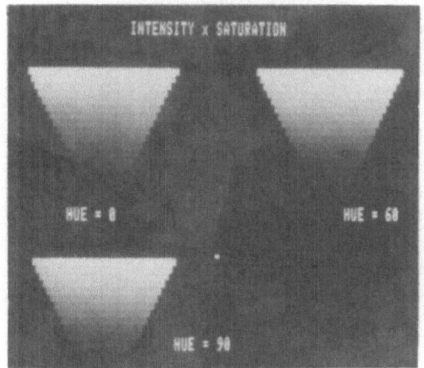

FIGURE 8
Saturation vs. Intensity
at H=0, H=60, H=120

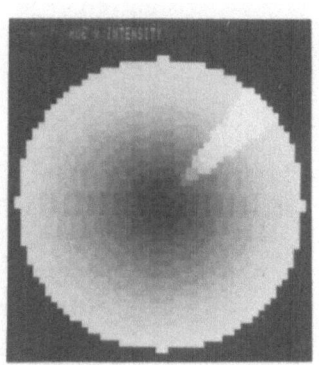

FIGURE 9
Hue vs. Intensity
n(H)=20, n(I)=12

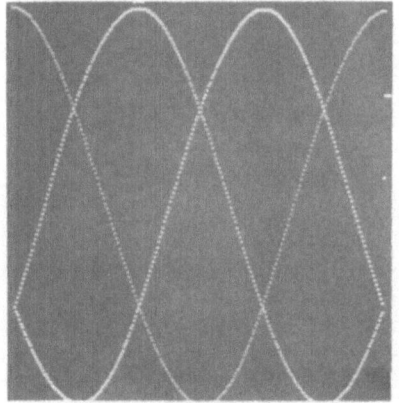

FIGURE 10
RGB color tables used
to display color wheel.

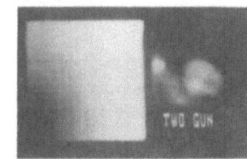

FIGURE 11
Two gun comparisons -
Ramp and MAA particles.

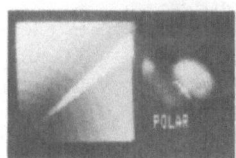

FIGURE 12
Polar comparisons -
Ramp and MAA particles.

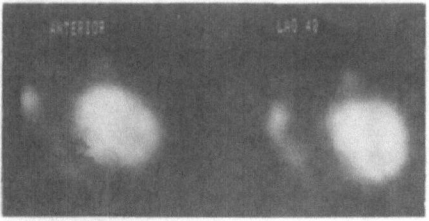

FIGURE 13
Normal MAA study.

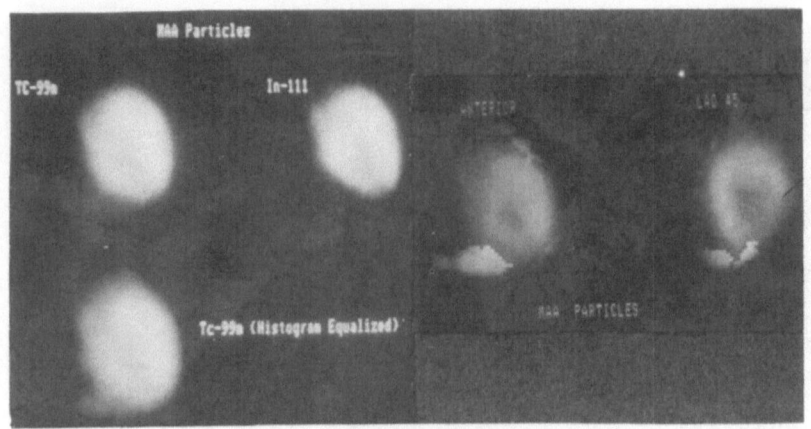

FIGURE 14
MAA study - LAD collateral
circulation to RV.

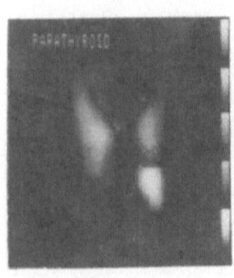

FIGURE 15
Parathyroid Adenoma.
n(H)=5, n(I)=49

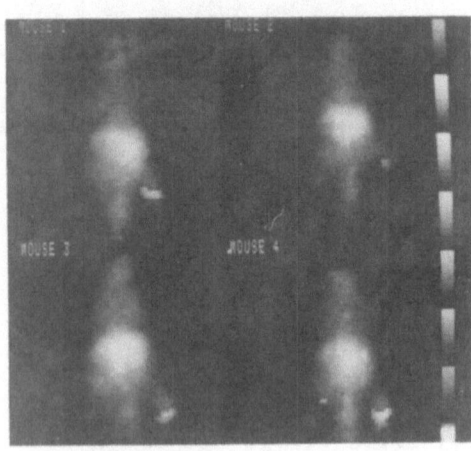

FIGURE 16
Monoclonal antibody study.
n(H)=7, n(I) = 31

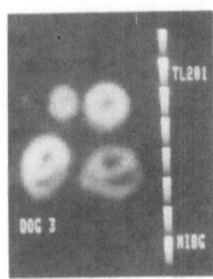

FIGURE 17
Myocardial sections.
Tl-201 vs. I-123 MIBG

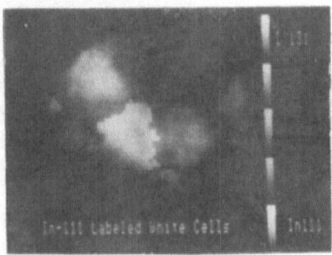

FIGURE 18A
In-111 white cells vs. I-131
hippuran. n(H)=5, n(I)=49

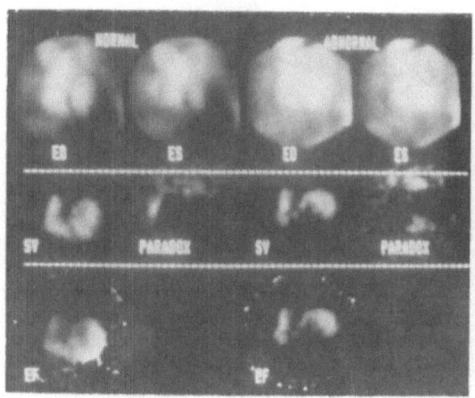

FIGURE 18B
Cardiac functional images -
Normal and abnormal studies.

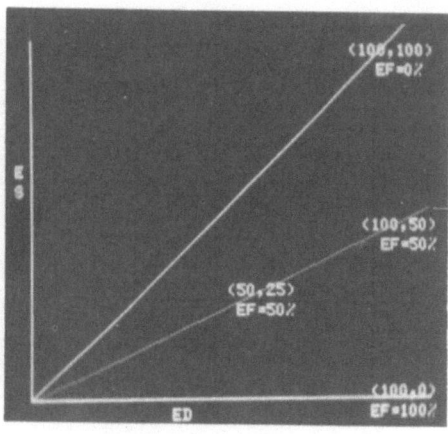

FIGURE 19
ED vs. EF pixel values.

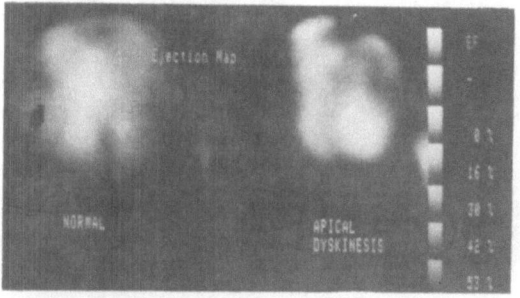

FIGURE 20.
Color EF maps -
Normal and abnormal studies.

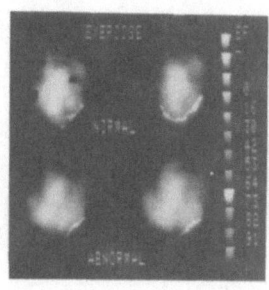

FIGURE 21
Exercise EF maps -
Normal and abnormal studies.

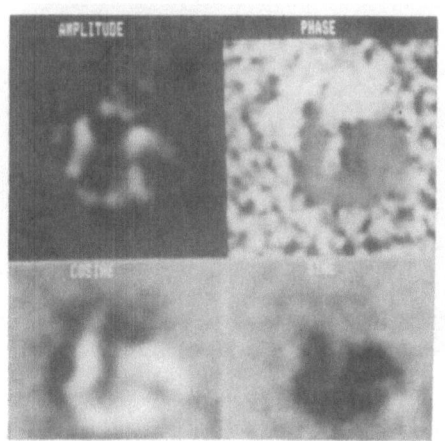

FIGURE 22
Top - Amplitude and phase.
Bottom - cosine and sine.

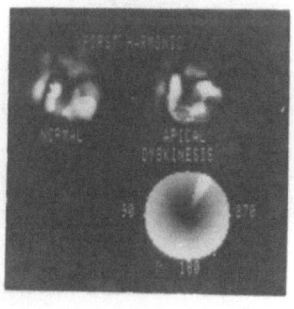

FIGURE 23
Phase x Amplitude image -
n(H) = 20, n(I) = 12

520

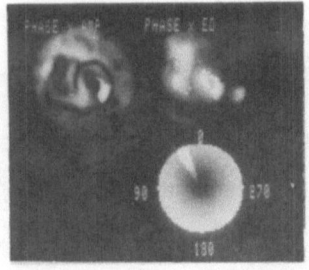

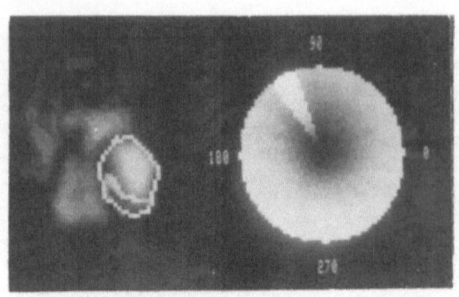

FIGURE 24
Left - Phase x Amplitude.
Right - Phase x ED blood pool.

FIGURE 25
Phase x Amplitude -
Late apex and septum.

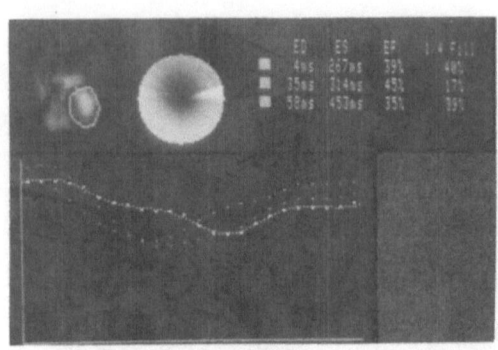

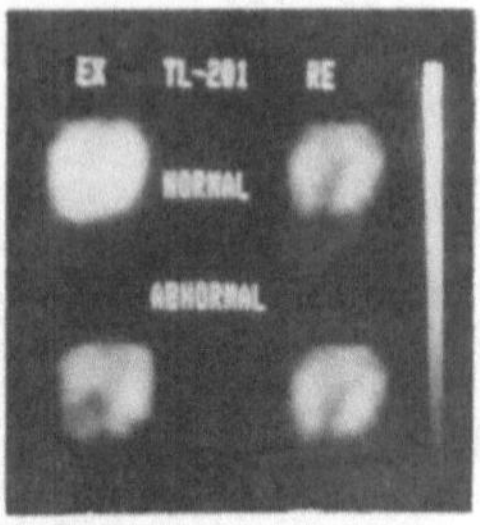

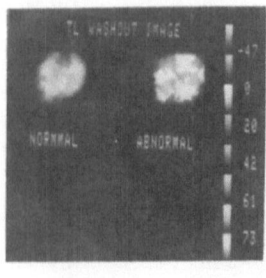

FIGURE 27
TL-201 EX and RE images -
Normal and abnormal.

FIGURE 26
3-harmonic curves fit to volume curves
of regions defined by first harmonic.

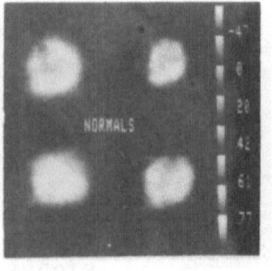

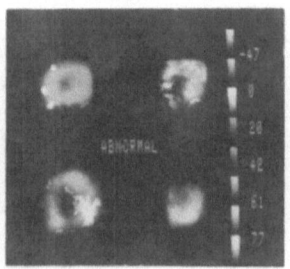

FIGURE 28
TL washout images -
Normal and abnormal

FIGURE 29
TL washout images -
4 normal studies.

FIGURE 30
TL washout images -
4 abnormal studies.

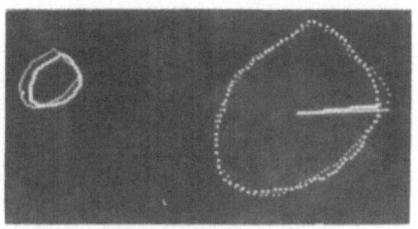

FIGURE 31
Registration of 2
ventricular outlines.

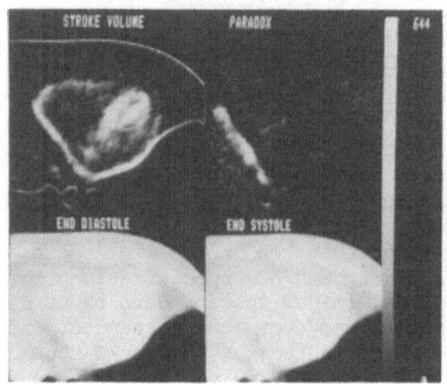

FIGURE 32
ED and ES slices of
cine CT study.

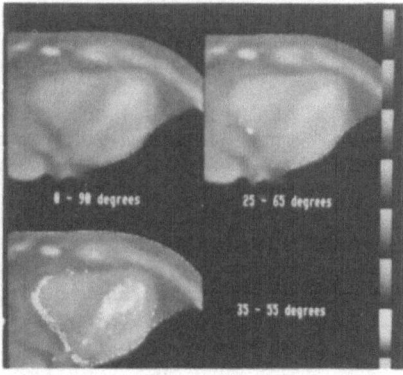

FIGURE 33
Polar comparison images
of cine CT study.

IMAGE DATA COMPRESSION TECHNIQUES APPLICABLE TO
IMAGE NETWORKS

A. Todd-Pokropek, C. Chan and R. Appledorn

1. INTRODUCTION

As the use of digitally acquired images increases in Medical Diagnosis, so there is also an increased requirement for Image Networks. At present, all images obtained in CT and MRI (magnetic resonance imaging), DSA (digital subtraction angiography), and most images in nuclear medicine and ultrasound exist in digital form. It is anticipated that when appropriate captors have been developed, most conventional radiology will also have the capability of being performed digitally. Image processing for enhancement, expert system aided diagnosis, and digital long term storage will then be possible on most medical images. However, such facilities do not in themselves improve medical care or decrease costs, and may be considered to be of limited value. To be exploited properly, it is necessary that access to such digital images, and the means to manipulate them, be widely available. This supposes an image network (with appropriate image workstations). Descriptions of particular systems are given in [1,2] and many other general references may be found in [3]

However, a major limitation in most conventional PACS (Picture Archiving and Communication System) networks is that they tend to be limited to a small geographical area. For example the draft NEMA/ACR specifications for an industry wide interface for radiological images specify data rates of ~80Mbits/sec [4]. Such rates cannot be maintained over long distances, and therefore cannot be used for a wide area network. Networks should therefore be designed such that images can be transmitted via a high speed network, throughout an extended 'campus', but also available via low speed bridges to clinics or individual General Practitioners. This implies the use of data compression.

A typical raw image is ~0.5Mbytes in size, although in conventional radiology images might be up to 16 times larger. At a data transmission rate of 19.2Kbaud then the time to transmit this typical image would be ~200 seconds. A highly desirable data compression ratio would be to reduce this time by a factor of 100, corresponding to ~0.1-0.2bits/pixel on average.

One approach has been attempted by the U.S. National Institutes of Health to provide remote radiological cover at a number of Veterans Administration Hospitals over (~9600 baud) telephone links by transmitting radiographs to a central site after image compression for interpretation [5]. Such studies indicate that a data compression ratio of about 10 (to achieve ~1bits/pixel) can be and must be achieved to make suitable use of data communication channels. Such techniques require considerable processing power at both transmitting and receiving station.

This paper will firstly consider data compression techniques in general, and them give some example of some specific methods considered to be of potential interest. An excellent general review is given by Jain [6], and also the chapter on data compression in Rosenfeld and Kak [7]. Both papers contain many further references to the data compression literature, which will not be included here. A recent review is that of M. Kunt et Al [8].

2. THE LIMITS OF DATA COMPRESSION- ENTROPY

Bmax, the maximum number of bits needed to be transmitted for an image (excluding identification information etc) is the number of pixels N x N assuming the image to be square multiplied by the number of bits per pixel Nmax. Thus a conventional CT image might have an upper limit Bmax of 512x512x16 bits, i.e. 0.5Mbytes or 4Mbits.

One value for the lower limit is defined by the entropy [6,7]. Let $p[i]$ be the probability that an pixel takes the value i then zero order entropy H_o is defined as

$$H_o = \sum_i p[i] \; log_2(p[i])$$

A typical value for a CT image is about 6bits per pixel [6]. Thus a data compression technique which achieves the limit supposed by zero order entropy could compress a CT image from 4M bits to about 1.5M bits and achieve a compression of just over a factor of 2. Huffman coding can come very close to achieving such compression [6].

For the rest of this paper, the efficiency of a data compression techniques will be considered only in terms of the average number of bits per pixel after compression (Npix). If a compression technique were to achieve Npix=1 on a CT image, then typically the total amount of data would be reduced by about 16 (e.g Nmax/Npix). However, the use of compression ratios can sometimes be rather misleading since they depend rather arbitrarily on the upper limit of size for the image.

Shannon's noiseless coding theorem states that it is possible to code without distortion a source of entropy H using H+epsilon data bits [6,7]. Thus zero order entropy appears to be the absolute lower limit for compression, given several constraints. Firstly, the data is assumed to be formed from independent Gaussian variables, or completely decorrelated. Secondly, it is assumed that the compression is to be completely reversible, that is, the original image can identically be reconstructed after expansion of the compressed image. However, firstly, most medical images have very considerable correlation between pixel values. Secondly, if the compressed image after expansion cannot be distinguished from the original image, although may not be identical, such a compression method would normally be considered acceptable. Both these facts lead to the exploitation of data compression methods which can give a value of bits per pixel very much less than that suggested from zero order entropy.

First order entropy is defined as

$$H_1 = \sum_{i_1, i_2} P[i_1, i_2] \; log_2 P[i_1, i_2]$$

where $P[i_1, i_2]$ is the condition probability of state i_1 given state i_2. Higher order entropies H_n are defined correspondingly using n states. Typical values quotes for H_1 and H_2 are 4 and 2 bits correspondingly. This gives some indication of the potential for compression by exploiting the correlation between pixels.

It is also of interest to see how entropy changes as a function of the variance (sigma^2) in an image, and on Nmax the maximum number of bits per pixel. This is illustrated in Fig 1 which was derived by simulating image

Fig 1. A graph where the entropy of a simulated image data set containing independent Gaussian distributed values is plotted against the standard deviation of these values for images where the maximum grey value was 16 and 256. Note that the entropy is almost independent of maximum value.

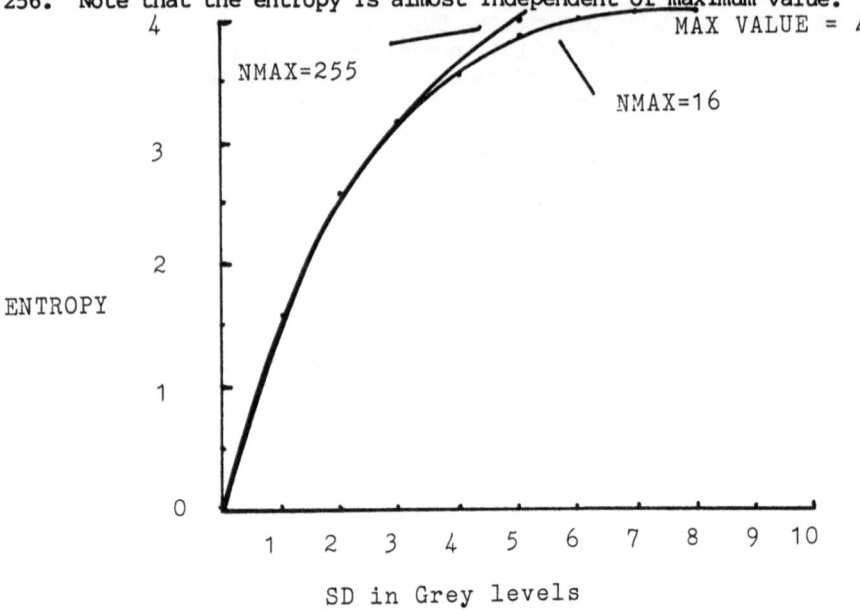

Fig 2. The layout of the number of bits to be used for each transform coefficient is shown, for a 16x16 DCT transform. The average number of bits per pixel is 2.18

```
16  12  11  10   9   8   8   7   6   5   4   4   4   4   4   4
12  10   9   9   8   7   7   6   5   4   4   3   0   0   0   4
11   9   8   7   7   6   6   5   4   3   3   0   0   0   0   0
10   9   7   7   6   5   5   4   3   3   0   0   0   0   0   0
 9   8   7   6   5   4   4   3   3   0   0   0   0   0   0   0
 8   7   6   5   4   3   3   3   0   0   0   0   0   0   0   0
 8   7   6   5   4   3   3   0   0   0   0   0   0   0   0   0
 7   6   5   4   3   3   0   0   0   0   0   0   0   0   0   0
 6   5   4   3   3   0   0   0   0   0   0   0   0   0   0   0
 5   4   3   3   0   0   0   0   0   0   0   0   0   0   0   0
 4   4   3   0   0   0   0   0   0   0   0   0   0   0   0   0
 4   3   0   0   0   0   0   0   0   0   0   0   0   0   0   0
 4   0   0   0   0   0   0   0   0   0   0   0   0   0   0   0
 4   0   0   0   0   0   0   0   0   0   0   0   0   0   0   0
 4   0   0   0   0   0   0   0   0   0   0   0   0   0   0   0
 4   4   0   0   0   0   0   0   0   0   0   0   0   0   0   0
```

data for independent Gaussian distributed data. Entropy is to a good approximation independent of Nmax. It is of course very dependent on sigma, only reaching useful values when sigma is very small. This provides support for expressing compression in terms of bits/pixel (Npix) rather than as a compression ratio.

The basic tool of data compression techniques is to eliminate the co-variance between pixels, and to transmit only the independent component, which are essentially the random variations between the expected image and the observed image. As might be expected, in medical images, such random variations are mostly (but not entirely) noise, Thus, if noise may be suppressed (which is therefore non-reversible), very efficient data compression can be achieved.

3. DECORRELATION OF PIXELS- THE KL TRANSFORM

It may be demonstrated that, in a certain sense, the Karhunen-Loeve (KL) transform is optimal in generating uncorrelated values from a set (an image of) correlated values [6,7]. This can be demonstrated from the definition of the KL transform. In the discrete case the transform is defined by the relationship

$$F(u,v) = \sum_m \sum_n f(m,n) \, \phi^{(u,v)*}(m,n)$$

where $f(m,n)$ is the original image, $F(u,v)$ is the transformed image and the basis functions [$\phi^{(u,v)}$] are a set of orthonormal matrices or eigenmatrices, of which $\phi^{(u,v)}(p,q)$ is the p,qth element. These eigenmatrices are given from the solution of

$$\sum_p \sum_q R(m,n,p,q) \, \phi^{(u,v)}(p,q) = \gamma_{uv} \, \phi^{(u,v)}(m,n)$$

where R is the autocorrelation function

$$R(m,n,p,q) = E\{ f(m,n) \, f(p,q) \}$$

$E\{\}$ indicates the expected value and $\gamma_{mn} = E\{/F(u,v)/^2\}$. In this case

$$E\{ F(u,v) \, F^*(u',v') \} = \emptyset \quad \text{and} \quad E\{ F(u,v) \} = \emptyset$$

$$\text{provided that} \quad E\{ f(m,n) \} = \emptyset, \quad u=u', \quad v=v',$$

which is the desired result.

Thus the KL transform can be used to generate a series of value $F(m,n)$ which have, in some sense, a minimum entropy, which is, in that sense, optimal for data compression. However, the use of the KL transform itself is image dependent and not very convenient and it is desirable to look for alternatives or approximations.

4. APPROXIMATIONS- THE DISCRETE COSINE TRANSFORM

One suitable approximation which has been described is the discrete cosine transform (DCT), defined as

$$F(u,v) = \frac{4\ c(u,v)}{N^2} \sum_n \sum_m f(m,n)\ \cos(\ (2m+1)\ u\ \pi\ /\ 2N)\ .\cos(\ (2n+1)\ v\ \pi\ /\ 2N\ )$$

where $c(u,v) = 0.5$ for $u=v=0$ and 1 elsewhere. It may be demonstrated that, for a small matrix size of 16x16, the basis functions of the DCT transform are very close to those of the KL transform [9] where

$$E\{\ f(m,n)\ f(p,q)\ \} = \exp(-alpha/m-p/)\ .\exp\ (-beta/n-q/)$$

that is the autocorrelation matrix is assumed to be separable and obeying an exponential model. It may be noted that such a model is often hypothesised when performing Wiener type filtering operations.

The advantages of using the DCT over the KL transform is primarily that of computational efficiency. The DCT can be implemented using a conventional FFT with appropriate weights. When the image is decomposed into blocks of size nxn (see below) the DCT also has a symmetry property over 2n which tends to reduce the so called blocking artefact.

5. DISCRETIZATION, ENCODING AND BLOCKING

Having performed a transformation, one is left with a series of real (continuous) values which are inappropriate for transmission; they need to be truncated with respect to discrete intervals, a process known as 'discretization'. The simplest form of such an operation is to convert the real numbers into integers. However, the range of values found after use of the transform have typically very different (dynamic) ranges. The fundamental is usually very large, but higher order coefficients fall off very rapidly. The choice of an appropriate encoding scheme can achieve significant gains in compression for given noise properties.

Normally, it is found very inefficient to manipulate the whole image (which might be of size 1Kx1K) in a single operations, and the image is usually treated as a series of blocks of size nxn, for example 16x16. Non square blocks may also be employed. However, it is important that after de-compression, the edges between blocks should not generate (blocking) artefacts; and that the selection of values be chosen to given good decorrelation after the transform. Di Paola chose a 1-D transform, selecting the values in zig-zag fashion [10]. In this study, a 2-D transform was also tested. An example of the encoding scheme used with a DCT transform is shown in Fig 2. This example shows number of bits used per pixel for a 16x16 block and an average number of 2.18 bits/pixel. To achieve greater compression, the coding scheme has to be modified as described below.

Optimal codes may be selected by studying the performance of the transform for many samples of image data. Essentially Huang and Schultheiss [11] have performed a constrained minimisation and obtained the result that

Fig 3. A histogram for a typical medical image showing the number of runs that were found plotted, against run length. Note that the number of long runs was rather few. For this reason, run length coding was not found to be very efficient.

Fig 4. The Gaussian pyramid for a radioisotope kidney scan is shown at each level, above, while below, the corresponding Laplacian pyramid is shown. Each level of the pyramid has been expanded, without interpolation, to the size of the original image, as a result of which individual pixels are visible.

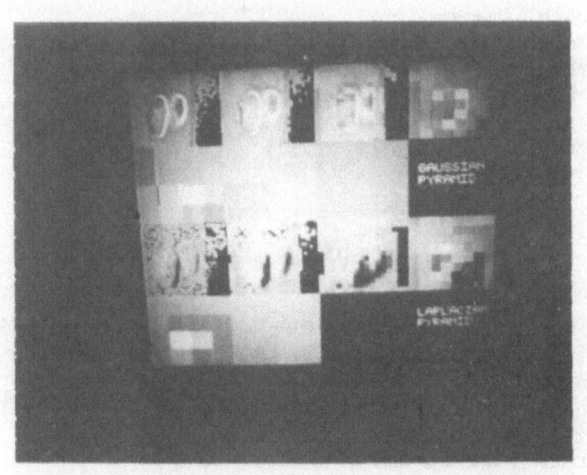

$$b(u,v) = b_{aver} - 0.5 \log_2 sigma^2(u,v)$$
$$- (1/2n^2) \sum_u \sum_v \log_2 sigma^2(u,v)$$

where $sigma^2(u,v)$ is the expected variance at the position u,v in the nxn transform. $b(u,v)$ is the number of bits to use to encode the data at that position and b_{aver} is the desired average number of bits/pixel.

6. RUN-LENGTH CODING AND PREDICTIVE DCPM CODING

Run length coding (RLC) is often suggested as a suitable data compression technique. In essence, when a pixel value is found to be repeated, RLC consists of recording the value of the pixel and the number of times that it occurs, rather than storing the complete sequence. Thus edges of images when uniformly zero may be largely eliminated, that is, replaced by a zero value and a count. Many improvements can be made, for example by using variable length bit codes to store changes rather than absolute values etc. Unfortunately, as shown in Fig 3, the run lengths observed in medical images tends to be very short, when edges are excluded [12]. Much of this is a result of random fluctuations associated with statistical noise.

Predictive coding is, in a way, a related technique. If one knows the expected form of the image, then one can record only the differences between that image, and the observed image [6,7]. Such differences might be expected to be very uncorrelated, and thus very efficient data compression could be achieved. In many respects, the use of the KL transform determines the form of such an 'expected image' by finding a set of basis matrices. Simpler techniques can and have been employed, for example, by predicting the value of the jth pixel horizontally in an image in terms of some linear combination of the previous j-1....j-i pixels. In this case, only the difference between the predicted value and the observed value is recorded, and compression results for the decrease in the number of bits required to store such a difference, with respect to that of the original pixel value.

7. PYRAMID CODING

A pyramid is defined (here) as a set of images G_L where each image is defined by means of some rule, for example summation of adjacent pixels, from the previous image in the pyramid G_{L-1}. The initial image G_0 is the raw data or original image.

Burt [13] has described a novel form of data compression using pyramids, and examples are also shown in [8]. A Gaussian pyramid can be constructed in terms of the REDUCE operation defined as

$$G_L = \text{REDUCE} [G_{L-1}]$$

such that

$$G_L(i,j) = \sum_{m,n = -2}^{+2} w(m,n) \ G_{L-1}(2i+m,2j+n)$$

where G_L is the result of performing the operation L times and G_0 is the original image, $w(m,n)$ is a suitable weighting function which is separable, normalised and symmetric. After each operation the size of G_L is reduced linearly by a factor of 2 (1/4 the number of pixels. Basically $w(m,n)$ is a Gaussian weighting function.

A similar operation EXPAND can be defined as

$$G_{L,K} = \text{EXPAND} \ [\ G_{L,K-1} \ ]$$

such that

$$G_{L,K}(i,j) = 4 \sum_{m,n = -2}^{+2} w(m,n) \ G_{L,K-1}((i+m)/2,(j+n)/2)$$

where only those elements for which i+m)/2 and j+n)/2 are integer are used. A Laplacian pyramid is defined as the set of images over L

$$\text{LAP}_L = G_L - \text{EXPAND} \ [\ G_{L+1} \ ]$$

where the subscripts L,L indicate that the corresponding image LAP_L has been expanded L times. and has the property that

$$G_{\emptyset} = \sum_L \text{LAP}_{L,L}$$

If $G_{\emptyset}$ is of size NxN the entire set of data in LAP is ~$4N^2/3$. Thus the operation of creating the Laplacian pyramid will slightly increase the amount of data (by 1/3). However, on 'discretization' the amount of data can be considerably reduced. The lowest level of the Laplacian pyramid contains mostly noise and can be encoded very coarsely. Higher order pyramids are each reduced in size by a factor of 4 and because of this are therefore less critical. They may then be, and indeed should be, encoded more finely. Burt [13] has suggested using bin sizes of 19,9,5,3 for the four lowest levels of the pyramid for an image with a maximum grey value of 255. Each level of the pyramid corresponds to the equivalent of the result of band pass filtering at progressively lower spatial frequencies. The image can be built up in reverse order, starting with the highest order (smallest) Laplacian pyramid levels, and progressively adding in lower orders containing finer detail. Thus provided the EXPAND operation can be performed rapidly by the display hardware, the image can be recovered in coarse resolution, and resolution progressively improved, while the observer is watching. This assumes that the expand operation can be performed rapidly in hardware.

An example of a Gaussian pyramid and the corresponding Laplacian pyramid is shown in Fig 4. Fig 5 shows the histograms for the distribution of pixels values in the orginal image and the first level of the Laplacian pyramid. Note that the histogram for the Laplacian pyramid is much more tightly distributed. Finally, examples of results of pyramid compression are shown in Figs 6 and 7.

8. THE 'S' TRANSFORM

A transform which does not appear to be directly related to compression is the 'S' transform [14]. However, there is an interesting application. Consider a vector of 4 input values [a,b,c,d] multiplied by a matrix [s] to give a vector of 4 output values such that

Fig 5. A graph showing the histogram of pixel values for the original
image of Fig 4, together with the histogram for the first level of the
Laplacian pyramid. The value for zero is indicated. The Laplacian data is
symmetrical about zero, while in the original data, no values below zero
existed, but extend up to quite large positive values. Thus the number of
symbols to be coded is far fewer, or alternatively, the standard deviation
is much smaller.

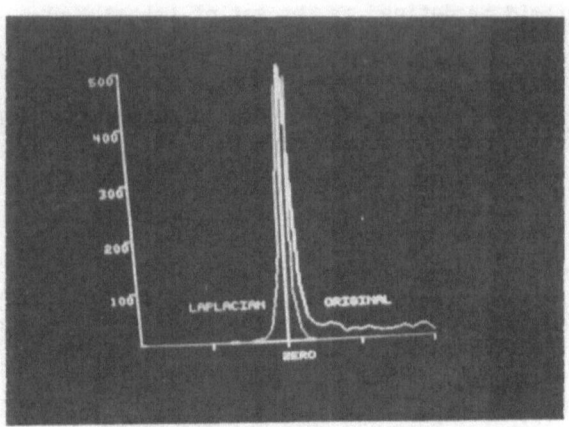

Fig 6. The result of data compression of the kidney scan as shown in Fig
4.   Above left is the original image, while above right is the image after
compression and de-compression. The difference image is shown to the same
scale, below left, while, below right, the difference image is shown with
the display scale expanded by a factor of 100.

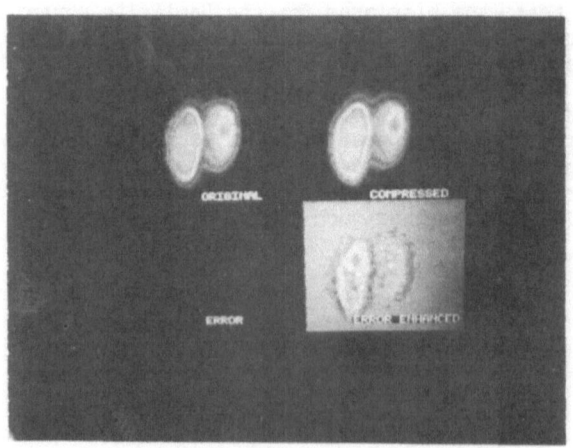

Fig 7. The result of data compression of an isotopic thyroid scan displayed in the same manner as in Fig 5.

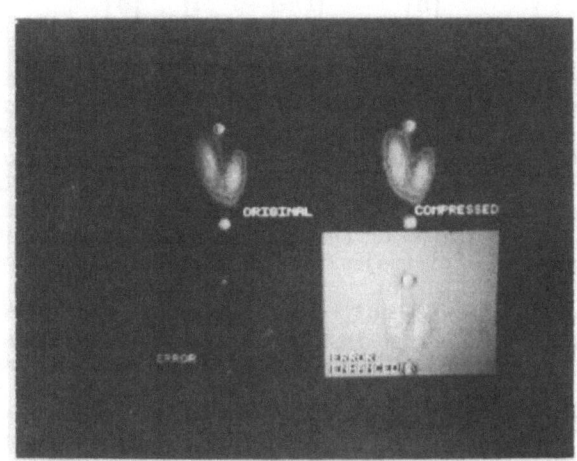

Fig 8. The use of the 'S' transform on a CT image. The original image is shown in the top left quadrant. The four images resulting from the first application of the 'S' transform are shown in the top right quadrant (only one image of the four is visible). The 'S' transformed results of each of the images in the top right quadrant are displayed in sub-quadrants of the bottom left quadrant, and so on recursively. Many of the images have little data and so are not visible.

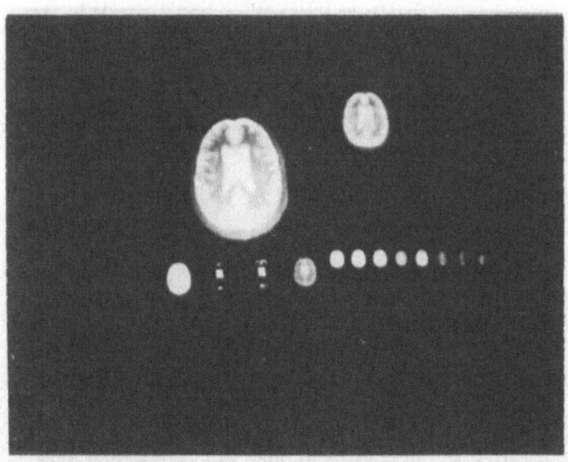

$$[s] = \begin{bmatrix} 1 & 1 & 1 & 1 \\ 1 & 1 & -1 & -1 \\ 1 & -1 & 1 & -1 \\ 1 & -1 & -1 & 1 \end{bmatrix}, \qquad \begin{bmatrix} e \\ f \\ g \\ h \end{bmatrix} = \begin{bmatrix} 1 & 1 & 1 & 1 \\ 1 & 1 & -1 & -1 \\ 1 & -1 & 1 & -1 \\ 1 & -1 & -1 & 1 \end{bmatrix} \begin{bmatrix} a \\ b \\ c \\ d \end{bmatrix}$$

then the following operation may be performed. Let the original image be treated as a set of 2x2 subregions. The 'S' transform is applied to each subregion to give 4 separate output values. The data may be regrouped such that the complete original NxN image is transformed into 4 N/2 x N/2 images, which may be called the e,f,g and h subimages. This may be repeated recursively to generate 16 N/4 x N/4 etc. Note that the so-called 'e' image is merely the 2x2 sum of the image used to generate it, and the set of 'e' images of 'e' images form a very conventional pyramid (quad tree).

The amount of data after each 'S' transform is constant. However, the 'e' image, as may be observed in Fig 8, is a low resolution copy of the original image. Thus, as described in the previous section, the technique may be employed to transmit firstly a low resolution copy of the original image, followed by additional data to restore the image (at leisure) to its full resolution. This is of considerable value in terms of improving the apparent response time of image transmission. The particular value and interest of the 'S' transform is that the kernel [s] is its own inverse, and can be implemented by addition and subtraction only, if necessary by a simple logic array. The 'S' transform is related to the Hadamard transform.

9. METHOD

Various data compression methods were tested, and applied to CT scans, and radioisotope scans. The size of the CT scans was 256x256, but the radioisotope scans were only 64x64. The total number of bit required after compression was noted, and converted to a average value per pixel. The image was then 'decompressed' and compared visually with the original image. A difference image was also generated, together with an estimate of the difference before and after compression.

Various distance measures where used: an L_2 norm of a least squares difference (in fact the RMS error), Chi-squared distance (squared distance divided by the variance), maximum error, and signal to noise ratio (SNR) [6,7]. There are two alternative definitions of SNR, essentially both in terms of the sum of the squared error SQERROR, such that

$$SQERROR = \sum_{m,n} (\, f(m,n) - f'(m,n) \,)^2 \; / N^2$$

$$SNR = 10 \log_{10} (\, SIG\,/\,SQERROR \,) \quad (dB)$$

where SIG is (firstly) the peak amplitude in the original image, or alternatively (secondly) the variance. Of all these many distance measures, none was considered to be ideal. Information theory based measures such as indicated by rate distortion theory were not estimated [15].

It is considered that the best method for testing the acceptability of a given amount of compression is to use an ROC based approach. As a (related) alternative, one could give observers a two alternative forced choice test, for example, by presenting the uncompressed and 'decompressed' images simultaneously, and asking the observed to decide which was which. An acceptable compression method is one where there is no significant degradation of the image such that an observer is unable to decide which was the original. The issue of noise reduction is important, in that it might be claimed that the image after data compression was (from the legal and ethical point of view) not the same as the original. This suggestion can be tested and evaluated by such ROC based tests.

10. RESULTS

In brief, the results obtained can essentially be summarised as follows:

1. Reversible noiseless data compression could not achieve useful amounts of data compression. Non-reversible data compression was able to achieve much greater compression without significant (e.g. noticeable) changes in compressed images. The best reversible data compression method achieved of the order of 2.5 average bits/pixel.

2. The use of run length coding were not helpful, with the exception of edge stripping, which, on its own, could at almost no cost remove 50% of the data. The best data compression was similarly about 2.5 average bits/pixel.

3. The DCT transform gave good results, down to ~1.5bits/pixel, but some blocking artefacts were noticed. A full DCT transform of large matrices was not considered practical.

4. The Laplacian pyramid coding approach was very encouraging, gave similar compression as the DCT, but did not generate blocking artefacts. It was found to be rather compute intensive. Using Huffmann coding data compression of ~1.0-1.5 average bits/pixel could be achieved.

Table 1 shows the amount of compression achieved using the DCT in average bits per pixel, together with the corresponding RMS error. Figs 6 and 7 shows the results of compression using the Laplacian pyramid method, showing the image before and after compression, and also showing the difference image displayed on the same scale and the difference image with the contrast increased by a factor of 100. Fig 9 shows an example of blocked DCT compression applied to a CT scan. Note the presence of some blocking artefacts.

534

Fig 9. The result of DCT transform coding of a CT scan. The compressed and de-compressed image is shown above, while the difference image is displayed (at higher contrast), below, to illustrate the blocking artefacts. The data compression achieved 2.4 average bits/pixel.

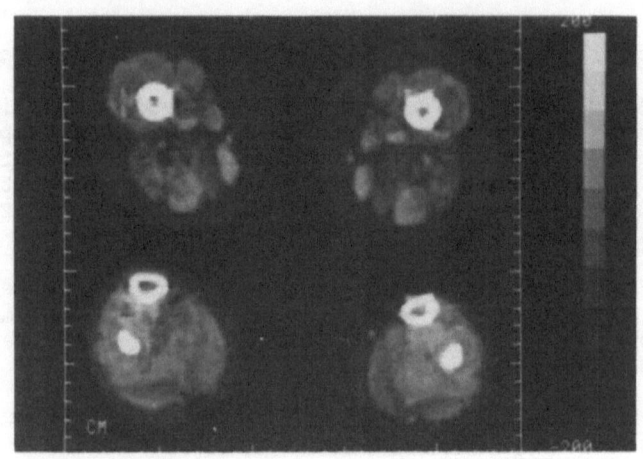

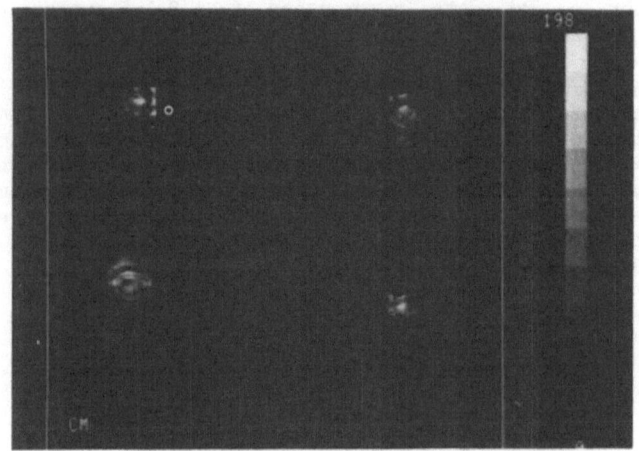

Table 1

| Ave. bits/pixel | RMS difference | |
	CT image	NM scan

The RMS difference between images before and after data compression as a function of the amount of compression achieved expressed as average bits/pixel, for a CT image and an radioisotope (NM) scan. images.

Ave. bits/pixel	CT image	NM scan
2.44	2.89	6.22
2.31	2.91	6.4
2.21	2.93	6.59
2.09	2.95	6.9
1.9	3.1	7.51
1.62	4.24	9.63

11. FUTURE EXTENSIONS

A dramatic improvement in the data compression efficiency can be achieve when considering not just single images but sets of images either in 3-D, or as in time. The compression previously discussed has been achieved by predicting structure in 2-D. Elimination of co-variance in the 3rd dimension should be able to produce results of up to a factor of ten better, but at the expense of a considerable increase in computational complexity and storage requirements. This could be achieved by a 3-D DCT block transform over a 16x16x16 volume. Other potential methods for improving compression are discussed in [8] where the use of a general contour-texture model for coding is recommended as a method for establishing the a-priori model of the image based on aspects determined from a knowledge of the human visual system.

The compression techniques employed tended to be rather heavy on computation time, requiring of the order of several seconds of time (~30 for a 256x256 matrix) on a PDP11/44. They must be made more efficient, for example by the use of appropriate hardware such as an array (vector) processor. It is estimated that sub-second compression techniques can be achieved. Both the DCT and the Laplacian techniques are suitable for handling in this manner. The interest in multi-resolution image processing makes it likely that suitable hardware for creating and manipulating pyramids may soon become available.

Perhaps one of the most attractive features of the pyramid coding method is that there is a similarity between the processing of such multiresolution image sequences, and one possible mechanism for visual perception. It may be that such a coding scheme is a 'natural' coding scheme in that there is a better mapping between the data structures and the manner in which they are handled by an observer. This potential needs to be further explored (as suggested in [8]).

12. CONCLUSION

The use of digital information in medical imaging can be exploited to a much greater extent if image data can be widely distributed. This seems to imply the use of low speed bridges for some time into the future such that compression techniques will be essential for their exploitation. A (near) loss-less coding scheme, or one which only removes noise, even if it achieves a tenfold reduction in the amount of data in images, is only desirable if the computational overheads can be made acceptable. This seems to imply that special purpose hardware must be used. It is intended to incorporate and test such data compression schemes in a practical hospital image network [16], currently under development.

REFERENCES

1. Ackerman LV, et al: Implementation of a broadband network in a diagnostic radiology department and large hospital. Radiology 153(P) 1984 abstract 249.
2. DHSS and NWTRHA: The creation of a film-less radiology department and hospital. STB/9/84, 1984.
3. SPIE 418 Picture Archiving and Communication Systems (PACSII) for Medical Applications (1983)
4. NEMA/ACR: Draft report, Digital imaging and communications standard, November 1984.
5. Gitlin JN: Managing medical images: current status and future expectations. In NATO ASI Physics and Engineering of Medical Imaging, ed Guzzardi R., Martinus Nijhoff, The Hague, in press.
6. Jain AK: Image data compression: a review. Proc IEEE 69, 1981, 349-406.
7. Rosenfeld A. and Kak AC: Digital Picture Processing 2nd Edition Academic Press, New York, 1982, Vol 1 Chapter 5.
8. Kunt M., Ikonomopoulos A. and Kocker M: Second-generation image coding techniques. Proc IEEE 73, 1985, 549-574.
9. Ahmed N., Natarajan T. and Rao KR: Discrete cosine transform, IEEE Trans Comput C-25, 1974, 90-93.
10. Di Paola R. and Todd-Pokropek AE: New developments in techniques for information processing in radionuclide imaging. In 'Medical radionuclide imaging' IAEA Vienna, 1981, 1 287-312.
11. Huang TTY, and Schultheiss PM: Block quantization of correlated Gaussian random variables, IRE Trans Commun. Syst CS-11, 1963, 289-297.
12. Chan CA: Data compression of medical images. MSc Dissertation, University College London 1984.
13. Burt PJ: The pyramid as a structure for efficient computation. In 'Multiresolution image processing and analysis', ed Rosenfeld A., Springer-Verlag Berlin, 1984, 6-37.
14. Lux P: A novel set of closed orthogonal functions for image coding. AEII, 31, 1977, 267-274.
15. Berger T: Rate distortion theory, a mathematical basis for data compression. Prentice-Hall, Englewood Cliffs, New Jersey, 1971.
16. Todd-Pokropek A. and Jameson G: Broadband link for the Bloomsbury district. Bloomsbury Internal Report 1985.

DESIGN CRITERIA FOR A DATA BASE MANAGEMENT SYSTEM FOR A PACS AT
GEORGETOWN UNIVERSITY HOSPITAL

F.H. FAHEY, P.C. WANG, S.K. MUN, P.L. CHOYKE, H.R. BENSON, A. DUERINCKX,
L.P. ELLIOTT

1. INTRODUCTON

In the radiology department, as with other industries, data have
been realized as a most valuable commodity. These data, which include
radiologic images, the radiology reports, and patient data available for
administrative purposes, are utilized by a variety of users such as
radiologists, referring physicians, technologists, and department
administators. The requests from these users differs greatly with
regard to what data they require, how the data will be used, and when it
will be needed. A major goal of a radiologic picture archival and
communication system (PACS) is to increase the availability of the data
to the users who require access to them. This is done by providing the
data in a digital form which can be readily communicated and archived
(1). In this manner, the PACS can be seen as a specific example of a
data base managements system (DBMS).

The PACS/DBMS should organize the data base in such a way as to
provide its users with the data they require in a timely and efficient
manner. The ability to integrate the variety of data into common data
base should lead to a more complete and relevant representation of the
available information. A PACS/DBMS is not only unique in the types of
data contained in the data base and its different users but also in the
volume of data that are entered into the system and transferred within
the system each day. Consideration of these characteristics leads to
the definition of functional criteria for the PACS/DBMS. This report
discusses the criteria that will be used in the design of a DBMS for a
PACS at Georgetown University Hospital.

The PACS for Georgetown is proposed to be implemented into three
phases (2). The first phase will involve the development of a
PACS/DBMS, the second phase will center around the inclusion of work
stations and remote viewing terminals, and the third will be the
completion of the system with full image and report distribution and
communication capability. A prerequisite of the PACS/DBMS is the
presence of a radiology information system (RIS). At Georgetown, the RIS
is part of the hospital information system (HIS). The relationship
between the RIS/HIS and the PACS/DBMS will be discussed in this report.
The eventual system will have three levels of storage: archive for long
term storage, intermediate storage for current cases, and local storage
to handle the data for a single review session.

2. DESCRIPTION OF THE DATA BASE

The data base will be comprised of two main types of data: image and
text. The radiologic image data are obtained on a number of different
imaging modalities with varying requirements of resolution. These would

include nuclear medicine, computed tomography (CT), nuclear magnetic resonance (NMR), ultrasound, digital angiography, along with conventional film-based radiology. The amount of spatial digitization necessary for any one of these types of images depends upon the inherent spatial resolution of the modality. A 64x64 digitization matrix may be adequate for many of the nuclear medicine images whereas 1000x1000 may not be sufficient for some bone radiographs. Intensity digitization is, in turn, related to the required contrast resolution. Levels of 8-12 bits per pixel seem to be adequate for the majority of the radiologic images. There will be three main types of text data within the data base: header block data for the image acquisition files, administrative data, and radiologic reports. The administrative data and the radiologic reports will be discussed in the section on the relationship between the RIS/HIS and the PACS/DBMS.

A communication standard is being formulated by the American College of Radiology and the National Electrical Manufacturers Association for use in the transmission of digital, radiologic image data.(3) This will be referred to in this report as the ACR-NEMA standard. This document describes a standard representation of image data and we have chosen to utilize this standard to describe our data representation. Adherence to this standard is a requirement for the PACS/DBMS described here.

The image data and associated information are contained within a "message" where a message is the minimum amount of data that can be transmitted between two pieces of radiologic equipment. The message is organized into "groups", where a group contains data, all of which is of a similar nature. For instance, the image, pixel data are stored in group 51 and data describing the structure of the image and how it should be displayed are in group 5. Text data, which could include the radiologic report, are located in group 101.

An image will typically be identified by numbers associated with the imaging procedure, the study, the series within the study, the acquisition within the series, and the image within the acquisition. This will identify the location of a particular image and the data within group 5 will define how those data are organized and how they should be displayed. There is enough data in group 5 to redisplay the image, just as it was at the time that it was reviewed by the radiologist. This is necessary for later comparison with new studies and for transmission of hardcopy versions of the data to referring physicians.

3. DATA STORAGE AND TRANSFER REQUIREMENTS

Design of appropriate storage and traffic control resources in the implementation of a PACS must be based upon accurate estimates of the number of transactions which will occur within the system. Because the amount of text data will be much smaller than the amount of image data under PACS, only image data will be considered in our estimation process. Workload statistics categorized by different procedures were gathered at Georgetown and have been published (4).

Currently our department permanently stores images on films. Each patient has a master film jacket which contains all the patient's films grouped by procedure type. A film library maintains the jackets and keeps track of film jacket transactions. The films are kept several years depending on the requirement by law and departmental policy.

The required archival storage in PACS is the same as in the film-based system. The storage requirement can be estimated by images produced every year multiplied by the number of years that records need to be stored. There were 943,000 images generated in 1984 at Georgetown (a 550 bed, teaching hospital) that is 988,800 Mbytes/year if a 1024x1024 spatial digitization per image and no data compression is assumed.

The intermediate storage includes newly generated images as well as some relevant previous images from archival storage for reference purposes. If it is assumed that same number of old images are needed for interpreting new images and the last seven day's images are stored, the intermediate storage requirement is then 55,000 Mbytes.

The total number of PACS transactions will equal the sum of the number of transactions between: 1) archival and intermediate storage, 2) intermediate storage and the work stations, and 3) the image generators and intermediate storage. Transactions between archival and intermediate storage will usually be scheduled and can be processed during off-peak times. The transactions include the relevant files in archive being brought to intermediate storage for reference to newly acquired images. It also includes the requests from physicians for consultation and teaching purposes. The estimated transaction is 2300 images per day at Georgetown. After a procedure has been interpreted by a radiologist and its report signed, the images and the report will be placed into archive. The number of such transactions is equal to the number of newly generated images each day, which is 3800 images. The data transmitted between intermediate storage and the work stations will demand transactions and should occur within the acceptable response time determined by the users: the radiologists and the referring physicians. The images typically will be newly generated images from different modalities and relevant images from previous studies. The estimated transactions are 7700. The estimated transactions from the image generating modalities to intermediate storage can be obtained from the workload statistics. The mean of the new images generated each day is 3800. The absolute maximum number of images per unit time is the total transactions if all the image generating equipment were producing images simultaneously. About 85% of this theoretical maximum could be assumed to be a practical maximum load. The sum of all the transactions is 17000 images or 18.4 Gbytes per day.

4. DATA SECURITY

In the PACS/DBMS, the lack of data security will not only lead to user mistrust of the system and therefore hinder the implementation of the PACS, but can also lead to serious medical and legal problems. System reliability, recoverability, and data access control will all be considered in this section.

With regards to data reliability, there are several facts to consider. The data must, firstly, be accurately digitized and stored, and secondly, once the data have been stored, they must be readily available to the user, particularly when the data pertain to medical decision making. The proper digitization of the image data is primarily dependent upon the acquisition computers and the film digitizers which may be considered outside the realm of the PACS/DBMS. Proper quality control and appropriate preventive maintenance performed on these devices should insure acceptable reliability in this regard. The proper archival of image data will also require the proper quality control of the hardware but will also require the proper entrance of patient identification data. Errors in such entrance can lead to misplaced data which may even be irretrievably lost. In a study of the reliability of a film-based PACS at Georgetown, 5.5% of the patient's film jackets were found to have incorrect record numbers.(5) Therefore, errors in the entrance of patient identification data must be checked prior to archival. This could be done by comparing these data with similar data contained in the RIS/HIS. Even with such precautions, errors will probably still occur, and thus these data should be correctable although only with proper authorization.

The film-based PACS at our institution was found to be remarkably reliable, yielding a 96% total exam retrieval, although significant delays in retrieval were encountered, particularly if the file was on loan, misplaced or lost, or older than 9 months.(5) The digital PACS is expected to lead to greater reliability and more timely access to the requested data. Down time of 12-24 hours for the intermediate and archival storage could probably be tolerated as long as such failure is rare. In the intermediate storage case, such down time could be made more tolerable by maintaining image data on the acquisition computer systems or as film for at least several days. Total system failure will not be tolerated although many of the subsystems may fail as long as these are not common occurrences.

Permanent losses of large amounts of data (e.g. corruption of an optical disk farm) will not be tolerated. To guard against permanent loss of archival data, a backup archival system will be required. This may either be a second, less expensive archive such as magnetic tape. Such a system could be also utilized during archival down time. Archive, itself, could be used as a backup for intermediate storage as well as local storage, both at the work stations and at the acquisition computers. Such a distributed memory system would lead to increased system recoverability.

The control of access to the data is necessary to both insure the integrity of the data base due to unauthorized modification of the data and also helps to protect the patient's right to privacy. Since the PACS will ultimately lead to the wide-spread access to the radiologic data, both within and outside the hospital, such control becomes an important yet complex task for the PACS/DBMS. Issues concerning who has access to radiologic data and when become matters of departmental policy rather being dominated by the physical constraints of the film-based system. It will no longer be sufficient to limit access to radiographs until after report generation because the images are on the alternator in the reading room. If the department wants to restrict access to images until after the report has been written, it will have to be because its a matter of policy and not because the film cannot be in two places at once.

Each user would require a password, credit card, or other such device in order to log on. Once on the system, the user's access to patient files will be limited depending upon the work station location, the user's status (resident, referring physician, attending radiologist, etc.), and the particular patient files being requested. The ability to modify, add, and delete data must also be controlled. Inadvertent deletion or modification of images should not be allowed. Many users will not be given the capabilities to delete or modify files and would be given "read only" privileges. While a file resides in intermediate storage, the attending radiologist would be allowed to perform certain image processing to create new, modified data files (these being flagged as such), although the raw data would also be preserved. The radiologist may also decide to eliminate certain irrelevant images or slices from the file prior to archival. However, once the radiologist has signed the report and it has been sent to archive, no further manipulation of the image data would be allowed.

5. PACS/DBMS FUNCTIONS

The PACS/DBMS should provide a number of features, some of which would be specific for a certain type of data (text versus image data), and many users will be limited in the features available to them. A list of the possible data base commands would include the following: file creation, addition, deletion, modification, retrieval, search, and data sort. For administrative uses of the data base most of these features would be necessary. Compilations of data lists to be used in managerial and administrative evaluations would require the use of many of these functions.

The list of fields that should be considered by the PACS/DBMS are listed below:

patient name	diagnosis
patient number	referring physician name
exam type (body part)	radiologist name
exam date	billing code
date of birth	report status
social security number	access code
exam number	pointers to other pertinent data

Thus a particular file should be accessible through the patient's name, or number. Also all of a particular radiologist's studies of a certain exam type on a certain date should be accessible through the system. These fields would allow the various users the ability to attain the data that is most meaningful for him/her.

6. RELATIONSHIP OF PACS/DBMS TO RIS/HIS

The PACS will not take the place of the RIS. In fact, the presence of an appropriate RIS is necessary prior to the installation of the PACS. The communication between the RIS and the PACS is extremely crucial in the appropriate handling of the information being processed by both systems. The RIS plays an integral role in the administration of the radiology department. As described by the Radiology Information System Consortium (RISC), it handles the following administrative tasks: patient registration, patient scheduling, file room management, report generation, among other tasks.(6) Much of the information utilized in patient registration and scheduling is also necessary for the management of the data within the PACS.

At Georgetown, the RIS is contained in the HIS, although one of several minicomputers maintained by HIS is devoted entirely to radiology, yielding a certain degree of independence from HIS also. Within RIS, there is a reverse, chronological list of patient activity, organized by patient name and number. A list of all procedures (and those scheduled but not performed) is maintained for each patient within the system. A patient is maintained on this list for a minimum of 5 years (10 years for CT, ultrasound, nuclear medicine, and special procedures). It is not necessary to have PACS/DBMS duplicate this feature, but these data should be accessible through the PACS/DBMS.

Another feature of the RIS/HIS is a film locator system. In this system, the location of each patient's master file and sub-folder is traced. This is accomplished with the use of light pens and bar codes. In this system, folders are traced and not the individual films. During the implementation of a PACS, when there is still a substantial film library, this system must be continued and possibly expanded to follow specific films. Eventually, this may not be needed as the films are replaced images stored on a digital archive. At this point, this feature may be modified to follow images within the PACS archive rather than in the film library. When a patient is scheduled for an exam, the PACS/DBMS can generate a "pull" of any pertinent past exams from the archive into intermediate memory. Extra-mural requests for hardcopy can also be initiated by the PACS/DBMS. It will not be necessary to send notices to borrowers of the images from the PACS.

At Georgetown, an automated radiologic report generation capability is currently incorporated into the RIS/HIS. A radiologic report typically contains one or two pages of text. Presently, "signed" reports (that is those signed as final by the radiologist) are maintained on the RIS for 2 to 3 weeks. In addition, all complete but unsigned reports are available. As part of the PACS/DBMS it is important to maintain these reports for as long as the images are archived. This implies that the report should be archived within the PACS in conjunction with the image file, in addition to being available on the RIS for 2-3 weeks. Thus when the report is signed, the images and the report should be sent to the archive. The two should be retrievable through the PACS/DBMS over the period of time that it is deemed necessary to archive the images.

7. SUMMARY

A set of functional, design criteria have been designed for a data base management system for a PACS at Georgetown University Hospital, a 550 bed teaching hospital. The workload statistics indicate that the digital archive must accommodate approximately 1000 Gbytes/year of uncompressed data. If the intermediate storage is to contain seven days worth of data, it must hold 50 Gbytes of data. The system must be able to handle the communication of 20 Gbytes of data per day.

The PACS/DBMS must comply with the ACR-NEMA standard with regard to hardware interface and data representation and identification. It must communicate with the RIS/HIS of the hospital and support the communication and archival of radiologic reports. The data within the system must be accessible by reference through a number of fields, such as patient name, patient number, exam type, radiologist's name, and physician's name.

The PACS/DBMS must have a high degree of security and reliability in order to insure the integrity of the data base. Permanent data loss must be avoided although limited, temporary loss may be tolerated. Data access must be controlled, both to insure security and to protect the patient's right to privacy. In short, the PACS/DBMS must be designed in such a way as to protect the integrity of the data base, to make the data readily available to all authorized users, to minimize data redundancy, and to control the organization of the data in order to provide the first three.

REFERENCES

1. Templeton, AW, et al.,"On-line and Long Term Digital Management

System", Radiographics, $\underline{5}$:121 (1985).

2. Mun, SK, <u>et al</u>.,"Design and Implementation of PACS at Georgetown University Hospital", SPIE Procedings, $\underline{555}$ (1985).

3. National Electrical Manufacturer's Association, Washington, DC

4. Wang, PC, <u>et al</u>., in preparation (1985).

5. Choyke, PL, <u>et al</u>.,"Reliability Issues in Digital Image Archiving" SPIE Procedings, $\underline{536}$ (1985).

6. <u>The DIN Report</u>, F. Hartel and J. Cerva, eds., MITRE Corp. (1985)

Design Considerations for a Neuroradiologic
Picture Archival and Image Processing Workstation

Donn S. Fishbein, MD

The design and implementation of a small scale image
archival and processing workstation for use in the study of
digitized neuroradiologic images will be described. The
system is designed to be easily interfaced to existing
equipment (presently PET, NMR and CT), function independent
of a central file server, and provide for a versatile image
processing environment. The aim of the project is to serve
the research needs of a small group of physicians, rather
than providing a department wide picture archival system.

A major design consideration is portability across
hardware, both to allow developed software to be used in
many environments, and to allow software projects to outlive
their original host hardware. Merely having a compiler for
the project language on a new machine does not ensure
portability, since most non-trivial programs depend upon the
operating system environment. Porting is simplified if the
compiler, system calls and file structure are identical on
both host and target machines. This requirement is largely
satisfied if an identical operating system exists for a
number of machines. The UNIX (System V) operating system
(1), available on various inexpensive yet powerful machines,
was chosen as satisfying the above conditions. Adherence to
the principle of portability allows better utilization of
program developers' time, since software can be utilized in
multiple settings on different hardware.

The UNIX operating system (2) has several
characteristics which make it a good choice for writing
portable software. The operating system kernel is
relatively small, with many functions normally associated
with the operating system performed by utilities, allowing
operation on machines with limited memory space. User
supplied routines can be substituted for many system
utilities, allowing greater control over the application
environment. It is written almost entirely in a high level
language (3), which makes porting the operating system to
new machines much easier, thus encouraging its wide
availability. At present it is available on machines
ranging from portable microcomputers to supercomputers, and

is supported by most major manufacturers.

To simplify design and allow integration of program modules from many sources, all code is written in a modular format. The concept of modularity extends to the user interface as well. The user is given considerable flexibility in piecing together existing programs to accomplish tasks which may not have been anticipated by the designer. This command line modularity is supported in part by an input-output mechanism of the UNIX operating system known as "pipes". This mechanism allows the output of one program to be used as the input to another program without any prearrangement or use of intermediate files. For example, if digitize, transform, and display are three programs which perform their named tasks, simply issuing the instruction

digitize | transform | display

to the command processor will arrange for "transform" to use the output of "digitize" as its input, and for "display" to use the output of "transform" as its input. The "|" character is a meta-command which establishes a "pipe". A program which reads its standard input and writes its standard output is suitable for use in a "pipeline", and can be thought of as a filter. Any of the three programs above may themselves consist of several program modules linked by pipes.

On a programming level, the use of pipes is supported by a single system call. An initial program, known as a parent, issues a pipe() call, which returns two file descriptors for reading and writing, respectively. The parent then spawns two children via a fork() and exec() call, passing to the children the pipe file descriptors. The children use the file descriptors as though they represented regular files; they need not even be aware that the descriptors reference pipes. The only departure from generality is that two programs communicating via a pipe must in general have a common ancestor. Internally the pipe is simply a FIFO (first-in first-out) buffer, with its "in" and out channels corresponding to the "read" and "write" file descriptors respectively. Pipes can be established by the use of the "|" metacharacter through the command processor (the "shell"), which then handles all the details of setting up the pipe. The opening of a pipe and the spawning of communicating processes is illustrated in the code fragment from the parent program shown below:

```
int fildes[2];
pipe (fildes);
proc_id1 = fork();
        if ( proc_id1 == 0 )
```

```
                execlp ("child1", fildes, arg1, arg2...);
        proc_id2 = fork();
                if ( proc_id2 == 0)
                    execlp ("child2", fildes, arg1, arg2...);
```

Although presenting few problems in theory, acquisition of data from imaging devices is one of the more cumbersome details of implementation. Because the system is intended to be easily implemented, both from a technical and administrative viewpoint, extensive modifications to existing imaging devices to allow for high speed local area networking was ruled out. Image transfer is done by means either of high speed serial ports or magnetic tape. Because the images of research interest are only a small subset of all images acquired, this method has not proved excessively cumbersome or time-consuming.

The cost of mass storage can make up a large percentage of the cost of an image processing workstation. The number of images which can be stored on-line is a major determinant of the usefulness of the system. To minimize cost and maximize storage capability, it is desirable to represent image data in as small a space as possible, using techniques of data compression. Only information preserving (error-free) techniques, in which the decoding algorithm is an exact inverse of the encoding process, were considered. The decoding algorithm must execute quickly enough so as to not delay viewing. The encoding algorithm, which presumably is executed much less frequently, and usually without a user awaiting its results, may take considerably longer to execute.

In storing radiologic images, several additional optimizations are possible. First, the image occupies somewhat less than the rectangular matrix it is displayed in. This is of little consequence if the background is uniform, since compression algorithms will reduce the storage requirement considerably. However, if the background is noisy, considerable gain can be made by first detecting the edges of the image, and storing only the image data. One may select a simple geometric shape with which to bound the image, or precede each line with an offset from the boundary of an enclosing rectangle and a count of the number of image pixels on the line. Within the margins of an image, data compression is often hampered by pixel-to-pixel variations due to noise. These variations are usually present in the lesser significant bits. If data compression is performed on each bit plane separately, significant compression can be achieved in the more significant bit planes. The primary algorithm used in this system for data compression within bitplanes is an adaptation of Huffman shift encoding (4). Applying the aforementioned techniques to typical 128 x 128 x 8 bit PET images, compression rates range from 40 to 85%.

In order to maximize storage capacity, the number of bits stored per pixel should be carefully considered, independent of any compression technique. The pixel representation on the scanning device may have been selected simply to conveniently fit the word length of the internal architecture of the associated computer. Simply duplicating the pixel representation used on the scanning device within the workstation without consideration as to the significance of the number of bits used can waste storage space with the representation of noise.

Software design accommodates frame buffers and graphic displays of varying resolution. At present images studied range in resolution from 128 x 128 to 512 x 512. The ability to display multiple images simultaneously greatly increases the usefulness of the system. As the price of graphic devices steadily declines, devices of higher display resolution can be added with minimal modification.

The image processing software is derived from several sources. A large library of standard image processing routines written for the UNIX operating system was ported to this environment with only minor changes. All code specific for local hardware such as frame buffers is isolated to a small number of low-level driver routines, and easily changed. Routines for image operations are in the form of filters, and perform simple manipulations (rotation, reflection, data-type conversion, compression), operations upon pixels, mask convolutions, digital transformations and filtering (5), edge detection, region drawing, noise generation, and computation of image statistics. Each image self-documents itself; the image header includes a history of the transformations to date. The system can accept the header as input and regenerate the final image based upon the transform history. Locally developed image transformations include routines for edge detection, anatomic region identification, and data compression.

Because the system is to be used primarily for research work, it is important that ready access be available to non-image data relating to the subject under study. A relational database system is tightly integrated into the design of the workstation for the storage of relevant clinical and research data. The database is also used to store numerical results from image processing routines, and keep track of available raw and processed images. The database offers subroutine calls to execute tasks not possible from its menu language; these subroutines are utilized extensively.

The user interface attempts to accommodate users of differing technical ability. The non-technical user can utilize menus, canned display formats, and presequenced image transforms, while the more sophisticated user can step around the interactive menu and specify actions in both a more precise and concise manner. Because of the use of pipelines and small, modular filters, new transforms are easily incorporated. One merely codes a program in any executable language and uses it in a pipeline; no change is required to existing software.

SUMMARY

Several considerations in the design of an picture storage and image processing have been discussed. The workstation is designed to serve the investigative needs of a neuroradiology department, rather than serve as an image archival system for an entire radiology department. Wherever possible, standard hardware and software are used, including but not limited to bus structure, operating system, and programming language. All software, with the exception of device specific drivers, is designed to be portable across differing hardware configurations. Interface to existing imaging equipment for image acquisition is flexible and easy to implement. Software routines are highly modular; likewise, the user is presented with a modular interface, allowing creation of new processing routines. An overall goal has been to keep hardware and software design straightforward, and not to exploit quirks of individual items, with an eye towards assuring portability and ease of maintenance.

REFERENCES

1. Ritchie DM, Thompson KL: The Unix Time-sharing System, The Bell System Technical Journal 57(6), 1978, 1905-29.
2. Kernighan BW, Pike R: The Unix Programming Environment. Englewood Cliffs, NJ: Prentice-Hall, 1984.
3. Kernighan BW, Ritchie DM: The C Programming Language. Englewood Cliffs, NJ: Prentice-Hall, 1978.
4. Huffman DA: A method for the construction of minimum redundancy codes, Proc. IRE 40(10), 1952, 1098-1101
5. Rosenfeld A, Kak AC: Digital Picture Processing. New York: Academic Press, 1982.

PARTICIPANTS

JOUAN ALEXANDRE
lab d'optique facultie de Science
Laboratory de Biophysique
Facultie de Medicine
2 Place St. Jacques
25030 Besonuge
FRANCE

C. ROBERT APPLEDORN
Div. of Nuclear Medicine
Indiana University School of Medicine
926 W. Michigan Street
Indianapolis, IN
U.S.A.

SIMON ROBERT ARRIDGE
Dept. Medical Physics
University College Hospital
Shropshire House, 11-20 Capper Street
London WC1
U.K.

STEPHEN BACHARACH
Dept. Nuclear Medicine
National Institutes of Health
Bldg. 10, Rm. 1C-401
Bethesda, MD 20205
U.S.A.

D.C. BARBER
Medical Physics
Royal Hallamshire Hospital
Sheffield S11 7EY
U.K.

WALTER BENCIVELLI
Clinical Physiology Institute
via SAV1 8-I56-100 PISA
ITALY

BERNARD BENDRIEM
Service Hospitalier Frederic Joliot
(C.E.A.)
Hopital D'orsay
S1L05 Orsay
FRANCE

YVES J.C. BIZAIS
Projet DIMI, Hopital Nord
44035 Nantes Cedex
FRANCE

SANDRA H. BLOOMBERG
University of North Carolina
4215 Trotter Ridge Road
Durham, NC 27707
U.S.A.

FRED L. BOOKSTRIN
University of Michigan
300 North Ingalls Bldg.
Ann Arbor, MI 48109
U.S.A.

AXEL BOSSUYT
AZ VVB
Laarbeeklaan 101
B-1080 Brussels
BELGIUM

A BERTRAND BRILL
Medical Department
Brookhaven National Laboratory
Upton, NY 11973
U.S.A.

ARTHUR BURGESS
Radiology Department
University of British Columbia
2211 Wesbrook Mall
Vancouver, BC V6T 2B5
CANADA

RICHARD CARSON
Department Nuclear Medicine
National Institutes of Health
Bldg. 10, Rm. 1C-401
Bethesda, MD 20205
U.S.A.

JORGE CARRASQUILLO
Department Nuclear Medicine
National Institutes of Health
Bldg. 10, Rm. 1C-401
Bethesda, MD 20205
U.S.A.

CHIN-TU CHEN
University of Chicago
FMI, Box 433, 5841 Maryland Ave.
Chicago, IL 60637
U.S.A.

LAWRENCE P. CLARKE
Dept. Radiology
College of Medicine
Univ. of South Florida
Box 17, 12901 N. 30th Street
Tampa, FL 33612
U.S.A.

ANNE CLOUGH
Dept. Radiology, Div. Nuclear Medicine
Arizona Health Sciences Center
Tucson, AZ 85724
U.S.A.

A. COLCHESTER
Dept. Neurology, St. George's Hospital
Cleves House, Cleves Lane
Upton Grey, New Basingstoke
Hampshire RG25 2RG
U.K.

FRANK DECONINCK
Vrije Universiteit Brussel
AS - VUB, Laarbeeklaan 101
1090 Brussel
BELGIUM

MICHEL DEFRISE
Vrije Universiteit Brussel
AZ-VUB, Laarbeeklaan 101
1090 Brussel
BELGIUM

CORNELIS N. DE GRAAF
Institute of Nuclear Medicine
Catharynesingel 101
3511 Utrecht
NETHERLANDS

MARGARET A. DOUGLAS
National Institutes of Health
Bldg. 12A, Rm. 2047
Bethesda, MD 20205
U.S.A.

JACQUES DU VERNOY
lab d'optique facultie de Science
Universite de Franche
Rouh de Gray
25030 Besongue
FRANCE

ROBERT L. EISNER
Dept. of Radiology
Emory University School of Medicine
1364 Clifton Road, N.E.
Atlanta, GA 30322
U.S.A.

PETER D. ESSER
Columbia University

FREDERIC H. FAHEY
Div. of Nuclear Medicine
Georgetown University Hospital
3800 Reservoir Road
Washington, DC 20007
U.S.A.

ISAAC FRAM
Siemens Gammasonics, Inc.
2000 Nuclear Drive
Des Plaines, IL 60018
U.S.A.

ALAN R. GARLINGTON, CAPT., USAF
Armed Forces Radiobiology
  Research Institute (AFRRI)
Building 42
Bethesda, MD 20814-5145
U.S.A.

E.M. GELDENHUYS
Dept. of Biophysics
University of Orange Free State
P.O. Box 339, UOFS, Bloemfontein 9300
REPUBLIC OF SOUTH AFRICA

MARIACARLA GILARDI
CNR Milando
CNR via Olgettina 60
20132 Milano
ITALY

MARCUS E. GLENN
Gov't. Aerospace Systems Div.
Harris Corporation
1021 Abada Ct., No. 101
Palm Bay, FL 32905

MICHAEL L. GORIS
Div. of Nuclear Medicine
Stanford University School of Medicine
Stanford, CA 94305
U.S.A.

MICHAEL V. GREEN
Dept. Nuclear Medicine
National Institute of Health
Bldg. 10, Rm. 1C-401
Bethesda, MD 20205
U.S.A.

JAMES D. HALE
Radiologic Imaging Laboratory
Univ. California - SF
400 Grandview
South San Francisco, CA 94080
U.S.A.

D. J. HAWKES
Dept. Medical Physics
St. George's Hospital
Blackshaw Road
London, SW17 0QT
U.K.

INGRID HOFMANN
University of Erlangen-Nuernberg
Martensstr. 3, 8520 Erlangen
F.R.G.

JULIE HORROCKS
Physics Department
Middlesex Hospital Medical School
Cleveland Street
London W
U.K.

A.S. HOUSTON
Dept. Nuclear Medicine
Royal Naval Hospital
Haslar, Gosport, Hants
U.K.

NOLA M. HYLTON
Radiologic Imaging Laboratory
Univ. California - SF
400 Grandview Drive
South San Francisco, CA 94080
U.S.A.

MICHAEL INSANA
Center for Devices
  and Radiological Health
Food & Drug Administration
HFZ-136, 5600 Fishers Lane
Rockville, MD 20857
U.S.A.

LLOYD G. KNOWLES
Applied Physics Laboratory
Johns Hopkins University
Johns Hopkins Road
Laurel, MD 20707
U.S.A

SYTSE KUIJK
Free University of Brussels
Laarbeeklaan 101
1090 Brussels
BELGIUM

INGER-LENA LAMM
Dept. Radiation Physics
Lund University Hospital
S-221 85 Lund
SWEDEN

HEINZ U. LEMKE
Technical University of Berlin
Sekr. CG FR 3-3, Franklinstrabe 28/29
D-1000 Berlin 10
WEST GERMANY

JEAN CLAUDE LIEHN
Institut Jean Godinot
1 rue du General Koenig
BP 171 F51056 Reims Cedex
FRANCE

LAWRENCE LIFSHITZ
Computer Science Department
Univ. of North Carolina at Chapel Hill
Chapel Hill, NC
U.S.A.

THOMAS A. LIVELY
Armed Forces Radiobiology
  Research Institute (AFRRI)
AFRRI, Bldg. 42
Bethesda, MD 20814-5145
U.S.A.

JORGE LLACER
Lawrence Berkeley Laboratory
Univ. of California
Bldg. 29, Lawrence Laboratories
Berkeley, CA 94720
U.S.A.

M.A. MAC LEOD
Dept. Nuclear Medicine
Royal Naval Hospital, Haslar
Gosport, Hants, PO122AA
U.K.

GERALD Q. MAGUIRE, JR.
Dept. Compute Science
Columbia University
520 W. 120th St.
New York, NY 10027
U.S.A.

B. M. MOORES
Dept. Medical Physics
Christie Hospital, Withington
Manchester M20 9BX
U.K.

E. MOVIUS
Armed Forces Radiobiology
  Research Institute (AFRRI)
AFRRI (RSDN) Bldg. 42
Bethesda, MD 20814-5145
U.S.A.

HIDEO MURAYAMA
Medical Department
Brookhaven National Laboratory
Upton, NY 11973
U.S.A.

MARILYN E. NOZ
Dept. of Radiology
New York University
550 First Avenue
New York, NY 10016
U.S.A.

DOUGLAS A. ORTENDAHL
University of California
400 Grandview Drive
South San Francisco, CA 94080
U.S.A.

BERNARD E. OPPENHEIM
Indiana Univ. School of Medicine
926 W. Michigan Street
Indianapolis, IN 46223
U.S.A.

WILLIAM O'CONNELL
Nuclear Medicine, S-455
Univ. of California, SF
San Francisco, CA 94143
U.S.A.

DENNIS L. PARKER
Univ. of Utah, LDS Hospital
325 Eighth Avenue
Sal Lake City, UT 84143
U.S.A.

DAN G. PAVEL
Univ. of Illinois Hospital
1740 W. Taylor, Rm. 2500
Chicago, IL 60612
U.S.A.

HUBERT A. PETITIER
Centre Hemodynamique
Hopital NORD
44035 Nantes Cedex
FRANCE

LAURENT PHILIPPE
Div. Nuclear Medicine
UCLA Medical Center
1000 W. Carson Street
Torrance, CA 90509
U.S.A.

STEPHEN M. PIZER
Computer Science Department, NWH 035A
Univ. North Carolina, Chapel Hill
Chapel Hill, NC
U.S.A.

DAVID L. PLUMMER
Dept. of Medical Physics
University of College London
11-20 Capper Street
London WC1E 6JA
U.K.

STEWART ROSENBERG
Service de Medicine Nuclaire
Hopital Trousseau
Chambray-les-Tours, 3F0441
FRANCE

R. WANDA ROWE
Division of Ophthalmology
North Shore University Hospital
300 Community Drive
Manhasset, NY 11030
U.S.A.

CHRISTIAAN SCHIEPERS
Nuclear Medicine
Albany Medical Center
New Scotland Avenue
Albany, NY 12208
U.S.A.

DIETER SCHLAPS
Inst. Fuer Nucklearmedizin, DKFZ
IM Neuenheimer Feld 280
D-6900 Heidelberg
FRG.

ROBERT SELZER
Jet Propulsion Laboratory
4800 Oak Grove Drive
Pasadena, CA 91109
U.S.A.

P.F. SHARP
Dept. of Medical Physics
Univ. of Aberdeen
Foresterhill, Aberdeen, AB9 2ZD
SCOTLAND

ROBERT D. SPELLER
Physics Department
Middelsex Hospital Medical School
London W1P 6DB
U.K.

SHARON STANSFIELD
CIS Department
Univ. of Pennsyvania
Philadelphia, PA 19104
U.S.A.

CHARLES E. SWENBURG
Armed Forces Radiobiology
  Research Institute (AFRRI)
AFRRI (RSNB), Bldg. 42
Bethesda, MD 20814-5145
U.S.A.

JERRY SYCHRA
Univ. of Illinois Hospital
1740 W. Taylor, Rm. 2500
Chicago, IL 60612
U.S.A.

EIICHI TANAKA
National Inst. of Radiological Sciences
9-1, Anagawa-4-chome
Chiba-shi, 260
JAPAN

A. TODD-POKROPEK
Dept. of Medical Physics
Universtiy College of London
Gower Street
London WC1
U.K.

DAVID TOWNSEND
Div. of Nuclear Medicine
Geneva University Hospital
Geneva
SWITZERLAND

S. RICHARD UNDERWOOD
Magnetic Resonance Univ
National Heart and Chest Hospitals
30 Britten Street
London SW3 6NN
U.K.

JOHN W. VAN GIESSEN
Delft Univ. of Technology
P.O. Box 356
2600 A.J. Delft
THE NETHERLANDS

JORIS VANREGEMORTER
Dept. Nuclear Medicine, AZ-VUB
Vrije Universiteit Brussel
Laarbeeklaan 101
1090 Brussels
BELGIUM

MAX A. VIERGEVER
Delft Univ. of Technology
P.O. Box 356
2600 A.J. Delft
THE NETHERLANDS

WERNER VON SEELEN
Institut of Biophysik
University Hainz
SAA RSH 21 Hainz
FRG

WALTER J. WILD
Optical Sciences Center
University of Arizona
Tuscon, AZ
U.S.A.

BARRY ZEEBERG
Nuclear Medicine Department
Nat'l. Institutes of Health
Building 10
Bethesda, MD 20205
U.S.A.

PROCEEDINGS OF PREVIOUS IPMI CONFERENCES.

INFORMATION PROCESSING IN SCINTIGRAPHY, Proceedings of the
3rd conference, Cambridge, Mass., 1973. Document number
CONF-730687, USERDA Technical Information Center, Oak
Ridge, Tennessee, 1975. Contact: National Technical
Information Service, U.S. Department of Commerce,
Springfield, Virginia 22161, U.S.A.

INFORMATION PROCESSING IN SCINTIGRAPHY, Proceedings of the
4th conference, Orsay, 1975. C.Raynaud and A.Todd-Pokropek,
Ed.. C.E.A., Service Hospitalier F.Joliot, 91406, Orsay,
France.

INFORMATION PROCESSING IN MEDICAL IMAGING, Proceedings of
the 5th conference, Nashville, Tennessee, 1977. A.B.Brill
and R.Price, Ed.. Document number ORNL/BCTIC-2. Contact
National Technical Information Service, U.S. Department of
Commerce, Springfield, Virginia 22161, U.S.A.

INFORMATION PROCESSING IN MEDICAL IMAGING, Proceedings of
the 6th conference, Paris, 1979. R. Di Paola and E. Kahn,
Ed.. Editions INSERM, Paris, France.

MEDICAL IMAGE PROCESSING, Proceedings of the 7th
International Meeting on Information Processing in Medical
Imaging, Stanford, California, 1981. M.L.Goris, Ed.,
Division of Nuclear Medicine, Stanford University,
Stanford, U.S.A.

INFORMATION PROCESSING IN MEDICAL IMAGING,
Proceedings of the 8th Conference, Brussels,
1983, F. Deconinck, Ed., Martinus Nijhoff
Publishers, Dordrecht 1984, ISBN 0-89838-677-2.